Manual of Psychiatric Care for the Medically Ill

Manual of Psychiatric Care for the Medically Ill

Edited by

Antoinette Ambrosino Wyszynski, M.D.
Clinical Associate Professor of Psychiatry
New York University School of Medicine
Faculty, the Psychoanalytic Institute
at New York University
New York, New York

Bernard Wyszynski, M.D.
Clinical Associate Professor of Psychiatry and
Assistant Professor of Neurology
Albert Einstein College of Medicine
Bronx, New York

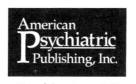

American Psychiatric Publishing, Inc.

Washington, DC
London, England

Manufactured in the United States of America on acid-free paper
09 08 07 06 05   5 4 3 2 1
First Edition

Typeset in Adobe's Palatino and Frutiger 55 Roman

American Psychiatric Publishing, Inc.
1000 Wilson Boulevard
Arlington, VA 22209-3901
www.appi.org

Library of Congress Cataloging-in-Publication Data
Manual of psychiatric care for the medically ill / edited by Antoinette Ambrosino Wyszynski,
    Bernard Wyszynski.—1st ed.
        p. ; cm.
    Includes bibliographical references and index.
    ISBN 1-58562-118-8 (spiralbound : alk. paper)
    1. Consultation-liaison psychiatry. 2. Mental illness—Chemotherapy.
  3. Medicine, Psychosomatic. 4. Psychopharmacology. 5. Psychotropic drugs.
  6. Sick—Mental health. I. Wyszynski, Bernard, 1954– II. Title.
    [DNLM: 1. Mental Disorders—therapy. 2. Mental Disorders—diagnosis.
  3. Psychophysiologic Disorders—diagnosis. 4. Psychophysiologic Disorders—therapy.
  5. Psychotropic Drugs—therapeutic use. WM 400 W995m 2004]
  RC455.2.C65W973 2004
  616.89—dc22

                                                                                2004052944

British Library Cataloguing in Publication Data
A CIP record is available from the British Library.

To our daughter Sofia, whose patience, good humor, and understanding made this book possible.

A.A.W.
B.W.

Contents

Chapter 1

   Antoinette Ambrosino Wyszynski, M.D.

Chapter 2

   Antoinette Ambrosino Wyszynski, M.D.

Chapter 3

   Antoinette Ambrosino Wyszynski, M.D.
   Melanie Schwarz, M.D.
   Bruce Rubenstein, M.D.
   Victor B. Rodack, M.D.
   Manuel Santos, M.D.

Chapter 4

   Antoinette Ambrosino Wyszynski, M.D.

Chapter 5

   Antoinette Ambrosino Wyszynski, M.D.
   Elyse D. Weiner, M.D.

Tables, Boxes, and Figures

Chapter 3. The Patient With Cardiovascular Disease

Chapter 4. The Patient With Kidney Disease

Chapter 5. The Patient With Pulmonary Disease

Chapter 6. The Patient With GI Symptoms and Psychiatric Distress

Chapter 7.   The Obstetrics Patient

Chapter 8.   The Patient Using Steroids

Chapter 9.   The HIV-Infected Patient

Chapter 11.   A Primer on Solid Organ Transplant Psychiatry

Chapter 12. Assessing Decisional Capacity and Informed Consent in Medical Patients: A Short, Practical Guide

Chapter 14. When Patients Ask About the Spiritual: A Primer

Locator for Worksheets, Forms, and Screening Instruments

Contributors

Salvatore V. Ambrosino, M.D.
Clinical Professor of Psychiatry, New York University School of Medicine, New York

Khleber Chapman Attwell, M.D., M.P.H.
Clinical Assistant Professor of Psychiatry, New York University School of Medicine, New York

Leonard Barkin, M.D.
Clinical Professor of Psychiatry, New York University School of Medicine; Training and Supervising Analyst, The Psychoanalytic Institute at New York University, New York

Brian D. Bronson, M.D.
Clinical Instructor of Psychiatry, New York University School of Medicine, New York

Bryan Bruno, M.D.
Clinical Assistant Professor of Psychiatry, New York University School of Medicine; Director of Inpatient and Emergency Psychiatry, Lenox Hill Hospital, New York

Linda Chuang, M.D.
Instructor of Psychiatry, New York University School of Medicine; Attending Psychiatrist, Division of Consultation-Liaison Psychiatry, Bellevue Hospital, New York

Nancy Forman, M.D.
Associate Director, Division of Consultation-Liaison Psychiatry, Bellevue Hospital, New York

Miriam Friedlander, M.D.
Fellow, Department of Psychiatry, Memorial Sloan-Kettering Cancer Center, New York

Carol F. Garfein, M.D.
Attending Psychiatrist, Zucker Hillside Hospital, North Shore–Long Island Jewish Health System, New York

Stanley Grossman, M.D.
Clinical Professor of Psychiatry, New York University School of Medicine; Training and Supervising Analyst, The Psychoanalytic Institute at New York University, New York

Ceri Hadda, M.D.
Attending Psychiatrist, Lenox Hill Hospital, New York

Silvia Hafliger, M.D.
Clinical Assistant Professor of Psychiatry and Attending Psychiatrist, Transplant Psychiatry, Center for Liver Disease and Transplantation, Columbia Presbyterian Medical Center, New York

Shari I. Lusskin, M.D.
Director of Reproductive Psychiatry and Clinical Assistant Professor of Psychiatry, Obstetrics, and Gynecology, New York University School of Medicine, New York

Victor B. Rodack, M.D.
Clinical Instructor of Psychiatry, New York University School of Medicine; Attending Psychiatrist, Division of Consultation-Liaison Psychiatry, Bellevue Hospital, New York

Bruce Rubenstein, M.D.
Clinical Assistant Professor of Psychiatry, New York University School of Medicine, New York

Manuel Santos, M.D.
Clinical Instructor of Psychiatry, New York University School of Medicine; Attending Psychiatrist, Division of Consultation-Liaison Psychiatry, Bellevue Hospital, New York

Victor Schwartz, M.D.
Clinical Assistant Professor of Psychiatry, New York University School of Medicine; Medical Director, New York University Counseling Service, New York

Melanie Schwarz, M.D.
Clinical Assistant Professor of Psychiatry, New York University School of Medicine; Attending Psychiatrist, Division of Consultation-Liaison Psychiatry, Bellevue Hospital, New York

Elyse D. Weiner, M.D.
Clinical Assistant Professor of Psychiatry, SUNY Downstate Medical Center, Brooklyn, New York; Director of Consultation-Liaison Psychiatry, Department of Veterans Affairs, New York Harbor Health Care System, Brooklyn, New York

Antoinette Ambrosino Wyszynski, M.D.
Clinical Associate Professor of Psychiatry, New York University School of Medicine; Faculty, The Psychoanalytic Institute at New York University, New York

Bernard Wyszynski, M.D.
Clinical Associate Professor of Psychiatry and Assistant Professor of Neurology, Albert Einstein College of Medicine, Bronx, New York

Patrick Ying, M.D.
Clinical Assistant Professor of Psychiatry and Associate Director of Outpatient Services, Department of Psychiatry, Tisch Hospital, New York University School of Medicine, New York

Van Yu, M.D.
Clinical Assistant Professor of Psychiatry, New York University School of Medicine; Attending Psychiatrist, Project for Psychiatric Outreach to the Homeless, New York

Preface

There were several reasons to write a basic, practical manual for managing psychiatric problems in medical patients. First, there has evolved a disturbing paradox in twenty-first-century medicine: do more, document more, but see patients for less time, or face the consequences. Lurking over the shoulder of most clinicians stands the visit-counting insurance reviewer with the length-of-stay guillotine. Prove that the patient needs services, and has the illness you say, or the patient is denied coverage and cannot see you. Even for academically based clinicians, the completeness of one's paperwork has trumped the "publish or perish" of one's papers.

Second, doctors-in-training are attempting to learn in the crossfire that pits cost-containment against patient care. They sometimes have at most two visits to make a diagnosis and implement a treatment plan—often for clinical syndromes they are encountering for the first time. The available textbooks on the psychiatric care of medical patients are invaluable references but tend to be encyclopedic. Our trainees have requested more concise "bedside" teaching materials for use when the patient—along with their opportunity to learn—is literally "here today, gone tomorrow."

It is tempting to decry "the state of modern medicine" and to rant that psychiatric treatment cannot be short-circuited to two visits. We have. And we do. But like percussing an acute abdomen when there is no CT scan, practicing psychiatry under the improbable conditions of twenty-first century managed care forces clinical focus, while we still try to heed the principle "Patient First." The patient may receive only that small slice of care. It must be made to help.

Complex predicaments sometimes can be solved by practical, short-term solutions. We have altered *A Case Approach to Medical-Psychiatric Practice* (A. Wyszynski and B. Wyszynski, American Psychiatric Press, 1996). The extensive literature reviews are replaced with summaries, Web addresses, checklists, and worksheets. A good template is worth a thousand diffusely worded progress notes or lecture materials; it focuses information-gathering, organizes the data, and ideally generates an outline, allowing you to document as you go. Our trainees find such templates to be helpful learning tools.

Succinctness and practicality are the goals of this manual. Medical updates are combined with strategies for managing issues arising in the psychiatric treatment of patients with cardiovascular, hepatic, renal or pulmonary disease, or gastrointestinal symptoms. A few conditions warranted their own chapters: delirium, pregnancy, HIV infection, hepatitis C, and steroid-induced psychiatric syndromes. We added "A "Primer on Solid Organ Transplant Psychiatry" because patients with transplanted organs are more commonly appearing in community hospitals. There is a chapter on assessing decisional capacity and informed consent. The final chapters are written as a short, practical guide to addressing general psychological issues occurring in medical patients. The final appendix contains study questions for selected issues arising in the psychiatric management of cardiovascular, hepatic, renal, pulmonary, and pregnant patients.

The *Manual of Psychiatric Care for the Medically Ill* is intended as a companion to the more comprehensive textbooks. We have excluded several topics in order to contain the size of the manual: neuropsychiatry, psycho-oncology, gynecology, somatization, and pain management. Consistent with our aim to provide practical, patient-focused strategies, staff-focused ("liaison") interventions are not included. Several excellent textbooks and concise guides have already been published specifically covering these areas.

We hope we have achieved our purpose in providing you with useful materials for your clinical practice.

Antoinette Ambrosino Wyszynski, M.D.
Bernard Wyszynski, M.D.
New York, New York, July 2004

■ SUGGESTED READINGS

Coffey CE, Cummings JL (eds): Textbook of Geriatric Neuropsychiatry, 2nd Edition. Washington, DC, American Psychiatric Press, 2000

Cummings J, Mega M (eds): Neuropsychiatry and Behavioral Neuroscience. New York, Oxford University Press, 2003

Dolin S, Padfield N, Pateman J, et al (eds): Pain Clinic Manual. Boston, MA, Butterworth-Heinemann, 2003

Hay D, Klein D, Hay L, et al (eds): Agitation in Patients With Dementia: A Practical Guide to Diagnosis and Management. Washington, DC, American Psychiatric Publishing, 2003

Holland JC, Breitbart W (eds): Psycho-oncology. New York, Oxford University Press, 1998

Holland JC, Lewis S: The Human Side of Cancer: Living With Hope, Coping With Uncertainty. New York, HarperCollins, 2000 [for patients]

Holland JC, Rowland JH (eds): Handbook of Psychooncology: Psychological Care of the Patient With Cancer. New York, Oxford University Press, 1999

Isaac A, Wise T: A low-frustration strategy for treating somatization. Current Psychiatry 2:33-50, 2003 [excellent "how-to" review article]

Leo RJ: Concise Guide to Pain Management for Psychiatrists. Washington, DC, American Psychiatric Publishing, 2003

Levenson JL (ed): The American Psychiatric Publishing Textbook of Psychosomatic Medicine. Washington, DC, American Psychiatric Publishing, 2005

Lishman W: Organic Psychiatry, 3rd Edition. London, Blackwell Scientific, 1998

Stern TA, Fricchione GL, Cassem BH, et al (eds): The Massachusetts General Hospital Handbook of General Hospital Psychiatry, 5th Edition. Philadelphia, PA, Mosby, 2004

Stotland NL, Stewart DE (eds): Psychological Aspects of Women's Health Care: The Interface Between Psychiatry and Obstetrics and Gynecology, 2nd Edition. Washington, DC, American Psychiatric Press, 2001

Stoudemire A, Fogel BD, Greenberg D (eds): Psychiatric Care of the Medical Patient. New York, Oxford University Press, 2000

Wise M, Rundell J (eds): The American Psychiatric Publishing Textbook of Consultation-Liaison Psychiatry: Psychiatry in the Medically Ill, 2nd Edition. Washington, DC, American Psychiatric Publishing, 2002

Yudofsky S, Hales R (eds): American Psychiatric Publishing Textbook of Neuropsychiatry, 4th Edition. Washington, DC, American Psychiatric Publishing, 2002

Acknowledgments

There are many people to thank for their contributions to this volume:

- Dr. Robert Cancro, Professor and Chair of the Department of Psychiatry at the New York University School of Medicine, for his ongoing encouragement and leadership.
- Dr. T. Byram Karasu, Silverman Professor and Chairman, Department of Psychiatry and Behavioral Sciences at Albert Einstein College of Medicine, Bronx, New York, for his support.
- Dr. Manuel Trujillo, Medical Director of Psychiatry at Bellevue Hospital in New York City, for his encouragement.
- Dr. Carol A. Bernstein, Director of Residency Training, Department of Psychiatry, New York University School of Medicine, for encouraging the development of the academic teaching program in consultation-liaison psychiatry and psychosomatic medicine, which served as the basis for this book.
- Drs. Victor Schwartz and Bruce Rubenstein, for their insightful help in revising the manuscript.
- Our chapter reviewers, for contributing their time and advice: Drs. Asher Aladjem, Jane Algus, Greg Alsip, Philip A. Bialer, Jonathan Brodie, David Ginsberg, Ze'ev Levin, Andrew Martin, Laura J. Miller, Eric Peselow, Michael J. Robinson, Benjamin Sadock, James Schluger, Manuel Trujillo, and Arthur Zitrin.
- Drs. Paul Appelbaum, E. Wesley Ely, Thomas Grisso, Donald Royall, and Paula Trzepacz, who generously assisted with the adaptation of testing instruments.
- Drs. Alice Medalia and David Erlanger for their guidance regarding neuropsychological test instruments.
- Dr. Karen Brewer's staff of the Public Services Department of the Frederick L. Ehrman Medical Library at New York University School of Medicine, especially Richard L. Faraino, Dorice L. Vieira, Joan Himmel, and the tireless staff of the Document Delivery Service.
- John McDuffie, Editorial Director of Books for American Psychiatric Publishing, Inc. (APPI), for his patience and help throughout the preparation of this manuscript.
- Roxanne Rhodes, Senior Editor in APPI Books, for her expert help navigating a daunting project.
- Finally, we thank the medical students and psychiatric residents we have taught, who have kept us thinking "Patient First" and whose questions have taught us how to teach.

Dedication

It has been said that a man is not appreciated in his own time. A remarkable exception to this is Dr. Robert Cancro, who for more than 25 years has served as Professor and Chair of the Department of Psychiatry at the New York University School of Medicine. Dr. Cancro has been an outstanding clinician, leader, and educator for nearly half a century. That most of the contributors to this volume have served as faculty or residents within the Department of Psychiatry at the New York University School of Medicine and at Bellevue Hospital Center during his tenure is a testimony to his exceptional talent.

Bellevue psychiatrists have cared for patients from every walk of life, every racial and ethnic group, every socioeconomic group, and almost every country in the world. It would be difficult to find another group of clinicians whose richness of wisdom and clinical experience would be better suited to contribute to a textbook addressing a practical approach to treating psychiatric problems occurring in medical patients. It is in this spirit that the contributors dedicate this volume in Dr. Cancro's honor.

Carol A. Bernstein, M.D.

Associate Professor of Psychiatry, Vice-Chair for Graduate Medical Education, and Director of Residency Training, Department of Psychiatry; Senior Assistant Dean for Graduate Medical Education, New York University School of Medicine, New York, New York

The Delirious Patient

Antoinette Ambrosino Wyszynski, M.D.

■ DEFINITION

Delirium is defined as a disturbance of consciousness accompanied by a change in cognition that cannot be better accounted for by a preexisting or evolving dementia (DSM-IV-TR; American Psychiatric Association 2000). Delirium is a global, diffuse disturbance of central nervous system functioning that affects consciousness, attention, and perception. The disturbance usually develops over a short time period (hours to days) and tends to fluctuate during the course of the day. Ability to focus, sustain, and shift attention is impaired, reducing the patient's awareness of his or her environment. The delirious patient is easily distracted, so questions must be repeated, and the patient may respond perseveratively to a previous question rather than shift attention to a new one. Perceptual disturbances often include hallucinations and delusions. Disruptions may also occur in sleep, psychomotor activity, and affective state. DSM-IV-TR criteria for delirium due to a general medical condition appear in Table 1–1.

■ CASE EXAMPLES

The following vignettes were chosen because they represent prototypical diagnostic and management dilemmas for the psychiatric consultant. A list of study questions for discussion follows the cases.

Case 1: Mrs. July 1st (The Prototypical Emergency Room "Everypatient")

It is July 1st, and all housestaff have assumed their new positions at the teaching hospital. A 75-year-old woman with "stable" breast cancer arrives at the medical emergency room at 9:00 A.M. with her family. Over the past week the family have been worried that she is "developing Alzheimer's" because of memory problems and agitation. Past psychiatric history is notable for mild depression, treated with paroxetine 20 mg daily, and sleep difficulties, for which she recently began taking trazodone 50 mg at bedtime.

The 1:00 P.M. nurse's note reads: "Quiet, resting comfortably. Alert, oriented ×3." Results of a complete blood count, tests for serum electrolyte levels, and urinalysis are pending. The oncologist approves the medical resident's request for magnetic resonance imaging (MRI) of the brain. The medical resident calls for psychiatry consultation at 4:05 P.M. because the patient has become agitated and has voiced suicidal ideation. The medical workup has been negative except for 5–10 white cells found in the urinalysis, without accompa-

Table 1–1.   DSM-IV-TR diagnostic criteria for delirium due to a general medical condition

A.   Disturbance of consciousness (i.e., reduced clarity of awareness of the environment) with reduced ability to focus, sustain, or shift attention.

B.   A change in cognition (such as memory deficit, disorientation, language disturbance) or the development of a perceptual disturbance that is not better accounted for by a preexisting, established, or evolving dementia.

C.   The disturbance develops over a short period of time (usually hours to days) and tends to fluctuate during the course of the day.

D.   There is evidence from the history, physical examination, or laboratory findings that the disturbance is caused by the direct physiological consequences of a general medical condition.

Coding note: If delirium is superimposed on a preexisting Vascular Dementia, indicate the delirium by coding 290.41 Vascular Dementia, With Delirium.

Coding note: Include the name of the general medical condition on Axis I, e.g., 293.0 Delirium Due to Hepatic Encephalopathy; also code the general medical condition on Axis III (see Appendix G for codes).

nying fever or pain. The consultation request reads: "Medically cleared. Please transfer to psychiatry for treatment of emotional instability and psychotic depression secondary to cancer." The psychiatric resident arrives at 5:00 P.M. and finds that the patient is visually hallucinating and disoriented. He knows that this is not a major depressive disorder, but he is not sure how to proceed.

Case 2: Mr. Sundowning (The Psychotic Patient in the Intensive Care Unit)

A 70-year-old-man begins supportive outpatient psychotherapy for phase-of-life issues. His medical history is notable for lung cancer 15 years ago, treated with surgery and chemotherapy. There is no evidence of disease at the time of referral. While in psychotherapy, he develops anxiety-like symptoms, which he attributes to the stressful material being discussed in psychotherapy about a serious childhood illness. The psychiatrist refers him back to the internist for evaluation. Unfortunately, medical workup reveals recurrent

lung cancer. The lung tumor advances rapidly, and the patient requires admission to the intensive care unit (ICU) because of progressive respiratory failure.

In the ICU, the patient communicates that he wants to die. The nurses note that he is sometimes OK, sometimes agitated, often "out of it." Their main complaint is that he "sundowns" (becomes more active and agitated in the evenings) and sometimes keeps the other patients up at night. They ask if this could be ICU psychosis stemming from sleep deprivation. Meanwhile, the medical intern needs advice on sedating the patient in order for him to cooperate with his scans.

Case 3: Ms. Psych-History-Clear-Scans-Please-Transfer (The Patient With Psychiatric History, Mental Status Changes, and Normal Imaging Studies)

A 66-year-old woman with a history of depression responsive to paroxetine 10 mg is admitted to the hospital septic from a urinary tract infection. As the infection resolves, the patient becomes less sedated and more blatantly psychotic. She develops the delusion that there is a gambling ring operating from beneath the hospital beds. Paroxetine is discontinued, and psychiatric consultation is requested several days later, after the sepsis resolves. At the time of consultation, the physical and neurological examinations are normal. The patient's urinalysis and bloodwork, including results of thyroid function tests and all serum electrolyte tests, are normal. She is afebrile. Results of MRI of the head, electroencephalography, and lumbar puncture are normal. Chest X ray, however, is notable for a midline mass. Bronchoscopy has been recommended, but the patient has refused. Arterial blood gases and pulmonary function test results are normal. The medical staff decides to defer further workup until her psychotic state clears.

The patient's family say they had noted that her "personality was different" over the previous 2 months, when she was more irritable and uncharacteristically "lost her temper over nothing." At times, she was suspicious that her next-door neighbor was sending mental messages to her about the Middle East conflict, and she would become agitated if anyone challenged her. She took no medications other than paroxetine, prescribed by her internist, and refused to see a psychiatrist. The family report that she has never been psychotic before and has no substance abuse history. She is a widowed attorney who retired from a successful law practice about 1 year ago. The medical staff notes that the patient has a schizophrenic first cousin, and the medical students ask if schizophrenia could account for her psychiatric presentation.

Mental status examination reveals no depressive content, but the patient is paranoid and delusional. There are no hallucinations. She is alert and oriented to person and time but thinks she is in a nursing home rather than a hospital. The patient performed within normal limits on the Mini-Mental State Examination (MMSE) but shows disruption of the sleep-wake cycle, perceptual disturbances, hallucinations, delusions, and psychomotor agitation that place her in the delirious range on the Delirium Rating Scale-Revised-98 (Trzepacz et al. 2001). On the Marie Three Paper Test (see p. 13), the patient is asked to manipulate three different-sized pieces of paper but becomes confused about the directions. She crumples the papers on several tries and puts them under the pillow without explanation. She has difficulty signing her name without duplicating the last letters of her surname.

Repeated bloodwork and second MRI of the head are normal. A second eletroencephalogram (EEG) performed 1 week after the first shows diffuse slowing.

Study Group Questions for Cases 1–3

1. What documentation would be helpful in the psychiatric assessment in each of the cases? (See pp. 288–301)
2. What conditions should be included in the differential diagnosis? (See p. 4, column 1)
3. What additional medical workup should be requested? (See p. 255)
4. How should each patient be managed while the additional workup is under way? (See pp. 14–22)
5. In Case 1, how should the consultant explain to the family that is concerned about Alzheimer's the differences between delirium and dementia? (See p. 4)
6. How would you respond to the question about ICU psychosis in Case 2? (See pp. 7–8)
7. What would you advise about the nighttime agitation in Case 2? Do you think sleep deprivation is etiologic or symptomatic? (See pp. 21–22)
8. What cancers are most likely to metastasize to the brain? (See p. 8)
9. How would you respond to the question about schizophrenia in Case 3? (See p. 4)
10. What do you propose as the etiology of the change in mental status examination results, given the normal metabolic and metastatic workup in Case 3? (See pp. 8–9)

■ DIAGNOSIS

Delirium is a potentially grave medical complication in the treatment of seriously ill patients. Many terms have been used for it over the years: organic brain syndrome, acute confusional states, confusion, acute dementia, acute brain failure, metabolic encephalopathy, reversible toxic psychosis, and ICU psychosis (Rabinowitz 2002). It is a common neuropsychiatric illness among medically compromised patients, with significant mortality and morbidity.

Delirium represents "acute brain failure," analogous in urgency to acute congestive heart failure or acute renal failure. *It is a medical emergency.* The delirious patient may initially present with psychiatric symptoms, such as psychosis, affective lability, and psychomotor disturbances. Such a patient is at risk for languishing on a psychiatric or medical-surgical service if the underlying physiological etiology of the disturbance is not recognized.

The following checklists and worksheets may be useful for your consultations:

- Appendix 1. "American Psychiatric Association Guidelines for Assessing the Delirious Patient: Checklist" (American Psychiatric Association 1999)
- Appendix 2. "Worksheet for Organizing Medical Chart Information: The Initial Psychiatric Consultation." It might be helpful to fill out this worksheet, using chart review and information gathered from staff and family, before seeing the patient.
- Appendix 3. "Decision Tree for Psychiatric Differential Diagnosis of Medically Ill Patients"
- Appendix 4. "'VINDICTIVE MADS'" [a mnemonic]: Differential Diagnosis of Mental Status Changes"
- Appendix 17. "Neuropsychiatric Effects of Electrolyte and Acid-Base Imbalance"

Presenting Features

Fluctuating consciousness is the crux of delirium, occurring in approximately 10%–15% of medical patients, with elderly patients at special risk (Rosen et al. 1994). Recovery is related inversely to age and duration of illness, with mortality rates of elderly patients ranging from 15% to 30% (Liston 1984; Rabins and Folstein 1982).

In Search of Delirium's "Hallmark"

In the universe of inappropriate consults, it is unlikely that psychiatrists will be called for bladder problems.

But one study (Francis et al. 1990) found that the most common behavioral marker for the delirious elderly patient was incontinence! Another study revealed that up to 30% of a sample of patients (age >50 years) with subsequently proven urinary tract infection initially presented with confusion (Barkham et al. 1996). (The etiology of delirium in Case 1, Mrs. July 1st, was a urinary tract infection.) *Delirium does not always present as blatant cognitive deficits or agitation.* It may be subtle and surreptitious in onset. For example, the placid medical-surgical patient is rarely the object of a "psych consult." However, many delirious patients appear calm and in no obvious distress, riding the wave of fluctuating brain impairment while the delirious process rumbles on below the surface.

"Unpredictable, fluctuating alertness and clouded sensory awareness" sound more recognizable on paper than they are at the bedside. Obvious cognitive problems occur in only about 30% of consultations. Other presentations are the rule: in 20% of consultations, anxiety or depression is the main feature; in 20%, hallucinations or delusions; and in another 20%, inappropriate behavior (e.g., irascibility, uncooperativeness, attempts to leave against medical advice) (Horvath et al. 1989; Nicholas and Lindsey 1995).

Because many requests for psychiatric consultation are for agitated patients who are later diagnosed with delirium, one may think of psychomotor agitation as delirium's "hallmark." It is not. The clinical emphasis on agitation is an artifact of the tendency to select agitated patients for referral to psychiatrists.

Delirium and Dementia

Diagnosis is challenging when delirium and dementia occur simultaneously, especially when the delirium is of the hypoactive type. Both disorders target the elderly. Both conditions attack cognition. Both produce behavioral disinhibition, particularly at night ("sundowning.") What distinguishes one from the other is the *state of consciousness*. The demented patient is usually consistently alert, albeit cognitively impaired. The alertness of the delirious patient is variable and shifts throughout the day. Longitudinal information helps establish the pattern and must be collected from the observations of friends, family, and staff. The Delirium Rating-Scale Revised-98 (Trzepacz et al. 2001) is a bedside screening instrument that has been shown to reliably discriminate between delirium and dementia. It is reproduced in Appendix 8.

The neuropsychiatry of dementia is a subspecialty in itself and exceeds the range of this handbook. Appendix 5 provides a quick guide to treating dementia-related behavioral problems in the medical setting and offers references for further reading.

Beware of Default Psychiatric Diagnoses

A psychiatric etiology may be proposed "by default" when no medical cause is obvious (e.g., "psychotic depression," insomnia-induced psychosis, and schizophrenia in Cases 1, 2, and 3 above, respectively). Maintain diagnostic vigilance when there is no straightforward explanation for the delirious state, particularly when the etiology seems "a little of this, a little of that." For example, the combination of a urinary tract infection and a low-grade fever may not be dramatic, but it can devastate the brain functioning of a debilitated patient, as in Case 1 above.

Observe over time. "Hit and run" consultation is fraught with potential mistakes. One cross-sectional interview may coincide with a lucid state, concealing the disordered sensorium. Collection of longitudinal data from many sources provides the best method for diagnosis.

Do not *"diagnose and vanish."* It is inappropriate to diagnose delirium and limit psychiatric involvement to an order for an antipsychotic. Delirious patients need ongoing psychiatric follow-up. If the initial psychiatric consultant cannot return to the bedside, follow-up should be signed out to a colleague who can monitor the patient and assist the staff with questions.

Risk Factors

When consulting on an inpatient with any of the following risk factors, it is clinically helpful to *assume delirium is present* until proven otherwise, regardless of the presenting psychiatric complaint (American Psychiatric Association 1999; Casarett and Inouye 2001; Inouye 2000; Lawlor et al. 2000; Liptzin 2000; Morita et al. 2001):

- Advanced age (especially >80 years)
- Severe illness (especially cancer)
- Dehydration
- Dementia
- Fever or hypothermia
- Substance abuse
- Azotemia
- Hypoalbuminemia
- Abnormal sodium levels
- Polypharmacy
- Visual or hearing impairment

■ ETIOLOGIES

There has been a shift away from conceptualizing delirium as an "imbalance" between two neurotransmitter systems and toward the view that delirium involves neuronal membrane dysfunction (Brown et al. 2000). In clinical practice, delirium is often a direct consequence of a general physiological stressor. *The goals of evaluation and treatment are to find the underlying cause of delirium and to correct it.* The seven "WHHHIMP" etiologies must be evaluated quickly because of their potential to permanently injury the central nervous system: **W**ernicke's encephalopathy, **H**ypoxia, **H**ypoglycemia, **H**ypertensive encephalopathy, **I**ntracerebral hemorrhage, **M**eningitis/encephalitis, and **P**oisoning.

Appendix 4, "'VINDICTIVE MADS': Differential Diagnosis of Mental Status Changes," lists the many diverse etiologies of delirium. (The acronym is a mnemonic for remembering the general categories of factors.) A few etiologies bear special emphasis in the psychiatric care of the medically ill because they occur commonly or masquerade as psychiatric illness.

Infection

Under the right circumstances, in a sufficiently vulnerable patient, bacteremia can induce mental status changes. For example, bacteremia was associated with encephalopathy in a prospective case series of 50 patients selected according to clinical and laboratory criteria for severe sepsis (Eidelman et al. 1996). Urinary tract infection (UTI)–associated bacteremia (confirmed by blood cultures) presented as confusion in 30% of a sample of patients over age 50 (Barkham et al. 1996). Only 20% had presented with new urinary symptoms. (The remaining sample of UTI patients presented with respiratory features, such as cough and dyspnea, with no pulmonary pathology.) Although the majority had pyuria, fewer than half of the urine samples arrived in the laboratory on the day of admission, delaying diagnosis. The mental status of Mrs. July 1st (Case 1 above) cleared entirely upon resolution of the UTI.

Note that UTIs and pneumonias are particularly common infections in older patients. The onset of confusion in an elderly or debilitated person *should trigger concerns about infection, regardless of setting* (Cassem et al. 2004).

Medications

Almost any medication can induce mental status changes in a sufficiently vulnerable patient, especially in elderly persons. In addition, a previously stable dose may cause toxicity in the setting of medical illness, particularly for drugs with a narrow therapeutic index (e.g., digitalis). Some notable offenders:

- Medications with anticholinergic side effects. The evaluation of the delirious patient should include examining medications with anticholinergic properties. For example, even two common over-the-counter medications, cimetidine (Tagamet) and ranitidine (Zantac), have anticholinergic properties, as does prednisone (Tune et al. 1992) (see Table 1–2).
- Corticosteroids and anabolic-androgenic steroids (see Chapter 8, "The Patient Using Steroids")
- Antihypertensives
- Antiarrhythmics. Digoxin, especially, can produce neuropsychiatric side effects, even at therapeutic serum concentrations (Brunner et al. 2000). Neuropsychiatric symptoms, which may be the first sign of digoxin toxicity, include disorientation, confusion, delirium, and hallucinations ("digitalis delirium"). Visual disturbances include white borders or halos on dark objects ("white vision") and disturbances of color vision, commonly with yellow or green coloration of objects, or, less frequently, red, brown, and blue vision. It has been said that the painter Vincent van Gogh chewed on digitalis leaves, prompting the colorful visual effects so characteristic of his painting. Although of dubious value as art history, this anecdote is a good way to remember digoxin toxicity. Digoxin has also been associated with inducing depression-like states at therapeutic serum levels (Eisendrath and Sweeney 1987; Schleifer et al. 1991; Song et al. 2001).
- Syndrome of inappropriate secretion of antidiuretic hormone (SIADH) and hyponatremia, which have been associated with mental status changes and may be precipitated by a number of medications, most notably selective serotonin reuptake inhibitors (SSRIs)
- Antibiotics, especially in high doses and intravenous form
- Any drug used to treat AIDS (see Chapter 9, "The HIV-Infected Patient")
- Anticonvulsants
- NSAIDS (nonsteroidal anti-inflammatory drugs) (see Jiang and Chang 1999; MacKnight and Rojas-Fernandez 2001; Sussman and Magid 2000)
- Histamine H_2 receptor antagonists (H_2-blockers) used to treat peptic ulcers and reflux esophagitis (Heckmann et al. 2000; Rodgers and Brengel 1998; Yuan et al. 2001)
- Herbal supplements (see Appendix 6)

Table 1–2.   Common drugs with significant anticholinergic effects

Antianginals
  Isosorbide dinitrate

Antiarrhythmics
  Disopyramide
  Procainamide
  Quinidine

Antiasthmatics
  Theophylline

Anticoagulants
  Warfarin

Antidepressants
  Amitriptyline
  Amoxapine
  Clomipramine
  Desipramine
  Doxepin
  Imipramine
  Maprotiline
  Nortriptyline
  Olanzapine
  Protriptyline
  Trimipramine

Antidiarrheals
  Diphenoxylate

Antihistamines
  Brompheniramine
  Chlorpheniramine
  Cyclizine
  Dimenhydrinate
  Diphenhydramine
  Hydroxyzine
  Meclizine

Antiparkinsonian agents
  Amantadine
  Benztropine
  Biperiden
  Ethopropazine
  Orphenadrine
  Procyclidine
  Trihexyphenidyl

Antiplatelet agents
  Dipyridamole

Antipsychotics
  Chlorpromazine
  Chlorprothixene
  Clozapine
  Loxapine
  Mesoridazine
  Pimozide
  Thioridazine

Antispasmodics
  Atropine
  Belladonna
  Clidinium
  Dicyclomine
  Glycopyrrolate
  Homatropine
  Hyoscine
  Hyoscyamine
  Mepenzolate
  Methscopolamine
  Oxybutynin
  Propantheline
  Scopolamine
  Tolterodine

Calcium channel blockers
  Nifedipine

Cardiac glycosides
  Digoxin

Corticosteroids
  Prednisolone

Diuretics
  Furosemide

H$_2$ antagonists
  Cimetidine
  Ranitidine

Narcotic analgesics
  Codeine

Sedatives
  Promethazine

Skeletal muscle relaxants
  Cyclobenzaprine

Source.   Robinson MJ, Owen JA (compiled from Bezchlibnyk and Jeffries 2002; McEvoy 2003; Repchinsky 2003; Tune et al. 1992; USP DI Editorial Board 2003). Used with permission.

A word on manipulating medication: If medications believed to be disrupting mental status, such as steroids, cannot be discontinued, two strategies may be helpful (Boland et al. 2000): 1) switch to a medication that is less lipophilic, and therefore less likely to penetrate the blood-brain barrier (e.g., among the β-blockers, atenolol [Tenormin] is a reasonable alternative to its more lipophilic cousin, propranolol [Inderal]), or 2) try lowering the medication to its minimally effective dose.

Withdrawal Syndromes

Withdrawal syndromes may be overlooked, particularly if the patient is delirious or critically ill and unable to give history. The presence of unexplained autonomic arousal (e.g., elevated vital signs) or seizures should bring up the possibility of withdrawal states. Symptoms of autonomic arousal may be masked by the patient's acute illness or by antihypertensive medication such as β-blockers. Try to obtain detailed alcohol and drug histories whenever possible.

Hypoxia

Check oxygen saturation in the workup of mental status changes. Hypoxia cannot be inferred from level of consciousness. It is a clinical myth that alertness is a sensitive indicator of oxygenation; alertness is preserved even in the setting of moderate hypoxemia (Grant et al. 1987). Usually only extreme hypoxia causes alertness to suffer in an obvious way. "Guesstimating" of a patient's level of oxygenation is fraught with error because hypoxic, cognitively impaired patients may appear perfectly "awake."

The rate at which hypoxia develops, rather than the absolute level of oxygen saturation, will determine the acute neuropsychiatric consequences of hypoxemia (Griggs and Arieff 1992; Lipowski 1990). In the setting of chronic hypoxia, for example, oxygen saturations as low as 60 mm Hg may produce few mental status changes, whereas abrupt declines from higher baselines usually result in delirium (Lipowski 1990). Even mild hypoxemia produces cognitive changes such as problems in abstraction, perceptual motor integration, and language function (Fix et al. 1982; Prigatano et al. 1983). The mental status examination results of "Mr. Sundowning" (Case 2 above) improved remarkably once his hypoxia was corrected.

Carbon dioxide retention produces anesthetic-like changes that resemble barbiturate intoxication. Whereas acute increases of PCO_2 to 70 mm Hg will produce confusional states, patients who are experiencing chronic hypercapnia may preserve alertness (Lipowski 1990).

Electrolyte Disturbances

Appendix 17 lists the neuropsychiatric effects of electrolyte and acid-base imbalance. Often, these present as subtle mental status changes that mimic primary Axis I conditions.

Surgical Factors

Delirium is particularly common postoperatively in elderly patients, with estimates as high as 30% (Dyer et al. 1995; van der Mast 1999; van der Mast and Roest 1996). Several associated risk factors have been described for "post-op delirium." They are summarized in Table 1–3.

Factors Mislabeled "ICU Psychosis"

Note that "ICU psychosis" is not included in the exhaustive differential diagnosis of delirium. In the context of an intact brain, the noise of the critical care environment should not precipitate psychosis. "ICU psychosis" has become a wastebasket term, cited when delirium is unsuspected or the etiology is unknown. Often, sleep deprivation is proposed as the etiology for psychosis occurring in ICU patients. However, this formulation confuses cause and effect. Delirium produces disruptions in sleep architecture, rather than the other way around.

One might hear examples of patients whose "ICU psychosis" "resolved" upon transfer out of the intensive care unit. Such observations are used in support of the ICU-psychosis causality theory. ICU patients tend to be sicker than other patients, predisposing them to delirium, with its characteristic mental status changes and sleep-wake cycle disturbances. However, the patient's medical improvement (marked by im-

Table 1–3. Generally accepted risk factors for postoperative delirium

Status	Risk factor
Preoperative	Advanced age
	Dementia
	Severity of preoperative illness
	Psychological symptoms, especially depression
	Family history of psychiatric illness
Postoperative	Lower limb ischemia
Surgical	Duration of surgery
	Increased perioperative infusion and transfusion requirements (vascular surgery)
	Type of surgery (aortic aneurysm surgery > vascular surgery)

Note. Based on the pooled findings of several studies (Marcantonio et al. 1998; Sasajima et al. 2000; Schneider et al. 2002). Not every study supported every risk factor.

proved mental status examination results and sleep architecture) is more likely to be causally related to improvement than is the transfer itself.

- *Bottom line: try to avoid the term "ICU psychosis."* Attributing neuropsychiatric changes to "noisy environments" derails thorough differential diagnosis and medical workup (McGuire et al. 2000). Noise reduction does not resolve delirium, but it does promote restful sleep. Check with nursing staff to ensure that nighttime sleep is as uninterrupted as possible. See also Box 1–3, a checklist of supportive interventions for the delirious patient ("SPOCCC"), later in this chapter.

Cancer

Although delirium occurs at a high rate in advanced cancer patients, it is reversible in approximately 50% of episodes (Lawlor et al. 2000). Reversibility of delirium in this population has been associated with the following precipitants: opioid analgesics, psychoactive medications, and dehydration.

Brain metastases may sometimes present as depressed mood, trembling, confusion, and forgetfulness in the absence of other demonstrable neurological symptoms. Differential diagnosis becomes difficult, and symptoms may be misattributed to a primary psychiatric etiology—particularly if there is a prior history of psychiatric illness or if the patient's premorbid personality has been considered "unstable" or "maladjusted." The most common primary cancer sites that metastasize to the brain are (in descending order of frequency):

- Lung, Breast, Melanoma (mnemonic: "Little Brain Mets"), colon, rectum, and kidney

Meningeal carcinomatosis is usually documented by lumbar puncture and the occurrence of relevant clinical findings (i.e., headache, focal weakness, seizures, ataxia, and signs of increased intracranial pressure). It usually presents with radiculopathies (particularly involving the cauda equina), cranial nerve palsies, and dementia. Mental and behavioral abnormalities may also occur. (Note that bacterial meningitis presents differently, with fever, stiff neck, and headache.)

Paraneoplastic Syndromes

Nonmetastatic neuropsychiatric syndromes may occur as rare, remote effects of cancer—"paraneoplastic" syndromes. When they produce mental status or behavioral phenomena, they are grouped together and

termed *paraneoplastic limbic encephalopathy* (PLE), also known as limbic encephalitis. In PLE, cancers occurring in remote parts of the body induce pathological changes in the limbic gray matter of the brain, even in the absence of metastases. Patients present in a variety of ways: with dementia-like alterations of recent memory and other intellectual functions; severe anxiety or depression; and/or psychosis (Amir and Galbraith 1992; Boylan 2000; Khan and Wieser 1994; Lishman 1998; McClure et al. 1999; Newman et al. 1990). Amnesia may be the sole neuropsychological abnormality in some patients (Bak et al. 2001). Catatonia has also been reported as the presenting symptom (Tandon et al. 1988).

A paraneoplastic etiology for the psychiatric symptoms is more likely to be suspected when there are accompanying focal neurological symptoms, such as ataxia, seizures, peripheral neuropathy, or opsoclonus (an eye movement abnormality). These may prompt a search for paraneoplastic-associated antibodies in the serum (see discussion of objective findings below).

Sometimes, however, PLE neuropsychiatric symptoms occur in isolation and may precede the diagnosis of cancer, obscuring the underlying etiology (Gultekin et al. 2000; Posner 2000; Zeimer 2000). Routine diagnostic tests, including MRI of the brain, may be initially normal, prompting the oft-heard, dreaded conclusion that the patient is "medically cleared" and should be transferred to psychiatry.

PLE in DSM-IV-TR would be classified as a psychiatric condition (delirium, psychosis, or dementia) "due to a general medical condition." PLE has been reported in association with many types of cancer, but it most frequently occurs with lung cancer; it also has been associated with testicular cancer, breast cancer, and viral encephalitis in immunocompromised patients (Almeras et al. 2001; Gultekin et al. 2000; Posner 2000; Sutton et al. 2000; Tattevin et al. 2001; Wainwright et al. 2001; Wani et al. 2001). PLE syndromes can persist even after successful resection of the tumor (Lishman 1998). Prognosis is generally poor.

Objective findings may include cerebrospinal fluid (CSF) pleocytosis, elevated CSF protein concentration, and generalized slowing on EEG (Fakhoury et al. 1999; Kassubek et al. 2001). It is believed that an autoimmune-mediated mechanism accounts for most paraneoplastic syndromes. Antibodies found in paraneoplastic syndromes are mostly polyclonal immunoglobulin G (IgG) that fixes complement (Posner 2000). These antibodies react with target neurological tissue as well as the underlying tumor. The most frequently found antineuronal antibodies are anti-Hu, anti-Ta, and anti-Ma (Gultekin et al. 2000). However, some patients with PLE test negative for these antibodies, complicating the diagnosis. Points to keep in mind:

- PLE may occur in the absence of documentable metabolic or metastatic neurological disease.
- A preexisting psychiatric history may divert attention away from the paraneoplastic etiology, especially when there are no focal neurological symptoms and laboratory and imaging tests are normal. Ms. Psych-History-Clear-Scans-Please-Transfer (Case 3 above) was found to have PLE.
- *Bottom line:* PLE should be considered in a patient who presents with psychosis, personality changes, or cognitive deficits. It should be included in the differential diagnosis of oncology patients who present with behavioral or mental status changes and negative findings on brain imaging studies.

Cardiovascular Disease

Rates of delirium are high among cardiac patients, particularly in those undergoing cardiac surgery and intraaortic balloon pump (IABP) therapy. Huffman et al. (2004, p. 561) devised the following list of risk factors for delirium that are of special relevance to cardiac patients:

- *Central nervous system hypoperfusion:* poor cardiac output due to congestive heart failure, myocardial infarction, or myocardial ischemia; cerebrovascular accident (ischemic or hemorrhagic, in the setting of anticoagulation); comorbid carotid disease; hypovolemia (due to dehydration or bleeding); hypotension relative to patient's baseline blood pressure
- *Medication-related causes:* digoxin toxicity, narcotic analgesics, benzodiazepines, anticholinergic medications, H_2-blockers (such as cimetidine, famotidine, nizatidine, ranitidine)
- *Other general medical conditions:* electrolyte abnormalities (especially hyponatremia with diuretic administration), hypertensive encephalopathy, hypoxia (during pulmonary edema), infections (e.g., pneumonia, urinary tract infections), alcohol withdrawal

Serotonin Syndrome

The antidepressant selective serotonin reuptake inhibitors (SSRIs) have become so routinely prescribed and easy to use in general medical practice that their drug-drug interactions may be overlooked. The potential deliriogenic role of serotonergic medications is impressive. The complications of combining a monoamine oxidase inhibitor with an SSRI have been well publicized. Less familiar, however, are the risks of inducing serotonin syndrome by the clinically "benign" action of increasing an SSRI in a vulnerable patient. Case reports of serotonin syndrome have been described in the addition to an SSRI regimen of trazodone (Desyrel) for sleep or buspirone (BuSpar) for anxiety. Over-the-counter cough syrups with dextromethorphan may precipitate serotonin syndrome, as may certain analgesics and the triptan family of migraine medications. There are occasional anecdotal reports of atypical antipsychotics being associated with this syndrome (Duggal and Fetchko 2002; Hamilton and Malone 2000; Mason et al. 2000). In one such report, the serotonin 5-HT$_2$ and 5-HT$_3$ receptor antagonism of olanzapine (Zyprexa) added to a mix of mirtazapine (Remeron) and tramadol (Ultram) was thought to have precipitated serotonin syndrome (Duggal and Fetchko 2002). A list of drugs potentiating serotonin in the central nervous system can be found in Table 1–4.

Serotonin syndrome resembles neuroleptic malignant syndrome (NMS) but has certain distinct features. Appendix 7 includes checklists for diagnosing serotonin syndrome and NMS.

In most case reports, serotonin syndrome was self-limited and responded to discontinuing serotonergic agents. In more severe cases, other interventions included respiratory and cardiovascular monitoring, intravenous hydration to prevent renal failure, a cooling blanket for hyperthermia, and anticonvulsants for myoclonus or seizures. The nonspecific serotonin antagonist cyproheptadine (Periactin; 4–24 mg/day) was the most consistently effective treatment in an exhaustive 2003 review of case reports of patients nonresponsive to discontinuation of serotonergic agents or general supportive measures (Mann et al. 2003). In this same review, other interventions such as benzodiazepines, dantrolene (Dantrium; a muscle relaxant), and propranolol (Inderal; the L-isomer is a serotonin antagonist) were markedly effective in some patients but equivocally so in others.

The 2003 volume by Mann et al. is a practical, in-depth guide to the differential diagnosis and treatment of the serious hyperthermic reactions encountered in the treatment of psychiatric disorders, including serotonin syndrome, NMS, neuroleptic-induced heatstroke, malignant catatonia, and hyperthermic reactions associated with other neuropsychiatric drugs.

Table 1–4.   Drugs potentiating serotonin in the central nervous system

Class	Potentiating drugs
Antidepressants	SSRIs (all), mirtazapine (Remeron), tricyclic antidepressants (all), nefazodone (Serzone), trazodone (Desyrel), venlafaxine (Effexor), MAOIs
Antiemetics	Granisetron (Kytril), ondansetron (Zofran)
Antiobsessionals	Clomipramine (Anafranil), fluvoxamine (Luvox)
Anxiolytics	Buspirone (BuSpar)
Antimigraine drugs	Dihydroergotamine (DHE-45), sumatriptan (Imitrex)
Antipsychotics, atypical	[Anecdotal case reports]
Mood stabilizers	Lithium
Opioids	Meperidine (Demerol), tramadol (Ultram), fentanyl (opioid agonist; anesthetic agent), dextromethorphan (in over-the-counter antitussives)
Stimulants	Amphetamines, cocaine
Miscellaneous	Bromocriptine (Parlodel), sibutramine (Meridia)

Note.   MAOI=monoamine oxidase inhibitor; SSRI=selective serotonin reuptake inhibitor.
Source.   Adapted from Mann et al. 2003. Used with permission.

■ BEDSIDE ASSESSMENT

It has been said that "the mental status examination is to the consultation-liaison psychiatrist what the cardiac examination is to the cardiologist or the neurological examination is to the neurologist" (Wise and Cassem 1990). However, a general psychiatric interview is often not enough to elicit subtle cognitive deficits, and general interviews may miss nonverbal deficits, giving the illusion of a normal exam. Neuropsychiatrists warn, however, about the pitfalls of informal bedside screening: simple tests yield simplistic results and cannot accurately reflect the complexities of cognition. Most bedside screening tests lack standardization and reliability. When they are interpreted out of context, the results may be misleading. False positives may overestimate pathology, leading to unnecessary testing and sometimes to treatment errors. False negatives may overlook pathology, resulting in the premature suspension of clinical evaluation because the patient has "passed" the bedside "test."

Despite these limitations, judicious bedside cognitive screening can improve the specificity of the psychiatric diagnostic interview in the medical setting. It can flag those patients requiring additional investigation by a specialist. Some suggestions follow.

- *Consider delirium to be public enemy #1.* Err on the side of the false positive: assume that cognition is disturbed and that delirium is the culprit until proven otherwise. A medical workup that disproves the assumption of delirium better serves the patient than a treatment plan that misses reversible pathology.
- *Remember dementia.* It may coexist with delirium, predate it, and confound its evaluation. Longitudinal history from caregivers is crucial.
- *Collaborate with a neurologist.* Keep in mind that asking "Do you think that encephalopathy may be contributing to the mental status abnormalities?" will be more meaningful to a neurologist than a request to "rule out delirium." Include the basics of the neurological examination in your bedside screening. Limiting "neurologic evaluation" to ordering MRIs and CT scans is inadequate. The EEG is not high-tech, but it flags cases of diffuse cerebral dysfunction in situations where tests for space-occupying lesions may be noncontributory (Jacobson and Jerrier 2000).
- *Diversify.* Assemble tests that tap different cognitive domains as part of regular screening of medical patients. Consider the results as indicators of potential vulnerability rather than as "hard data." Pursue questions with ongoing follow-up, and request additional consultation when you feel it is appropriate.
- *Observe.* Continue to monitor those patients whose symptoms do not meet full syndromal status. Although not as grave, subsyndromal delirium still predicts a poor medical outcome (Levkoff et al. 1996).

Establishing good rapport improves the accuracy of mental status interviews. (See Box 1–1 for practical suggestions for bedside manner in the general hospital setting.)

Box 1–1. Practical suggestions for bedside manner in the general hospital setting

1. Sit down. Offer to do something tangible for the patient.

Ideally, pull up a chair up to the bedside and conduct the interview sitting down. Physicians who sit with patients are usually perceived to have been present for much longer than those who remain standing. Sitting down conveys that the consultant has time to spend with the patient.

Offer to do something concretely helpful, such as bringing a drink of water, adjusting a pillow, getting the patient's eyeglasses. Sick people appreciate obvious, nurturing actions. This is a way to establish rapport quickly.

2. Shake hands. Smile at the patient.

Even if you are not usually a warm person, act as if you were! Unless clinically inappropriate, a handshake and a smile can be reassuring and reduce the sense of threat that a patient may feel when seeing a psychiatrist. Both gestures humanize the often sterile, frightening medical setting.

3. Begin by telling the patient what you know about his or her situation.

Rather than ask the patient to tell the story from the beginning, start by summarizing the key elements in the patient's history, in simple language. Ask the patient to correct any misinformation. This spares the patient the ritual of once again repeating information, and it allows for correcting misperceptions and providing new information.

4. Find out the patient's most pressing immediate concerns.

Preoccupied patients are difficult to engage. Explore whether the patient has an undisclosed fear or concern.

5. Ask what the patient thinks about the illness.

Ask in detail about the patient's understanding regarding the nature, cause, and prognosis of the illness or injury. What are the patient's specific concerns? For example: "Even though your doctors are still trying to discover your problem, what have you thought yourself about what is making you sick?"

6. Ask about the patient's life and family.

Find out the details about the patient's family, major social roles (such as occupation), and the impact of the current illness. These questions might be phrased as "Who are the important people in your family? How are they coping with your being in the hospital? What impact is your illness having on life outside the hospital?"

7. Ask about the patient as a person.

The patient role can be demoralizing and isolating. Many seriously ill people feel useless, and think that their caregivers do not appreciate them as "as people" or recognize the contributions they made when they were well. Ask about the patient's personal characteristics, activities, and achievements. Find appropriate (not forced) opportunities to acknowledge them.

8. Acknowledge the patient's plight.

It can be comforting to hear from an authority figure, "If I were facing all that you have told me about, I might feel very similarly." The patient should be told that it is very natural—and expected—to react emotionally when bearing severe pain, confronting death, experiencing major medical problems, or contending with disability.

9. Involve the patient as an ally in the mental status examination.

Try to avoid the abrupt shift from gathering history to the embarrassed statement, "I just need to ask you a few questions that we ask everybody." Many patients interpret the mental status exam as a search for serious mental problems or evidence that the patient is "crazy," and such a shift can reinforce that impression. Instead, try to cull as much as you can from naturalistic observations made during the course of the interview.

If formal testing is necessary, try to enlist the patient as an ally with an explanation about how the patient stands to benefit (e.g., "Sometimes medical conditions cause problems with memory and thinking. Could you help me figure out if this is happening with you? If it is, we can investigate the cause and do something to help you. I have some tests of concentration, memory, and thinking. As your treatment goes along, we can follow these tests, just as we do with blood tests.") This approach relieves the patient from feeling like a "specimen" with the consultant as grand inquisitor.

10. Leave the patient with something concrete.

Give the patient feedback, and ask for feedback. Offer a revised formulation, or confirm that the original one was correct. Say what you intend to do with the information: e.g., share it with the primary physician, recommend certain diagnostic or treatment interventions, return for further interviews, suggest medications. If you intend to return, try to be specific about when the patient should expect you.

Source.   Adapted from Yager J: "Specific Components of Bedside Manner in the General Hospital Psychiatric Consultation: 12 Concrete Suggestions." *Psychosomatics* 30:209–212, 1989.

■ BEDSIDE SCREENING INSTRUMENTS

There are many bedside screening instruments, but only a few are standardized. Box 1–2 lists the standardized bedside screening instruments. Copies of the actual test instruments are provided in this volume whenever possible.

Mini-Mental State Examination (MMSE)

The MMSE is the most widely used bedside screening instrument of cognition. It taps orientation, registration, memory, attention, calculation, recall, visuospatial function, and language. A score of 20 or less out of 30 suggests significant cognitive difficulties but is not specific as to etiology (Folstein et al. 1975). Advantages of the MMSE include quick administration, little

Box 1–2. **Bedside assessment tests of cognitive function**	
Test	**Description**
Mini-Mental State Examination (MMSE)	Assesses orientation, registration, memory, attention, calculation, recall, visuospatial function, and language. A score ≤20/30 occurs with significant cognitive difficulties but is not specific as to etiology. ADVANTAGES: Quick administration, little practice effect, can track cognitive fluctuations over time. DISADVANTAGES: Low sensitivity for detecting delirium. AVAILABILITY: Psychological Assessment Resources, Inc. (http://www.parinc.com; or http://www.minimental.com, accessed June 2004)
Delirium Rating Scale-Revised-98 (DRS-R-98)	A 16-item clinician-rated scale with 13 severity items and 3 diagnostic items. ADVANTAGES: Specifically, sensitively, and reliably measures delirium symptoms. AVAILABILITY: Appendix 8.
Abbreviated Cognitive Test for Delirium (CTD)	Derived from the original CTD, the abbreviated version consists of five subtests: Orientation, Attention 1 and 2, Memory 1 and 2, Comprehension 1 and 2, and Vigilance 1 and 2. ADVANTAGES: Quick administration, responses nonverbal (pointing, nodding head, raising hand). AVAILABILITY: See Hart et al. 1996, 1997.
Confusion Assessment Method (CAM) and CAM for the Intensive Care Unit (CAM-ICU)	CAM: High sensitivity and specificity for detecting delirium. AVAILABILITY: Appendix 9. CAM-ICU: Substitutes nonverbal tasks for verbal responses, allowing assessment of mechanically ventilated patients (Ely et al. 2001). AVAILABILITY: http://www.icudelirium.org (accessed May 2004)
Memorial Delirium Assessment Scale (MDAS)	Developed as a brief, reliable tool for assessing delirium severity among medically ill populations. ADVANTAGES: Rates delirium severity and tracks the changes over time. Cutoff score of 13 distinguishes "moderate" and "severe" delirium. DISADVANTAGES: May miss "mild" evidence of delirium, so best used in conjunction with a more sensitive instrument (Breitbart et al. 1997). AVAILABILITY: Appendix 10.
Trail Making Test (TMT)	In Part A, patient connects numbered circles in sequence (1–2–3–4...) as quickly as possible. In Part B, patient completes a number-letter connection task (1-A-2-B-3...). ADVANTAGES: Highly sensitive to detecting delirium. DISADVANTAGES: High rate of false positives and limited reliability. AVAILABILITY: Psychological Assessment Resources, Inc. (http://www.parinc.com)
Symbol Digit Modalities Test (SDMT)	Patient has 90 seconds to pair specific numbers with given geometric figures on a reference page. ADVANTAGES: High sensitivity, quick administration, little practice effect, can track cognitive fluctuations over time. AVAILABILITY: Western Psychological Services (http://www.wpspublish.com).

practice effect, and the ability to track cognitive fluctuations over time. Disadvantages include insensitivity to delirium and thought disorders. The MMSE may overestimate the cognitive deficits of patients who have stable focal deficits such as aphasia, dyslexia, or dyscalculia.

The MMSE is widely available online (search: "Folstein Mini-Mental State Exam"). Alternatively, it can be purchased from Psychological Assessment Resources, Inc. (http://www.parinc.com). Updated normative data for age and education are now available. The newly revised test forms are convenient and appropriate for inclusion in medical charts.

Delirium Rating Scale Revised-98 (DRS-R-98)

The DRS-R-98 (Appendix 8) is probably the most widely used instrument for bedside screening and research in delirium (Trzepacz et al. 2001). This instrument is a 16-item clinician-rated scale divided into two sections: 3 diagnostic items for initial ratings and a 13-item severity scale for repeated measurements. The scores from both groups of questions are added together to arrive at a total score. Total scores in excess of 18 are highly suggestive of the presence of delirium.

The severity items allow ratings for gradations of symptom intensity, and specific characteristics can be noted on the score sheet. Items cover language, thought processes, two motoric presentations, and five components of cognition. The test is a revision of the Delirium Rating Scale, a widely used delirium rating instrument that specifically, sensitively, and reliably measures delirium symptoms. The DRS-R-98 has been shown to be a valid and reliable symptom severity scale for delirium. It is also useful in serial measurements of delirium in treatment research.

■ OTHER INSTRUMENTS AND INFORMAL ASSESSMENT STRATEGIES

Box 1–2 also describes the Confusion Assessment Method (CAM; Appendix 9) and CAM-ICU, Memorial Delirium Assessment Scale (MDAS; Appendix 10), Trail Making Test (TMT), and Symbol Digit Modalities Test (SDMT).

Every clinician should have one or two informal bedside strategies to supplement the more structured instruments. Some of the more easily administered tests in critically ill patients are described below.

Handwriting

Impairment of writing (dysgraphia) is one of the most sensitive indicators of delirium (Aakerlund and Rosenberg 1994; Wallesch and Hundsalz 1994). For example, in a classic study, 33 of 34 acutely confused patients demonstrated clumsily drawn letters, reduplication of strokes (in letters like *M* and *W*), inability to align letters properly, problems with upward-downward letter orientation, and misspellings (Chedru and Geschwind 1972). Clearing of the delirium was associated with resolution of the dysgraphia.

Constructional Ability: The 10-Point Clock Test

The degree of difficulty in drawing a clock face correlates with nonspecific cognitive dysfunction and electroencephalographic slowing (Manos and Wu 1998). (See instructions for administration and scoring of the 10-Point Clock Test at http://www.seniorpsychiatry.com/pages/articles/10ptclocktest.html; accessed June 2004.)

Reitan-Indiana Aphasia Screening Test

This test aids in discriminating between hemispheric lesions; patients with left hemispheric deficits can copy the designs but cannot write, whereas patients with right hemispheric lesions can write but often cannot reproduce the designs (Lezak 1983). A shortened version of a more extensive screening test consists of four tasks:

a. Copy a square, a Greek cross (+), and a triangle without lifting pencil from paper.
b. Name each copied figure.
c. Spell each name.
d. Repeat "He shoute   ~ " then explain its meaning and writ

Marie Three Pa

The patient is give
per and asked to
the examiner, ta
ground, and tak
his or her own

Left-Right

The patient
right hand

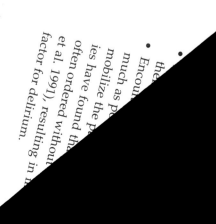

on your right ear"; "place your right hand on your right elbow." These tasks not only assess left-right confusion but also tax the patient's ability to understand and manipulate information. The unimpaired patient will realize that the last request is impossible, whereas confused patients will either attempt it or perseveratively repeat the first two tasks.

■ DECISION-MAKING CAPACITY AND INFORMED CONSENT

One of the most important components of the bedside assessment of cognition is the determination of decision-making capacity. Often, it is when the patient refuses a medical procedure or diagnostic test that an underlying cognitive disturbance such as delirium is discovered. See Chapter 12 in this volume, "Assessing Decisional Capacity and Informed Consent in Medical Patients: A Short, Practical Guide."

■ SUPPORTIVE INTERVENTIONS

The following supportive interventions are derived from the intervention studies of Inouye and colleagues (Inouye 2000; Inouye et al. 1999). See also Box 1–3, a checklist of supportive interventions for the delirious patient ("SPOCCC").

- Review medication lists regularly, minimizing psychoactive medications whenever possible.
- Provide patients with frequent reorientation and a schedule of their activities.
- Emphasize interpersonal contact and communication, using reorientation strategies, simple instructions and explanations, and frequent eye contact. Family members and caregivers should be shown how to provide this type of ongoing support.
- Allow patients to participate in their care and decision making as much as possible.
- Reduce sensory deficits by providing patients with their eyeglasses and/or hearing aids.
- Encourage mobility, self-care, and independence as possible; try to minimize devices that immobilize patient (e.g., bladder catheters). Studies show that bed rest or minimal activity is rarely with clinical justification (Lazarus et al. ...) ... immobility, a leading risk

- Avoid physical restraints, if possible, because of the potential adverse effects of immobility and increased agitation and the potential to cause injury.
- Use clocks, calendars, and orienting objects from home (e.g., personal tokens, family photographs, and religious items).
- Keep room and staff changes to a minimum.
- Encourage a quiet environment with low-level lighting to calm the delirious patient.
- Check with nursing staff to ensure that nighttime sleep is as uninterrupted as possible.
- Consider nonpharmacological approaches for relaxation, such as music, relaxation tapes, and massage, which can enhance sleep and reduce agitation (McDowell et al. 1998). See also the American College of Critical Care Medicine practice guideline "The Use of Physical Restraints and Pharmacologic Therapies to Maintain Patient Safety in the Intensive Care Unit" (Maccioli et al. 2003), available at: http://www.sccm.org/professional_resources/guidelines/table_of _contents/index.asp.

■ PHARMACOLOGICAL INTERVENTIONS

When agitation accompanies delirium in the medical setting, short-term use of antipsychotics remains the treatment of choice. No clear guidelines exist for the specific choice of antipsychotic agent. Haloperidol (Haldol) alone or in combination with lorazepam (Ativan) remains the most widely used treatment for the agitation of delirium (Ely et al. 2004). However, the atypical antipsychotics have gained use for delirium, particularly for patients at risk for extrapyramidal side effects. For example, a recent survey regarding the treatment of delirium in elderly persons revealed no consensus on a first-line drug but did yield several high "second-line" ratings, including haloperidol, risperidone, quetiapine, and olanzapine (Alexopoulos et al. 2004).

- For delirium, the goal of psychiatric treatment is twofold:
  1. To completely calm (not obtund) an agitated, delirious patient at the outset (rather than partially control or barely keep up with agitation over several days) so that the etiology of the delirium can be diagnosed and corrected (Cassem et al. 2004)
  2. To normalize sleep disruption (which is a consequence of delirium, not a cause of it)

Box 1–3. **A checklist of supportive interventions for the delirious patient ("SPOCCC")**	
Category	**Intervention**
SUPPORT	The delirious patient is confused, not comatose; listen to concerns and provide reassurance. Research shows that delirium is often remembered as a frightening experience (Breitbart et al. 2002a).
PROTECT	Agitation and confusion may cause danger to self or others. Use mittens and restraints, applying the fewest restraints possible.
ORIENT	Reorient frequently, using calendars, television. Enlist the help of family members.
CALM	Limit noise from alarms and equipment; maintain semblance of day-night cycle; perform nonessential care during the day (to reduce nighttime disruptions).
COMMUNICATE	Encourage interactions with family and staff to help orient the patient. Use writing if speaking is not possible; use letterboard, hand, or blink signals if patient is unable to write.
COMFORT	Provide adequate pain control; try to mobilize from bed to chair; permit rest and limit unnecessary awakenings; invite family members to stay with patient to reduce suspiciousness and paranoia.

Source. Adapted from Boland R, Goldstein M, Haltzman S: "Psychiatric Management of Behavioral Syndromes in Intensive Care Units," in *Psychiatric Care of the Medical Patient.* Edited by Stoudemire A, Fogel B, Greenberg D. New York, Oxford University Press, 2000, p 303.

Pharmacologic Treatment of Delirium: General Principles

Box 1–4 outlines the principles for treating delirium with pharmacologic agents.

Day 1: Acute Phase Treatment

The strategy for treating delirium is to calm the patient completely during the first day, later slowly tapering the medication as the delirium clears. For highly agitated patients, the choice of medications may be limited to those with intramuscular forms. On Day 1, medication is titrated against agitation in a stepwise fashion. Avoid obtunding the patient.

Torsades de pointes: Reports of arrhythmia and sudden death correlating with the use of antipsychotics have been the focus of increased attention. These agents (and other psychotropics, particularly the tricyclic antidepressants) produce prolongation of the QT interval of the electrocardiogram. This effect, termed *acquired long QT syndrome,* predisposes to the malignant ventricular arrhythmia *torsades de pointes* ("twisting of points"; i.e., a twisting or a 180-degree rotation of the axis of ectopic beats). Torsades de pointes (TDP) may degenerate into ventricular fibrillation, which is fatal if left untreated. Thioridazine (Mellaril) has earned the dubious distinction of being the most cardiotoxic antipsychotic because of this potential side effect. (In 1994, a gene that codes for a cardiac ion channel sub-

unit with the unlikely name *Human Ether-a-Go-Go related gene,* or *HERG,* was found to be responsible for congenital long QT syndrome. This finding supported the notion that pharmacologic inhibition of cardiac potassium channels was a possible mechanism for acquired long QT syndrome. Several reviews are available on this topic (Glassman 2002; Glassman and Bigger 2002; Taylor 2003; Witchel et al. 2003). (See also Chapter 3 in this volume, "The Patient With Cardiovascular Disease.")

Vital signs should be checked regularly and the patient screened for other risk factors for TDP (see Appendix 11). In particular:

- QTc interval >450 ms (proceed cautiously); >500 ms (consider other medications)
- Check and correct electrolyte abnormalities (goal: $K^+ > 4$ mEq/L, $Mg^{++} > 2$ mEq/L) (Huffman et al. 2004)

After the patient is completely calm, but not overly sedated, write standing orders for the antipsychotic to be given at regular intervals (every 4–6 hours, "hold for excessive sedation") over the next 24 hours. Administer most of the medication at bedtime, in order to normalize sleep and medicate the "sundowning" behavior occurring with sleep cycle disruptions. Dose estimates should be based on what happened with the patient's medications the day before, seeking to maintain antipsychotic blood levels while avoiding oversedation.

Box 1–4. **General principles for treating delirium**

Goals: 1) To completely calm agitation. 2) To normalize sleep.

DAY 1: *GOAL:* SEDATE, DO NOT OBTUND.
Assess before medication, if possible:
- Check vital signs.
- TDP risk factors (see Appendix 11), particularly:
    - Obtain baseline QTc interval (goal: <450 ms). If baseline QTc shows prolongation ≥450 ms, or ≥25% over baseline, get cardiology consultation and consider other options (e.g., lorazepam).
    - Check and correct electrolyte abnormalities, serum potassium and magnesium (goal: K^+>4 mEq/L, Mg^{++}>2 mEq/L).

Dose 1: Titrate antipsychotic to severity of agitation (see Tables 1–7 and 1–8).
↓
Wait 15–30 minutes.
↓
Dose 2: If patient is still agitated, repeat the antipsychotic at ≥ dose 1.
↓
Wait another 15–30 minutes.
↓
Dose 3 and thereafter: Repeat antipsychotic at ≥dose 2, over next few hours, until patient is no longer agitated.

Sample recommendations (assuming the patient has been successfully sedated):
STANDING MEDICATION: "Antipsychotic [estimate milligrams based on previous dosages required] every 4–6 hours and at bedtime over next 24 hours."
AS-NEEDED MEDICATION: "Antipsychotic every 1–2 hours as needed for agitation [a small dose permitting staff to fine-tune medication based on agitation]. Call psychiatric consultation again at Beeper X if agitation is increasing."
PARAMETERS: "Hold medication for excessive sedation."
 "Hold medication for blood pressure < [fill in parameter] or pulse > [fill in parameter]."
MONITORING: "One-to-one supervision [if patient is a danger to self or others]."
 "Please obtain the following the next morning: ECG; serum K^+, Ca^{++}, Mg^{++}."

DAY 2: *GOAL:* MAINTAIN SEDATION.
Recheck:
- Vital signs.
- TDP risk factors (see Appendix 11), particularly:
    - Check QTc interval (goal: <450 ms). If baseline QTc shows prolongation ≥450 ms, or ≥25% over baseline, get cardiology consultation, reduce dose, or discontinue antipsychotic.
    - Check and correct electrolyte abnormalities, serum potassium and magnesium (goal: K^+>4 mEq/L, Mg^{++}>2 mEq/L).

Calculate: Day 1 grand total of all medication required to sedate patient (i.e., stat+standing+prn).
Reassess: Reexamine mental status and medical course, ideally first thing in the morning and then at intervals throughout the day.

Sample recommendations:
STANDING MEDICATION: "Repeat Day 1 grand total, in divided doses, morning, afternoon, evening, with the largest at bedtime" [e.g., if Day 1 grand total was 15 mg, recommend 3 mg three times during the day and 6 mg at bedtime].
AS-NEEDED MEDICATION: (same as Day 1)
PARAMETERS: (same as Day 1)
MONITORING: (same as Day 1)

DAYS 3–7: *GOAL:* SLOWLY TAPER THE ANTIPSYCHOTIC.
- Titrate to mental status findings (e.g., reduce dose by 50% every 24 hours).
- Recheck vital signs and TDP risk factors.

Some Notes:
- Premature or abrupt discontinuation of medication may cause delirium to relapse.
- Reduce standing Day 2 doses in fragile patients with impaired hepatic metabolism.
- Convert parenteral medications to oral form as soon as possible.
- Withdraw bedtime medication last, in order to normalize sleep-wake cycle.
- If using haloperidol, monitor for akathisia mimicking worsening agitation.

Table 1–5. Steps to prevent suicidal behavior

People who commit suicide are agitated, depressed, anxious, and distressed.
* Treat agitation, anxiety, and depression immediately and aggressively.
* Stabilize current or potential medications.
* Provide early psychiatric consultation for mental status changes or abnormalities.

External support acts as a deterrent to suicide.
* Encourage family support and involvement if possible.
* Discourage impersonality, distance, and apathy in staff, who may serve as "family equivalents."

Suicidal patients often give prior indications of intent by word or behavior.
* Encourage staff communication.
* Seek psychiatric consultation about the patient's suicide potential early.

Suicidal patients may be less able to tolerate pain.
* Treat pain aggressively and consider a psychiatric overlay when pain seems out of proportion to its cause.

Practical safeguards are effective, especially in deterring impulsive suicides.
* "Safety-proof" patient rooms and bathrooms (e.g., place stops on windows; eliminate overhead bars; limit time alone in the bathroom).

The intervention of hospital staff is crucial in preventing suicides.
* The most important antisuicidal measures are the sensitivity and alertness of the staff to the suicidal danger as well as the indication of interest and concern for the patient as a person.

Source.   Adapted from Bostwick JM: "Suicidality," in *The American Psychiatric Publishing Textbook of Consultation-Liaison Psychiatry: Psychiatry in the Medically Ill,* 2nd Edition. Edited by Wise MG, Rundell JR. Washington, DC, American Psychiatric Publishing, 2002, pp. 127–148. Used with permission.

Table 1–6. Specific psychiatric interventions to prevent suicidal behavior in medical-surgical patients

---

* Identify and eliminate factors driving an agitated delirium.
* Diagnose and treat alcohol withdrawal.
* Explore and neutralize rageful emotions stemming from a marital crisis.
* Offer comfort and support in the face of a life-threatening illness.
* Effect a reunion between the suicidal patient and estranged family members or friends.
* Implement a referral plan for ongoing inpatient or outpatient psychiatric treatment of major depression or other psychiatric disorders.

Source.   Reprinted from Bostwick JM: "Suicidality," in *The American Psychiatric Publishing Textbook of Consultation-Liaison Psychiatry: Psychiatry in the Medically Ill,* 2nd Edition. Edited by Wise MG, Rundell JR. Washington, DC, American Psychiatric Publishing, 2002, pp. 127–148. Used with permission.

As-needed (prn) antipsychotic medications written so that small quantities may be given every 1–2 hours permit the staff to fine-tune the antipsychotic dosage, guided by symptomatology. Include orders to check vital signs regularly before administering the medication, and to "hold for excessive sedation" so

that the patient does not become obtunded. Standing orders are intended to assist the staff but *cannot substitute for regular bedside visits* during acute phase treatment. If using the high-potency conventional antipsychotic haloperidol, monitor for the occurrence of akathisia mimicking worsening agitation.

For patients in the acute phase of treatment for delirium, consider one-to-one supervision to avoid injury to self or others. Table 1–6 and Table 1–7 show suggestions for preventing suicidal behavior in the medically ill.

Day 2

Assuming that the patient has remained calm, add the sum of all doses of administered antipsychotic medication (stat+standing+prn) from the day before. Administer the same number of milligrams over the next 24 hours in divided doses, reserving the largest single dose for bedtime. It may be necessary to reduce the standing doses of antipsychotic for elderly patients and for medically fragile patients with impaired hepatic metabolism. Conversely, it may be necessary to increase the antipsychotic if the patient becomes agitated again. To repeat, *the goal is to calm the agitated, delirious patient completely.*

Try to convert parenteral medications to the oral form as soon as possible. Intramuscular injections have limitations, such as erratic absorption in cachectic patients, discomfort, and elevation of muscle enzymes (e.g., creatine phosphokinase [CPK]). In immunocompromised patients, thrombocytopenia and the risk of infection at injection sites may limit the number of intramuscular doses.

Days 3–7

After confusion has cleared and the patient is lucid, continue the antipsychotic, but taper over the next several days (e.g., one strategy is to reduce the dose by 50% every 24 hours). If the medication is discontinued abruptly or prematurely, there is the risk that the delirium may relapse (Wise et al. 2002). The bedtime dose of antipsychotic (or of a potentiating agent such as lorazepam [Ativan]) should be the last to be withdrawn for patients with disrupted sleep-wake cycles.

Specific Agents

Table 1–7 and Table 1–8 summarize the recommended doses of haloperidol and the atypical antipsychotics for the treatment of delirium. A brief description of each type of strategy follows.

Haloperidol

Haloperidol has been the most widely studied neuroleptic for treating delirium. It is a high-potency dopamine-blocking agent with few anticholinergic side effects and minimal cardiovascular or pulmonary side effects. Clinical improvement appears to be due to a combination of haloperidol's sedative and antipsychotic properties. The other conventional antipsychotics, the phenothiazines (e.g., chlorpromazine, thioridazine) are less desirable because of hypotensive effects, anticholinergic side effects (which may complicate delirium), and their tendency to produce QTc widening, which predisposes to TDP.

Intramuscular haloperidol is useful for acutely agitated patients. However, repeated intramuscular injections are painful and may confirm the delirious patient's often paranoid concerns. Most delirium protocols call for conversion to an oral equivalent once the patient has been adequately sedated. Parenteral haloperidol is approximately twice as potent as the oral form (e.g., 10 mg iv or im is equivalent to 5 mg po).

Intravenous haloperidol offers several advantages over the intramuscular form: 1) quicker onset of action, 2) fewer extrapyramidal side effects, and 3) shorter mean half-life (14 hours) compared with the intramuscular (21 hours) or oral (24 hours) forms. It is now

Table 1–7. Initial haloperidol doses for the treatment of delirium

Level of agitation	Initial adult dose of haloperidol[a,b] (po, im, iv[c,d])	
	Young or healthy	Elderly or frail
Mild	0.5–1.0 mg	0.5 mg
Moderate	2.0–5.0 mg	1.0 mg
Severe	5.0–10.0 mg	2.0 mg

[a]May repeat at regular intervals, but not before 30 minutes, until the patient is calmer.
[b]Small doses of intravenous (iv) lorazepam (e.g., initially, 1 mg of iv lorazepam over 1 minute; repeated again after 30 minutes if agitation persists) may be useful in patients who have not responded to haloperidol alone.
[c]10 mg im or iv is equivalent to 5 mg po.
[d]Flush iv line with 2 mg of normal saline before using iv form.
Source. Wise et al. 2002.

commonly used in intensive care settings without psychiatric consultation. Before intravenous haloperidol is administered, the iv line should be flushed with 2 mL of normal saline (particularly if the patient is receiving heparin or phenytoin, which may cause precipitates). Patients receiving epinephrine drips may receive intravenous haloperidol. However, the use of a pressor other than epinephrine (e.g., norepinephrine) will avoid unopposed β-adrenergic activity in patients who have receive large intravenous haloperidol doses (Cassem and Hackett 1991). The maximum dose of intravenous haloperidol has not been established; Cassem et al. (2004) reported giving single bolus doses of 200 mg, and up to 1,600 mg total has been given in a 24-hour period (Tesar et al. 1985). A continuous infusion of haloperidol has also been used (Fernandez et al. 1988).

Haloperidol and torsades de pointes: There have been several case reports of intravenous haloperidol–induced TDP, although the oral form rarely causes TDP. A 1998 case-control study reviewed all critically ill adult patients in the medical, cardiac, and surgical intensive care units who received intravenous haloperidol over the course of 1 year (Sharma et al. 1998). Of the 223 consecutive critically ill patients who received intravenous haloperidol, 8 (3.6%) developed TDP, which appeared to be:

- Dose related (intravenous haloperidol ≥35 mg), in 78% of cases
- Associated with rapid haloperidol infusion (≤6 hr)
- Preceded by significant QTc prolongation (>500 ms) in 84% of cases

Table 1–8. Atypical antipsychotics for the treatment of mild to severe agitation in delirium

Agent	Initial dose (oral preparation)	As-needed dose (prn)
Risperidone (Risperdal)	0.25–0.5 mg twice daily	0.25–0.5 mg every 4 hours; up to 4 mg/day
Olanzapine (Zyprexa)[a]	2.5–5.0 mg at bedtime	Increase in divided doses; up to 20 mg/day
Quetiapine (Seroquel)	25–50 mg twice daily	25–50 mg every 4 hours; up to 600 mg/day
Ziprasidone (Geodon)[b,c]	Not extensively tested in delirium	
Aripiprazole (Abilify)	Not extensively tested in delirium	
Clozapine (Clozaril)	AVOID	

[a]Available in an orally disintegrating tablet, Zydis.
[b]Prolongs QTc interval in a dose-related fashion; induces orthostatic hypotension associated with dizziness, tachycardia, and syncope. Use cautiously in patients with cardiovascular disease or predisposed to hypotension (e.g., dehydration, hypovolemia).
[c]Contraindications: known history of QT interval prolongation or combination with other drugs that prolong QT interval.
Source. Data from Wise et al. 2002, Schwartz and Masand 2002.

Spontaneous restoration of sinus rhythm upon haloperidol discontinuation occurred in some but not all TDP patients. Several patients required both electrical cardioversion and pharmacological intervention. All patients survived their hospital stay and were discharged.

TDP has been reported to occur also with oral haloperidol (Fayer 1986; Henderson et al. 1991; Kriwisky et al. 1990; Zee-Cheng et al. 1985) at low doses (Jackson et al. 1997), in the absence of QT prolongation (Perrault et al. 2000) and without other discernible predisposing factors (O'Brien et al. 1999).

Recommendations for using haloperidol in critically ill delirious patients: The above data have led to the following recommendations for using haloperidol—in any form—for the treatment of delirium (Huffman et al. 2004; Sharma et al. 1998):

1. Obtain baseline QTc interval (goal: ≤450 ms).
2. Obtain baseline serum calcium, magnesium, and potassium levels (goal: $K^+ > 4$ mEq/L, $Mg^{++} > 2$ mEq/L).
3. Continuously monitor QTc for at-risk critically ill patients, especially if they receive intravenous haloperidol ≥35 mg/24 hours, are quickly tranquilized (≤6 hours), or have one or several of the risk factors listed in Appendix 11 (Sharma et al. 1998).
4. If baseline QTc shows prolongation to >450 ms, or >25% over baseline, get cardiology consultation, reduce dose, or discontinue haloperidol (American Psychiatric Association 1999).

In summary, although clinicians should be aware of this potentially lethal complication, it should not deter them from using intravenous haloperidol to treat acute agitation in the critically ill patient with a normal QTc (Hassaballa and Balk 2003).

Benzodiazepines

Benzodiazepines with active metabolites should be avoided in the setting of delirium. The slow, progressive accumulation of active metabolites occurring with long-acting agents like diazepam (Valium; t½=20–100 hours) or chlordiazepoxide (Librium; t½=30–100 hours) produces cumulative CNS toxicity in delirious patients, especially the elderly.

Benzodiazepines without active metabolites may be used in combination with antipsychotics to sedate agitated, delirious patients. As discussed in Chapter 2 of this volume, these agents can be remembered by the mnemonic *CLOT*:

- **C**lonazepam (Klonopin; po)
- **L**orazepam (Ativan; po, im, or iv)
- **O**xazepam (Serax; po)
- **T**emazepam (Restoril; po)

Lorazepam's flexible means of administration (oral, intramuscular, and intravenous) and wide therapeutic index allow it to be safely used in the medical setting. Lorazepam is primarily eliminated through conjugation with glucuronic acid. It does not rely on hepatic oxidation by the cytochrome enzyme system. When combined with an antipsychotic, lorazepam lowers the required dosage, reducing the likelihood of adverse, dose-related side effects. Although lorazepam by itself has a place in treating the agitated psychotic patient who is *not* delirious (Battaglia et al. 1997; Bienek et al. 1998; Foster et al. 1997), delirious patients fare better with combination therapy (Breitbart et al. 1996).

Midazolam (Versed) is a benzodiazepine administered intravenously for sedation prior to medical procedures and as an adjunct to anesthesia. It has several advantages for treating delirium in the ICU, such as rapid onset and short half-life (1–4 hours). It is among the recommended medications for use in agitated, mechanically ventilated patients, according to the American College of Critical Care Medicine (Jacobi et al. 2002). There are several case reports demonstrating efficacy for treating aggressivity, violence, and hyperarousal (Bond et al. 1989; Mendoza et al. 1987). Drawbacks, however, include the potential for respiratory depression, apnea, hypotension, and prolonged half-life in the setting of liver dysfunction and systemic illness. The narrower therapeutic index of midazolam in comparison with lorazepam increases the risk of iatrogenic overdose and toxicity. Lorazepam is the safer option for the treatment of delirium for patients not on mechanical ventilation.

Droperidol (Inapsine) is a butyrophenone used as an adjunct to anesthesia. The FDA has approved it for intravenous administration. Droperidol is not as commonly used as haloperidol for delirium, but it has a place in many emergency departments for sedation, analgesia, and antiemesis (Chambers and Druss 1999; Richards et al. 1998).

Compared with haloperidol, droperidol has more rapid onset of action (within 5 minutes), a shorter duration of action (2–4 hours), and a lower incidence of extrapyramidal side effects. Sedation is its most common clinical effect. It is a far more potent α-adrenergic antagonist than haloperidol and is more likely to produce hypotension, particularly when it is combined with other agents. These are potential problems for the medically ill. Although droperidol is more quickly acting than haloperidol, the two agents are equivalent at 1 hour (Thomas et al. 1992).

In 2001, the FDA issued a black box warning (the strongest type of warning label for an FDA-approved drug) that droperidol, even at low doses, could cause QT prolongation and/or TDP. Since that time, it has been questioned whether the black box warning was justified; the cases on which the warning was based are confounded by factors such as polypharmacy, alcohol intoxication, suicide attempts, general anesthesia, multiorgan dysfunction, and sepsis (Bailey et al. 2002). A review of the literature for the years 1960–2002 also concluded that droperidol is safe for use as a sedative in acutely agitated or violent patients in an emergency department setting when used in 5-mg intramuscular doses (Shale et al. 2003)

Atypical Antipsychotics

The atypical antipsychotics are increasingly used as alternatives to haloperidol and lorazepam. A 2002 re-

view of the literature (Schwartz and Masand 2002) made the delirium-specific recommendations that are summarized in Table 1–8 .

Medications may be discontinued 7–10 days after patients return to baseline with cleared sensorium and alleviation of delirium symptoms, particularly after restoration of the sleep-wake cycle.

Risperidone: Several case reports of the use of risperidone specifically with delirious patients have shown few side effects and good efficacy with 0.5–1.0 mg of risperidone twice daily (Sipahimalani and Masand 1997a, 1997b). Of concern was a series of three elderly patients whose delirium may have been precipitated or exacerbated by risperidone (Ravona-Springer et al. 1998), although the patients were also on other medications. Delirium remitted when all medications, including risperidone, were discontinued.

A prospective open trial of risperidone was carried out in 10 patients with delirium (Horikawa et al. 2003). At a low dose of 1.7 mg/day, on average, risperidone was effective in 80%, and the effect appeared within a few days. There were no serious adverse effects. However, sleepiness (30%) and mild drug-induced parkinsonism (10%) were observed; the symptom of sleepiness was a reason for not increasing the dose.

Finally, a prospective, multicenter, observational 7-day study in five university hospitals enrolled 64 patients (62.5% male [n=40]; mean age 67.3 years) hospitalized due to a medical condition who met criteria for delirium according to DSM-IV (Parellada et al. 2004). Fifty-six patients received 7 days of treatment or less, and eight patients continued treatment for more than 7 days. Risperidone was administered at the time of diagnosis, and treatment was maintained according to clinical response. Response to treatment was defined as a reduction in Delirium Rating Scale score to below 13 within the first 72 hours. Results indicated that risperidone (mean dose 2.6 mg/day at day 3) was effective in 90.6% (58/64) of the patients and significantly improved all symptoms measured by the scales from baseline to day 7. It was concluded that low-dose risperidone had proved to be safe and effective in the treatment of symptoms of delirium in medically hospitalized patients.

Olanzapine: One controlled study found that oral olanzapine was as effective as haloperidol in controlling delirium-associated agitation, with fewer extrapyramidal side effects and less sedation (Sipahimalani and Masand 1998). An open, prospective trial of olanzapine for the treatment of delirium in a sample of hospitalized cancer patients also showed it to be safe and efficacious (Breitbart et al. 2002b). The most common side effect was sedation. No patients on olanzapine therapy developed extrapyramidal side effects. The most powerful predictor of poor response to this medication was age over 70 years. The authors suggested that a dose of about 5 mg/day is reasonable to start for treating delirium. In a randomized, prospective study of delirious patients, olanzapine was found to be equivalent to haloperidol in efficacy and to be accompanied by fewer side effects (Skrobik et al. 2004). (No side effects were noted in the olanzapine group, whereas the use of haloperidol was associated with extrapyramidal side effects.)

Olanzapine is more than 160 times more antihistaminic than diphenhydramine (Benadryl). Note that new-onset diabetes mellitus and diabetic ketoacidosis have been reported in olanzapine-treated patients, although no reports of these complications specifically in delirious patients have appeared.

Quetiapine has been safely and effectively used at low doses (25–50 mg) for the management of delirium (Schwartz and Masand 2000; Torres et al. 2001). A case report on two middle-aged hospitalized patients with delirium poorly controlled by haloperidol and risperidone showed good treatment response to quetiapine (Al-Samarrai et al. 2003). Another study reported on 12 older patients with delirium who were treated with quetiapine. The mean duration for stabilization was 5.91±2.22 days, and the mean dose was 93.75±23.31 mg/day. None of the 12 patients developed extrapyramidal symptoms (Kim et al. 2003). Another 12 patients with delirium were treated with flexible doses of open-label quetiapine (dosage, mean±SD, 44.9±31.0 mg/day) and achieved remission of delirium several days after starting treatment (duration until remission 4.8±3.9 days) (Sasaki et al. 2003). Twenty-two Korean inpatients with delirium who were administered prospectively received a flexible dose of quetiapine (Pae et al. 2004). The DRS-R-98 and Clinical Global Impression Scale Severity scores, assessed pre- and post-treatment, were significantly reduced (by 57.3% and 55.1%, respectively).

Ziprasidone has a tendency to prolong QTc in a dose-related fashion and induces orthostatic hypotension, associated with dizziness, tachycardia, and syncope (mechanism: α_1 antagonism). However, at this writing ziprasidone had not been associated with TDP or sudden death. Use caution in patients who have cardiovascular disease and who have conditions that would predispose an individual to hypotension (such as dehydration and hypovolemia). Contraindications include known history of QT prolongation, and combination with other drugs that prolong the QT interval

(Glassman and Bigger 2002). One case report on the use of ziprasidone in delirium in a patient with HIV and cryptococcal meningitis (Leso and Schwartz 2002) showed effective clearing of delirium, but with resulting QTc prolongation. The patient may have been predisposed to this side effect because of hypokalemia and hypomagnesemia secondary to amphotericin B therapy.

Clozapine: Although clozapine is helpful in chronically psychiatrically ill psychotic patients, serious potential medical side effects, such as seizures and agranulocytosis, limit its usefulness in delirium.

Aripiprazole: There are not enough data to comment on the safety of aripiprazole in delirium.

Other Agents

The American College of Critical Care Medicine has published practice guidelines on the use of analgesics and sedatives in the critically ill adult (Jacobi et al. 2002). They include medications such as the short-acting benzodiazepine midazolam (Versed) and propofol (Diprivan; an anesthetic agent). These guidelines can be accessed at the Web site http://www.sccm. org/ professional_resources/guidelines/table_of _contents/ index.asp.

■ MANAGEMENT OF INSOMNIA AND SUNDOWNING

Delirium usually is accompanied by disruptions in sleep architecture, often causing "sundowning." The patient who was lethargic and sleeping by day becomes alert, agitated, and restless at night, often with no memory for the event. Because intensive care units are noisy, disruptive places, it is reasonable to associate noise, sleep deprivation, and delirium. However, it is the encephalopathic process, not the incidental noise, that disrupts sleep architecture. A recent study corroborated that noise and patient-care activities accounted for only a minority of arousals and awakenings in the ICU, a finding that suggested "the operation of other factors" in sleep disruption of patients hospitalized in the ICU (Gabor et al. 2003). (See earlier section on "ICU psychosis.")

Normalizing sleep-wake cycle disturbances has high therapeutic priority. No one agent has been proven to be consistently superior to others in treating insomnia in the medically ill (Krahn and Richardson 2000). The following points are relevant:

- Most of the antipsychotic medication used to resolve delirium should be given at bedtime, in order to normalize sleep.
- Respiratory depression is a potential problem with most benzodiazepine hypnotic medications.
- The ultrashort half-life of the hypnotic triazolam (Halcion) has been associated with amnestic and dissociative episodes as well as rebound insomnia (i.e., middle-of-the-night awakening that occurs when the hypnotic effect wears off before morning). Rebound insomnia may predispose patients to get out of bed in the dark, increasing the vulnerability to falls.
- Long-acting benzodiazepines with active metabolites (e.g., diazepam [Valium] and chlordiazepoxide [Librium]) may contribute to obtundation and confusion, particularly if they are used over a period of days or weeks.
- The nonbenzodiazepine medications zolpidem (Ambien) and zaleplon (Sonata) specifically target the receptors mediating sleep, so they have fewer effects than the benzodiazepines on motor and respiratory function. There are no controlled studies on their use in delirious patients.
- Barbiturates cause both rapid eye movement (REM) suppression and respiratory depression. Avoid using them in delirious patients.
- Anticholinergic and antihistaminic medications such as diphenhydramine (Benadryl) and phenothiazines such as chlorpromazine (Thorazine) potentially worsen the confusion of delirium. Avoid using them as hypnotics in delirious patients.

Limiting noise when possible, maintaining a semblance of a day-night cycle (e.g., dim lights at night), providing all routine care during the day, and scheduling oral medications in a way that will minimize nighttime awakenings are useful nonpharmacologic strategies. Appendix 13 lists commonly used drugs with sedative-hypnotic properties.

■ REFERENCES

Aakerlund L, Rosenberg J: Writing disturbances: an indication for postoperative delirium. Int J Psychiatry Med 24:245–257, 1994

Alexopoulos GS, Streim J, Carpenter D, et al: Using antipsychotic agents in older patients. J Clin Psychiatry 65 (suppl 2):1–105, 2004

Almeras C, Soussi N, Molko N, et al: Paraneoplastic limbic encephalitis, a complication of the testicular cancer. Urology 58:105, 2001

Al-Samarrai S, Dunn J, Newmark T, et al: Quetiapine for treatment-resistant delirium. Psychosomatics 44:350–351, 2003

American Psychiatric Association: Practice Guideline for the Treatment of Patients With Delirium. Am J Psychiatry 156 (suppl):1–20, 1999

American Psychiatric Association: Diagnostic and Statistical Manual of Mental Disorders, 4th Edition, Text Revision. Washington, DC, American Psychiatric Association, 2000

Amir J, Galbraith R: Paraneoplastic limbic encephalopathy as a nonmetastatic complication of small cell lung cancer. South Med J 85:1013–1014, 1992

Bailey P, Norton R, Karan S: The FDA droperidol warning: is it justified? (letter) Anesthesiology 97:288–289, 2002

Bak T, Antoun N, Balan K, et al: Memory lost, memory regained: neuropsychological findings and neuroimaging in two cases of paraneoplastic limbic encephalitis with radically different outcomes. J Neurol Neurosurg Psychiatry 71:40–47, 2001

Barkham TM, Martin FC, Eykyn SJ: Delay in the diagnosis of bacteraemic urinary tract infection in elderly patients. Age Ageing 25:130–132, 1996

Battaglia J, Moss S, Rush J, et al: Haloperidol, lorazepam, or both for psychotic agitation? A multicenter, prospective, double-blind, emergency department study. Am J Emerg Med 15:335–340, 1997

Bezchlibnyk KZ, Jeffries JJ: Clinical Handbook of Psychotropic Drugs. Toronto, ON, Hogrege & Huber, 2002

Bienek S, Ownby R, Penalver A, et al: A double-blind study of lorazepam versus the combination of haloperidol and lorazepam in managing agitation. Pharmacotherapy 18:57–62, 1998

Boland R, Goldstein M, Haltzman S: Psychiatric management of behavioral syndromes in intensive care units, in Psychiatric Care of the Medical Patient. Edited by Stoudemire A, Fogel B, Greenberg D. New York, Oxford University Press, 2000, pp 299–314

Boylan L: Limbic encephalitis and late-onset psychosis (letter). Am J Psychiatry 157:1343–1344, 2000

Breitbart W, Marotta R, Platt MM, et al: A double-blind trial of haloperidol, chlorpromazine, and lorazepam in the treatment of delirium in hospitalized AIDS patients. Am J Psychiatry 153:231–237, 1996

Breitbart W, Rosenfeld B, Foth F, et al: The Memorial Delirium Assessment Scale. J Pain Symptom Manage 13:128–137, 1997

Breitbart W, Gibson C, Tremblay A: The delirium experience: delirium recall and delirium-related distress in hospitalized patients with cancer, their spouses/caregivers, and their nurses. Psychosomatics 43:183–194, 2002a

Breitbart W, Tremblay A, Gibson C: An open trial of olanzapine for the treatment of delirium in hospitalized cancer patients. Psychosomatics 43:175–182, 2002b

Brown T, Stoudemire A, Fogel B, et al: Psychopharmacology in the medical patient, in Psychiatric Care of the Medical Patient. Edited by Stoudemire A, Fogel B, Greenberg D. New York, Oxford University Press, 2000, pp 329–372

Brunner G, Zweiker R, Krejs GJ: A toxicological surprise. Lancet 356:1406, 2000

Casarett D, Inouye S: Diagnosis and management of delirium near the end of life. Ann Intern Med 135:32–40, 2001

Cassem N, Murray G, Lafayette J, et al: Delirious patients, in Massachusetts General Hospital Handbook of General Hospital Psychiatry, 5th Edition. Edited by Stern T, Fricchione G, Cassem N. Philadelphia, PA, Mosby, 2004, pp 119–134

Chambers R, Druss B: Droperidol: efficacy and side effects in psychiatric emergencies. J Clin Psychiatry 60:664–667, 1999

Chedru F, Geschwind N: Writing disturbances in acute confusional states. Neuropsychologia 10:343–353, 1972

Duggal H, Fetchko J: Serotonin syndrome and atypical antipsychotics (letter). Am J Psychiatry 159:672–673, 2002

Dyer C, Ashton C, Teasdale T: Postoperative delirium. Arch Intern Med 155:461–465, 1995

Eidelman LA, Putterman D, Putterman C, et al: The spectrum of septic encephalopathy: definitions, etiologies, and mortalities. JAMA 275:470–473, 1996

Eisendrath S, Sweeney M: Toxic neuropsychiatric effects of digoxin at therapeutic serum concentrations. Am J Psychiatry 144:506–507, 1987

Ely EW, Margolin R, Francis J, et al: Evaluation of delirium in critically ill patients: validation of the Confusion Assessment Method for the Intensive Care Unit (CAM-ICU). Crit Care Med 29:1370–1379, 2001

Ely EW, Stephens RK, Jackson JC, et al: Current opinions regarding the importance, diagnosis, and management of delirium in the intensive care unit: a survey of 912 healthcare professionals. Crit Care Med 32:106–112, 2004

Fakhoury T, Abou-Khalil B, Kessler R: Limbic encephalitis and hyperactive foci on PET scan. Seizure 8:427–431, 1999

Fayer SA: Torsades de pointes ventricular tachyarrhythmia associated with haloperidol (letter). J Clin Psychopharmacol 6:375–376, 1986

Fernandez F, Holmes V, Adams F, et al: Treatment of severe, refractory agitation with a haloperidol drip. J Clin Psychiatry 49:239–241, 1988

Fix A, Golden C, Daughton D, et al: Neuropsychological deficits among patients with COPD. Int J Neurosci 16:99–105, 1982

Folstein MF, Folstein SE, McHugh PR: "Mini-Mental State": a practical method for grading the cognitive state of patients for the clinician. J Psychiatr Res 12:189–198, 1975

Foster S, Kessel J, Berman M, et al: Efficacy of lorazepam and haloperidol for rapid tranquilization in a psychiatric emergency room setting. Int Clin Psychopharmacol 12:175–179, 1997

Francis J, Martin D, Kapoor W: A prospective study of delirium in hospitalized elderly. JAMA 263:1097–1101, 1990

Gabor JY, Cooper AB, Crombach SA, et al: Contribution of the intensive care unit environment to sleep disruption in mechanically ventilated patients and healthy subjects. Am J Respir Crit Care Med 167:708–715, 2003

Glassman A: Clinical management of cardiovascular risks during treatment with psychotropic drugs. J Clin Psychiatry 63:12–17, 2002

Glassman A, Bigger J Jr: Prolongation of QTc interval and antipsychotics (letter). Am J Psychiatry 159:1064, 2002

Grant I, Prigatano G, Heaton R, et al: Progressive neuropsychologic impairment and hypoxemia. Arch Gen Psychiatry 44:999–1006, 1987

Griggs R, Arieff A: Hypoxia and the central nervous system, in Metabolic Brain Dysfunction in Systemic Disorders. Edited by Arieff A, Griggs R. Boston, MA, Little, Brown, 1992, pp 39–54

Gultekin S, Rosenfeld M, Voltz R, et al: Paraneoplastic limbic encephalitis: neurological symptoms, immunological findings and tumour association in 50 patients. Brain 123:1481–1494, 2000

Hamilton S, Malone K: Serotonin syndrome during treatment with paroxetine and risperidone (letter). J Clin Psychopharmacol 20:103–105, 2000

Hart R, Levenson J, Sessler C, et al: Validation of a cognitive test for delirium. Psychosomatics 37:533–546, 1996

Hart R, Best A, Sessler C, et al: Abbreviated cognitive test for delirium. J Psychosom Res 43:417–423, 1997

Hassaballa HA, Balk RA: Torsade de pointes associated with the administration of intravenous haloperidol: a review of the literature and practical guidelines for use. Expert Opin Drug Saf 2:543–547, 2003

Heckmann JG, Birklein F, Neundorfer B: Omeprazole-induced delirium. J Neurol 247:56–57, 2000

Henderson R, Lane S, Henry JA: Life-threatening ventricular arrhythmia (torsades de pointes) after haloperidol overdose. Hum Exp Toxicol 10:59–62, 1991

Horikawa N, Yamazaki T, Miyamoto K, et al: Treatment for delirium with risperidone: results of a prospective open trial with 10 patients. Gen Hosp Psychiatry 25:289–292, 2003

Huffman J, Stern T, Januzzi J: The psychiatric management of patients with cardiac disease, in Massachusetts General Hospital Handbook of General Hospital Psychiatry, 5th Edition. Edited by Stern T, Fricchione G, Cassem N. Philadelphia, PA, Mosby, 2004, pp 547–569

Horvath T, Siever L, Mohs R, et al: Organic mental syndromes and disorders, in Comprehensive Textbook of Psychiatry, 5th Edition. Edited by Kaplan H, Sadock B. Baltimore, MD, Williams & Wilkins, 1989, pp 599–641

Inouye SKF: Prevention of delirium in hospitalized older patients: risk factors and targeted intervention strategies. Ann Med 32:257–263, 2000

Inouye SK[F], Bogardus ST Jr, Charpentier PA, et al: A multicomponent intervention to prevent delirium in hospitalized older patients. N Engl J Med 340:669–676, 1999

Jackson T, Ditmanson L, Phibbs B: Torsade de pointes and low-dose oral haloperidol. Arch Intern Med 157:2013–2015, 1997

Jacobi J, Fraser G, Coursin D, et al: Clinical practice guidelines for the sustained use of sedatives and analgesics in the critically ill adult. Crit Care Med 30:119–141, 2002

Jacobson S, Jerrier H: EEG in delirium. Semin Clin Neuropsychiatry 5:86–92, 2000

Jiang H, Chang D: NSAID drugs with adverse psychiatric reactions: five case reports. Clin Rheumatol 18:339–345, 1999

Kassubek J, Juengling FD, Nitzsche EU, et al: Limbic encephalitis investigated by ^{18}FDG-PET and 3D MRI. J Neuroimaging 11:55–59, 2001

Khan N, Wieser H: Limbic encephalitis: a case report. Epilepsy Res 17:175–181, 1994

Kim KY, Bader GM, Kotlyar V, et al: Treatment of delirium in older adults with quetiapine. J Geriatr Psychiatry Neurol 16:29–31, 2003

Krahn L, Richardson J: Sleep disorders in the medically ill, in Psychiatric Care of the Medical Patient. Edited by Stoudemire A, Fogel B, Greenberg D. New York, Oxford University Press, 2000, pp 683–697

Kriwisky M, Perry GY, Tarchitsky D, et al: Haloperidol-induced torsades de pointes. Chest 98:482–484, 1990

Lawlor P, Gagnon B, Mancini I, et al: Occurrence, causes, and outcome of delirium in patients with advanced cancer: a prospective study. Arch Intern Med 160:786–794, 2000

Lazarus B, Murphy J, Colletta E, et al: The provision of physical activity to hospitalized elderly patients. Arch Intern Med 151:2452–2456, 1991

Leso L, Schwartz T: Ziprasidone treatment of delirium. Psychosomatics 43:61–62, 2002

Levkoff S, Liptzin B, Cleary P, et al: Subsyndromal delirium. Am J Geriatr Psychiatry 4:320–329, 1996

Lezak M: Neuropsychological Assessment, 2nd Edition. New York, Oxford University Press, 1983

Lipowski Z: Delirium: Acute Confusional States. New York, Oxford University Press, 1990

Liptzin B: Clinical diagnosis and management of delirium, in Psychiatric Care of the Medical Patient. Edited by Stoudemire A, Fogel B, Greenberg D. New York, Oxford University Press, 2000, pp 581–596

Lishman W: Organic Psychiatry, 3rd Edition. London, Blackwell Scientific, 1998

Liston E: Diagnosis and management of delirium in the elderly patient. Psychiatric Annals 14:109–118, 1984

Maccioli G, Dorman T, Brown B, et al: Clinical practice guidelines for the maintenance of physical patient safety in the intensive care unit: use of restraining therapies—American College of Critical Care Medicine Task Force 2001–2002. Crit Care Med 31:2665–2676, 2003

MacKnight C, Rojas-Fernandez CH: Celecoxib- and rofecoxib-induced delirium (letter). J Neuropsychiatry Clin Neurosci 13:305–306, 2001

Mann S, Caroff S, Keck P, et al: Neuroleptic Malignant Syndrome and Related Conditions, 2nd Edition. Washington, DC, American Psychiatric Publishing, 2003

Manos P, Wu R: The ten point clock test: a quick screen and grading method for cognitive impairment in medical and surgical patients. Int J Psychiatry Med 24:229–244, 1998

Marcantonio E, Goldman L, Orav E, et al: The association of intraoperative factors with the development of postoperative delirium. Am J Med 105:380–384, 1998

Mason PJ, Morris VA, Balcezak TJ: Serotonin syndrome: presentation of 2 cases and review of the literature. Medicine (Baltimore) 79:201–209, 2000

McClure FS, Gladsjo JA, Jeste DV: Late-onset psychosis: clinical, research, and ethical considerations. Am J Psychiatry 156:935–940, 1999

McDowell J, Mion L, Inouye S: A non-pharmacologic sleep protocol for hospitalized older patients. J Am Geriatr Soc 46:700–705, 1998

McEvoy G (ed): AHFS Drug Information 2003. Bethesda, MD, American Society of Health-System Pharmacists, 2003

McGuire BE, Basten CJ, Ryan CJ, et al: Intensive care unit syndrome: a dangerous misnomer. Arch Intern Med 160:906–909, 2000

Morita T, Tei Y, Tsunoda J, et al: Underlying pathologies and their associations with clinical features in terminal delirium of cancer patients. J Pain Symptom Manage 22:997–1006, 2001

Newman N, Bell I, McKee A: Paraneoplastic limbic encephalitis: neuropsychiatric presentation. Biol Psychiatry 27:529–542, 1990

Nicholas L, Lindsey A: Delirium presenting with symptoms of depression. Psychosomatics 36:471–479, 1995

O'Brien JM, Rockwood RP, Suh KI: Haloperidol-induced torsade de pointes. Ann Pharmacother 33:1046–1050, 1999

Pae C-U, Lee S-J, Lee C-U, et al: A pilot trial of quetiapine for the treatment of patients with delirium. Hum Psychopharmacol 19:125–127, 2004

Parellada E, Baeza I, de Pablo J, et al: Risperidone in the treatment of patients with delirium. J Clin Psychiatry 65:348–353, 2004

Perrault LP, Denault AY, Carrier M, et al: Torsades de pointes secondary to intravenous haloperidol after coronary bypass grafting surgery. Can J Anaesth 47:251–254, 2000

Posner J: Primary and secondary tumors of the central nervous system: paraneoplastic syndromes, in Neurology in Clinical Practice, 3rd Edition. Edited by Bradley WG, Daroff R, Fenichel G, et al. Boston, MA, Butterworth-Heinemann, 2000, pp 1299–1307

Prigatano G, Parsons O, Wright E, et al: Neuropsychological test performance in mildly hypoxemic patients with COPD. J Consult Clin Psychol 51:108–116, 1983

Rabinowitz T: Delirium: an important (but often unrecognized) clinical syndrome. Curr Psychiatry Rep 4:202–208, 2002

Rabins P, Folstein M: Delirium and dementia: diagnostic criteria and fatality rates. Br J Psychiatry 140:149–153, 1982

Ravona-Springer R, Dolberg OT, Hirschmann S, et al: Delirium in elderly patients treated with risperidone: a report of three cases (letter). J Clin Psychopharmacol 18:171–172, 1998

Repchinsky C (ed): Compendium of Pharmaceuticals and Specialties, the Canadian Drug Reference for Health Professionals. Ottawa, ON, Canadian Pharmacists Association, 2003

Richards J, Derlet R, Duncan D: Chemical restraint for the agitated patient in the emergency department: lorazepam versus droperidol. J Emerg Med 16:567–573, 1998

Rodgers PT, Brengel GR: Famotidine-associated mental status changes. Pharmacotherapy 18:404–407, 1998

Rosen J, Sweet R, Mulsant B, et al: The Delirium Rating Scale in a psychogeriatric inpatient setting. J Neuropsychiatry Clin Neurosci 6:30–35, 1994

Sasajima Y, Sasajima T, Uchida H, et al: Postoperative delirium in patients with chronic lower limb ischemia: what are the specific markers? Eur J Vasc Endovasc Surg 20:132–137, 2000

Sasaki Y, Matsuyama T, Inoue S, et al: A prospective, open-label, flexible-dose study of quetiapine in the treatment of delirium. J Clin Psychiatry 64:1316–1321, 2003

Schleifer S, Slater W, Macari-Hinson M, et al: Digitalis and beta-blocking agents: effects on depression following myocardial infarction. Am Heart J 121:1397–1402, 1991

Schneider F, Boehner H, Habel U, et al: Risk factors for postoperative delirium in vascular surgery. Gen Hosp Psychiatry 24:28–34, 2002

Schwartz TL, Masand PS: Treatment of delirium with quetiapine. Prim Care Companion J Clin Psychiatry 2:10–12, 2000

Schwartz TL, Masand PS: The role of atypical antipsychotics in the treatment of delirium. Psychosomatics 43:171–174, 2002

Shale J, Shale C, Mastin W: A review of the safety and efficacy of droperidol for the rapid sedation of severely agitated and violent patients. J Clin Psychiatry 64:500–505, 2003

Sharma ND, Rosman HS, Padhi ID, et al: Torsades de pointes associated with intravenous haloperidol in critically ill patients. Am J Cardiol 81:238–240, 1998

Sipahimalani A, Masand PS: Treatment of delirium with risperidone. International Journal of Geriatric Psychopharmacology 1:24–26, 1997a

Sipahimalani A, Masand PS: Use of risperidone in delirium: case reports. Ann Clin Psychiatry 9:105–107, 1997b

Sipahimalani A, Masand PS: Olanzapine in the treatment of delirium. Psychosomatics 39:422–430, 1998

Skrobik YK, Bergeron N, Dumont M, et al: Olanzapine vs haloperidol: treating delirium in a critical care setting. Intensive Care Med 30:444–449, 2004

Song Y, Terao T, Shiraishi Y, et al: Digitalis intoxication misdiagnosed as depression—revisited (letter). Psychosomatics 42:368–369, 2001

Sussman N, Magid S: Psychiatric manifestations of nonsteroidal anti-inflammatory drugs. Primary Psychiatry 7:26–30, 2000

Sutton I, Winer J, Rowlands D, et al: Limbic encephalitis and antibodies to Ma2: a paraneoplastic presentation of breast cancer. J Neurol Neurosurg Psychiatry 69:266–268, 2000

Tandon R, Walden M, Falcon S: Catatonia as a manifestation of paraneoplastic encephalopathy. J Clin Psychiatry 49:121–122, 1988

Tattevin P, Schortgen F, de Broucker T, et al: Varicella-zoster virus limbic encephalitis in an immunocompromised patient. Scand J Infect Dis 33:786–788, 2001

Taylor DM: Antipsychotics and QT prolongation. Acta Psychiatr Scand 107:85–95, 2003

Tesar G, Murray B, Cassem N: Use of high-dose intravenous haloperidol in the treatment of agitated cardiac patients. J Clin Psychopharmacol 5:344–347, 1985

Thomas H Jr, Schwartz E, Petrelli R: Droperidol versus haloperidol for chemical restraint of agitated and combative patients. Ann Emerg Med 21:407–413, 1992

Torres R, Mittal D, Kennedy R: Use of quetiapine in delirium: case reports. Psychosomatics 42:347–349, 2001

Trzepacz PT, Mittal D, Torres R, et al: Validation of the Delirium Rating Scale-Revised-98: comparison with the Delirium Rating Scale and the Cognitive Test for Delirium. J Neuropsychiatry Clin Neurosci 13:229–242, 2001

Tune L, Carr S, Hoag E, et al: Anticholinergic effects of drugs commonly prescribed for the elderly: potential means for assessing risk of delirium. Am J Psychiatry 149:1393–1394, 1992

USP DI Editorial Board (eds): USP Dispensing Information, Vol 1: Drug Information for the Health Care Professional. Greenwood Village, CO, MICROMEDIX Thompson Healthcare, 2003

van der Mast RC: Postoperative delirium. Dement Geriatr Cogn Disord 10:401–405, 1999

van der Mast RC, Roest F: Delirium after cardiac surgery: a critical review. J Psychosom Res 41:13–30, 1996

Wainwright M, Martin P, Morse R, et al: Human herpesvirus 6 limbic encephalitis after stem cell transplantation. Ann Neurol 50:612–619, 2001

Wallesch C, Hundsalz A: Language function in delirium: a comparison of single word processing in acute confusional states and probable Alzheimer's disease. Brain Lang 46:592–606, 1994

Wani M, Dar J, Khan M, et al: Paraneoplastic limbic encephalitis associated with bronchogenic carcinoma: a case report. Neurol India 49:185–187, 2001

Wise M, Cassem N: Psychiatric consultation to critical-care units, in American Psychiatric Press Review of Psychiatry, Vol 9. Edited by Tasman A, Goldfinger SM, Kaufmann CA. Washington, DC, American Psychiatric Press, 1990, pp 413–432

Wise M, Hilty D, Cerda G, et al: Delirium (confusional states), in The American Psychiatric Publishing Textbook of Consultation-Liaison Psychiatry: Psychiatry in the Medically Ill, 2nd Edition. Edited by Wise MG, Rundell JR. Washington, DC, American Psychiatric Publishing, 2002, pp 257–272

Witchel H, Hancox J, Nutt D: Psychotropic drugs, cardiac arrhythmia, and sudden death. J Clin Psychopharmacol 23:58–77, 2003

Yuan RY, Kao CR, Sheu JJ, et al: Delirium following a switch from cimetidine to famotidine. Ann Pharmacother 35:1045–1048, 2001

Zee-Cheng C, Mueller C, Seifert C, et al: Haloperidol and torsades de pointes (letter). Ann Intern Med 102:418, 1985

Zeimer H: Paraneoplastic limbic encephalitis should not be overlooked as a possible cause of delirium in cancer patients (letter). Arch Intern Med 160:2866, 2000

Chapter

2

The Patient With Hepatic Disease, Alcohol Dependence, and Altered Mental Status

Antoinette Ambrosino Wyszynski, M.D.

The patient with altered mental status and alcohol dependence is diagnostically challenging. It is tempting to attribute psychiatric symptoms, when they occur, to "DTs" (delirium tremens), but the differential diagnosis spans a range of entities, including some unrelated to alcohol withdrawal. Alcohol withdrawal can be an unexpected complication for patients in the hospital, where abstinence is enforced by lack of availability. Withdrawal symptoms may be mistaken for anxiety unless the clinician suspects withdrawal as the underlying etiology. Unrecognized alcohol withdrawal is particularly dangerous in surgical patients, causing up to a threefold increase in postoperative mortality (Sonne and Tonnesen 1992; Spies et al. 1996). Sometimes alcohol withdrawal occurs with reduction of intake rather than with cessation (e.g., the patient is not feeling well and cuts back his or her drinking). Table 2–1 shows the stages of alcohol withdrawal.

There is a case vignette in the Study Guide (Appendix 19 in this volume) that illustrates the diagnostic and management dilemmas confronting the psychiatric consultant. A list of study questions for discussion follows the case.

■ AIDS TO DIAGNOSIS AND TREATMENT

Diagnostic categories for psychiatric conditions associated with alcohol dependence are listed below; DSM-IV-TR diagnostic nomenclature (American Psychiatric Association 2000) is shown in parentheses.

- The following conditions are deliria and are therefore medical emergencies: delirium tremens (alcohol withdrawal delirium); hepatic encephalopathy (delirium due to hepatic insufficiency); Wernicke's encephalopathy (delirium due to thiamine deficiency).
- The following are alcohol withdrawal states: uncomplicated alcohol withdrawal; delirium tremens

Table 2–1. Stages of alcohol withdrawal

Stage	Symptoms	Management options
I	Shaking, elevated pulse, increased blood pressure, agitation	Outpatient management
II	All of stage I symptoms plus hallucinations with insight	Outpatient management if patient reverts to stage I in 3 hours
III	All of stage I symptoms plus a temperature above 38.3°C (101°F) and hallucinations without insight	Intensive inpatient treatment with close monitoring

Source.   Adapted from Mayo-Smith MF: "Management of Alcohol Intoxication and Withdrawal," in *Principles of Addiction Medicine,* 2nd Edition. Edited by Graham AW, Schultz TK. Chevy Chase, MD, American Society of Addiction Medicine, 1998. Reprinted by permission of the publisher.

(alcohol withdrawal delirium); alcoholic hallucinosis (alcohol withdrawal with perceptual disturbances or alcohol-induced psychotic disorder).

- Residual conditions occurring because of heavy alcohol use include chronic alcoholic hallucinosis (alcohol withdrawal with perceptual disturbances [chronic] or alcohol-induced psychotic disorder [chronic]); Korsakoff's syndrome (alcohol-induced persisting amnestic disorder); minimal encephalopathy (no specific DSM-IV-TR term; 294.9 cognitive disorder not otherwise specified [NOS] [e.g., mild neurocognitive disorder], 294.8 amnestic disorder NOS, or 294.8 dementia).

- Other causes of mental status changes in the setting of alcohol dependence include subdural hematoma, electrolyte imbalance, hypoxia, and hypoglycemia.

The Patient Placement Criteria of the American Society of Addiction Medicine include assessment of the following key criteria: 1) acute intoxication or withdrawal potential; 2) biomedical conditions or complications; 3) emotional/behavioral conditions or complications; 4) treatment acceptance/resistance; 5) relapse potential; and 6) recovery environment (Mee-Lee et al. 2001). However, this chapter will focus on approaching those conditions that present diagnostic and treatment dilemmas for the consulting psychiatrist. The following tools should be helpful in determining diagnosis and planning treatment:

- Table 2–2. "Differential Diagnosis and Psychiatric Treatment of the Delirious Psychotic Patient With Cirrhosis"
- Box 2–1. "Diagnostic Workup of the Cirrhotic, Psychotic Patient"
- Figure 2–1. "CIWA-Ar: Addiction Research Foundation Clinical Institute Withdrawal Assessment for Alcohol—Revised." Although used primarily in detoxification centers, this instrument can be

adapted for use in the medical setting (Foy et al. 1988). Symptoms (e.g., nausea, tremor, sweats, anxiety, agitation, and sensory disturbances) are graded on a point scale, and the clinician then devises a treatment plan based on the total score.

We have included the following alcohol screening questionnaires:

- Figure 2–2. "CAGE Questions"
- Figure 2–3. "Alcohol Use Disorders Identification Test (AUDIT)"
- Figure 2–4. "Michigan Alcoholism Screening Test (MAST)"

Also included are two examples of alcohol withdrawal regimens:

- Figure 2–5. "Management of Alcohol Withdrawal: Symptom-triggered Medication Regimen"
- Figure 2–6. "Management of Alcohol Withdrawal: Structured Medication Regimens"

Psychopharmacology in hepatic failure is discussed at the end of the chapter and graphically displayed in

- Figure 2–7. "Psychopharmacology in Liver Failure"

■ PSYCHIATRIC CONDITIONS ASSOCIATED WITH ALCOHOL DEPENDENCE

Warning: Although each syndrome is described below in pure form, alcohol intoxication is likely to complicate the clinical presentation in real life. For example, the patient in the early stages of hepatic encephalopathy may also present acutely intoxicated.

Box 2–1.	**Diagnostic workup of the cirrhotic, psychotic patient**
General workup of delirium	See Appendix 1: American Psychiatric Association Guidelines for Assessing the Delirious Patient.
Liver function tests	Chronic, severe liver disease may cause "liver burnout," resulting in relatively *normal* serum enzyme levels and only modest hyperbilirubinemia. All syndromes discussed in this chapter can coexist with liver function test results that fall within normal limits.
Ammonia levels	The diagnosis of hepatic encephalopathy is usually one of exclusion; an elevated serum ammonia level in a delirious patient with hepatic insufficiency is highly suggestive of the diagnosis. Limitations: 1) sample must be arterial; 2) sample must be iced and immediately analyzed; 3) about 10% of encephalopathic patients have normal blood ammonia levels (Lipowski 1990).
Electroencephalogram	The EEG cannot distinguish among etiologies of psychiatric syndromes in the delirious cirrhotic patient but can help identify "psychiatric" presentations with a covert neurological cause. The earliest changes are slowing of alpha rhythm and appearance of 4- to 7-cps theta waves, most prominent in the frontal and temporal regions (Lockwood 2000). These changes are nonspecific for etiology, but they may precede obvious changes in mental status and may correlate with severity grades of neuropsychiatric abnormalities.

Progression of delirium: As consciousness is progressively impaired, alpha activity is replaced by theta waves. Eventually, triphasic waves appear, portending a poor prognosis. (Triphasic slow waves also occur in other conditions, such as head injury, subdural hematomas, uremia, cerebral anoxia, infection, and electrolyte abnormalities.) In a conscious patient demonstrating stigmata of liver disease, mental status changes, and no other findings, these changes are highly suggestive of delirium that is progressing to coma. |
| **Cerebrospinal fluid** | *Hepatic encephalopathy:* Lumbar puncture, including opening pressure, is usually normal, although increased protein may accompany evolution to coma.

DTs, alcoholic hallucinosis, Wernicke-Korsakoff syndrome: no distinctive CSF findings. |
| **Imaging studies** | Chronic alcoholic patients are at high risk for head trauma. CT and MRI scans help identify structural etiologies for mental status changes, such as subdural hematomas. Imaging studies are of limited value in discriminating among metabolic causes of psychiatric symptoms. Sometimes medical workup is abandoned prematurely and the patient deemed "medically cleared" if results of imaging studies are negative. *Think metabolic* until there is another proven etiology. |

Delirium Tremens

Presentation

The most frequent cause of psychotic symptoms in alcoholic individuals is DTs, which occur in about 15% of alcohol-dependent patients. However, the occurrence and content of vivid visual hallucinations are not specifically diagnostic. DTs usually begin 24–72 hours after the last drink; 90% of affected patients show symptoms within the first 7 days of abstinence. *Note:* The onset of delirium tremens may be delayed by the administration of anesthetic agents that cross-react with alcohol during surgery or other medical procedures; thus, some surgical patients may have delayed withdrawal or DTs during the postoperative period.

The prodrome, as in any delirium, may begin with sleep-cycle disturbances, restlessness, and fear. The patient startles easily, has vivid nightmares, and frequently awakens panicked from sleep. Restlessness and anxiety increase as the illness progresses. The degree of impaired consciousness varies widely among individuals and may shift from moment to moment in the same patient. The typical picture is of a hyperalert-hyperactive delirium with prominent psychotic fea-

Table 2–2.   Differential diagnosis and psychiatric treatment of the delirious psychotic patient with hepatic encephalopathy

Type of syndrome	Diagnosis (DSM-IV-TR terminology)	Mental status examination findings
WITHDRAWAL	**Alcohol hallucinosis** (alcohol withdrawal with perceptual disturbances or alcohol-induced psychotic disorder)	Sensorium intact; prominent auditory hallucinations, usually voices, often threatening; presentation may resemble schizophrenia. Hallucinations>delusions. May progress to delirium.
	Alcohol withdrawal	Irritability, anxiety, malaise; transient hallucinations or illusions (poorly formed); depressed mood or irritability. May progress to delirium.
	Alcohol withdrawal seizures ["rum fits"]	Loss of consciousness; postictal confusion. May be complicated by progression to DTs.
DELIRIUM	**Delirium tremens** (alcohol withdrawal delirium)	#1 cause of psychosis in this population. Confusion; disorientation; perceptual disturbances, often hallucinatory and threatening, but thematically variable.
	Hepatic encephalopathy (delirium due to hepatic insufficiency)	Confusion>psychosis. Change in personality may be part of delirious prodrome. Diagnosis of exclusion.
	Wernicke's encephalopathy (delirium due to thiamine deficiency)	Confusion>psychosis. Change in personality may be part of delirious prodrome.
DEMENTIA	**Korsakoff syndrome/ Korsakoff "psychosis"** (alcohol-induced persisting amnestic disorder)	Not a true "psychosis," but a confabulatory state; retrograde and anterograde amnesia are cardinal features. Frontal lobe symptoms (apathy, inertia, loss of insight). 3 A's (alert, amiable, amnestic).

Note.   CNS=central nervous system; DTs=delirium tremens; EtOH=beverage alcohol; GI=gastrointestinal; WNL=within normal limits.
[a]Figure 2–2: CAGE questions.
[b]Figure 2–3: Alcohol Use Disorders Identification Test.

Relationship to alcohol	Physical examination findings	Psychiatric treatment
Usually within 48 hours or less after heavy EtOH ingestion in person with EtOH dependence. Screen with CAGE,[a] AUDIT,[b] MAST.[c] May become a chronic hallucinatory state.	Often WNL. Use CIWA-Ar[d] screening tool.	Antipsychotic medication. Risperidone (Risperdal) may have some advantage
Symptoms peak 24–48 hours after last drink, usually disappear within 5–7 days unless DTs develop. Screen with CAGE[a], AUDIT[b], MAST[c].	Tremulousness; nausea, vomiting; autonomic hyperactivity; insomnia; headache. Use CIWA-Ar[d] screening tool.	Choose detox regimen.[e]
Symptoms peak 7–38 hours after last drink. Screen with CAGE,[a] AUDIT,[b] MAST.[c]	Generalized tonic-clonic seizures; urinary incontinence; possible focal signs. Brain excitability secondary to withdrawal of CNS depressant (EtOH). Use CIWA-Ar[d] screening tool.	Choose detox regimen.[e]
Gradual onset after 2–3 days; peaks 4–5 days after last drink; first episode usually after 5–15 years of heavy drinking.	Marked autonomic hyperactivity (tachycardia, sweating); stigmata of delirium. Use CIWA-Ar[d] screening tool.	*Medical emergency!* Use supportive measures. Choose detox regimen.[e]
Onset may be temporally independent of EtOH intake. Precipitants: benzodiazepines, phenothiazines, constipation, GI bleeding.	Pyramidal and extrapyramidal motor signs predominate over sensory; may fluctuate in parallel with psychotic symptoms. Liver function test results may be "normal." Normal serum ammonia in 10%.	*Medical emergency!* Avoid meds that undergo oxidative hepatic metabolism. Choose detox regimen.[e]
Onset may be temporally independent of EtOH intake	Ophthalmoplegia (6th cranial nerve palsy); cerebellar ataxia; often followed by Korsakoff residua (see below).	*Medical emergency!* Thiamine 100 mg iv (po poorly absorbed) with $MgSO_4$ 1–2 mL in 50% solution prior to glucose loading.
Not temporally related to EtOH ingestion; however, usually the consequence of many years of EtOH dependence.	Stigmata of EtOH dependence possible; may have history of Wernicke's encephalopathy.	No effective treatment; as with other dementias, institutionalization often needed. Provide supportive treatment.

[c]Figure 2–4: Michigan Alcoholism Screening Test.
[d]Figure 2–1: CIWA-AR: Addiction Research Foundation Clinical Institute Withdrawal Assessment for Alcohol—Revised.
[e]Figures 2–5 and 2–6: examples of medication regimens.

tures. Consciousness is rarely profoundly abnormal except in the terminal stages, but progressive disorientation and confusion may presage impending deterioration (Lishman 1998).

Men develop DTs more commonly than women do. The syndrome usually occurs in alcoholic patients with a 5- to 15-year history of drinking who suddenly decrease their blood alcohol levels and also have major physical illness. Table 2–3 lists risk factors for delirium tremens.

Table 2–3.   Risk factors for delirium tremens

Comorbid medical illness (e.g., electrolyte abnormalities, infection, or poorly controlled cardiovascular, pulmonary, or renal disease)

Delirium tremens by history

Blood alcohol level>300 mg/dL on presentation

Alcohol withdrawal seizures upon presentation

Older age

Source.   Adapted from Saitz R: "Introduction to Alcohol Withdrawal." *Alcohol Health and Research World* 22:5–12, 1998.

The visual hallucinations of DTs have been described as vivid, colorful, Lilliputian in size, and in constant movement. Although apprehension and fear are typical affective responses, the hallucinations may sometimes be amusing or playful in nature, resulting in affective states that are shifting and labile. Delusions are usually fragmented, transitory, and as changeable as the hallucinations. The patient is often markedly suggestible, enhancing the likelihood of illusions and confabulations. The psychotic symptoms in DTs, unlike those in alcoholic hallucinosis, usually occur in the presence of cognitive deficits and other symptoms of delirium.

Treatment

DTs are the most serious of the alcohol withdrawal syndromes. Deaths due to DTs may be from infections, fat emboli, or cardiac arrhythmia associated with electrolyte abnormalities (hypercalcemia, hypokalemia, hyponatremia, and hypophosphatemia), alcoholic ketoacidosis, hyperpyrexia, poor hydration, rhabdomyolysis, and hypertension. Other complications include pancreatitis, gastritis, upper gastrointestinal (GI) bleeds, and hepatitis.

DTs constitute a *medical emergency* and do not remit spontaneously, unlike uncomplicated alcohol withdrawal. These patients are gravely ill and require intensive inpatient care, including intravenous hydration and benzodiazepines for sedation (e.g., diazepam 5–10 mg iv every 15–20 minutes until sedation is achieved).

Pharmacotherapy replaces alcohol with a cross-tolerant sedative drug, which then can be tapered in a controlled manner. Benzodiazepines are the drugs of choice because they are as effective as and less toxic than the alternatives—phenothiazines, barbiturates, and paraldehyde. The long half-lives of benzodiazepines with active metabolites—such as diazepam (Valium) and chlordiazepoxide (Librium)—allow drug levels to decline slowly over many days, creating a gradual withdrawal with relatively few abstinence symptoms. (One survey found that some hospitals still provide beverage alcohol for the prevention or treatment of alcohol withdrawal delirium, and that among the specialties, it is surgeons who order alcohol for their patients [Rosenbaum and McCarty 2002].)

Avoid diazepam and chlordiazepoxide until the risk of hepatic encephalopathy has been eliminated, because they can hasten the deterioration into coma through the accumulation of CNS-depressing metabolites. Instead, choose an agent that has no active metabolites, such as lorazepam (Ativan), over diazepam or chlordiazepoxide for treating withdrawal symptoms in this context. The disadvantage of more frequent dosing required with lorazepam is outweighed by its relative safety in this setting (see Figure 2–5 and Figure 2–6 for medication regimens).

Although benzodiazepines are the current standard of care, some of the newer strategies for the treatment of alcohol withdrawal include the use of valproic acid (Depakote, Depakene) (Myrick et al. 2000, 2001; Reoux 2001).

Restraining paranoid patients may increase their agitation; a quiet environment will minimize agitation and allow the sedative medications to be more effective.

Hepatic Encephalopathy

Presentation and Diagnosis

Hepatic encephalopathy (HE; also termed *delirium of hepatic insufficiency*) is sometimes the hardest condition to diagnose as a cause of mental status changes in cirrhotic patients, particularly if the patient's recent history of alcohol intake—and therefore vulnerability to alcohol withdrawal—is unknown.

The prodrome of HE is initially indistinguishable from DTs and may cue the clinician to prescribe the long-acting benzodiazepines used for DTs, thus iatrogenically hastening HE's progression to coma.

HE is a *medical emergency,* rapidly progressing from the early prodromal signs, which are neurobehavioral, to deepening confusion and coma. Sometimes if the risk of alcohol withdrawal is long past and the imaging study of the brain is normal, the clinician's attention may be diverted away from further investigating medical causes for the mental status changes. The opportunity for meaningful intervention may be lost; HE is potentially reversible only if it is treated promptly.

Most authors emphasize the variable nature of HE. Unlike delirium tremens (which presents with agitated delirium, tremor, and unmistakable changes in vital signs) or Wernicke's encephalopathy (which has sudden onset and often distinct neurological features), the prodrome of HE may escape detection unless the clinician retains a high index of suspicion for its occurrence. The profile of at-risk patients easily allows them to present first to the psychiatric emergency room, where their symptoms may resemble primary psychiatric illness or be mistaken for alcohol intoxication or uncomplicated withdrawal. The diagnosis *depends on clinical suspicion,* confirmed by history, clinical features, and laboratory findings that exclude other etiologies. Hepatic encephalopathy is a diagnosis of exclusion *(Blei et al. 2001; Ferenci et al. 2002), and* it may be misdiagnosed because it presents with psychiatric symptoms in its early stages that overlap with other syndromes:

> While it may seem redundant to state that successful treatment [of hepatic encephalopathy] can only follow a correct diagnosis, this is worth emphasizing because of the high frequency with which relatively subtle alterations of mental capacity may be missed, unless thorough examinations are conducted…. Decrements in mental capacity may be subtle and range from slight inattentiveness in a high-level executive to failure to eat usual meals at a shelter in a destitute alcoholic. (Lockwood 1992, p. 177)

Etiology

The most important factor in the pathogenesis of HE is the adverse effect on brain function of nitrogenous substances derived from the gut. These compounds enter systemic circulation because of hepatocellular dysfunction and/or shunting of portal venous blood into the systemic circulation so that liver metabolism is largely bypassed. As a result, toxic substances absorbed from the intestine are deprived of detoxification by the liver and produce metabolic abnormalities in the CNS. *The neuropsychiatric disturbances are similar*

regardless of the underlying liver pathology (e.g., hepatocellular failure, portal hypertension, surgical portocaval anastomosis).

Ammonia is the substance most often incriminated in the pathogenesis of HE, and recovery is often accompanied by declining blood ammonia levels. Detection of elevations in arterial ammonia level is helpful, but accurate readings are not easy to achieve, for several reasons. First, the sample must be arterial; venous ammonia levels may be high because applying a tourniquet predisposes to muscle ischemia and therefore to increased venous ammonia levels (Lockwood 2000). Second, ammonia may be produced within the blood sample itself if the sample is not iced and immediately analyzed. Finally, the results must be interpreted in clinical context; about 10% of encephalopathic patients have normal blood ammonia levels (Lipowski 1990).

Abnormalities in glutamatergic, serotonergic, GABA (γ-aminobutyric acid)–ergic, and catecholamine pathways have been proposed (Blei 1999). Increased CNS GABA may reflect the failure of the liver to extract precursor amino acids efficiently and may contribute to the potentially lethal impact of benzodiazepines, barbiturates, and chloral derivatives. Benzodiazepine-like substances have been hypothesized to arise from a specific bacterial population in the colon. It appears that ammonia itself may contribute to increased GABAergic neurotransmission in liver failure. Manganese may deposit in basal ganglia, inducing extrapyramidal symptomatology. There have also been investigations into other products of colonic bacterial metabolism, such as neurotoxic fatty acids, phenols, and mercaptans.

Precipitants

Precipitants of HE include the following:

- Increased nitrogen load: gastrointestinal bleeding, excess dietary protein, azotemia, constipation
- Electrolyte imbalance: hypokalemia, alkalosis, hypoxia, hypovolemia
- Drug use: narcotics, tranquilizers, sedatives, diuretics
- Miscellaneous: infection, surgery, superimposed acute liver disease, progressive liver disease

Staging

Several staging systems are used clinically and in research. Table 2–4 organizes neuropsychiatric abnormalities associated with hepatic encephalopathy.

Table 2–4.   Neuropsychiatric abnormalities associated with hepatic encephalopathy

Sphere	Severity of encephalopathy		
	Grade 1 (mild)	**Grade 2 (moderate)**	**Grade 3 (severe)**
Consciousness	Alert; trivial lack of awareness, short attention span	Slight blunting	Lethargic, somnolent
Behavior	Personality change, fatigue, abnormal sleep pattern	Slight lethargy, disinhibition	Bizarre behavior, paranoia
Affect	Irritable, depressed	Anxious, angry	Blunted
Cognition	Selective visuospatial abnormalities	Impaired	Too severely impaired to test reliably
Neurological examination	Tremor, asterixis, hyperactive reflexes, Babinski's reflex	Blunted consciousness, slurred speech	Dilation of pupils, nystagmus

Grade 0:   Overtly normal in all spheres.

Grade 4:   Coma, intact oculocephalic and pupillary light reflexes, no response to noxious stimuli

Source.   Adapted from Lockwood A: "Toxic and Metabolic Encephalopathies," in *Neurology in Clinical Practice,* 3rd Edition. Edited by Bradley W, Daroff R, Fenichel G, et al. Boston, MA, Butterworth-Heinemann, 2000, p. 1477. Used with permission.

Grade 1–2.   This stage presents as often subtle changes in personality, mood, psychomotor activity, and cognition. Sleep-cycle disturbances may result in nighttime wandering and confusion reminiscent of that in patients with dementia. Symptoms may be more apparent to the patient's family and friends than to the physician. The electroencephalogram (EEG) is usually normal at this point, and it is easy to overlook the underlying medical etiology. In their classic paper detailing the neuropsychiatric changes associated with hepatic disease, Summerskill et al. (1956) described several patients who had been given psychiatric diagnoses (anxiety state, hysterical ataxia, depression) and were admitted to a psychiatric hospital. Liver disease was not immediately evident in these patients; neuropsychiatric symptoms were the presenting feature in eight of the series of 17. Only three of the 17 were jaundiced, seven had hepatomegaly, and five showed little evidence of hepatic dysfunction. Fetor hepaticus, splenomegaly, palmar erythema, spider nevi, finger clubbing, and loss of body hair were the symptoms most useful in supporting the diagnosis.

It is now well established that *personality changes,* even without liver function test abnormalities, may be the initial presenting feature of hepatic failure and that interepisode personality characteristics similar to those of frontal lobe syndromes may endure (Lishman 1998). Affective changes that have been described range from depression to euphoria (Murphy et al. 1948) and at times include paranoid reactions.

Grade 2–3.   In this stage, the EEG is abnormal (often with theta waves of 5 to 7 cps) but nonspecific. There is worsening of cognitive function, and psychiatric symptoms, such as paranoid ideation, inappropriate behavior, mood disturbances (ranging from irritability to apathy or euphoria), and perceptual distortions, are present. It is here that the differential diagnosis based on gross symptomatology most obviously overlaps with DTs. There may be frank visual hallucinations. For example, a patient's report of vivid, panoramic scenes of frightening bears and wolves (Summerskill et al. 1956) would easily lead the clinician to diagnose DTs unless the suspicion for HE remained high. A long-acting benzodiazepine would be contraindicated because of the risk of progressive obtundation leading to coma. A regimen using frequent doses of a short-acting agent such as lorazepam is preferable. Aggressive intervention is crucial to prevent progression to the next phase.

Asterixis (liver flap)—a transient loss of wrist extensor postural tone when the hands are outstretched—often occurs at this point. It is assessed by asking the patient to extend the hands or dorsiflex the wrists. Note that it is easy to miss when the patient's arms are restrained. Asterixis is not specific for a hepatic etiology; it also occurs in other conditions, such as uremia, pulmonary disease, and malnutrition.

Grade 3–4.   Unless HE is treated, the patient's consciousness can rapidly deteriorate from alertness to drowsiness and eventually to stupor and coma. Mortality and morbidity are high.

Neurological abnormalities may worsen or remit from day to day, often in parallel with the variation in psychiatric symptoms. Motor symptoms predominate over sensory findings. There may be fluctuating rigidity of the trunk and limbs, grimacing and suck and grasp reflexes, exaggeration or asymmetry of tendon reflexes, Babinski signs, and focal or generalized seizures (Victor and Martin 1991). Pyramidal and extrapyramidal symptoms and signs can occur, such as dysarthria, ataxia, gross tremor, limb rigidity, hyperreflexia, and clonus. Asterixis occurs at some point in almost every patient but is nonspecific and may be seen in other encephalopathic conditions. Other neurological abnormalities include constructional apraxia, dysphasia with perseverative speech disturbances, blurred vision, diplopia, and nystagmus (Lishman 1998).

The most striking neuropathological finding in patients who die in hepatic coma is a diffuse increase in the number and size of protoplasmic astrocytes (Alzheimer type II astrocytes) in the deep layers of the cerebral cortex and in the lenticular nuclei, with little or no alteration in the nerve cells or other parenchymal elements (Victor and Martin 1991).

Treatment

The treatment of HE, like that of any delirium, involves therapy of the underlying condition. Most psychotic symptoms and behavioral abnormalities will improve with medical treatment. Specific treatment aims at correcting the precipitating factors and eliminating nitrogenous products from the intestine. In the setting of acute GI bleeding, blood in the bowel is evacuated with enemas and laxatives in order to reduce the nitrogen load. Protein ingestion is reduced to 1 gram per kilogram. Every effort is made to prevent constipation. Ammonia absorption is decreased with lactulose (a nonabsorbable disaccharide), and intestinal ammonia production by bacteria is reduced with the antibiotic neomycin.

Because atypical antipsychotics such as risperidone have minimal extrapyramidal side effects, they are rapidly replacing haloperidol, particularly in chronically ill HE patients such as those awaiting liver transplantation (S. Hafliger, personal communication, July 2, 2003). Intramuscular and intravenous administration of haloperidol, on the other hand, has the advantage of bypassing problems with absorption and first-pass metabolism, thereby increasing bioavailability. All benzodiazepines have the potential to exacerbate the hypothesized increased GABAergic tone accompanying the hepatic delirium. Disturbances of

sleep architecture usually accompany the delirium of HE, as they do any delirium. The hypnotic agent zolpidem (Ambien) has been associated with precipitating or worsening HE in vulnerable patients (S. Hafliger, personal communication, July 2, 2003).

When benzodiazepines are necessary for coexisting withdrawal syndromes, consider administering those that do not undergo oxidation in the liver, such as lorazepam (Ativan) or oxazepam (Serax) (Cozza et al. 2003). Unlike diazepam and chlordiazepoxide, these agents undergo glucuronidation, have no active metabolites, and are largely unaffected by parenchymal liver disease. Lorazepam has the advantage of availability in oral, intramuscular, and intravenous forms.

Flumazenil (Romazicon) binds to the GABA-A receptor and antagonizes the neuroinhibitory effects of the endogenous benzodiazepines thought to be present in patients with HE. A large clinical trial of 560 patients showed that an intravenous bolus of flumazenil improved mental state in about 15% of patients compared with 3% of placebo-treated control subjects (Blei et al. 2001). Flumazenil (1mg bolus iv) is recommended for patients with HE and suspected benzodiazepine intake.

Chlorpromazine (Thorazine) can exacerbate hepatotoxicity and induce cholestasis. The other phenothiazines (e.g., thioridazine, trifluoperazine) are also undesirable because of hypotensive effects, anticholinergic side effects (which may complicate delirium and induce constipation), and their tendency to produce QTc widening, which predisposes to torsades de pointes (as discussed in Chapter 1 of this volume, "The Delirious Patient").

Other medications with anticholinergic properties that may induce constipation and exacerbate HE in susceptible individuals include tricyclic antidepressants and diphenhydramine (Benadryl).

Wernicke's Encephalopathy (Delirium Due to Thiamine Deficiency)

Presentation

Like hepatic encephalopathy, Wernicke's encephalopathy (WE) may occur independently of alcohol intake. In DSM-IV-TR terminology, the diagnosis is delirium due to thiamine deficiency. WE is typically a global confusional state that has been termed a quiet, or "hypokinetic," delirium (Victor et al. 1989). Patients demonstrate profound fatigue, apathy, impaired awareness and responsiveness, and derangements of perception and memory. These symptoms cause WE to resemble hepatic encephalopathy but make it easier to distinguish from delirium tremens. WE occurs less frequently than DTs.

Victor and colleagues (1989) have described these patients in detail: "[Patients were usually] inert and impassive, and they seemed detached and indifferent to everything and everybody in their environment and without any interest in their illness. Inattention was a conspicuous abnormality so that it was often difficult to engage the patient in a simple conversation" (p. 40).

Focal neurological findings are characteristic; ocular abnormalities occur in more than 95% of patients with WE. The most common findings are nystagmus and ophthalmoplegia (i.e., gaze paresis), including sixth-nerve palsies producing lateral rectus weakness or various forms of conjugate gaze paresis. Sixth-nerve palsy is not characteristic of DTs, hepatic encephalopathy, or alcoholic hallucinosis. Classically, WE has an abrupt onset of oculomotor disturbances, cerebellar ataxia, and mental confusion. Progression to frank stupor and coma has been reported in 10% to 80% of cases of WE, depending on the source of data (Nakada and Knight 1984).

Presence of confabulation is neither unique nor necessary for the diagnosis of WE or Korsakoff's syndrome (see section below). Peripheral neuropathy is common in alcoholic individuals but is not part of this syndrome.

Etiology

Wernicke's encephalopathy is a *medical emergency. Thiamine deficiency* plays a central role in its development, causing a diffuse decrease in cerebral glucose utilization, with resulting neurotoxicity. WE most often is associated with alcoholism, but it can occur in any condition that causes thiamine deficiency (e.g., thyrotoxicosis, upper GI obstruction, severe anorexia, hyperemesis gravidarum, malabsorption syndrome, hemodialysis, prolonged intravenous feeding) (Parkin et al. 1991). Although the etiology of WE is not always related to alcohol withdrawal, some Wernicke's patients may coincidentally develop DTs, and some patients with DTs may develop WE.

Neuropathological findings in WE include punctate lesions in the periventricular, periaqueductal regions of the brain stem and diencephalon; periventricular lesions of the dorsomedial nucleus of the thalamus, the hypothalamus, the mammillary bodies, the reticular activating system, the periaqueductal areas of the midbrain, and the floor of the fourth ventricle;

and loss of tissue and edema in the mammillary bodies (Victor and Ropper 2001).

Approximately 80% of patients who survive Wernicke's encephalopathy develop the Korsakoff amnestic syndrome (alcohol-induced persisting amnestic disorder, described below). However, many Korsakoff patients have no known history of prior WE.

Treatment

Treatment involves medical management of the delirium and parenteral thiamine 100 mg initially, with upward titration until ophthalmoplegia resolves. Oral thiamine is not always well absorbed.

Korsakoff's Syndrome/Psychosis (Alcohol-Induced Persisting Amnestic Disorder)

Presentation

Korsakoff's psychosis, the original term for *alcohol-induced persisting amnestic disorder,* is a misnomer: psychotic symptoms such as delusions and hallucinations are not typical, although they can occur in the encephalopathic phase of the illness (i.e., the Wernicke delirium component). Certainly, however, the subsequent confabulation and evasiveness stemming from the memory deficits can seem like conviction about the unreal.

> Typically the patient gives a reasonably coherent but entirely false account of some recent event or experience, usually in relation to his own activities and often in response to suggestion by the examiner....The common "momentary type" [of confabulation] is brief in content, has reference to the recent past, and has to be provoked. The content can often be traced to a true memory, which has become displaced in time or context. Much rarer is the "fantastic type" in which a sustained and grandiose theme is elaborated, usually describing farfetched adventures and experiences, which clearly could not have taken place at any time. This form tends to occur spontaneously even without a provoking stimulus. (Lishman 1998, p. 31)

Confabulation has been traditionally accepted as an integral feature of the Korsakoff syndrome (which has also been referred to as *confabulatory psychosis*), but it is neither consistently present nor essential for the diagnosis. Be sure to distinguish confabulation from delusions.

Neuropsychology

Not all types of memory are equally affected by the Korsakoff amnestic syndrome. For example, patients can learn their way around the hospital ward and can acquire knowledge of simple ward routines. (This type of learning is called *procedural memory.*)

Amnesia.   Both retrograde amnesia (impairing memory of material learned before the onset) and anterograde amnesia (impairing new learning and memorization) occur. Remote memories are better preserved than recent ones.

Intact attention, faulty retention.   Attention and perception of new material are intact (digit span is normal), but retention is faulty. For example, patients are able to repeat three simple bits of information and understand what is wanted, but cannot retain the bits after distraction or learn them despite many repetitions. Memorization problems extend to all aspects of new learning: the names of persons and objects, nonsense syllables, a line of poetry, a card game, and all but the simplest motor tasks. "It seemed not to matter whether the information to be acquired was highly emotional or purely cognitive in nature, or by what sensory avenue the information was presented" (Victor et al. 1989, p. 43).

Intact remote memory.   In addition, the impairment of past memory is never complete. Patients may retain islets of information with varying degrees of accuracy but without their proper temporal sequence. A telescoping of events characteristically occurs (e.g., a patient who had been in a state mental hospital for 6 years reported that he had been there for only a few days). The descriptions by Victor and colleagues (1989) remain among the most vivid in the literature:

> We were quite unable to discern the factor(s) that governed what was forgotten and what was remembered. This aspect of the memory disorder seemed to follow no distinctive or consistent pattern. A patient might not recall seemingly important or emotionally charged events…but at the same time might be able to recall seemingly casual items or ones in which he or she was not personally involved…. Similar inconsistencies were noted in regard to new memories. (Victor et al. 1989, p. 45)

Apathy.   Korsakoff amnestic patients in the chronic stages of the illness are apathetic and placid, lack motivation, and show bland affect. Korsakoff patients might admit to memory defects, but without insight about the seriousness of their amnesia. "It was our impression that the patients were difficult to anger or to frighten, and although their emotional reactions were more or less appropriate, they were difficult to arouse" (Victor et al. 1989, p. 45). This apathy is in contrast to the *catastrophic reaction,* consisting of hyperemotionality, restlessness, uncooperativeness, anxiety, tearfulness, and irritability, that occurs with left-hemisphere lesions.

Distinction from Alzheimer-type dementia.   Unlike senile dementia of the Alzheimer type, Korsakoff syndrome is not a progressive *global dementia.* Although sensory, motivational, and visuospatial difficulties may occur, they are less prominent than the disordered memory and learning. Alertness is preserved, with intact awareness of the patient's surroundings and without serious defects in social behavior. Also preserved are vocabulary, general language facility, long-standing motor skills and social habits, and the ability to recognize people known long before the illness. Apraxia and agnosia are not typical features, nor is aphasia; Korsakoff patients have normal speech and are able to write from dictation, copy figures, and draw simple objects like a clock from memory.

Treatment

There is no effective treatment other than supportive management of dementia. Some patients will improve with time, but it is not possible to predict in the acute phase who will get better and who will not. Patients often require institutionalization or sheltered settings (Kopelman 1995).

Minimal Encephalopathy

Many cirrhotic patients without overt delirium suffer from subtle neuropsychological deficits that have been termed *minimal encephalopathy* (formerly *latent* or *subclinical encephalopathy*). Diagnostic neuropsychological testing focuses on the following areas of difficulty: motor speed and accuracy, visual perception, visuospatial orientation, visual construction, concentration, attention, and, to a lesser extent, memory (Weissenborn et al. 2001). The clinical neurological examination and the EEG are not particularly helpful because they may be normal.

Performance skills, such as short-term visual memory and reaction times, are more often impaired than verbal skills, which may be normal. This type of impairment may interfere with a patient's daily activities such as driving or operating machinery. These findings have practical impact. For example, one study found that among cirrhotic patients, 73% of those who were blue-collar workers experienced impaired earning capacity in the presence of minimal

HE. In addition, 80% of the white-collar workers were fit for work even in the presence of minimal HE because of the preservation of verbal abilities in this condition, whereas only 40% of the blue-collar workers met work fitness criteria (Weissenborn et al. 2001).

DSM-IV-TR gives no specific instructions on how to code minimal encephalopathy. Depending on the clinical findings, it may fit into 294.9 cognitive disorder not otherwise specified (NOS) (e.g., mild neurocognitive disorder), 294.8 amnestic disorder NOS, or 294.8 dementia NOS.

Treatment

There is no effective treatment other than supportive management of dementia.

Alcohol Withdrawal

Presentation

Symptoms of uncomplicated alcohol withdrawal include coarse tremors of the hands or tongue; nausea or vomiting; malaise; autonomic nervous system hyperactivity, manifested by tachycardia, sweating, and elevated blood pressure; anxiety; irritability; insomnia; and nightmares. Peak symptoms occur 24–48 hours after the last drink and, in uncomplicated cases, subside within 5–7 days, even without treatment. Uncomplicated alcohol withdrawal may progress to DTs or resolve spontaneously. The following instruments may be helpful in diagnosing alcohol withdrawal:

- Figure 2–1. CIWA-Ar: Addiction Research Foundation Clinical Institute Withdrawal Assessment for Alcohol–Revised
- Alcohol screening questionnaires: Figure 2–2, Figure 2–3, and Figure 2–4 (CAGE questions, Alcohol Use Disorders Identification Test [AUDIT], and Michigan Alcoholism Screening Test [MAST])

Treatment

A preset dosing schedule of benzodiazepines that is tapered over several days with hydration has long been the treatment of choice for alcohol withdrawal. Figure 2–5 and Figure 2–6 present two sample regimens for the management of alcohol withdrawal. Figure 2–5 is a symptom-triggered regimen with short- and long-acting benzodiazepine options. Figure 2–6 is a structured medication regimen. Symptom-triggered dosing reduces medication doses by a factor of four and shortens symptom duration by a factor of about six (Saitz et al. 1994).

Note that any regimen for treating uncomplicated alcohol withdrawal should include the following:

- Thiamine 100 mg im immediately and then 100 mg po daily
- Folic acid 1 mg po daily
- Multivitamin one daily

Alcohol Withdrawal Seizures

Alcohol withdrawal seizures are also sometimes called "rum fits." They typically begin 7–48 hours after cessation of drinking, with more than 60% of seizures occurring 17–24 hours after the last drink. Alcoholic patients presenting with their first seizure or focal seizures should have a workup for structural lesions (e.g., subdural hematoma). Seizures in alcoholic individuals usually do *not* indicate epilepsy and do not require prolonged anticonvulsant therapy, although patients with preexisting seizure disorders are at greater risk for alcohol withdrawal seizures. Alcohol withdrawal seizures are frequently self-limited and require only supportive care. To help distinguish simple alcohol withdrawal seizures from the more serious DTs, remember that withdrawal seizures almost always occur with a clear sensorium (Chang and Steinberg 2001).

Alcoholic Hallucinosis

Presentation

Alcoholic hallucinosis (alcohol withdrawal with perceptual disturbances or alcohol-induced psychotic disorder) is a relative rare psychiatric disorder, although one group reported that 7.4% of their patients (48 of 643 patients) met DSM-III and ICD-10 criteria for alcoholic hallucinosis (Tsuang et al. 1994). Auditory, visual, and/or tactile hallucinations are its main symptoms. Usually, auditory hallucinations predominate.

Unlike DTs or the other deliria, alcoholic hallucinosis *occurs in a clear sensorium*, without confusion, psychomotor hyperactivity, or intense autonomic reactivity. These symptoms help to distinguish it from other alcohol-associated syndromes. When delusional elaborations occur, they typically *result from* the hallucinatory experiences and usually do not precede them or arise in their absence. Onset is classically within 48 hours of drinking cessation but can occur during drinking bouts. Like DTs, the visual hallucinations may be of small animals, such as rodents and insects, characteristically moving rapidly on the walls, floor, or ceiling (Lishman 1998). Visual disturbances such as blurring, flashes, and spots often accompany visual hallucinations. Tinnitus is common, sometimes pre-

Patient_____ Date_____ Time_____ Pulse_____ Blood pressure_____

NAUSEA AND VOMITING Ask "Do you feel sick to your stomach? Have you vomited?" 0 No nausea and no vomiting 1 Mild nausea with no vomiting 2 3 4 Intermittent nausea with dry heaves 5 6 7 Constant nausea, frequent dry heaves, and vomiting	**TREMOR** Arms extended and fingers spread apart. Observation. 0 No tremor 1 Not visible but can be felt fingertip to fingertip 2 3 4 Moderate, with patient's arms extended 5 6 7 Severe, even with arms not extended
PAROXYSMAL SWEATS Observation. 0 No sweating 1 Barely perceptible sweating, palms moist 2 3 4 Beads of sweat obvious on forehead 5 6 7 Drenching sweats	**ANXIETY** Ask "Do you feel nervous?" Observation. 0 No anxiety, at ease 1 Mildly anxious 2 3 4 Moderately anxious, or guarded, so anxiety is inferred 5 6 7 Equivalent to acute panic states as seen in severe delirium or acute schizophrenic reactions
AGITATION Observation. 0 Normal activity 1 Somewhat more than normal activity 2 3 4 Moderately fidgety and restless 5 6 7 Paces back and forth during most of the interview or constantly thrashes about	**TACTILE DISTURBANCES** Ask "Have you any itching, any pins and needles sensations, any burning, any numbness, or do you feel bugs crawling on or under your skin?" Observation. 0 None 1 Very mild itching, pins and needles, burning, or numbness 2 Mild itching, pins and needles, burning, or numbness 3 Moderate itching, pins and needles, burning, or numbness 4 Moderately severe hallucinations 5 Severe hallucinations 6 Extremely severe hallucinations 7 Continuous hallucinations
AUDITORY DISTURBANCES Ask "Are you more aware of sounds around you? Are they harsh? Do they frighten you? Are you hearing anything that is disturbing to you? Are you hearing things you know are not there?" Observation. 0 Not present 1 Very mild harshness or ability to frighten 2 Mild harshness or ability to frighten 3 Moderate harshness or ability to frighten 4 Moderately severe hallucinations 5 Severe hallucinations 6 Extremely severe hallucinations 7 Continuous hallucinations	**VISUAL DISTURBANCES** Ask "Does the light appear to be too bright? Is its color different? Does it hurt your eyes? Are you seeing anything that is disturbing to you? Are you seeing things you know are not there?" Observation. 0 Not present 1 Very mild sensitivity 2 Mild sensitivity 3 Moderate sensitivity 4 Moderately severe hallucinations 5 Severe hallucinations 6 Extremely severe hallucinations 7 Continuous hallucinations
HEADACHE, FULLNESS IN HEAD Ask "Does your head feel different? Does it feel like there is a band around your head?" Do not rate for dizziness or light-headedness. Otherwise, rate severity. 0 Not present 1 Very mild 2 Mild 3 Moderate 4 Moderately severe 5 Severe 6 Very severe 7 Extremely severe	**ORIENTATION AND CLOUDING OF SENSORIUM** Ask "What day is this? Where are you? Who am I?" 0 Oriented and can do serial additions 1 Cannot do serial additions or is uncertain about date 2 Disoriented for date by no more than 2 calendar days 3 Disoriented for date by more than 2 calendar days 4 Disoriented for place and/or person

CIWA-Ar SCORE _____   Treat if score >8–10
(Goal <8–10 over 24 hours)

Figure 2–1. CIWA-Ar: Addiction Research Foundation Clinical Institute Withdrawal Assessment for Alcohol—Revised.

Source. Adapted from Sullivan JT, Sykora K, Schneiderman J, et al: "Assessment of Alcohol Withdrawal: The Revised Clinical Institute Withdrawal Assessment for Alcohol Scale (CIWA-Ar)." *British Journal of Addiction* 84:1353–1357, 1989. Available online: http://addiction-medicine.org/files/15doc.html.

C	Have you ever felt the need to **c**ut down on your use of alcohol?
A	Has anyone **a**nnoyed you by criticizing your use of alcohol?
G	Have you ever felt **g**uilty because of something you've done while drinking?
E	Have you ever taken a drink to steady your nerves or get over a hangover (**e**ye-opener)?

Figure 2–2. CAGE questions.

Note. Two or more "yes" responses represent a positive screen for alcohol abuse and dependence. However, the CAGE is nonspecific regarding pattern of alcohol intake and the distinction between past and current drinking problems. It also cannot detect gradations of alcohol problems (e.g., hazardous or harmful drinking).

dating the appearance of auditory hallucinations and persisting even after they clear. The auditory hallucinations often begin as simple sounds (buzzing, roaring, bells) and gradually take on vocal form, usually the voices of friends or enemies that malign, threaten, or reproach the patient (Lishman 1998; Victor 1992). The voices may be of a command nature. Patients tend to preserve insight that the hallucinations are imaginary (Lishman 1998).

In the majority of cases, the symptoms remit within a few hours to days. However, one review suggested that approximately 10% to 20% of patients develop *chronic* alcoholic hallucinosis with persisting auditory hallucinations, independent of further alcohol intake (Glass 1989). The chronic psychosis of alcoholic hallucinosis may make it indistinguishable from schizophrenia on the basis of psychopathological or clinical symptoms alone (Soyka 1994). It had been thought that the disorder was part of the schizophrenic spectrum. Family and genetic studies have failed to support this hypothesis.

Among individuals with primary alcoholism, those who consume more drugs and/or alcohol seem to be at an increased risk for developing alcoholic hallucinosis (Tsuang et al. 1994).

Diagnostic Coding

Preservation of insight in the patient with alcoholic hallucinosis affects the assignment of a diagnosis in DSM-IV-TR. When the patient shows intact reality testing (i.e., knows that his or her hallucinations are induced by the substance and do not represent external reality), the diagnosis for alcoholic hallucinosis becomes *alcohol withdrawal with perceptual disturbances.* If hallucinations occur in the absence of intact reality testing, consider a diagnosis of *alcohol-induced psychotic disorder, with hallucinations.*

Treatment

Antipsychotic drugs are the treatment of choice for the psychotic symptoms of alcoholic hallucinosis, although these agents do not ameliorate the chronic condition. However, Soyka et al. (1997) reported on a 33-year-old patient with a 6-year history of auditory hallucinations that persisted despite abstinence from alcohol and continuous neuroleptic therapy with haloperidol decanoate (2 mL every 3 weeks). Gradual switchover to risperidone 6 mg in divided doses resulted in compete disappearance of symptoms, which was maintained at 8-week follow-up. The authors speculated that because both dopaminergic and serotonergic dysfunction may play a role in the development of hallucinations in alcoholic individuals, the combined dopamine D_2 and serotonin 5-HT$_2$ receptor-blocking properties of risperidone may make it a particularly effective antipsychotic in alcoholic hallucinosis.

■ PSYCHOPHARMACOLOGY IN HEPATIC FAILURE

Pharmacokinetic changes may affect the mechanism and timing of a drug's absorption, distribution, metabolism, or excretion. Most psychotropic medications—other than lithium—are primarily metabolized by the liver. Hepatic insufficiency significantly affects medication clearance. Considerations affecting psychopharmacology in liver failure are diagrammed in Figure 2–7. The following are a few highlights.

Phase I Metabolism

Phase I metabolism alters compounds by oxidation, reduction, or hydrolysis to prepare them for excretion or for further (Phase II) reactions. Most Phase I oxidation reactions occur by means of the cytochrome P450 system. Phase I activity is decreased in parenchymal liver disease. Most psychotropic drugs are metabolized by Phase I reactions and thus have their clearance decreased by cirrhosis, which reduces the activity and levels of liver enzymes. Exceptions: 1) medications that bypass Phase I metabolism and proceed directly to phase II metabolism (e.g., by conjugation; see below); 2) psychotropic medications that bypass hepatic metabolism entirely, such as lithium and gabapentin (Neurontin), and are metabolized by the kidneys.

Cytochromes are a group of hepatic enzymes that are important in oxidative drug metabolism. Several subgroups (isoenzymes) of cytochrome P450 have been identified. At least two of them—2D6 and 3A4—may be inhibited by medications commonly used in both psychiatric and other medical practice. The

---

(Each of the 10 questions is given 0 to 4 points. A score of 8 or more out of 40 identifies an alcohol use disorder.)

1. How often do you have a drink containing alcohol?

   (0) never   (1) monthly or less   (2) 2–4x/month   (3) 2–3x/week   (4) ≥4x/week

2. How many drinks containing alcohol do you have on a typical day when you are drinking?

   (0) 1 or 2   (1) 3 or 4   (2) 5 or 6   (3) 7 to 9   (4) ≥10

3. How often do you have ≥6 drinks on one occasion?

   (0) never   (1) less than monthly   (2) monthly   (3) weekly   (4) daily or almost daily

4. How often during the last year, have you found that you were not able to stop drinking once you had started?

   (0) never   (1) less than monthly   (2) monthly   (3) weekly   (4) daily or almost daily

5. How often during the last year have you failed to do what was normally expected from you because of drinking?

   (0) never   (1) less than monthly   (2) monthly   (3) weekly   (4) daily or almost daily

6. How often during the last year have you needed a drink in the morning to get yourself going after a heavy drinking session?

   (0) never   (1) less than monthly   (2) monthly   (3) weekly   (4) daily or almost daily

7. How often during the last year have you had a feeling of guilt or remorse after drinking?

   (0) never   (1) less than monthly   (2) monthly   (3) weekly   (4) daily or almost daily

8. How often during the last year have you been unable to remember what happened the night before because you had been drinking?

   (0) never   (1) less than monthly   (2) monthly   (3) weekly   (4) daily or almost daily

9. Have you or someone else been injured as a result of your drinking?

   (0) no   (1) yes, but not in the last year   (4) yes, during the last year

10. Has a relative, friend, or a physician or other health care worker been concerned about your drinking or suggested you cut down?

    (0) no   (1) yes, but not in the last year   (4) yes, during the last year

---

Figure 2–3. Alcohol Use Disorders Identification Test (AUDIT).

Source. Reprinted from Saunders JB, Aasland OG, Babor TG, et al: "Development of the Alcohol Use Disorders Identification Test (AUDIT): WHO Collaborative Project on Early Detection of Persons With Harmful Alcohol Consumption, II." *Addiction* 88:791–804, 1993. Used with permission.

monograph by Cozza et al. (2003) is one of the most comprehensible and comprehensive explanations of P450 drug interaction principles. A few crucial points:

- "3A4 is the workhorse of the P450 system" (Cozza et al. 2003), accounting for more than 50% of all drug oxidation in the human liver. Large numbers of substrates, inhibitors, and inducers affect the 3A4 isoenzyme. There is great variability in how well 3A4 functions in individuals.
- 2D6 was the first P450 isoenzyme to be extensively studied, and it remains particularly important in understanding psychotropic drug interactions. It

has polymorphic forms; that is, individuals may be classified in one of several genotypes: homozygous or heterozygous extensive ("normal") metabolizers (EMs); homozygous poor metabolizers (PMs); and ultraextensive metabolizers (UEMs), who have duplicate or multiple copies of the *2D6* gene.

- Delayed 2D6 drug metabolism is likely in PMs, resulting in the accumulation of the parent drug and more side effects. The risk of toxicity increases if enzyme activity is further inhibited (e.g., by adding a selective serotonin reuptake inhibitor [SSRI] to an antiarrhythmic agent or a tricyclic antidepressant). PMs are particularly common among

	YES (points)	NO (points)
Do you enjoy a drink now and then?	0	
1. Do you feel you are a normal drinker? (By normal we mean you drink less than or as much as most people)		(2)
2. Have you ever awakened in the morning after some drinking the night before and found that you could not remember part of the evening?	(2)	
3. Does your wife, husband, a parent, or other near relative ever worry or complain about your drinking?	(1)	
4. Can you stop drinking without a struggle after one or two drinks?		(2)
5. Do you ever feel guilty about your drinking?	(1)	
6. Do friends and relatives think you are a normal drinker?		(2)
7. Do you ever try to limit your drinking to certain times of the day or to certain places?	(0)	
8. Have you ever attended a meeting of Alcoholics Anonymous?	(2)	
9. Have you gotten into physical fights when drinking?	(1)	
10. Has your drinking ever created problems between your and your wife, husband, a parent, or other relative?	(2)	
11. Has your wife, husband, a parent, or other family members ever gone to anyone for help about your drinking?	(2)	
12. Have you ever lost friends because of your drinking?	(2)	
13. Have you ever gotten into trouble at work or school because you were drinking?	(2)	
14. Have you ever lost a job because of drinking?	(2)	
15. Have you ever neglected your obligations, your family, or your work for two or more days in a row because you were drinking?	(2)	
16. Do you drink before noon fairly often?	(1)	
17. Have you ever been told you have liver trouble? Cirrhosis?	(2)	
18. After heavy drinking, have you ever had severe shaking or delirium tremens (DTs)? heard voices or seen things that really weren't there?	(5) (2)	
19. Have you ever gone to anyone for help about your drinking?	(5)	
20. Have you ever been in a hospital because of your drinking?	(5)	
21. Have you ever been a patient in a psychiatric hospital or on a psychiatric ward of a general hospital where drinking was part of the problem that resulted in hospitalization?	(2)	
22. Have you ever been seen at a psychiatric or mental health clinic or gone to a doctor, social worker, or clergyperson for help with an emotional problem in which drinking played a part?	(2)	
23. Have you ever been arrested for drunk driving, driving while intoxicated, or driving under the influence of alcoholic beverages? (If YES, how many times? ___) (2 pts per arrest)	( )	
24. Have you ever been arrested, or taken into custody, even for a few hours, because of other drunken behavior? (If YES, how many times? ___) (2 pts per arrest)	( )	
SCORING Alcoholism: ≥ **5 points likely** **4 points suggestive** **<3 points unlikely**	**TOTAL POINTS**	

Figure 2–4. Michigan Alcoholism Screening Test (MAST).

Source.   Reprinted from Selzer M: "The Michigan Alcoholism Screening Test: The Quest for a New Diagnostic Instrument." *American Journal of Psychiatry* 127:1653–1658, 1971. Used with permission.

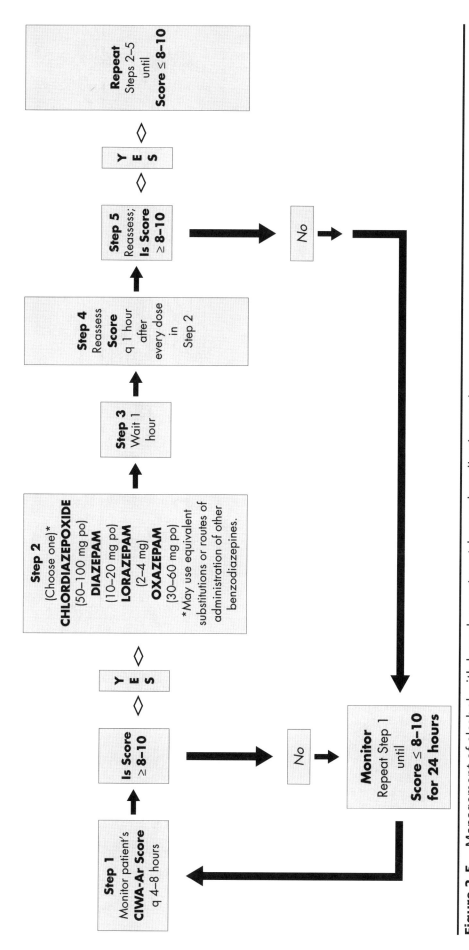

Figure 2–5. Management of alcohol withdrawal: symptom-triggered medication regimen.

Source. Adapted from recommendations by Mayo-Smith MF: "Management of Alcohol Intoxication and Withdrawal," in *Principles of Addiction Medicine,* 2nd Edition. Edited by Graham AW, Schultz TK. Chevy Chase, MD, American Society of Addiction Medicine, Inc., 1998, p. 437; and Prater CD, Miller KE, Zylstra RG: "Outpatient Detoxification of the Addicted or Alcoholic Patient." *American Family Physician* 60:1667–1674, 1999.

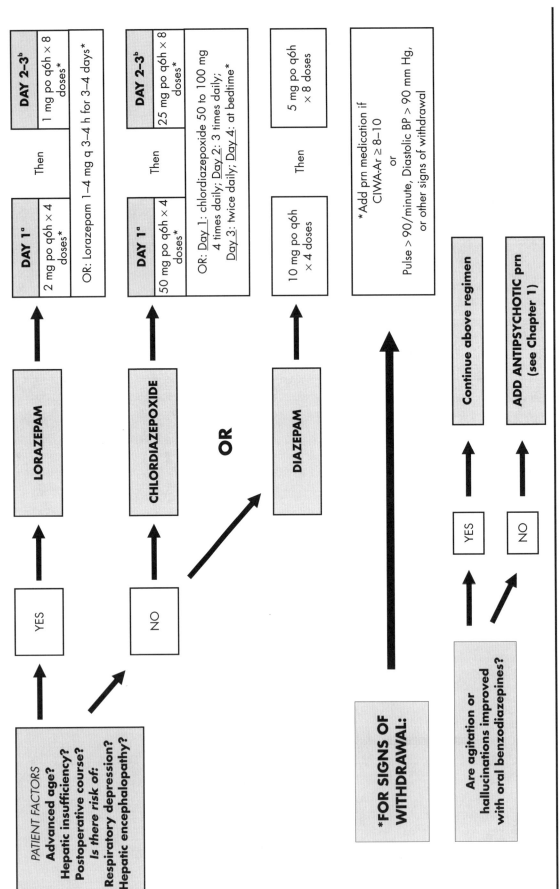

Figure 2–6. Management of alcohol withdrawal: structured medication regimens.

[a]Plus thiamine 100 mg immediately and then 100 mg po daily; folic acid 1 mg po daily; multivitamin 1 per day.

[b]Extend to Day 4 or 5 as needed, guided by symptoms of withdrawal.

Source. Adapted from recommendations by Mayo-Smith MF: "Management of Alcohol Intoxication and Withdrawal," in *Principles of Addiction Medicine*, 2nd Edition. Edited by Graham AW, Schultz TK. Chevy Chase, MD, American Society of Addiction Medicine, Inc., 1998, p. 437; and Prater CD, Miller KE, Zylstra RG: "Outpatient Detoxification of the Addicted or Alcoholic Patient." *American Family Physician* 60:1667–1674, 1999.

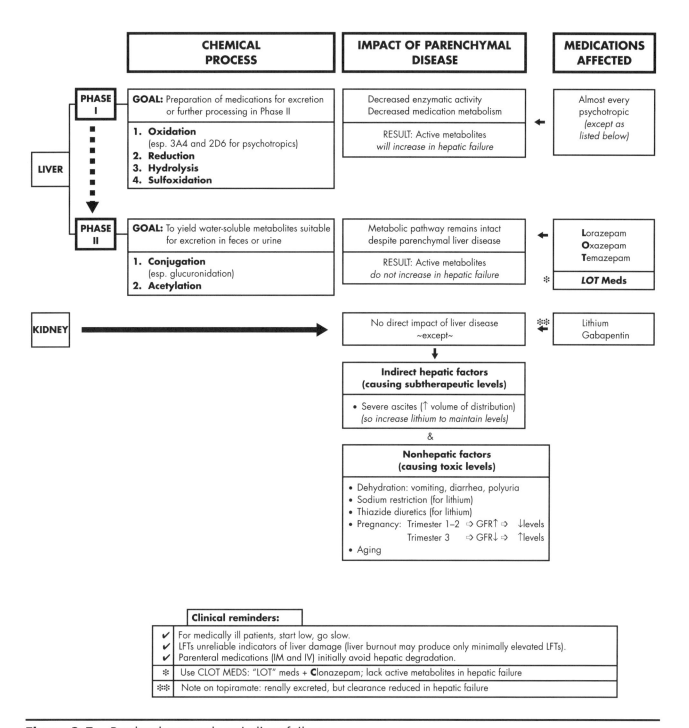

Figure 2–7.   Psychopharmacology in liver failure.
Abbreviations: GFR=glomerular filtration rate; LFTs=liver function tests.

Asians, Pacific Islanders, Africans, and African Americans.

• EMs may be pharmacologically "converted" to PMs by medications that inhibit 2D6. Certain SSRIs are inhibitors of cytochrome 2D6 and may produce drug-drug interactions. (SSRIs are much weaker inhibitors of 3A4.)

• Other enzyme systems also have an impact on me-

tabolism and include the uridine diphosphate glucuronosyltransferases.

The case approach is a practical way of learning the principles of this complicated topic and is provided in a casebook by Sandson (2003). Useful Web sites for help with P450 interactions are http://www.Drug-Interactions.com and http://mhc.com/Cytochromes (accessed June 2004).

Phase II Metabolism

Phase II metabolism consists of several conjugation and acetylation pathways that usually result in the compound's inactivation. The Phase II reactions usually produce highly polar, water-soluble medications that are suitable for renal excretion. Most psychotropics undergo Phase I and Phase II metabolism. Exceptions:

- Lithium and gabapentin (renally excreted)
- Topiramate (not extensively metabolized and primarily eliminated unchanged in the urine. In hepatically impaired subjects, the clearance of topiramate may be decreased; the mechanism underlying the decrease is not well understood. The manufacturer recommends caution for use in hepatically impaired patients; Ortho-McNeil Pharmaceutical, June 2003).
- A subset of benzodiazepines: lorazepam (Ativan), oxazepam (Serax), and temazepam (Restoril) (mnemonic: the "LOT" medications). The LOT medications undergo conjugation by glucuronidation, which remains intact despite hepatic failure.

Note: After oxidation in Phase I, the acetylation of clonazepam (Klonopin) is also relatively preserved in the setting of hepatic failure, producing no active metabolites. This characteristic makes it a better choice than diazepam when a long-acting benzodiazepine is needed. (Mnemonic for medications that are safe in hepatic failure: "CLOT" medications; see Figure 2–7).

Things get even more complicated, because the rate of hepatic metabolism is also dependent on either 1) the rate of delivery of the drug to the hepatic metabolizing enzymes, in which liver blood flow is rate limiting, or 2) the intrinsic capacity of hepatic enzymes to metabolize the substrate, in which the enzyme's saturation capacity is rate limiting. Both the rate of delivery and metabolic capacity may be impaired in cirrhosis—the former by extrahepatic shunting, the latter by decreased enzyme activity.

- *Low-clearance drugs* (e.g., diazepam, chlorpromazine) have the rate-limiting characteristics of low affinity, slower metabolism, and enzyme saturation.
- *High-clearance drugs* (e.g., haloperidol) are not enzyme dependent, but flow dependent, and they are metabolized as quickly as they can reach the liver (Leipzig 1990). High-clearance drugs undergo significant first-pass metabolism—that is, by the end of an orally administered drug's first pass through

the liver, only a small fraction of the parent compound remains to enter the circulation. Therefore, high-clearance drugs such as haloperidol are normally administered orally at 2 to 4 times the parenteral dose to compensate for extensive first-pass metabolism and to achieve equivalent blood levels and clinical response. Alternatively, intramuscular and intravenous administration of drugs avoids initial hepatic degradation, allowing direct entry into the systemic circulation.

■ CLINICAL IMPLICATIONS

- "Start low, go slow" when using most medications in cirrhotic patients.
- If there is a need to use benzodiazepines in cirrhotic patients, stick with the "CLOT" benzodiazepines. (clonazepam, lorazepam, oxazepam, temazepam).
- There is accumulating experience on the safe use of atypical antipsychotics in liver failure, particularly in liver transplantation centers. (See Chapter 11 in this volume, "A Primer on Solid Organ Transplant Psychiatry.")
- *Chlorpromazine (Thorazine) is contraindicated* because it can exacerbate hepatotoxicity and induce cholestasis.
- *The only antidepressant that should be avoided* is nefazodone (Serzone), because of its black box warning about unpredictable, potentially fatal liver failure.
- Even for medications that are excreted by the kidneys, such as lithium, when ascites accompanies cirrhosis the water composition of the body increases, requiring dose adjustments (increases) to accommodate the increased volume of distribution.

■ REFERENCES

American Psychiatric Association: Diagnostic and Statistical Manual of Mental Disorders, 4th Edition, Text Revision. Washington, DC, American Psychiatric Association, 2000

Blei A: Hepatic encephalopathy, in Oxford Textbook of Hepatology. Edited by Bircher J, Benhamou J, McIntyre N, et al. Oxford, UK, Oxford University Press, 1999, pp 765–786

Blei A, Cordoba J, The Practice Parameters Committee of the American College of Gastroenterology: Hepatic encephalopathy. Am J Gastroenterol 96:1968–1976, 2001

Chang P, Steinberg M: Postoperative medical complications: alcohol withdrawal. Med Clin North Am 85:1191–1212, 2001

Cozza KL, Armstrong SC, Oesterheld JR: Concise Guide to Drug Interaction Principles for Medical Practice: Cytochrome P450s, UGTs, P-Glycoproteins, 2nd Edition. Washington, DC, American Psychiatric Publishing, 2003

Daeppen J, Gache P, Landry U, et al: Symptom-triggered vs fixed-schedule doses of benzodiazepine for alcohol withdrawal: a randomized treatment trial. Arch Intern Med 162:1117–1121, 2002

Ferenci P, Lockwood A, Mullen K, et al: Hepatic encephalopathy—definition, nomenclature, diagnosis, and quantification: final report of the working party at the 11th World Congresses of Gastroenterology, Vienna, 1998. Hepatology 35:716–721, 2002

Foy A, March S, Drinkwater V: Use of an objective clinical scale in the assessment and management of alcohol withdrawal in a large general hospital. Alcohol Clin Exp Res 12:360–364, 1988

Glass I: Alcoholic hallucinosis: a psychiatric enigma, 2: follow-up studies. Br J Addict 84:151–164, 1989

Kopelman M: The Korsakoff syndrome. Br J Psychiatry 166:154–173, 1995

Leipzig R: Psychopharmacology in patients with hepatic and gastrointestinal disease. Int J Psychiatry Med 20:109–139, 1990

Lipowski Z: Delirium: Acute Confusional States. New York, Oxford University Press, 1990

Lishman W: Organic Psychiatry, 3rd Edition. London, Blackwell Scientific, 1998

Lockwood A: Hepatic encephalopathy, in Metabolic Brain Dysfunction in Systemic Disorders. Edited by Arieff A, Griggs R. Boston, MA, Little, Brown, 1992, pp 167–182

Lockwood A: Toxic and metabolic encephalopathies, in Neurology in Clinical Practice, 3rd Edition. Edited by Bradley W, Daroff R, Fenichel G, et al. Boston, MA, Butterworth-Heinemann, 2000, pp 1475–1493

Mee-Lee D, Shulman G, Fishman M, et al: ASAM Patient Placement Criteria for the Treatment of Substance-Related Disorders, 2nd Edition—Revised (ASAM PPC-2R). Chevy Chase, MD, American Society of Addiction Medicine, 2001

Myrick H, Brady KT, Malcolm R: Divalproex in the treatment of alcohol withdrawal. Am J Drug Alcohol Abuse 26:155–160, 2000

Myrick H, Brady KT, Malcolm R: New developments in the pharmacotherapy of alcohol dependence. Am J Addict 10 (suppl):3–15, 2001

Nakada T, Knight R: Alcohol and the central nervous system. Med Clin North Am 68:121–131, 1984

Parkin A, Blunden J, Rees J, et al: Wernicke-Korsakoff syndrome of nonalcoholic origin. Brain Cogn 15:69–82, 1991

Reoux JP, Saxon AJ, Malte CA, et al: Divalproex sodium in alcohol withdrawal: a randomized double-blind placebo-controlled clinical trial. Alcohol Clin Exp Res 25:1324–1329, 2001

Rosenbaum M, McCarty T: Alcohol prescription by surgeons in the prevention and treatment of delirium tremens: historic and current practice. Gen Hosp Psychiatry 24:257–259, 2002

Saitz R, Mayo Smith M, Roberts M, et al: Individualized treatment for alcohol withdrawal: a randomized double-blind controlled trial. JAMA 272:519–523, 1994

Sandson NB: Drug Interactions Casebook: The Cytochrome P450 System and Beyond. Washington, DC, American Psychiatric Publishing, 2003

Sonne N, Tonnesen H: The influence of alcoholism on outcome after evacuation of subdural haematoma. Br J Neurosurg 6:125–130, 1992

Soyka M: Alcohol dependence and schizophrenia: what are the interrelationships? Alcohol Alcohol Suppl 2:473–478, 1994

Soyka M, Wegner U, Moeller H-J: Risperidone in treatment-refractory chronic alcohol hallucinosis. Pharmacopsychiatry 30:135–136, 1997

Spies C, Nordmann A, Brummer G, et al: Intensive care unit stay is prolonged in chronic alcoholic men following tumor resection of the upper digestive tract. Acta Anaesthesiol Scand 40:649–656, 1996

Summerskill W, Davidson E, Sherlock S, et al: The neuropsychiatric syndrome associated with hepatic cirrhosis and an extensive portal collateral circulation. Q J Med 25:245–266, 1956

Tsuang J, Irwin M, Smith T, et al: Characteristics of men with alcoholic hallucinosis. Addiction 89:73–78, 1994

Victor M: The effects of alcohol on the nervous system, in Medical Diagnosis and Treatment of Alcoholism. Edited by Mendelson J, Mello N. New York, McGraw-Hill, 1992, pp 201–262

Victor M, Martin J: Nutritional and metabolic diseases of the nervous system, in Harrison's Principles of Internal Medicine, 12th Edition. Edited by Wilson J, Braunwald E, Isselbacher K, et al. New York, McGraw-Hill, 1991, pp 2045–2054

Victor M, Ropper A: Adams and Victor's Principles of Neurology, 7th Edition. New York, McGraw-Hill, 2001

Victor M, Adams RD, Collins GH: The Wernicke-Korsakoff Syndrome and Related Neurological Disorders Due to Alcoholism and Malnutrition (Contemporary Neurology Series, Vol 30, 2nd Edition). Philadelphia, PA, FA Davis, 1989

Weissenborn K, Ennen JC, Schomerus H, et al: Neuropsychological characterization of hepatic encephalopathy. J Hepatol 34:768–773, 2001

Chapter

3

The Patient With Cardiovascular Disease

Antoinette Ambrosino Wyszynski, M.D.
Melanie Schwarz, M.D.
Bruce Rubenstein, M.D.
Victor B. Rodack, M.D.
Manuel Santos, M.D.

■ THE PSYCHE AND CARDIAC MORBIDITY

Depression (Barefoot and Schroll 1996; Ford et al. 1998; Lett et al. 2004) and anxiety (Strik et al. 2003) appear to be independent risk factors for the development of coronary artery disease. Subsyndromal depressive symptoms also correlate with an increased risk of cardiovascular mortality (Frasure-Smith et al. 1995). Even more impressively, negative mood appears to predict long-term cardiac-related mortality following myocardial infarction (MI), independently of cardiac disease severity (Frasure-Smith and Lesperance 2003a, 2003b).

The mechanism for this effect remains unclear. Depression and anxiety may predispose to increased cardiac disease and mortality by affecting physiological and behavioral factors. For example, depressed patients experience elevated platelet activation, predis-

posing them to thromboembolic events. They also experience stress-induced immune activation and hypercortisolemia leading to decreased insulin resistance, showing increases in endogenous steroid production, catecholamine release, blood pressure, and coronary vasoconstriction. Behaviorally, depression is associated with higher incidence of treatment nonadherence and unhealthy lifestyle habits, failure to maintain modified behavior patterns learned during cardiac rehabilitation, and nonreturn to normal functioning after the acute cardiac illness.

Although there is substantial evidence for a relationship between depression and adverse clinical outcomes, it is surprising that no definitive data confirm that treating comorbid depression improves clinical cardiac outcomes for depressed coronary artery disease (CAD) patients. The Enhancing Recovery in Coronary Heart Disease Patients (ENRICHD) trial was the largest controlled trial of psychotherapy ever completed (Berkman et al. 2003). In this study, investigators enrolled 2,481 post–MI patients from 73 hospitals in eight U.S. cities in a 6-month course of weekly cognitive-behavioral therapy versus usual care. Three-quarters of the study patients had depression, and the remainder were included because of low perceived social support (LPSS). The goal was to determine whether treating depression and LPSS would reduce mortality and recurrent infarction. The intervention produced small, statistically significant decreases in depression symptoms and small, significant increases in perceived support. Disappointingly, these differences did not translate into any benefit in event-free survival during a mean follow-up of 29 months. The intervention improved depression and social isolation, although the relative improvement in the psychosocial-intervention group compared with the usual-care group was less than expected because of substantial improvement in usual-care patients.

Comment: Although treatment of depression in cardiovascular patients does not appear to affect disease progression, it does improve quality of life and should be given high therapeutic priority (see Table 3–1).

■ SUDDEN DEATH

The interaction of stress, anxiety, and depression with cardiac illness and sudden death is well recognized. Components of global type A behavior, such as hostility and competitiveness, seem to predispose certain individuals to coronary artery disease (Yoshimasu et al. 2002) and might even affect treatment response to medication (Rutledge et al. 1999). Yet pain does not necessarily accompany myocardial ischemia, prompting the term *silent ischemia.* Intervals of mental stress may silently induce cardiac events, often without the patient's awareness. For example, eight patients with known CAD were monitored for 4 hours and then subjected to both exercise and mental stress (Vassiliadis et al. 1998). Five had ischemic responses to exercise, with two of the five experiencing no chest pain. Mental stress produced transient episodes of left ventricular dysfunction in all patients, but these episodes were uniformly painless, occurred at low heart rates, and usually were accompanied by ST-segment changes. These data corroborate many previous studies that concluded that mental stress plays a major role in provoking silent ischemia.

There are practical implications of these findings. *Chest pain does not always occur* to alert cardiac patients that they are at physiological risk from their emotional states. What then is the best way to manage the anxiety that arises in certain forms of psychotherapy, given that its physiological signals may be silent? Clearly, chest pain is not reliably present as a warning to the patient that the material is—psychologically and physiologically—"too much."

Adding anxiolytic medication, biofeedback, or behavioral relaxation strategies may buffer some of the physiological impact of psychotherapy, allowing it to progress more safely in certain patients. As always, gauging the appropriate level of a psychological intervention is partly science, often art—largely a matter of clinical judgment regarding dosing, timing, and tact. When intense emotional content emerges, it must be thoughtfully managed relative to its potential cardiophysiological impact.

The Myocardial Infarction and Depression-Intervention Trial (MIND-IT) is under way in the Netherlands to investigate whether antidepressant treatment can improve the cardiac prognosis for patients with depressive disorder after MI (van den Brink et al. 2002). In the meantime, the International Consensus Group on Depression and Anxiety in General Medicine has made the recommendations summarized in Table 3–1.

■ DIAGNOSTIC AND MANAGEMENT DILEMMAS

Diagnosing Depression in the Medically Ill

Several problems complicate the accurate diagnosis of depression in medical patients:

- Overlap between psychological reactions to life-threatening illness and the onset of a depressive syndrome
- Misassumptions that depressive states are "normal" in response to medical illness
- Unreliability of vegetative symptoms (e.g., weight loss, fatigue, weakness, anorexia) in diagnosis
- Overlap with the effects of impaired cognitive functioning secondary to the medical illness itself

See Appendix 15 for suggestions about diagnosing depression in the medically ill.

Chest Pain: Panic Disorder or Angina?

Chest pain is one of the most frequent chief complaints at medical clinics, and the medical workup is often negative. As many as 25% of patients with chest

Table 3–1. Recommendations of the International Consensus Group on Depression and Anxiety in General Medicine

1. Depression and anxiety are risk factors for cardiovascular morbidity and mortality. They should be the focus of treatment intervention, in the same manner that other accepted risk factors, such as hypertension, elevated cholesterol, and obesity, are treated aggressively.

2. Screening of patients for depression and anxiety should take place routinely in primary care.

3. Treatment of depression with safe medication improves quality of life and may potentially improve cardiovascular risk profile (through behavioral change, lessening the physiological effect of stress, etc.)

4. There are well-controlled data to support the safety of treatment intervention with selective serotonin reuptake inhibitors (SSRIs) in the cardiovascular patient with concomitant depression and/or anxiety. Such treatment offers low risk and potentially high gain. SSRIs are the preferred medications for depression and anxiety comorbid with cardiovascular disease, on the basis of efficacy and cardiovascular safety data.

5. Treatment of depression with cognitive-behavioral therapy is potentially of great clinical and heuristic interest.

Source. Ballenger J, Davidson J, Lecrubier Y, et al.: "Consensus Statement on Depression, Anxiety, and Cardiovascular Disease." *Journal of Clinical Psychiatry* 62:24–27, 2001.

pain simulating coronary artery disease who come to hospital emergency departments are found to have panic disorder, with even higher rates among those who present for outpatient evaluation of their chest pain. A 2003 meta-analysis of studies published between 1970 and 2001 revealed five variables that correlated with higher rates of panic disorder among patients who presented with chest pain (Huffman and Pollack 2003): 1) absence of CAD , 2) atypical quality of chest pain, 3) female gender, 4) younger age, and 5) high level of self-reported anxiety.

There is a cohort of patients with coexisting panic disorder and coronary artery syndromes, but this group has not been studied extensively. Rates of panic disorder appear to be approximately four times greater in individuals with coronary artery disease than in the general population, but this statistic requires confirmation. It is difficult to conduct meaningful prevalence studies in patients with comorbid panic disorder and CAD, because chest pain may be due to an acute coronary syndrome, a panic attack, or both

(Huffman and Pollack 2003). The atypical presentations of MI in women—the population with the higher rates of panic disorder—may further complicate diagnosis (Mark 2000).

Pacemaker Syndrome or Panic Disorder?

There is considerable overlap between symptoms of the pacemaker syndrome and panic disorder (Peters et al. 1990). The pacemaker syndrome is in the differential diagnosis of panic-like symptoms occurring in pacemaker patients. Patients with this syndrome present with postural hypotension, dizziness, syncope, dyspnea, chest pain, neck pulsations, lassitude, and weakness (Ellenbogen et al. 1997; Lamas et al. 2002).

The symptoms of pacemaker syndrome are attributable to a loss of atrial contribution to ventricular systole; a vasodepressor reflex initiated by atrial contractions against a closed tricuspid valve; and systemic and pulmonary venous regurgitation due to atrial contraction against a closed atrioventricular (AV) valve. Sinus activity and atrial contraction occur at the same time as ventricular pacing and ventricular contraction, resulting in symptoms. Low cardiac output produces light-headedness, lethargy, hypotension, diaphoresis, apprehension, and palpitations. Treatment involves adjusting the programming of the pacemaker.

Correlation of the clinical symptoms with abnormal findings on Holter monitoring confirms the diagnosis of pacemaker syndrome.

Implantable Cardioverter-Defibrillators: "Things That Go Bang in the Night"

There is a growing literature on the adverse psychological effects of implantable cardioverter-defibrillators (ICDs) in patients who have malignant ventricular arrhythmias (Hamner et al. 1999). Reactions have included anxiety, depression, and severe sleep disorders, including phantom shocks that occur at night without evidence of ICD discharge. There have also been reports that the total number of ICD shocks can predict depressive symptoms in patients without a psychiatric history. Device failure involving full-power ICD discharges might lead to a full-blown anxiety disorder or panic attack (Goodman and Hess 1999).

A pilot study was published involving five ICD patients (ages 61–74 years) having frequent ICD shocks who had a diagnosis of comorbid panic disorder with agoraphobia and depression (Kuijpers et al. 2002). Patients were treated with a combination of a selective serotonin reuptake inhibitor (paroxetine 20 mg) and a behavior program (consisting of education on the nature of panic attacks, guidance on how to cope with them, and a counteraction avoidance behavior with gradual exposure). Four of five patients treated with combination therapy experienced no discharge of the ICD during a 6-month follow-up. The total number of ventricular premature beats decreased significantly after treatment. There was also clear psychiatric improvement.

Neuropsychiatric Effects of Cardiac Medications

As mentioned in Chapter 1 on delirium, almost any medication can induce mental status changes in a sufficiently vulnerable patient, especially in elderly persons. Medications used in the cardiovascular setting are notable offenders. For example, a previously stable dose may cause toxicity in the setting of medical illness, particularly for drugs with a narrow therapeutic index (e.g., digoxin).

Digoxin, especially, can produce neuropsychiatric side effects, even at therapeutic serum concentrations (Brunner et al. 2000). Neuropsychiatric symptoms, which may be the first sign of digoxin toxicity, include disorientation, confusion, delirium, and hallucinations ("digitalis delirium"). Visual disturbances include white borders or halos on dark objects ("white vision") and disturbances of color vision, commonly with yellow or green coloration of objects, or, less frequently, red, brown, and blue vision. It has been said that the painter Vincent van Gogh chewed on digitalis leaves, prompting the colorful visual effects so characteristic of his painting. Although of dubious value as art history, this anecdote is a good way to remember digoxin toxicity. Digoxin has also been associated with inducing depression-like states at therapeutic serum levels (Eisendrath and Sweeney 1987; Schleifer et al. 1991; Song et al. 2001).

Several factors make cardiac patients in the general hospital particularly vulnerable to delirium. Those factors are reviewed in Chapter 1, "The Delirious Patient."

■ NONPHARMACOLOGICAL MANAGEMENT OF DEPRESSION AND ANXIETY IN THE SETTING OF CARDIOVASCULAR DISEASE

Although this chapter concentrates on medication management, cardiac rehabilitation programs have

become the key to secondary prevention after myocardial events, reducing mortality and improving exercise tolerance, functional capacity, blood pressure, and symptoms of angina and dyspnea as well as psychosocial functioning (Wenger et al. 1995). Components of most rehabilitation programs include exercise training, risk factor modification, education, medical surveillance, vocational rehabilitation, and psychological counseling (McGee et al. 1999). Psychopathology and gender difference may affect how cardiac rehabilitation is utilized (Grace et al. 2002a, 2002b).

The cognitive-behavioral model for psychotherapy is the most thoroughly researched in this population and has become the standard. Cognitive-behavioral psychotherapy is highly effective in improving quality of life and reducing the frequency of subsequent coronary events.

Sometimes inadvertent reactions on the part of the medical practitioner and staff may provoke anxiety in the patient and interfere with appropriate management, as noted by Levenson (1993):

> Physicians old enough to be at risk for coronary disease will tend to identify with some of their cardiac patients. Although this could potentially enhance their ability to empathize with patients, it may lead them instead to distance themselves. If patients are very frightened by their heart disease, physicians may withdraw to avoid their own resonant anxiety. If patients are strong deniers, physicians unconsciously worried about their own mortality may collude in the denial, distancing themselves not only from the patients but from the disease as well. (p. 541)

Countertransference reactions to cardiac patients are not limited to older doctors (Levenson 1993):

> Younger physicians are more likely to err in the other direction. Enthusiastically launching an attack on risk factors, they may become almost messianic in their approach to the patient. Concerned over some patients' denial of illness, they may try to overcome their defenses directly. Benevolently, even feeling morally obligated to do so, the physician may attempt to "reason with" (i.e., scare) the patient by reciting a litany of disastrous consequences if the patient will not stop smoking, lose weight, and so on. This usually increases the patient's anxiety, in turn increasing the need to deny illness. Frustrated, the physician may then become angry, communicating (sometimes nonverbally) to the patient that the disease is self-induced, the result of an indulgent, undisciplined, and self-destructive lifestyle. (p. 542)

See also "The Seriously Ill Patient: Physician Factors in the Doctor-Patient Relationship," Chapter 15 in this volume.

■ ANXIOLYTICS

Patients must feel they can verbalize certain concerns without their doctors necessarily "jumping" to medicate them. Be sure to assess the patient's need for control; some will resist taking medications, particularly antianxiety medications, because they fear the drugs will make them feel "foggy" or "doped up." People have different, often anxious interpretations about the recommendation for anxiolytics. These reactions are not always dismissed by assurances that "the pill will make you feel better." When properly explained to the patient and the dosages carefully titrated, however, benzodiazepines improve comfort and could potentially reduce morbidity in coronary patients. Clinical benefits derive from their central anxiolytic effects as well as their ability to mute *physiological* responses to sympathetic arousal. Potential complications include habituation, tolerance, respiratory depression, and oversedation.

Buspirone (BuSpar) is a nonbenzodiazepine anxiolytic that avoids the complications of benzodiazepine use. It has no anticholinergic or α-adrenergic properties. Delayed onset of action is a problem with buspirone. One strategy is to start it simultaneously with a benzodiazepine or a sedating neuroleptic and then taper the other agent after buspirone begins to have an effect (Halperin 2002).

Note that alprazolam (Xanax) is popularly prescribed by internists. However, episodes of hypomania and mania have been reported in association with the use of alprazolam in patients with depression (Pharmacia & Upjohn Company, 2001). Dependence and withdrawal reactions, including seizures, also have been problems reported with alprazolam.

■ ANTIDEPRESSANTS

The list of available antidepressant medications keeps growing. Table 3–2 summarizes some considerations regarding use of commonly available antidepressants in patients with cardiovascular disease. A detailed discussion follows.

Selective Serotonin Reuptake Inhibitors (SSRIs)

The growing literature on major depressive disorder and cardiovascular morbidity clearly shows that depression is bad for cardiovascular health. SSRIs have become the first-line agents in treatment of depressed cardiac patients.

The SADHART Study

The 2002 publication of the Sertraline Antidepressant Heart Attack Randomized Trial (SADHART) (Carney and Jaffe 2002; Glassman et al. 2002; Shapiro et al. 1999) justified the rationale for what has become clinical practice since the release of fluoxetine (Prozac) in 1988.

The SADHART study was a randomized, double-blind, placebo-controlled trial conducted in 40 outpatient cardiology centers and psychiatry clinics in the United States, Europe, Canada, and Australia. Enrollment began in April 1997 and follow-up ended in April 2001. A total of 369 patients with major depressive disorder were randomly assigned to receive sertraline (Zoloft) or placebo. The investigators concluded that sertraline is a safe and effective treatment for recurrent depression in patients with recent MI or unstable angina when there are no other life-threatening medical conditions. Compared with placebo, sertraline had no statistically significant effects on any of the following measures: mean left ventricular ejection fraction, treatment-emergent ventricular premature complex runs, and QTc interval prolongation greater than 450 milliseconds at end point. The incidence of severe cardiovascular adverse events was 14.5% with sertraline and 22.4% with placebo. Limitations of the study included the following: 1) treatment was initiated an average of 34 days following acute MI; the safety of the drug in the early post-MI period remains unclear; 2) patients who received sertraline were carefully screened; individuals were excluded from this trial if they had a second medical condition that was deemed too risky or if alcohol dependence, drug abuse, or schizophrenia was present; 3) the sample size was not large enough to permit identification of rare adverse events or drug-drug interactions; and 4) sertraline was the only SSRI antidepressant agent tested in this trial.

When Is It Safe to Intervene Post-MI With an Antidepressant?

It is not possible based on current knowledge to answer the question of how long to wait post-MI before starting an SSRI. In the past, 6 weeks (the approximate healing time for myocardial tissue) was considered a reasonable interval before starting the cardioactive tricyclic antidepressants after uncomplicated MI (Stoudemire and Fogel 1987). Although waiting 6 weeks to begin an SSRI seems unnecessary, be alert to the risks of adding more medications soon after MI. Risk factors include further ischemic events, heart block,

Table 3–2.   Choosing antidepressants in patients with cardiovascular disease

Medication	Notes
SSRIs	Post-MI: sertraline safe. All SSRIs interact with warfarin and disrupt anticoagulation regimens. Rare but potential side effects: bradycardia, syncope, atrial fibrillation. Caution in patients with sick sinus syndrome and new-onset atrial fibrillation.
Bupropion (Wellbutrin, Zyban)	Post-MI: no data. Data: safe in patients with CV disease. Monitor BP in hypertensive patients.
Venlafaxine (Effexor)	2nd-line medication in CV disease because of dose-related effects on heart rate and diastolic BP, particularly at doses > 300 mg/day.
Mirtazapine (Remeron)	Post-MI: data pending. Potential side effects: ↑ weight, ↑ appetite, ↑ serum cholesterol. Orthostatic hypotension infrequent.
Psychostimulants	Clinically significant adverse CV effects: relatively uncommon with low doses, careful titration. Dose-related side effects: tremor, activation, anxiety, headache, nausea. Relative contraindications: substance abuse history, vulnerability to psychosis. Use with caution: history of ventricular tachycardia, recent MI, uncontrolled congestive heart failure, hypertension, or tachycardia. Absolute contraindications: glaucoma, motor tics, Tourette's syndrome, MAOI ingestion within past 14 days. *Sample Regimen:* (Assuming that vital signs are not adversely affected, push until there are demonstrable effects, i.e., improved mood or irritability.) Day 1: 2.5 mg methylphenidate (bid, before breakfast and after lunch, but not later than 3:00 P.M., to minimize insomnia); monitor vital signs over 4 hours. Days 2–4: If initial dose tolerated but with no response, successively increase the medication over the next 2–3 days (e.g., by 2.5 mg at each dose), monitoring vital signs:
Nefazodone (Serzone)	No significant CV effects in healthy subjects. Black box warning about hepatotoxicity.

Note.   BP = blood pressure; CV = cardiovascular; MAOI = monoamine oxidase inhibitor; MI = myocardial infarction; SSRI = selective serotonin reuptake inhibitor.

unstable congestive heart failure, and orthostatic hypotension. Huffman et al. (2004) anecdotally reported prescribing SSRIs in post-MI patients earlier than 1 month after the MI. However, for most patients who become depressed post-MI, they recommended a more conservative approach: follow-up with a psychiatrist or primary care physician within 2 to 3 weeks; if the patient remains depressed, begin sertraline or another antidepressant. Earlier prescription of antidepressants in the hospital (in coordination with cardiology) is recommended in the following circumstances (Huffman et al. 2004):

- Depression with suicidal ideation
- Development of depressive symptoms during hospitalization in a patient with a history of severe depression
- Severe depression that inhibits participation in rehabilitation or self-care

Roose has warned that in the context of sinus node disease, SSRIs in combination with β-blockers may predispose to arrhythmias (S. Roose, personal communication, September 2002).

The decision to start an antidepressant should be a psychiatric one. However, the post-MI timing for antidepressants is best decided in collaboration with a cardiologist.

Do All SSRIs Behave Like Post-MI Sertraline?

The SADHART study demonstrated that sertraline was safe in a specific, medically cleared population of patients who had recovered for at least 30 days after MI. Do all SSRIs behave similarly? Certainly, SSRI-associated cardiovascular problems occur rarely. Nonetheless, there do seem to be subtle differences among the SSRIs, both in their drug-drug interactions and in their overdose data. For example, whereas isolated case reports of bradycardia and presyncope are scattered throughout the SSRI literature, the unique occurrence of SSRI-associated QTc interval prolongation was reported in a case of an overdose of citalopram (trade name: Celexa) of approximately 400 mg in a healthy 21-year-old woman (Catalano et al. 2001). Although one case does not make a trend, it does raise concerns that "all SSRIs are not created equal." Clinicians should remain vigilant about using new medications in medically ill patients until enough experience has accumulated.

A quick review of the SSRIs and drug-drug interactions follows.

SSRIs, Cytochromes, and Secondary Cardiovascular Toxicity

Although the SSRIs themselves have favorable cardiovascular profiles, their impact on the oxidative metabolism of other medications is not always as trouble free. Two cytochrome P450 subgroups, 2D6 and 3A4, may be inhibited by medications commonly used in both psychiatric and medical practice. Many SSRIs are inhibitors of cytochrome 2D6 and may produce important drug-drug interactions. (SSRIs are much weaker inhibitors of 3A4.) *The Drug Interaction Casebook: The Cytochrome P450 System and Beyond* (Sandson 2003) is a practical review of this complicated topic. We also recommend *Concise Guide to Drug Interaction Principles for Medical Practice: Cytochrome P450s, UGTs, P-Glycoproteins* (Cozza et al. 2003).

Useful Web sites for help with P450 interactions are http://www.Drug-Interactions.com and http://www.mhc.com/Cytochromes (accessed June 2004). See also Table 3–3 for a list cardiac drug–psychotropic drug interactions.

SSRIs and Warfarin (Coumadin)

SSRIs disrupt anticoagulant control when they are added to previously stable regimens of warfarin. Warfarin is primarily metabolized by the 2C9 isoenzyme, with contributions from 2C19, 2C8, 2C18, 1A2, and 3A4 (Cozza et al. 2003). Protein-binding and vitamin K interrelationships further complicate warfarin metabolism. Warfarin's narrow therapeutic window makes monitoring drug-drug interactions particularly important. *Nearly every psychotropic drug interacts with warfarin* (Cozza et al. 2003), including the SSRIs. It is necessary to monitor anticoagulation (prothrombin time and international normalized ratio) for patients receiving an SSRI on warfarin.

Miscellaneous Agents

Bupropion (Wellbutrin, Zyban)

Bupropion is a norepinephrine and dopamine reuptake inhibitor. It has no significant effect on serotonin reuptake or on histaminergic, muscarinic, α-adrenergic, serotonergic, or dopaminergic receptors. Since its release in the 1980s, bupropion has kept its favorable cardiovascular side effect profile, characterized by low incidence of clinically significant changes in blood pressure, heart rate, and cardiac conduction (Belson et al. 2002). The most clinically relevant side effect has been hypertension, in some cases severe and requiring acute treatment. Hypertension occurs in patients with and without evidence of preexisting hypertension, receiving bupropion alone or in combination with nicotine replacement therapy for smoking cessation treatment.

Table 3–3. A short list of cardiac drug–psychotropic drug interactions

Psychotropic drug	Interacts with cardiac drug
Most psychotropics	Warfarin (Coumadin)
Buspirone (BuSpar)	Diltiazem (Cardizem)
Desipramine (Norpramin)	ACE inhibitors: captopril (Capoten), enalapril (Vasotec), ramipril (Altace), etc.
Fluoxetine (Prozac)	Carvedilol (Coreg), digoxin, nifedipine (Procardia), propafenone (Rythmol)
Fluvoxamine (Luvox)	Quinidine, metoprolol (Lopressor), propranolol (Inderal)
Lithium	Amiloride (Midamor)
Nefazodone (Serzone)	Atorvastatin (Lipitor), lovastatin (Mevacor, Altocor), pravastatin (Pravachol)
Paroxetine (Paxil)	Flecainide (Tambocor)
Psychostimulants (methylphenidate [Ritalin], dextroamphetamine [Dexedrine])	Warfarin (Coumadin), pressor agents such as clonidine (Catapres), adrenergic blockers such as doxazosin (Cardura), terazosin (Hytrin), prazosin (Minipress)

Source. Adapted from Strain JJ, Karim A, Caliendo G, et al: "Cardiac Drug–Psychotropic Drug Update." *General Hospital Psychiatry* 24:283–289, 2002.

Two studies specifically addressed the use of bupropion in patients with cardiovascular disease (Roose et al. 1987, 1991). Bupropion had no significant effects on ejection fraction in patients with left ventricular dysfunction. Although bupropion was associated with a rise in supine blood pressure, it did not significantly affect cardiac conduction and only rarely was associated with clinically significant blood pressure changes.

Bupropion appears to be cardiovascularly safe in overdose. Seizures—not CNS depression—complicate bupropion overdose. There is no clinical experience establishing the safety of bupropion in patients with a recent history of MI or unstable heart disease.

There is a small risk for treatment-emergent hypertensive events with the immediate-release (IR) formulation. Wellbutrin SR sustained-release tablets pose less risk for this side effect.

Venlafaxine (Effexor)

Venlafaxine inhibits the reuptake of both serotonin and norepinephrine and is a weak inhibitor of dopamine reuptake. It has no significant affinity for muscarinic, histaminergic, or adrenergic receptors in vitro.

Venlafaxine is associated with dose-related sustained increases in blood pressure in some patients (Bahk et al. 2001). A meta-analysis of blood pressure data from the premarketing trials of 3,744 patients concluded that venlafaxine does not appear to have adverse effects on the control of blood pressure for patients with preexisting hypertension or elevated pretreatment supine diastolic blood pressure (Thase 1998). There are no data to suggest that concurrent administration of an antihypertensive agent adds additional or special risks for patients taking venlafaxine.

Recommendations: 1) regularly monitor blood pressure of patients receiving venlafaxine, particularly at doses of 300 mg/day; 2) consider dose reduction or treatment discontinuation for patients experiencing sustained increase in blood pressure.

In medically healthy patients, the incidence of treatment-emergent conduction abnormalities (including QTc) with venlafaxine does not differ from that with placebo. No specific data in patients with recent history of MI or unstable heart disease exist at this time. However, because of venlafaxine's dose-related effects on heart rate, the manufacturer recommends caution in vulnerable patients (e.g., patients with hyperthyroidism, heart failure, or recent MI.)

Mirtazapine (Remeron)

Mirtazapine affects central presynaptic α_2-adrenergic autoreceptors and increases norepinephrine and serotonin activity. Antihistaminic side effects (drowsiness, sedation, and dry mouth), increased appetite, and weight gain occur with mirtazapine, but no significant changes in blood pressure or pulse usually occur. There is one study (Smulevich et al. 2001) on the use of mirtazapine in patients with comorbid ischemic heart disease. In 34 patients who completed the study receiving 30 mg/day of mirtazapine, no clinically significant electrocardiographic changes occurred at the end of 6 weeks. Blood pressure also remained stable. Case reports of overdose with mirtazapine have shown minimal cardiovascular toxicity (Velazquez et al. 2001). Currently, the Myocardial Infarction and Depression-Intervention Trial (MIND-IT) is under way in the Netherlands to investigate whether antidepressant treatment can improve the cardiac prognosis for patients with depressive disorder after myocardial infarction (van den Brink et al. 2002). First-choice treatment consists of placebo-controlled treatment with mirtazapine. One of the study objectives will be to evaluate the effectiveness, tolerability, and safety of mirtazapine in this population.

An advantage for patients who cannot ingest anything by mouth is the Remeron SolTab, which is an orally disintegrating tablet.

Nefazodone (Serzone)

Nefazodone both inhibits serotonin reuptake and antagonizes serotonin 5-HT$_2$ receptors. It does produce clinically significant fatigue, dizziness, blurred vision, and lightheadedness. It does not appear to affect the electrocardiogram (ECG). Nefazodone should be used only as a second-line agent in the medically ill because of the black box warning about unpredictable, potentially fatal liver failure.

Trazodone (Desyrel)

Trazodone is a triazolopyridine derivative. Although originally marketed as the antidepressant Desyrel, trazodone is still widely used as a hypnotic. It has few, if any, anticholinergic effects and thus does not increase heart rate. However, in doses required for an antidepressant effect (above 200 mg), there have been problems with conduction abnormalities, ventricular arrhythmias, and orthostatic hypotension. Priapism is a rare but serious side effect of trazodone in males.

Psychostimulants

The psychostimulants have been used since the pre-SSRI era for treating depressed medically ill patients when anorexia, apathy, and profound hopelessness interfere with medical management. Sometimes the wait required for conventional antidepressants to take effect is too long; the depressed medical patient who is languishing—refusing to eat, drink, or cooperate with tests or rehabilitation—needs an antidepressant effect, quickly (Pereira and Bruera 2001). In these situations, psychostimulants are invaluable. They are safe, usually well tolerated, short-acting, and quick to work. Short-term use of stimulants improves energy and appetite for medically ill individuals with anergic depressions, particularly during the wait for conventional antidepressants to "kick in." There is now an extensive literature on their use in medical and surgical inpatients, including persons living with HIV, stroke patients, the terminally ill, cancer patients, elderly persons, and those in chronic care facilities. Even in the setting of cardiovascular disease, the psychostimulant methylphenidate (Ritalin) was safely used in the pre-SSRI era when it was slowly, carefully titrated.

Indications and Contraindications

Little clinical debate remains regarding the appropriateness of psychostimulants as a short-term strategy for treating depression in the medically ill. There is no U.S. Food and Drug Administration (FDA) approval, however, for using these medicines as antidepressants. Clinically, psychostimulants are used to obtain a rapid antidepressant response for the medically ill with the following guidelines (Huffman et al. 2004):

- To improve energy (particularly if anergia is negatively affecting rehabilitation)
- To improve appetite (if patient demonstrates minimal oral intake)
- To improve cognition (particularly if cognitive impairment is affecting the patient's capacity to participate in medical decisions)

Relative contraindications call for caution in prescribing of psychostimulants. Some authors consider a history of ventricular tachycardia, recent MI, uncontrolled congestive heart failure, hypertension, or tachycardia to be a relative contraindication to psychostimulants (Huffman et al. 2004). However, these conditions are not absolute contraindications for the use of methylphenidate (Ritalin) (product information, Novartis Pharmaceuticals, January 2001).

Other relative contraindications include:

- A history of substance abuse
- A previous history of an acute psychotic illness

Absolute contraindications include:

- Diagnosis of glaucoma
- Diagnosis of motor tics
- A personal or family history of Tourette's syndrome
- Concurrent ingestion of monoamine oxidase inhibitors (MAOIs), or within 14 days following discontinuation of MAOIs
- For dextroamphetamine (Dexedrine): advanced arteriosclerosis, symptomatic cardiovascular disease, moderate to severe hypertension, hyperthyroidism (product information, GlaxoSmithKline, January 2002).

Formulations and Dosage

Several forms of psychostimulants are currently available, but not all have been tested in medically fragile individuals. Long-acting preparations may interfere with sleep, so they should be used judiciously. Table 3–4 shows dosing guidelines for various agents.

The following detailed instructions were taken from a 1991 chapter by Ned Cassem, who had extensive experience with using psychostimulants in cardiovascular patients before SSRIs became available.

1. The starting dose in fragile cardiovascular patients is 2.5 mg of either dextroamphetamine (given once before breakfast) or methylphenidate (given twice a day, usually before breakfast and after lunch, but usually not later than 3:00 P.M., in order not to produce insomnia), with careful monitoring of vital signs over the next 4 hours. (Stimulants can produce sinus tachycardia.)
2. If the patient has tolerated the initial dose without problems but also without demonstrable response, slowly increase the dose over the next 2 or 3 days, monitoring vital signs.
3. Assuming that vital signs are not adversely affected, push the medication over the course of several days until there are demonstrable effects: either improved mood or irritability.
4. Do not abandon the trial before the patient has experienced some medication-related response.
5. Persistent insomnia and only partial resolution of depressive symptoms on an adequate trial of psychostimulants are indications for trying another antidepressant.

Table 3–4.   Currently available psychostimulants

| | | Dose ranges (mg) (reduce if medically ill) | | |
| | | Starting | Maintenance | |
Generic name	Trade name	Starting	Maintenance	Half-life (hours)
Dextroamphetamine	Dexedrine	5–10	5–30	8–12
	Adderall[a]	5–10	5–10	8–12
Methylphenidate				
Immediate release	Ritalin	5–10	5–60	1–3[b]
Sustained release[c]	Ritalin-SR[c]	20	20–60	4–5[b]
Extended release[c]	Concerta[c]	18	18–54	3.5[b]
Modafinil	Provigil	100–200	100–400	15
Pemoline	Cylert	2nd-line medication, due to unpredictable hepatotoxicity		

[a]A combination of two amphetamines and two dextroamphetamine compounds.
[b]Represents plasma half-life; concentrations in the brain exceed those of plasma.
[c]Consider shorter-acting form in medically fragile patients.
Source.   Adapted from Fait ML, Wise MG, Jachna JS, et al.: "Psychopharmacology," in *The American Psychiatric Publishing Textbook of Consultation-Liaison Psychiatry: Psychiatry In the Medically Ill,* 2nd Edition. Edited by Wise MG, Rundell JR. Washington, DC, American Psychiatric Publishing, 2002, p. 956. Used with permission.

Side Effects and Drug-Drug Interactions

Side effects of psychostimulants are dose related. Possible CNS side effects include tremor, activation, a feeling of anxiety, and headache. These side effects may worsen or precipitate delirium in vulnerable patients. Gastrointestinal effects may include nausea. Adverse effects on heart rate, blood pressure, and appetite are rare with low-dose, carefully titrated psychostimulants. Although tolerance and abuse are potential complications, they are rare in medical patients and may be minimized by carefully selecting patients without substance abuse histories or vulnerability to psychosis.

Note that the psychostimulants are also used to potentiate the SSRIs. Other important drug interactions are with antihypertensives, vasopressors, and warfarin. Psychostimulants are contraindicated with MAOIs.

Tricyclic Antidepressants and Monoamine Oxidase Inhibitors

Before the 1988 introduction of fluoxetine, clinicians debated whether to choose a tricyclic antidepressant (TCA) or a monoamine oxidase inhibitor (MAOI) for a depressed cardiovascular patient, or to "do nothing" because it seemed safer. Rare was the medical patient who accepted electroconvulsive therapy (ECT) as a credible option. Today, the cardiovascular safety and efficacy of the SSRIs and bupropion offer clinical advantages. Tricyclics and MAOIs are unwieldy, requiring careful titration, monitoring drug-drug and drug-

food interactions, blood levels, serial ECGs, and blood pressure determinations.

TCAs and MAOIs have retained their place in contemporary psychopharmacology because some depressions respond only to these agents. In addition, the TCAs maintain a role in treating other conditions, such as panic disorder, attention deficit disorder, headache, pain, and obsessive-compulsive disorder. MAOIs are still used for "atypical depressions," characterized by rejection sensitivity, anxiety, hypersomnia, and increased appetite.

Table 3–5 summarizes the cardiovascular side effects of TCAs and MAOIs.

Electroconvulsive Therapy

The autonomic changes associated with seizure activity, such as transient tachycardia and blood pressure changes (which vary in type over the course of the seizure) are the primary risks of ECT for patients with cardiovascular disease. Cardiac arrhythmias are most likely to occur during the seizure, when the sympathetic reaction predominates, predisposing to tachycardia-related cardiac ischemia. The adverse impact of an induced seizure on preexisting cardiac arrhythmias can be minimized with adequate precautions.

ECT affects the cardiovascular system in two physiological phases (Guttmacher and Goldstein 1988):

1. *Parasympathetic phase:* Marked parasympathetic discharge produces increased vagal tone, resulting

Table 3–5. Summary of cardiovascular side effects of tricyclic antidepressants (TCAs) and monoamine oxidase inhibitors (MAOIs)

	Disadvantage	Screen for	Remedy
TCAs			
Conduction	Prolongs QTc interval	QTc>440 ms	OK to use in setting of bundle branch block if patient has a pacemaker; if no pacemaker, use a selective serotinin reuptake inhibitor (SSRI) or bupropion (Wellbutrin, Zyban).
Rate	Produces sinus tachycardia, which can increase myocardial demand	Baseline pulse	If careful monitoring is available or if patient has a pacemaker, OK to use. If not, use an SSRI or bupropion.
Rhythm	Can potentiate quinidine-like antiarrhythmic medications	Use of quinidine-like antiarrhythmics	Use an SSRI or bupropion.
Blood pressure	Produces orthostatic hypotension, especially in the setting of congestive heart failure	Preexisting baseline hypotension, even if patient is clinically asymptomatic	Nortriptyline (Pamelor, Aventyl) is the TCA least likely to produce this side effect.
Other	Anticholinergic side effects (dry mouth, ileus, constipation, bowel/bladder dysfunction)		
MAOIs			
Conduction	None		
Rate	None		
Rhythm	None		
Blood pressure	Most common effect: severe orthostatic hypotension; less frequently: hypertensive crisis in the presence of dietary tyramine	Baseline blood pressure, even if patient is clinically asymptomatic; regular blood pressure monitoring while on medications; careful check of drug-drug interactions	Warn about how to counter orthostatic symptoms (dangle feet, rise slowly, etc.) and how to recognize hypertensive symptoms (throbbing headache with palpitations, sweating, nausea, vomiting). Give printed instructions on low-tyramine diet and over-the-counter medications to avoid.
Other	No anticholinergic side effects		

in profound bradycardia in healthy subjects. Patients with cardiovascular disease are at risk for developing sinus arrest or conduction disturbances during this phase, although the routine use of anticholinergic agents has prevented cardiovascular complications caused by parasympathetic discharge.

2. *Sympathetic phase:* The phase of parasympathetic discharge is followed by one dominated by sympathetic discharge during the seizure. This phase is associated with hypertension, tachycardia, and, frequently, ventricular and other arrhythmias. Patients with all types of cardiovascular diseases are at risk during this period.

Appendix 14 lists the practice guidelines of the American Psychiatric Association for the use of ECT in medical illness.

■ ANTIPSYCHOTICS

We will briefly review some of the issues that are pertinent to prescribing antipsychotics in patients with cardiovascular disease. More extensive reviews have been published (Glassman 2002; Goodnick et al. 2002; Piepho 2002). Suggestions for managing cardiovascular risk in patients receiving antipsychotics are summarized in Table 3–6.

Cardiovascular Risk Factors

Alpha-1-Adrenergic Blockade

Alpha-1-adrenergic blockade results in the following clinical problems:

- Orthostatic hypotension
- Dizziness (both secondary to and independent of orthostatic hypotension)
- Increased cardiac workload stemming from drops in blood pressure, producing anginal episodes in susceptible patients
- Increased rate of injury from falls secondary to dizziness

These side effects are most prominent with the phenothiazines, such as chlorpromazine (Thorazine), which patients with cardiovascular disorders should avoid. Haloperidol (Haldol) largely bypasses problems with α_1-adrenergic blockade. Atypical antipsychotics, which are more likely to produce these problems early in treatment (Piepho 2002; Stanniland and Taylor 2000), as a class are safe and effective in patients with medical illness, particularly in elderly persons. Clozapine (Clozaril) is an exception; it should be used with caution because of its dual impact on blood pressure and dizziness, along with dose-related changes in the QTc interval, increased risk of myocarditis, and bone marrow suppression.

Table 3–6. Suggestions for managing cardiovascular risk in patients on antipsychotics

1. Ask whether anyone in the patient's family has ever suddenly died or been subject to syncope (sudden episodes of unconsciousness, sometimes symptomatic of TDP and long QT syndrome).
2. Obtain personal or family history of cardiovascular disease, diabetes, hypertension, syncope, or sudden death.
3. Obtain baseline electrocardiogram for older patients or those with cardiovascular risk factors.
4. Obtain baseline fasting plasma glucose levels, glycated hemoglobin (HbA1c), and fasting lipid profile with all antipsychotics. Perform follow-up monitoring every 6 months. Obtain fasting insulin assessment in at-risk patients. (These are slightly different recommendations made by a consensus conference; see p. 62.)
5. Check baseline weight, with regular follow-up with all antipsychotics.
6. Monitor drug-drug interactions that slow conduction and heighten TDP risk, particularly in females (Roe et al. 2003).
7. If the potential therapeutic efficacy of a drug overrides potential cardiovascular or metabolic concerns, carefully document risk-benefit considerations.

Specific antipsychotics:

1. Consider alternatives to ziprasidone in any patient with QTc > 450 ms, significant cardiovascular disease, or family history of long QT syndrome (unless there is a compelling reason to use ziprasidone, such as treatment failure with other drugs).
2. Consider alternatives to olanzapine and clozapine if a patient already has cardiovascular risk factors, such as weight gain, diabetes, or an unfavorable lipid profile.

Note.   TDP = torsades de pointes.
Source.   Adapted from data in Czobor et al. 2003 and Glassman 2002.

QT Prolongation

Quick review: There are two parts to the electrical action of the heart: *depolarization,* occurring before the peak of the cardiac wave that produces the contraction of the myocardium, and *repolarization,* the recharging of the heart for the next beat, during which the heart muscle relaxes. The *QT interval* is the time during which the electrical system in the heart repolarizes. This interval is "corrected" according to a formula (the Bazett formula) that accounts for the heart rate, to produce the rate-corrected QT interval (QTc). A long QTc interval can be congenital or drug induced (the latter type is termed *acquired long QT syndrome*). A prolonged QTc identifies those patients at risk for potentially fatal arrhythmias, particularly torsades de pointes (TDP; "twisting of points," a 180-degree rotation of the axis of ectopic beats). TDP may degenerate into ventricular fibrillation and sudden death. Appendix 11 lists risk factors for TDP.

- In general, a QTc of 440 ms is considered the average upper limit of normal.
- An interval of 500 ms or more is a signal to change the treatment method (Glassman 2002).

In 1994, a gene that codes for a cardiac ion channel subunit with the unlikely name *Human Ether-a-Go-Go–related gene,* or *HERG,* was found to be responsible for congenital long QT syndrome. This finding supported the notion that pharmacological inhibition of cardiac potassium channels was a possible mechanism for acquired long QT syndrome. One review has summarized this data particularly well (Witchel et al. 2003).

The importance of acquired long QT syndrome as a side effect was highlighted during the approval process of ziprasidone (Geodon), which prolongs the QT interval. The FDA requested that the manufacturer compare the impact of ziprasidone on QTc with that of the other antipsychotics. "Study 054" compared ziprasidone, haloperidol (Haldol), quetiapine (Seroquel), risperidone (Risperdal), olanzapine (Zyprexa), and thioridazine (Mellaril) (Pfizer Inc 2000). The study subjects were young males with schizophrenia who had baseline QTc intervals in the normal range. ECGs were taken at baseline and at the highest tolerated dose of each drug, with and without the addition of a metabolic inhibitor. A summary of relevant findings follows.

Thioridazine and mesoridazine. Thioridazine produced the greatest mean change in QTc, maintaining its long distinction as the most cardiotoxic of the antipsychotics and finally earning its FDA black box warning. Since the 1960s, there have been cautionary reports about thioridazine and its chemical cousin mesoridazine because of their association with TDP and sudden death. Neither medication is a wise choice for medically ill patients, particularly those with cardiovascular illness, given the availability of safer alternatives.

Ziprasidone. Ziprasidone also caused QTc prolongation, particularly under conditions of metabolic inhibition. About 13% of patients on ziprasidone (compared with 20% of patients on thioridazine) experienced QTc prolongation of greater than 60 ms, which is considered a threshold for ventricular arrhythmias. Its performance in Study 054 placed it between thioridazine (highest risk) and the other antipsychotics (lower risk: quetiapine, risperidone, olanzapine, haloperidol).

Other antipsychotics. Other antipsychotics also produced changes in the baseline QTc, including the "gold standard" antipsychotic, haloperidol. However, these changes were well below those of thioridazine and ziprasidone. Of the low-risk group, only patients on *quetiapine* (15%) had a QTc prolongation of greater than 60 ms under conditions of metabolic inhibition. Quetiapine-induced prolongation of the QTc interval is clinically relevant mainly in overdose.

Since the Pfizer study was published, several reviews have sounded the alarm that *most* antipsychotics carry some risk of QTc prolongation and sudden death (Taylor 2003; Witchel et al. 2003).

Hyperglycemia and Hypercholesterolemia

Atypical antipsychotics have been associated with hyperglycemia and hypercholesterolemia in several case reports and uncontrolled studies. In the first prospective, randomized trial, clozapine, olanzapine, and haloperidol were associated with an increase in plasma glucose levels, while clozapine and olanzapine were associated with an increase in cholesterol levels (Czobor et al. 2003). The mean changes in glucose and cholesterol levels remained within clinically normal ranges, but approximately 14% of the patients (six given clozapine, four given olanzapine, three given risperidone, and one given haloperidol) developed abnormally high glucose levels (>125 mg/dL) during the course of their study treatment. Changes in glucose levels were independent of weight increases in this study, despite significant weight gain (highest for olanzapine, followed by clozapine and risperidone.) In the small subset of patients who had preexisting diabetes ($n=7$), no adverse effect on glucose metabolism occurred with antipsychotic treatment.

Chlorpromazine and thioridazine are the conventional neuroleptics most closely associated with diabetes mellitus (DM), although less so than olanzapine and clozapine. Haloperidol has been reported to increase insulin resistance, producing higher fasting glucose levels in schizophrenic patients as well as obese women.

The American Diabetes Association, American Psychiatric Association, American Association of Clinical Endocrinologists, and North American Association for the Study of Obesity convened a consensus development conference in 2003 regarding antipsychotic drugs and diabetes (American Diabetes Association et al. 2004). The panel found that different antipsychotic agents vary in their association with weight gain, risk of diabetes mellitus, and worsening lipid profile:

- Clozapine and olanzapine are associated with the most weight gain, highest risk for DM, and greatest propensity to worsen lipid profiles.
- Risperidone and quetiapine are associated with weight gain; they have discrepant results on their risk of DM, and a negative impact on lipid profiles.
- Aripiprazole and ziprasidone are associated with minimal to no weight gain, and no increased risk of DM or worsening lipid profiles.

The panel has issued a consensus statement regarding the monitoring of patients receiving antipsychotic pharmacotherapy. The following should be documented and assessed:

- Personal history of obesity, diabetes mellitus, dyslipidemia, hypertension, cardiovascular disease (at baseline)
- Family history of obesity, diabetes mellitus, dyslipidemia, hypertension, cardiovascular disease (at baseline)
- Weight and height for body mass index calculation (at baseline; every 4 weeks for the first 12 weeks; then quarterly for the duration of treatment)
- Waist circumference (at baseline; then annually for the duration of treatment)
- Blood pressure (at baseline; after the first 12 weeks; then annually for the duration of treatment)
- Fasting plasma glucose (at baseline; after the first 12 weeks; then annually for the duration of treatment)
- Fasting lipid profile (at baseline; after the first 12 weeks; then every 5 years for the duration of treatment)

Clinicians should also be alert to the development of diabetic ketoacidosis (see Worksheet, Appendix 18), which includes rapid onset of the following symptoms:

- Polyuria, polydipsia
- Weight loss
- Nausea, vomiting
- Dehydration
- Rapid respiration
- Clouding of sensorium

Specific Agents

Clozapine (Clozaril)

Clozapine presents potential problems for medically ill patients because of the risk of significant bone marrow suppression, particularly of granulocytes, requiring weekly complete blood counts. Dose-related cardiovascular side effects include tachycardia and orthostatic hypotension, probably secondary to clozapine's anticholinergic effects (Gupta et al. 2001). ECG abnormalities (nonspecific ST-segment and T-wave changes) are common but usually benign (Kang et al. 2000). Of more concern are the dose-related changes in the QTc interval (Kang et al. 2000). Clozapine has been associated with increasing plasma glucose and cholesterol levels in a prospective controlled study (Czobor et al. 2003). In addition, it carries a 1,000- to 2,000-fold increased risk of fatal and nonfatal myocarditis and cardiomyopathy (Phan and Taylor 2002; Wooltorton 2002). Myocarditis is accompanied by eosinophilia, indicating a possible immunoglobulin E–mediated hypersensitivity reaction. A Web site providing more information on the cardiovascular complications of clozapine is at http://www.hc-sc.gc.ca/hpfb-dgpsa/tpd-dpt/clozaril_pa_e.html (accessed June 2004).

Risperidone (Risperdal)

Although it has not been extensively studied in medical patients, the side effect profile of risperidone is generally favorable. Occasional orthostatic hypotension occurs with risperidone at the beginning of treatment, accompanied by dizziness and tachycardia. These side effects may be problematic for medically fragile patients, particularly those with cardiovascular problems. There have been occasional reports of syncope due to risperidone's α_1-receptor–blocking properties. Risperidone does not appear to prolong the QTc interval when administered at usual clinical doses. Risperidone did not increase plasma glucose or cholesterol levels in a prospective controlled study (Czobor et al. 2003).

Olanzapine (Zyprexa)

Orthostatic hypotension sometimes occurs early in treatment with olanzapine. However, olanzapine does not appear to differ from placebo with regard to cardiovascular events. In Study 054, olanzapine did not significantly prolong the QTc interval in medically healthy schizophrenia patients (Pfizer Inc 2000). Consider alternatives to olanzapine for patients with other cardiovascular risk factors, such as diabetes, overweight, or hypercholesterolemia, because olanzapine has been associated with increasing plasma glucose and cholesterol levels in a prospective controlled study (Czobor et al. 2003) (see previous section).

Quetiapine (Seroquel)

Orthostatic hypotension associated with dizziness, tachycardia, and syncope may appear during the initial dose-titration period, probably reflecting quetiapine's α_1-adrenergic antagonist properties. Limiting the initial dose to 25 mg bid minimizes the risk of orthostatic hypotension. In Study 054, 15% of patients on quetiapine had a QTc prolongation of greater than 60 ms under conditions of metabolic inhibition (Pfizer Inc 2000). Quetiapine-induced prolongation of the QTc interval is clinically relevant mainly in overdose. This medication has the advantage of producing few anticholinergic side effects.

Ziprasidone (Geodon)

Ziprasidone has a tendency to prolong QTc in a dose-related fashion, as noted in the preceding section (Pfizer Inc 2000), and it induces orthostatic hypotension associated with dizziness, tachycardia, and syncope (mechanism: α_1 antagonism). Use caution for patients with cardiovascular disease and in settings that predispose to hypotension (e.g., dehydration, hypovolemia). *Contraindications:* known history of QT prolongation; combination with other drugs that prolong QTc interval (Glassman and Bigger 2002).

Haloperidol (Haldol)

Study 054 confirmed that haloperidol is unlikely to produce ECG changes or cardiac abnormalities. However, haloperidol has caused TDP, particularly when administered intravenously. Prolonged QT intervals, dilated cardiomyopathy, and a history of alcohol abuse predispose to this arrhythmia. (For discussion of TDP, see Chapter 1, "The Delirious Patient," and Appendix 11, "Risk Factors for Torsades de Pointes," in this volume.)

Aripiprazole (Abilify)

There are too few data to permit comment on the safety of aripiprazole in cardiovascular disease.

Phenothiazines

Phenothiazines produce α_1-adrenergic blockade and QT prolongation, making them poor choices for patients with cardiovascular illness.

Chlorpromazine, thioridazine, and mesoridazine can produce significant postural hypotension, as well as systolic drops, even while the patient is lying flat. Intramuscular administration or coadministration with other medications that lower blood pressure will magnify this effect. *Caution:* Even restrained patients incapable of changing position may still "bottom out" their blood pressure if given intramuscular phenothiazines. Trifluoperazine (Stelazine) has less hypotensive action than chlorpromazine or thioridazine.

As discussed in previous sections, thioridazine is the most cardiotoxic antipsychotic. Thioridazine has earned an FDA black box warning because of its effect on QTc and its association with sudden death.

■ MOOD STABILIZERS

Note that mania may be precipitated by antidepressant treatment in vulnerable patients. See also Appendix 16, "Screening Worksheet for Bipolar Spectrum Disorders."

Specific Agents
Lithium

Unlike the medications that affect ventricular conduction, lithium inhibits conduction within the atrium. Monitor for symptoms such as dyspnea, paroxysmal tachycardia, dizziness, and fainting, as well as abnormalities in resting pulse. The most common ECG effect of therapeutic levels of lithium in healthy patients is T-wave flattening or inversion, which is benign and reversible (Brady and Horgan 1988; Bucht et al. 1984).

Sinus node dysfunction and first-degree AV block occur infrequently but are the most common cardiac problems secondary to lithium pharmacotherapy (Lai et al. 2000; Terao et al. 1996). These problems usually occur when there is a vulnerable conduction system (DasGupta and Jefferson 1994). As with all medications, special care should be taken with elderly patients and those with preexisting atrial conduction disturbances.

Use in congestive heart failure. Use lithium at reduced dosages in the setting of congestive heart failure. In moderate to severe congestive heart failure, diminished renal blood flow may produce prerenal azotemia secondary to decreased cardiac output. This situation may cause lithium toxicity by inhibiting lithium clearance. Decrease lithium dose to compensate.

Use after myocardial infarction. No data suggest that lithium should be stopped after a myocardial infarction, although some consider the acute MI period a temporary contraindication to lithium (DasGupta and Jefferson 1990). It seems most prudent to wait to prescribe medications until a post-MI patient has been stabilized. Carefully monitor drug-drug interactions.

Table 3–7. Clinically significant drug interactions with lithium

Potential problem	Drug combination with lithium	Notes
Lithium toxicity	Thiazide diuretics	Mechanism: ↑ Na^+ and K^+ excretion ⇒ ↑ lithium resorption Management: ↓ lithium dose (by 50% per 50-mg dose of hydrochlorothiazide) Fewer problems with xanthine derivatives, aldosterone antagonists, loop diuretics, potassium-sparing diuretics
	Analgesics	Inhibit renal clearance by interference with a prostaglandin-dependent mechanism in the renal tubule
	Nonsteroidal anti-inflammatory drugs and cyclooxygenase-2 (COX-2) inhibitors (celecoxib [Celebrex], rofecoxib [Vioxx])	Fewer problems with aspirin, phenylbutazone (Butazolidin), and sulindac (Clinoril)
	Antimicrobials	Increased lithium levels associated with tetracycline, metronidazole, and parenteral spectinomycin
Subtherapeutic lithium	Methylxanthines (e.g., aminophylline [Phyllocontin, Truphylline], theophylline [Theo-Dur])	Increased renal clearance of lithium causes lowered serum levels
	Acetazolamide (Diamox)	Increased renal clearance of lithium resulting from alkalinization of urine. (Also occurs with sodium bicarbonate.)
Cardiac toxicity	Antiarrhythmic drugs	Carefully monitor, with regular ECGs Increased risk of arrhythmias with hypokalemia or digitalis toxicity, even at therapeutic serum lithium levels β-Blockers with lithium: synergistic bradycardia
	Hydroxyzine (Vistaril, Atarax)	Increased cardiac repolarization
Neurotoxicity	Neuroleptics	Worsened extrapyramidal side effects; rarely, neuroleptic malignant syndrome
	Calcium channel blockers	Verapamil (Calan) and diltiazem (Cardizem) associated with idiopathic neurotoxicity, despite normal or inconsistently altered lithium levels
	Neuromuscular blocking anesthetics	Prolonged muscle paralysis; mechanism unclear (e.g., succinylcholine, pancuronium, decamethonium)
Endocrine toxicity	Antithyroid medications	Lithium interferes with the production of thyroid hormones; synergistic effect with antithyroid medications (e.g., propylthiouracil [PTU] and methimazole [Tapazole])

Source. Adapted from Lenox RH, Manji HK: "Lithium," in *The American Psychiatric Press Textbook of Psychopharmacology*, 2nd Edition. Edited by Schatzberg AF, Nemeroff CB. Washington, DC, American Psychiatric Press, 1998, p. 406; and Alpert J, Fava M, Rosenbaum J: "Psychopharmacologic Issues in the Medical Setting," in *Massachusetts General Hospital Handbook of General Hospital Psychiatry*, 5th Edition. Edited by Stern T, Fricchione G, Cassem N. Philadelphia, PA, Mosby, 2004, pp. 248–249.

Drug interactions. It is safest to assume that a medication (especially a newly released one) produces psychiatric sequelae or interacts with psychotropics until the contrary is proven. Table 3–7 lists clinically significant drug interactions with lithium.

Carbamazepine (Tegretol)

Carbamazepine has a tricyclic structure similar to that of the TCAs and has quinidine-like effects on the heart. Patients older than 40 years and those having known cardiac risk factors should have a pretreatment ECG before receiving this medication (Stoudemire and Moran 1998). Consider alternative therapy if there is evidence of heart block or AV conduction delay. Repeat the ECG after reaching therapeutic serum carbamazepine levels. Reduce or discontinue drug if disturbances of AV conduction occur. Carbamazepine has a number of drug-drug interactions, particularly because it induces enzymes (Cozza et al. 2003), including antiarrhythmics, antihypertensives, and warfarin.

Valproic Acid (Depakote, Depakene)

Valproic acid does not have adverse cardiac effects. Its most common side effects are transient gastrointestinal symptoms (anorexia, nausea, vomiting), neurological symptoms (tremor, sedation, ataxia), and asymptomatic serum hepatic transaminase elevations. The most serious potential side effect of valproic acid is hepatotoxicity, which can lead to liver failure and death. This is a rare, idiosyncratic side effect, unrelated to dosage, and is more common in children who take multiple anticonvulsants.

Other Mood Stabilizers

Lamotrigine (Lamictal), topiramate (Topamax), zonisamide (Zonegran), and gabapentin (Neurontin) have variable effectiveness as mood stabilizers. None is cardiotoxic.

■ REFERENCES

American Diabetes Association, American Psychiatric Association, American Association of Clinical Endocrinologists, et al: Consensus development conference on antipsychotic drugs and obesity and diabetes. J Clin Psychiatry 65:267–272, 2004

Bahk WM, Pae CU, Chae JH, et al: Even low-dose treatment of venlafaxine may provoke recurrence of hypertension in an Asian patient? (letter) Gen Hosp Psychiatry 23:232–234, 2001

Barefoot J, Schroll M: Symptoms of depression, acute myocardial infarction, and total mortality in a community sample. Circulation 93:1976–1980, 1996

Belson M, Kelley T, Ilina N: Bupropion exposures: clinical manifestations and medical outcome. J Emerg Med 23:223–230, 2002

Berkman LF, Blumenthal J, Burg M, et al: Effects of treating depression and low perceived social support on clinical events after myocardial infarction: the Enhancing Recovery in Coronary Heart Disease Patients (ENRICHD) randomized trial. JAMA 289:3106–3116, 2003

Brady H, Horgan J: Lithium and the heart: unanswered questions. Chest 93:166–169, 1988

Brunner G, Zweiker R, Krejs GJ: A toxicological surprise. Lancet 356:1406, 2000

Bucht G, Smigan L, Wahlin A, et al: ECG changes during lithium therapy: a prospective study. Acta Med Scand 216:101–104, 1984

Carney R, Jaffe A: Treatment of major depression following acute myocardial infarction (editorial). JAMA 288:750–751, 2002

Cassem N: Depression, in Massachusetts General Hospital Handbook of General Hospital Psychiatry, 3rd Edition. Edited by Cassem N. St. Louis, MO, Mosby-Year Book, 1991, pp 237–268

Catalano G, Catalano M, Epstein M, et al: QTc interval prolongation associated with citalopram overdose: a case report and literature review. Clin Neuropharmacol 24:158–162, 2001

Cozza KL, Armstrong SC, Oesterheld JR: Concise Guide to Drug Interaction Principles for Medical Practice: Cytochrome P450s, UGTs, P-Glycoproteins, 2nd Edition. Washington, DC, American Psychiatric Publishing, 2003

Czobor P, Volavka J, Citrome L, et al: Changes in glucose and cholesterol levels in patients with schizophrenia treated with typical or atypical antipsychotics. Am J Psychiatry 160:290–296, 2003

DasGupta K, Jefferson J: The use of lithium in the medically ill. Gen Hosp Psychiatry 12:83–97, 1990

DasGupta K, Jefferson J: Treatment of mania in the medically ill, in Psychotropic Drug Use in the Medically Ill, Vol 21. Edited by Silver P. New York, Karger, 1994, pp 138–162

Eisendrath S, Sweeney M: Toxic neuropsychiatric effects of digoxin at therapeutic serum concentrations. Am J Psychiatry 144:506-507, 1987

Ellenbogen KA, Gilligan DM, Wood MA, et al: The pacemaker syndrome: a matter of definition. Am J Cardiol 79:1226–1229, 1997

Ford DE, Mead LA, Chang PP, et al: Depression is a risk factor for coronary artery disease in men: the precursors study. Arch Intern Med 158:1422–1426, 1998

Frasure-Smith N, Lesperance F: Depression: a cardiac risk factor in search of a treatment (editorial). JAMA 289:3171, 2003a

Frasure-Smith N, Lesperance F: Depression and other psychological risks following myocardial infarction. Arch Gen Psychiatry 60:627–636, 2003b

Frasure-Smith N, Lesperance F, Talajic M: Depression and 18-month prognosis after myocardial infarction. Circulation 91:999–1005, 1995

Glassman AH: Clinical management of cardiovascular risks during treatment with psychotropic drugs. J Clin Psychiatry 63 (suppl 9):12–17, 2002

Glassman AH, Bigger JT Jr: Prolongation of QTc interval and antipsychotics (letter). Am J Psychiatry 159:1064, 2002

Glassman AH, O'Connor CM, Califf RM, et al: Sertraline treatment of major depression in patients with acute MI or unstable angina. JAMA 288:701–709, 2002

Goodman M, Hess B: Could implantable cardioverter defibrillators provide a human model supporting the learned helplessness theory of depression? Gen Hosp Psychiatry 21:382–385, 1999

Goodnick P, Jerry J, Parra F: Psychotropic drugs and the ECG: focus on the QTc interval. Expert Opin Pharmacother 3:479–498, 2002

Grace SL, Abbey SE, Shnek ZM, et al: Cardiac rehabilitation, I: review of psychosocial factors. Gen Hosp Psychiatry 24:121–126, 2002a

Grace SL, Abbey SE, Shnek ZM, et al: Cardiac rehabilitation, II: referral and participation. Gen Hosp Psychiatry 24:127–134, 2002b

Gupta S, Masand P, Gupta S: Cardiovascular side effects of novel antipsychotics. CNS Spectr 6:912–918, 2001

Guttmacher LB, Goldstein MG: Treatment of the cardiac-impaired depressed patient, part II: lithium, carbamazepine, and electroconvulsive therapy. Psychiatr Med 6:34–51, 1988

Halperin P: Heart disease, in The American Psychiatric Publishing Textbook of Consultation-Liaison Psychiatry: Psychiatry in the Medically Ill, 2nd Edition. Edited by Wise MG, Rundell JR. Washington, DC, American Psychiatric Publishing, 2002, pp 536–545

Hamner M, Hunt N, Gee J, et al: PTSD and automatic implantable cardioverter defibrillators. Psychosomatics 40:82–85, 1999

Huffman J, Pollack M: Predicting panic disorder among patients with chest pain: an analysis of the literature. Psychosomatics 44:222–236, 2003

Huffman J, Stern T, Januzzi J: The psychiatric management of patients with cardiac disease, in Massachusetts General Hospital Handbook of General Hospital Psychiatry, 5th Edition. Edited by Stern T, Fricchione G, Cassem N. Philadelphia, PA, Mosby, 2004, pp 547–569

Kang UG, Kwon JS, Ahn YM, et al: Electrocardiographic abnormalities in patients treated with clozapine. J Clin Psychiatry 61:441–446, 2000

Kuijpers P, Honig A, Wellens H: Effect of treatment of panic disorder in patients with frequent ICD discharges: a pilot study. Gen Hosp Psychiatry 24:181–184, 2002

Lai CL, Chen WJ, Huang CH, et al: Sinus node dysfunction in a patient with lithium intoxication. J Formos Med Assoc 99:66–68, 2000

Lamas GA, Lee KL, Sweeney MO, et al: Ventricular pacing or dual-chamber pacing for sinus-node dysfunction. N Engl J Med 346:1854–1862, 2002

Lett HS, Blumenthal JA, Babyak MA, et al: Depression as a risk factor for coronary artery disease: evidence, mechanisms, and treatment. Psychosom Med 66:305–315, 2004

Levenson J: Cardiovascular disease, in Psychiatric Care of the Medical Patient. Edited by Stoudemire A, Fogel B. New York, Oxford University Press, 1993, pp 539–555

Mark D: Sex bias in cardiovascular care. JAMA 283:659–661, 2000

McGee HM, Hevey D, Horgan JH: Psychosocial outcome assessments for use in cardiac rehabilitation service evaluation: a 10-year systematic review. Soc Sci Med 48:1373–1393, 1999

Pereira J, Bruera E: Depression with psychomotor retardation: diagnostic challenges and the use of psychostimulants. J Palliat Med 4:15–21, 2001

Peters J, Alpert M, Beitman B, et al: Panic disorder associated with permanent pacemaker implantation. Psychosomatics 31:345–347, 1990

Pfizer Inc: Study Report of Ziprasidone Clinical Pharmacology Protocol 2000. Rockville, MD, U.S. Food and Drug Administration, Center for Drug Evaluation and Research, Division of Cardiorenal Drug Products Consultation, 2000

Phan KL, Taylor SF: Clozapine-associated cardiomyopathy (letter). Psychosomatics 43:248, 2002

Piepho R: Cardiovascular effects of antipsychotics used in bipolar illness. J Clin Psychiatry 63 (suppl 4):20–23, 2002

Roe C, Odell K, Henderson R: Concomitant use of antipsychotics and drugs that may prolong the QT interval. J Clin Psychopharmacol 23:197–200, 2003

Roose S, Glassman A, Giardina E, et al: Cardiovascular effects of imipramine and bupropion in depressed patients with congestive heart failure. J Clin Psychopharmacol 7:247–251, 1987

Roose S, Dalack G, Glassman A, et al: Cardiovascular effects of bupropion in depressed patients with heart disease. Am J Psychiatry 148:512–516, 1991

Rutledge T, Linden W, Davies R: Psychological risk factors may moderate pharmacological treatment effects among ischemic heart disease patients. Canadian Amlodipine/Atenolol in Silent Ischemia Study (CASIS) investigators. Psychosom Med 61:834–841, 1999

Sandson N: Drug Interactions Casebook: The Cytochrome P450 System and Beyond. Washington, DC, American Psychiatric Publishing, 2003

Schleifer S, Slater W, Macari-Hinson M, et al: Digitalis and beta-blocking agents: effects on depression following myocardial infarction. Am Heart J 121:1397–1402, 1991

Shapiro PA, Lesperance F, Frasure-Smith N, et al: An open-label preliminary trial of sertraline for treatment of major depression after acute myocardial infarction (the SADHAT Trial). Sertraline Anti-Depressant Heart Attack Trial. Am Heart J 137:1100–1106, 1999

Smulevich A, Drobijev M, Ilina N: Mirtazapine in the treatment of depression in patients with ischaemic heart disease (abstract). Eur Neuropsychopharmacol 11:S205, 2001

Song Y, Terao T, Shiraishi Y, et al: Digitalis intoxication misdiagnosed as depression—revisited. Psychosomatics 42:368–369, 2001

Stanniland C, Taylor D: Tolerability of atypical antipsychotics. Drug Saf 22:195–214, 2000

Stoudemire A, Fogel B: Psychopharmacology in the medically ill, in Principles of Medical Psychiatry. Edited by Stoudemire A, Fogel B. Orlando, FL, Grune & Stratton, 1987, pp 79–112

Stoudemire A, Moran M: Psychopharmacology in the medically ill patient, in The American Psychiatric Press Textbook of Psychopharmacology, 2nd Edition. Edited by Schatzberg AF, Nemeroff CB. Washington, DC, American Psychiatric Press, 1998, pp 931–959

Strik JJ, Denollet J, Lousberg R, et al: Comparing symptoms of depression and anxiety as predictors of cardiac events and increased health care consumption after myocardial infarction. J Am Coll Cardiol 42:1801–1807, 2003

Taylor D: Antipsychotics and QT prolongation. Acta Med Scand 107:85–95, 2003

Terao T, Abe H, Abe K: Irreversible sinus node dysfunction induced by resumption of lithium therapy. Acta Psychiatr Scand 93:407–408, 1996

Thase M: Effects of venlafaxine on blood pressure: a meta-analysis of original data from 3744 depressed patients. J Clin Psychiatry 59:502–508, 1998

van den Brink RH, van Melle JP, Honig A, et al: Treatment of depression after myocardial infarction and the effects on cardiac prognosis and quality of life: rationale and outline of the Myocardial Infarction and Depression-Intervention Trial (MIND-IT). Am Heart J 144:219–225, 2002

Vassiliadis IV, Fountos AI, Papadimitriou AG, et al: Mental stress-induced silent myocardial ischemia detected during ambulatory ventricular function monitoring. Int J Card Imaging 14:171–177, 1998

Velazquez C, Carlson A, Stokes KA, et al: Relative safety of mirtazapine overdose. Vet Hum Toxicol 43:342–344, 2001

Wenger N, Froeliche E, Smith L: Cardiac rehabilitation as secondary prevention. Clinical Practice Guideline 96–0673. Rockville, MD, U.S. Department of Health and Human Services, Public Health Service, Agency for Health Care Policy and Research, and National Heart, Lung and Blood Institute, 1995

Witchel H, Hancox J, Nutt D: Psychotropic drugs, cardiac arrhythmia, and sudden death. J Clin Psychopharmacol 23:58–77, 2003

Wooltorton E: Antipsychotic clozapine (Clozaril): myocarditis and cardiovascular toxicity. CMAJ 166:1185–1186, 2002

Yoshimasu K, Washio M, Tokunaga S, et al: Relation between type A behavior pattern and the extent of coronary atherosclerosis in Japanese women. Int J Behav Med 9:77–

The Patient With Kidney Disease

Antoinette Ambrosino Wyszynski, M.D.

■ NEUROPSYCHIATRIC DISTURBANCES IN PATIENTS WITH KIDNEY DISEASE

Neuropsychiatric Presentations of Renal Failure

Psychiatric consultation on a nephrology service can be complex, given all the medical and psychological variables that potentially influence mental status. A good assumption, however, is that the affective sequelae of renal failure typically will mimic depressive syndromes. There is often symptomatic overlap (i.e., malaise, apathy, fatigue, lethargy, memory disturbances) between depression and early renal failure. Progression of renal insufficiency usually causes frank delirium, with alterations in consciousness, disorientation, disruption in memory function, and psychotic symptoms. Mania does occur secondary to uremia, dialysis encephalopathy, or infection during dialysis, but much less commonly than depressive states (Wilson 2000).

Predictors of Neuropsychiatric Disturbance

Blood Urea Nitrogen (BUN)

Nephrology patients usually have a bewildering array of abnormal blood chemistries. It is often tempting to blame psychiatric symptoms on shockingly high BUN levels or to wonder how the patient maintains consciousness at all. Although BUN reflects the degree of renal impairment and loosely correlates with neuropsychiatric disturbance, the *absolute* urea level is not tightly related to the degree of neuropsychiatric impairment.

- Rather than be distracted by BUN values that seem to be incompatible with mentation, clinicians should pay attention to the *rate* of BUN change. This measure correlates more closely with mental status phenomena than does absolute BUN.

- See Appendix 17: "Neuropsychiatric Effects of Electrolyte and Acid-Base Imbalance."

Electroencephalogram (EEG)

The EEG usually becomes abnormal within 48 hours of the onset of renal failure. These abnormalities may persist for up to 3 weeks after the start of dialysis. Loss of organized alpha activity and diffuse slowing occur but are nonspecific and appear in other delirious states, such as delirium due to hepatic failure (hepatic encephalopathy) (Lockwood 2000).

Creatinine Clearance

BUN does not always reliably measure kidney function because BUN level depends on hydration status as well as protein intake and catabolism. For example, elderly or debilitated individuals may have relatively low BUN levels, which falsely suggest normal renal function despite significant renal insufficiency. Although creatinine levels are better measures, they may also be misleading because creatinine in its steady state depends on muscle mass as well as kidney function. Creatinine clearance is the most useful clinically available measure of renal function. If oliguria is present in the setting of acute renal failure, creatinine clearance can be estimated as less than 10 mL per minute (Aronoff et al. 1999).

Dialysis-Related Neuropsychiatric Syndromes

CNS abnormalities occur frequently among uremic patients. Although no one etiological metabolic factor predominates, contributants include anemia, endocrinopathy, hypertension, and cardiovascular disease. Acute changes in mental status require careful workup to rule out cerebral hemorrhage, seizure disorder, and dialysis disequilibrium. Anticoagulant therapy (to maintain patency of the shunts) and abnormal platelet function (secondary to chronic renal disease) predispose dialysis patients to subdural hematomas.

- Changes in mental status, when accompanied by symptoms of increased intracranial pressure or focal neurological signs, require *emergency* evaluation.

Disequilibrium Syndrome

Dialysis disequilibrium is an acute delirious state that occurs during or soon after hemodialysis. It is caused by overly vigorous correction of azotemia, leading to osmotic imbalance and rapid shifts in pH. The development of cerebral edema probably results in the symptomatology (Lockwood 2000). It is a transient disorder characterized by headaches, nausea, muscular cramps, irritability, agitation, drowsiness, and seizures. Psychosis may also appear (Aminoff 2000). The symptoms usually occur in the third to fourth hour of dialysis but may also arise 8–48 hours after completing a dialysis run.

Dialysis Dementia

Dialysis dementia, also termed *dialysis encephalopathy*, is a progressive and fatal syndrome. It occurs rarely, usually in patients who have been dialyzed for *at least 1 year*. The syndrome begins with speech disturbance, such as stuttering, which progresses to dysarthria and dysphasia, at times with periods of muteness. The dementia becomes global, with preservation of normal consciousness. The symptoms progress to focal and generalized myoclonus, focal and generalized seizures, personality changes, delusions, and hallucinations (Aminoff 2000).

Studies of dialysis dementia most consistently implicate aluminum toxicity in its pathogenesis. The aluminum content of brain gray matter in dialysis dementia patients has been reported to be 11 times the normal content. Prevention of dialysis dementia centers on avoiding aluminum toxicity from the dialysis fluid and the aluminum salts used to regulate serum phosphate levels. These preventive measures have made dialysis dementia rare.

Early cases are sometimes reversible by instituting chelation therapy with deferoxamine. If left untreated, the symptoms gradually become more persistent and eventually permanent. Once established, the syndrome is usually steadily progressive over a 1- to 15-month period. Death usually occurs within 6–12 months of onset of symptoms.

■ PSYCHOPHARMACOLOGY IN RENAL FAILURE

Fortunately, despite the physiological complexities of renal failure, a glance at Appendix 12, "Guidelines for Adult Psychotropic Dosing in Renal Failure," shows that few psychotropics require dose adjustments. Of those that do, the most notable is lithium.

Patients in renal failure theoretically do not require dose adjustments of most psychotropics. However, these patients become *clinically* quite vulnerable to adverse side effects at medication doses that healthy patients easily tolerate. The empirical *rule of two-thirds* advises lessening the side effect risk by using two-thirds of a normal dose as an upper limit, even though renal failure does not necessarily lead to blood levels in the toxic range.

For example, a healthy patient might comfortably tolerate a fluoxetine dose of 60 mg a day. A patient in renal failure of the same body mass does not pharmacokinetically require a dose adjustment. However, chronic disease is likely to have taken its toll, heightening the vulnerability to adverse side effects on the same dose. The rule of two-thirds advises using only 40 mg of fluoxetine ($2/3 \times 60$ mg) to compensate for this effect.

Cohen et al. (2004) observed that in their experience, the majority of patients with end-stage renal disease (ESRD) both tolerate and require ordinary doses of most psychotropic medications. If toxicity is present, it is usually apparent, and they cautioned more against undermedicating patients than against overmedicating them.

For the clinician, tracing the metabolism of psychotropics in renal failure can be extremely confusing, complicated by specifics of renal as well as nonrenal factors. The easiest-to-trace blood protein, albumin, simply decreases in renal failure, but unfortunately it is not the sole binder of psychotropics. This chapter reviews the practical consequences of these physiological changes for the renal patient. Often, dosing of psychotropics in ESRD patients requires trial and error.

Factors Affecting Psychotropic Drug Metabolism in Kidney Failure

Absorption

The small-bowel absorption of some medications decreases in renal failure, despite intact hepatic metabolism. Excess urea, which has a gastric alkalinizing effect, may be responsible for this problem. Antacids may interfere with gastric absorption of psychotropic medication.

Hepatic Metabolism

Hepatic metabolism changes variably in renal failure. For example, glucuronidation by the liver may actually *increase*. One cannot predict a medication's fate without specifics of its particular metabolism.

Volume of Distribution

Patients with ESRD often have other chronic medical problems, such as muscle wasting, ascites, edema, and dehydration, that affect the volume of distribution of a medication and require dose changes to maintain desired blood levels. Factors and dose adjustments are shown in Table 4–1.

Table 4–1. Factors affecting volume of distribution (VOD)

Clinical situation	Effect on VOD	Effect on medication blood levels	Dosing strategy to compensate
Ascites, edema	↑	↓	↑ dose to avoid dilution
Dehydration, muscle wasting	↓	↑	↓ dose to avoid toxicity

Proteins and Protein Binding

Most psychotropic medications (all except lithium and gabapentin) are lipophilic (lipid soluble), are strongly protein affinitive, and are not excreted by the kidneys. Lithium and gabapentin are hydrophilic (water soluble), are not protein bound, and are excreted unchanged by the kidneys. These factors affect 1) the ratio of free (unbound) to bound drug, 2) the dialyzability of the drug, and 3) the renal clearance of the drug. Details of these changes have been reviewed elsewhere (Wyszynski and Wyszynski 1996).

- *Bottom line:* Dialysis almost completely removes hydrophilic medications (i.e., lithium and gabapentin), but not lipophilic medications (i.e., most psychotropics).

Antidepressants

Although the most experience has accumulated with the tricyclic antidepressants, selective serotonin reuptake inhibitors (SSRIs) are considered first-line antidepressants (Levy and Cohen 2000; Wuerth et al. 2001). Fluoxetine has been the most widely studied of this group. In depressed patients on dialysis ($N=12$), fluoxetine administered as 20 mg once daily for 2 months produced steady-state fluoxetine and norfluoxetine plasma concentrations comparable with those seen in patients with normal renal function (Eli Lilly & Co, January 2003). Although the possibility exists that renally excreted metabolites of fluoxetine may accumulate to higher levels in patients with severe renal dysfunction, use of a lower or less frequent dose is not routinely necessary in renally impaired patients. However, the rule of two-thirds cautions about the *heightened sensitivity to side effects with standard medication doses* and includes the sensible advice to "start low, go slow." Elderly patients and those with concurrent medical problems should be treated with special caution. A few notes follow.

Sertraline (Zoloft) is also widely prescribed in this population. A clinical study comparing pharmacokinetics in healthy volunteers and in patients with renal impairment ranging from mild to severe (requiring dialysis) indicated that the pharmacokinetics and protein binding are unaffected by renal disease (Pfizer Inc, 2003).

Because citalopram (Celexa) is extensively metabolized, excretion of unchanged drug in urine is a minor route of elimination. No dosage adjustment is necessary for patients with mild or moderate renal impairment (Forest Pharmaceuticals, Inc, 2002). Until adequate numbers of patients with severe renal impairment have been evaluated during chronic treatment with citalopram, however, it should be used with caution in such patients.

Paroxetine (Paxil) and Venlafaxine (Effexor)

Lower the doses of paroxetine and venlafaxine for patients in renal failure. Fortunately, these are the only antidepressants that require dose changes in the setting of ESRD. It is not clear why changed dosing is required, but it is probably as a consequence of the changes in protein binding of these medications (see Appendix 12).

Warfarin (Coumadin) and Selective Serotonin Reuptake Inhibitors

Monitor warfarin and SSRIs. Most dialysis patients are on anticoagulant therapy to maintain patency of the shunts. SSRIs (including citalopram [Celexa] and escitalopram [Lexapro]) disrupt anticoagulant control when they are added to previously stable regimens of warfarin. (On warfarin, see Chapter 3 in this volume, "The Patient With Cardiovascular Disease," p. 55.)

Medications That Lower Seizure Threshold

Monitor seizure threshold. The electrolyte imbalances that occur in ESRD may predispose to seizures, and this tendency could be exacerbated by medications that lower the seizure threshold. For example, bupropion (Wellbutrin) has active metabolites that are al-

most completely excreted through the kidney. Their accumulation in ESRD may make patients more vulnerable to seizures.

Medications With a Narrow Therapeutic Index

Several medications prescribed to the ESRD population (e.g., tacrolimus [Prograf], sildenafil [Viagra], and cyclosporine [Sandimmune, Gengraf, Neoral]) are subject to inhibition of cytochrome P450 3A4 by psychotropic medications such as nefazodone, fluvoxamine, fluoxetine/norfluoxetine, sertraline, paroxetine, and valproic acid (weak inhibitors).

Electroconvulsive Therapy

There is no contraindication to using electroconvulsive therapy for ESRD patients.

Psychostimulants

There is no literature on using psychostimulants in the setting of ESRD.

Anxiolytics

Lorazepam (Ativan) and oxazepam (Serax) are preferred in ESRD because they have inactive metabolites. As shown in Appendix 12, ESRD almost quadruples the half-lives of these drugs (Aronoff et al. 1999).

Proceed cautiously when prescribing these agents. Neither lorazepam nor oxazepam is removed by dialysis, because they are highly protein bound. Other benzodiazepines with inactive metabolites include clonazepam (Klonopin) and temazepam (Restoril). Dialysis patients are more sensitive to the sedative, memory, and psychomotor effects of alprazolam (Xanax), which does have active metabolites (even though its half-life remains unchanged in renal failure).

The half-lives of many other benzodiazepines remain unchanged in ESRD, but these drugs are less desirable because of their active metabolites. Agents of this type include diazepam (Valium), chlordiazepoxide (Librium), clorazepate (Tranxene), prazepam (Centrax), halazepam (Paxipam), and flurazepam (Dalmane).

Buspirone (BuSpar) is metabolized by the liver and excreted by the kidneys. A pharmacokinetic study in patients with impaired hepatic or renal function demonstrated increased plasma levels and a lengthened half-life of buspirone. Therefore, the administration of buspirone to patients with severe hepatic or renal impairment is not recommended by the manufacturer (Bristol-Myers Squibb Company, November 2003). In addition, dizziness is a common adverse side effect of buspirone. Because buspirone-induced dizziness may accentuate dizziness secondary to the postural hypotension that often occurs in ESRD patients, buspirone doses should be carefully titrated in this population (Cohen et al. 2004).

Appendix 12 lists the dosing guidelines for other benzodiazepines, anxiolytics, and sedative-hypnotics in more detail.

Sedative-Hypnotics

Insomnia, restless legs syndrome, and sleep apnea syndrome occur frequently in ESRD (Sabbatini et al. 2002; Springer 2000). Zaleplon (Sonata) or zolpidem (Ambien) may be used in ESRD (see Appendixes 12 and 13).

Antipsychotics

Studies are not available on using atypical antipsychotics in the specific setting of renal failure, and "considerable wariness" is advised until we know more (Cohen et al. 2004, p. 44). Brief mention has been made of using risperidone and olanzapine (Levy 2000). However, the association of olanzapine with causing or aggravating diabetes mellitus (a common comorbidity for many ESRD patients) is of concern (Cohen et al. 2004, p. 44). Recent recommendations are to avoid ziprasidone (Geodon) if possible in this population, because of vulnerability to electrolyte shifts in ESRD and ziprasidone's tendency to prolong the QTc interval (Cohen et al. 2004).

The *rule of two-thirds* advises lowering doses by one-third to compensate for heightened sensitivity to side effects. The following material was gathered from the manufacturers:

Risperidone (Risperdal)

In patients with moderate to severe renal disease, clearance of the sum of risperidone and its active metabolite decreased by 60% compared with that in young healthy subjects. Risperidone doses should be reduced in patients with renal disease. The manufacturer recommends initial doses of 0.5 mg bid, with dose increases of no more than 0.5 mg bid (Janssen 2002). Wait at least 1 week before increasing the medication above 1.5 mg bid for the following patients: elderly or debilitated patients, those with severe renal or hepatic impairment, and patients either predis-

posed to or at risk for hypotension. Elderly or debilitated individuals, and individuals with renal impairment, may have less ability to eliminate risperidone than other adults, so patients need to be titrated cautiously and carefully monitored. For a once-a-day dosing regimen in the elderly or debilitated person, the manufacturer recommends that the patient be titrated on a twice-a-day regimen for 2–3 days at the target dose and then switched to a once-a-day dosing.

Olanzapine (Zyprexa)

According to the manufacturer, because olanzapine is highly metabolized before excretion and only 7% of the drug is excreted unchanged, renal dysfunction alone is unlikely to have a major impact on its pharmacokinetics (Eli Lilly & Co, 2003). The pharmacokinetic characteristics of olanzapine were similar in patients with severe renal impairment and normal subjects, indicating that dose adjustment based on the degree of renal impairment is not required. The association of olanzapine with inducing or exacerbating diabetes mellitus is of concern. (See also Chapter 3, "The Patient With Cardiovascular Disease," pp. 61–62.)

Quetiapine (Seroquel)

According to the manufacturer, patients with severe renal impairment (GFR [glomerular filtration rate]=10–30 mL/min) had a 25% lower mean clearance than normal subjects (GFR>80 mL/min, $n=8$), but plasma quetiapine concentrations in the subjects with renal insufficiency were comparable to those of unimpaired subjects receiving the same dose (AstraZeneca, 2002, 2003). According to the manufacturer, there is no need for dose adjustment in these patients.

Ziprasidone (Geodon)

Because ziprasidone is highly metabolized, with less than 1% of the drug excreted unchanged, renal impairment alone is unlikely to have a major impact on its pharmacokinetics. The pharmacokinetics of ziprasidone following 8 days of 20 mg bid dosing were similar among subjects with varying degrees of renal impairment ($n=27$) and subjects with normal renal function, indicating that dose adjustment based on the degree of renal impairment is not required (Pfizer Inc, 2002). Ziprasidone is not hemodialyzed. One of the components of intramuscular ziprasidone (cyclodextrin) is cleared by renal filtration and has not yet been systematically evaluated in patients with renal impairment. Intramuscular ziprasidone should therefore be used cautiously with patients with impaired renal function. Moreover, the vulnerability of ESRD patients to electrolyte shifts may heighten the risk of developing fatal arrhythmias secondary to QT prolongation by ziprasidone.

Clozapine (Clozaril)

No data could be located on the use of clozapine in renal failure. Because of a life-threatening risk of agranulocytosis, clozapine should be reserved for the treatment of severely ill schizophrenic patients who do not show an acceptable response to adequate courses of standard antipsychotic drug treatment. Other side effects of clozapine include seizures, myocarditis, and cardiovascular side effects, such as orthostatic hypotension (with or without syncope). Respiratory arrest and cardiac arrest during initial treatment have occurred in patients who were also receiving benzodiazepines or other psychotropic drugs.

Aripiprazole (Abilify)

According to the manufacturer, no dose adjustments are required in patients with renal impairment (Bristol-Myers Squibb, 2003). No other information is available at this time.

Conventional Antipsychotics

Haloperidol (Haldol) does not require modifications based on GFR (Aronoff et al. 1999); doses should be reduced empirically to minimize side effects such as sedation. Haloperidol is not dialyzable. It has been used safely in the setting of ESRD.

Phenothiazines are not strictly contraindicated but should be used cautiously because of potential sedation, anticholinergic and cardiovascular toxicity, urinary retention, and orthostatic hypotension. They do *not* accelerate the progression of renal failure. Like haloperidol, phenothiazines are not dialyzable. They are not as well tolerated as haloperidol in medically fragile populations.

Medications to Treat Extrapyramidal Symptoms

Akathisia is often treated with propranolol, which needs no dosing change in renal failure. We could locate no information on using benztropine mesylate (Cogentin) in patients with compromised renal function. Amantadine (Symmetrel) dose must be adjusted for

GFR; there is a two- to threefold increase in half-life when creatinine clearance falls below 40 mL/min. Half-life averages 8 days in patients on chronic maintenance hemodialysis. Amantadine is removed in negligible amounts by hemodialysis (Endo Pharmaceuticals, 2000).

Although GFR concerns do not require that dose adjustments be made for diphenhydramine (Benadryl), side effects such as dry mouth and sedation are poorly tolerated in ESRD patients.

Lithium and the Kidney

Since the mid-1960s, in a confusing array of papers, the literature has alternately supported and refuted lithium's capacity to do renal harm. It has been difficult to control for confounding factors, such as the duration of affective illness and lithium treatment, the occurrence of transient episodes of toxicity in unmonitored patients, and the coadministration of other psychotropics. Without knowing the statistics for renal insufficiency in patients with bipolar disorder who have never taken lithium, one cannot distinguish between lithium-induced renal failure and otherwise-occurring renal failure.

A practical summary follows with a selected list of review papers (Bendz et al. 2001; Gitlin 1999; Johnson 1998; Schou 2001). Box 4–1 lists strategies for managing the potential risk of lithium-induced renal insufficiency.

Lithium-Associated Renal Dysfunction

Reports of kidney damage appeared particularly in the late 1970s to mid-1980s, pointing to tubulointerstitial damage. Reports of histopathological damage secondary to lithium have been infrequent in the literature appearing between 1993 and 2002, particularly considering the widespread use of lithium. The consensus seems to be that a very small group of patients may develop lithium-induced renal insufficiency (possibly in combination with other medical factors) in the form of interstitial nephritis. However, lithium is not harmful for the majority of patients, particularly at low to moderate plasma levels and in the short term, with careful monitoring. It has been proposed that change in serum lithium level may more powerfully predict recurrence of bipolar disorder than the presence of lithium levels greater than 0.8 mEq/L (Perlis et al. 2002). It is possible that renal risk can be minimized with lower doses and plasma levels. The safety of lithium becomes more controversial in the setting of long-term use, at higher serum levels, or under conditions of casual monitoring.

Box 4–1.	**Strategies for minimizing risk of lithium-induced renal insufficiency**

1. Perform baseline measurements of BUN, creatinine, electrolytes, and thyroid function.

2. Perform baseline measurements of creatinine clearance and 24-hour urine volume for patients at risk for renal insufficiency (e.g., diabetic patients, hypertensive patients, drug and alcohol abusers).

3. Minimize episodes of lithium toxicity, which increase risk of developing renal dysfunction (see Tables 4–2 and 4–3).

4. Routinely measure creatinine every 6 months. If creatinine level rises to **>1.6 mg/100 mL,** request medical consultation. Consider switching to another mood stabilizer.

5. Check electrolyte and lithium levels during titration, and then periodically, to detect NDI. It is possible to administer a diuretic to correct NDI in lithium-treated patients.

6. Routinely ask about urine output. Polyuria and nocturia are relatively sensitive indicators of renal concentrating capacity. Thirst is a less reliable measure.

7. If polyuria develops: Assess 24-hour urine volume and consult with a nephrologist; retarget to lithium levels **0.5–0.8 mEq/L,** and monitor for psychiatric relapse.

Note. BUN=blood urea nitrogen; NDI=nephrogenic diabetes insipidus.

Risk Factors

The following risk factors appear to be associated with lithium-induced renal impairment:

- Lithium intoxication (more frequent episodes associated with greater risk)
- Lithium doses and plasma levels at high end of "normal" (levels>1.0 mEq/L associated with greater risk)
- Concomitant use of other medications
- Chronic physical illness
- Increasing age (*Note:* renal function diminishes with age, independently of lithium use)

Renal Side Effects of Lithium

Lithium adversely affects renal tubular function, causing deficits in urine concentrating ability. Polyuria (24-hour urine volume >3,000 mL) is a frequent side effect and may occur at any time during administration of lithium. It is a consequence of diminished sensitivity of the collecting tubule to antidiuretic hormone (ADH), interfering with production of concentrated urine. Polyuria has been considered a benign condition, the reversible result of a pharmacodynamic disturbance without histopathological changes. It sometimes can progress to nephrogenic diabetes insipidus (NDI). Lithium accumulation in collecting tubule cells, blocking ADH, is the most common cause of NDI. This effect is usually temporary, but 5%–10% of patients develop irreversible NDI. If the patient is rechallenged with lithium, diabetes insipidus is likely to recur but is treatable.

In contrast, an effect of lithium on glomerular function is rare, so that routine urinalysis for protein is not necessary.

Table 4–2. Clinical factors that change lithium clearance

Clinical factor	Mechanism
Cirrhosis with ascites Congestive heart failure Dehydration (fever, vomiting, diarrhea, unconsciousness) Low-sodium diet Nephrotic syndrome	Sodium retention leading to lithium retention and potential toxicity
Excessive caffeine in diet[a] High-sodium diet[b]	Increased lithium clearance, with potential subtherapeutic levels, due to mechanisms described in notes below

[a]Via afferent arteriolar vasodilation.

[b]Via activation of renal sodium-excreting mechanisms.

Source. Adapted from data in Thomsen K, Schou M: "Avoidance of Lithium Intoxication: Advice Based on Knowledge About the Renal Lithium Clearance Under Various Circumstances." *Pharmacopsychiatry* 32:83–86, 1999.

Table 4–3.   Medications that affect lithium levels

Potential adverse effect	Medication
Lithium toxicity	Angiotensin-converting enzyme (ACE) inhibitors
	Amiloride (Midamor)
	β-Blocking agents
	Cyclosporine (Sandimmune)
	Loop diuretics
	Methyldopa
	Nonsteroidal anti-inflammatory drugs (NSAIDs)
	Spironolactone (Aldactone)
	Thiazide diuretics
	Verapamil (various brands)
Subtherapeutic lithium level	Calcium entry blockers (e.g., isradipine [DynaCirc], nifedipine [Adalat, Procardia])

Source.   Adapted from data in Thomsen K, Schou M: "Avoidance of Lithium Intoxication: Advice Based on Knowledge About the Renal Lithium Clearance Under Various Circumstances." *Pharmacopsychiatry* 32:83–86, 1999.

Lithium in the Setting of Renal Failure and Dialysis

Lithium is contraindicated in acute renal failure. It may, however, be administered in *chronic* renal failure, in conservative doses, with careful monitoring of serum levels and renal function.

For patients with renal insufficiency, not on dialysis:

1. Obtain an estimate of GFR from the nephrologist.
2. Estimate the pre–renal failure maintenance lithium dose and target level.
3. Look up the dose adjustment in Appendix 12 of this volume (Table 4–4 is an excerpt).

For patients on dialysis:

1. Assume that lithium is 100% excreted via the kidneys. Therefore, if GFR=0, lithium clearance=0, so that serum lithium level remains essentially stable between dialysis runs.

2. Assume that lithium is 100% dialyzed. Therefore, postdialysis lithium=0.
3. Administer lithium after each dialysis run.
4. Lithium is either given in the dialysate during peritoneal dialysis or administered as a single oral dose after each hemodialysis treatment (DasGupta and Jefferson 1994).
5. Assuming that GFR=0 for anuric patients, interdialysis lithium levels should be consistent because of lack of kidney function and therefore lack of lithium clearance.
6. Obtain an assay of serum lithium levels before dialysis begins, several times per week initially, and then monthly, maintaining the lowest levels that are effective to prevent a manic relapse.

Case Example

Ms. Manic-Uremic is a 65-year-old woman who presents already in renal failure (BUN 62, creatinine 5.5), off lithium, and with recurrent manic episodes. Her management is brittle, responsive only to lithium 900 mg/day to achieve a level of 1.0 mEq/L. Several months ago, her internist discontinued lithium because of her rising creatinine level. She is not yet on dialysis. The patient has given consent to start lithium because she has been unresponsive to all other mood stabilizers.

Questions (see also Study Guide, Appendix 19)

1. How do you calculate Ms. Manic-Uremic's current lithium dose during the time that she remains off dialysis, assuming that her BUN and creatinine levels remain relatively stable?
2. After Ms. Manic-Uremic does begin hemodialysis, how do you calculate the amount of lithium she needs and how do you administer it?
3. The patient's husband brings her to your office on a Monday afternoon, directly after dialysis. She is confused and disoriented. He is worried that she is experiencing toxicity from lithium, and he is "afraid to give her more." How valid are his concerns? You learn that lithium was withheld by the dialysis team after the Monday afternoon dialysis run.

Table 4–4.   Adjustments of lithium maintenance dose in renal failure

	Half-life (hours)		GFR (mL/min)		
	Normal	ESRD	>50	10–50	<10
Lithium	14–28	40	No dose adjustment	↓ dose to 50%–75%	↓ dose to 25%–50%

Note.   ESRD=end-stage renal disease; GFR= glomerular filtration rate.

4. Let's say Ms. Manic-Uremic requires an antidepressant. Which antidepressants will not require dose adjustment for renal failure?

Answers

1. The nephrologist has given an estimated GFR of 50. Ms. Manic-Uremic's pre–renal failure lithium requirement was 900 mg/day to mount a therapeutic level of 1.0 mEq/L. According to Table 4–4, her new dose should be reduced to 50%–75% of the usual, or (50% of 900 mg)=450 mg to (75% of 900 mg)=675 mg. Her new dose should be somewhere between 450 mg and 675 mg of lithium. One would start low and test serum levels until the appropriate therapeutic level was reached.

2. Let's assume that after the first dialysis run of the week, Monday, Ms. Manic-Uremic's lithium level is 0. Administer a test dose of lithium initially (e.g., 150 mg) and ask the dialysis team to test lithium level on Wednesday morning, prior to dialysis. Because we have assumed that an essentially anuric patient does not clear lithium, the serum level attained after one 150-mg dose on Monday afternoon should remain constant until Wednesday morning's dialysis. Once the level is confirmed, you may either raise the dose or keep it the same. Let's say the level is 0.3 mEq/L on Wednesday morning. You might instruct the patient to try 300 mg of lithium after her dialysis run on Wednesday afternoon, testing the level on Friday morning before dialysis. You would repeat this procedure until an appropriate level per dose was achieved.

3. The likelihood of lithium toxicity after a dialysis run is nonexistent if lithium was withheld after dialysis, because lithium is 100% dialyzed. The differential diagnosis of acute mental status changes in dialysis patients should include dialysis disequilibrium syndrome, intracranial bleeds, and seizure disorder.

4. Paroxetine and venlafaxine specifically require dose changes in renal failure. All other antidepressants listed in Appendix 12 do not.

Other Mood Stabilizers

The most helpful information on the use of mood stabilizers other than lithium in renal failure comes from the epilepsy literature (Asconape 2002). Several important notes follow.

Carbamazepine (Tegretol)

Carbamazepine has been associated with hyponatremia. Usually hyponatremia is transient, mild (defined as sodium levels of 125–135 mEq/L), and asymptomatic, only rarely leading to serious consequences or discontinuation of the drug. Chronic hyponatremia most commonly causes confusion, lethargy, dizziness, weakness, headache, and nausea. The mechanism by which carbamazepine induces hyponatremia is not completely understood. Typically, patients present with the syndrome of inappropriate secretion of antidiuretic hormone (SIADH). The risk of carbamazepine-induced SIADH increases with old age, with renal failure, and with the coadministration of antipsychotics or antidepressant drugs (Asconape 2002). Periodic monitoring of sodium levels is recommended during the first 3 months of therapy with carbamazepine, especially in patients with risk factors for hyponatremia. Complex partial seizures in the setting of renal failure have been treated effectively with carbamazepine.

Valproic Acid (Depakote, Depakene)

Valproic acid is hepatically metabolized. A slight reduction (27%) in the unbound clearance of valproic acid has been reported in patients with renal failure (creatinine clearance <10 mL/min); however, hemodialysis typically reduces valproic acid concentrations by about 20% (Abbott Laboratories, 2002). Therefore, no dosage adjustment appears to be necessary in patients with renal failure. Protein binding in these patients is substantially reduced; thus, monitoring total concentrations may be misleading.

Gabapentin (Neurontin)

Gabapentin is excreted almost exclusively by the kidneys, with negligible liver metabolism. Doses must be modified according to GFR, although there are few drug-drug interactions (see Appendix 12).

Topiramate (Topamax)

Topiramate is almost 90% eliminated directly through the kidneys when not used with other enzyme-inducing medications (Asconape 2002). When enzyme inducers are present, about 30% of the drug is eliminated by hepatic biotransformation. Dose adjustments are necessary in renal insufficiency.

■ COPING WITH END-STAGE RENAL DISEASE

Every chronic medical illness is stressful, but the strain of end-stage renal disease is particularly exhausting;

there is no physical or psychological respite. Work, family, meals, leisure, finances, sexuality, life expectancy—chronic renal failure invades them all. Perhaps more than any other chronic disease, ESRD imposes unremitting, multifaceted deprivation. To comply with low-sodium, low-potassium, low-protein, and low-fluid diets, patients must eliminate almost all fruits and vegetables, ration only small amounts of meats and fish, and endure strict fluid restrictions. Family members often hover in disapproval when the patient's compliance wavers, creating misunderstandings and tension. Vacations must be planned around the availability of satellite dialysis units, with the attendant anxiety about relying on unknown doctors, unfamiliar staff, and the knowledge that even moderate dietary "cheating"—surely forgivable for any dieter on vacation—can lead to medical catastrophe.

Illness Intrusiveness and Quality of Life

Illness intrusiveness refers to an illness's direct or indirect interference with important facets of an individual's life. Examples of direct interference are the physiological effects of irreversible renal failure itself, the consequences of the treatment regimen, and/or the presence of nonrenal complications, such as cardiovascular disease. Examples of indirect interference include attitudinal shifts by family and friends that influence a patient's adjustment to his or her disease.

Illness intrusiveness may be particularly potent in its effect on general psychosocial well-being, which in turn affects adherence to a treatment regimen and thus ultimately affects morbidity. The quality of life in ESRD also depends on several nonrenal variables, most notably psychosocial support (Daneker et al. 2001; Kimmel 2000, 2001; Kimmel et al. 1998b; Shidler et al. 1998). One classic study examined illness intrusiveness in 200 ESRD patients receiving different treatments (hemodialysis, continuous abdominal peritoneal dialysis [CAPD], or renal transplantation) (Devins et al. 1990). Interference in life domains greatly differed across treatments, correlating significantly with the following: treatment time requirements; uremic symptoms; intercurrent nonrenal illnesses, such as infection and anemia; fatigue; and difficulties in daily activities.

Fewer negative life events, richer social networks, paid employment, and higher annual family income also correlated with well-being. The occurrence of negative stressful, nonrenal life events significantly increased perceived illness intrusiveness. The authors (Devins et al. 1990) proposed that

the co-occurrence of independent stressful life events potentiates the intrusions imposed by ESRD, augmenting their impact on lifestyles, activities, and interests. Alternatively, such co-occurrences may simply compromise the individual's ability to cope with the demands of the illness situation—for example, either by competing for available attention, energies, and efforts or by amplifying the overall perception of the magnitude of intrusions to be negotiated. (p. 135)

Note that the burden of ESRD was not equivalent across all life domains. The two domains that were especially affected, regardless of treatment modality, were 1) physical well-being and diet, and 2) work and finances. Less adversely affected were marital and family relations, recreation, and social relationships outside the family. Life domains such as self-improvement/self-expression, religious expression, and community and civic activities were least affected.

It is important to include family members in psychological and psychosocial interventions; ESRD usually has a profound effect on families (Daneker et al. 2001).

Dialysis Stressors

The demands of dialysis are stressful; this is no trivial procedure, however "routine" it may be. The quality-of-life literature comparing hemodialysis and CAPD is too extensive to review. A few points of information, however, will be helpful:

- Hemodialysis circulates the blood extracorporeally and may produce major complications, such as stroke and cardiac emergencies. It requires 4–6 hours daily three times a week, usually for 4-hour sessions.
- In CAPD, dialysis solution remains in the peritoneal cavity except during drainage periods, followed by reinstallation of fresh solution five times a day. After each exchange cycle, all tubing is disconnected, the chronic indwelling catheter is capped, and the patient is free to go about daily activities. Exchanges typically occur four to five times daily, requiring 30–60 minutes each, or continuously throughout the night. CAPD is self-administered. The most common medical complication is peritonitis.

There are often body-image problems with CAPD due to the abdominal distention caused by the fluid in the abdominal cavity, but CAPD has the advantage over hemodialysis of improved patient independence.

Home hemodialysis and CAPD appear to be psychologically superior to hospital-based treatments. Renal transplantation exceeds both of these options in terms of restoring psychosocial quality of life (Fujisawa et al. 2000) and is discussed in Chapter 11, "A Primer on Solid Organ Transplant Psychiatry," in this volume.

Anemia is quite prevalent in ESRD and can severely limit rehabilitation. Recombinant erythropoietin given for the anemia of chronic renal failure significantly improves the quality of life for dialysis patients. Better energy level, improved psychological well-being, and enhanced sexual functioning have been reported when physiological hemoglobin levels are maintained in hemodialysis patients (McMahon et al. 2000). Erythropoietin therapy avoids the adverse effects of transfusion but has been associated with hypertension, thrombosis of vascular access, and hyperkalemia.

Depression and Anxiety

To say that dialysis patients experience anxiety and depression is to state the obvious. Worry and dysphoria may invade everything—self-esteem, prognosis, sexual performance, ability to cope with dialysis stressors, and the expectations of staff and family. Patients who have a premorbid history of psychiatric disorders have a particularly difficult time.

Prevalence estimates of depression in ESRD patients have varied widely. Methodological problems have included variations in assessment instruments; differences in diagnostic criteria; and sample heterogeneity for disease type (e.g., systemic lupus erythematosus [SLE], hypertension), for duration of renal failure, and for treatment type.

A 1998 study examined the risk of psychiatric hospitalization among dialysis patients compared with individuals who had diabetes mellitus, ischemic heart disease, cerebrovascular disease, or peptic ulcer disease (Kimmel et al. 1998a). Hospitalization with psychiatric disorders was 1.5 to 3.0 times higher for renal failure patients compared with other chronically ill patients. Depression, dementia, and drug-related disorders were especially common. Men, African Americans of both genders, and younger patients were more likely to be hospitalized with a psychiatric disorder. The adjusted risk of hospitalization for peritoneal dialysis patients was lower compared with hemodialysis patients.

Uremia itself produces depression-like symptoms (irritability, decreased appetite and libido, insomnia, apathy, fatigue, poor concentration) that may be misattributed to a primary psychiatric condition. In addition, ESRD patients may be affected by other medical conditions that mimic depressive states or cause secondary mood disorders, such as anemia, electrolyte disturbances, alterations of endocrine function (especially from hyperparathyroidism), or underlying systemic disease (e.g., SLE). Intriguingly, a few studies have explored the effects of depression on survival in dialysis patients, showing that depression may be as powerful as medical risk factors in predicting outcome (Kimmel et al. 2000).

ESRD patients often report nonspecific physical complaints, such as fatigue, sleep disturbance, headache, nausea, and dyspnea. As in other medically ill populations, the nonvegetative symptoms of depression (e.g., depressed mood, suicidal ideas, guilt, loss of interest, discouragement) best distinguish ESRD patients with and without affective illness. Sexual dysfunction has been reported to occur frequently in patients with ESRD maintained on dialysis, even in the absence of affective illness (Camsari et al. 1999). Dialysis patients of both genders experience a marked decrease in libido and frequency of sexual intercourse once they become uremic, with some showing abnormal hypothalamic-pituitary functioning. For women dialysands, there may be diminished capacity for orgasm. For men, there is a high prevalence of physiologically based impotence, a reduction of testosterone, and decreased spermatogenesis. Antihypertensive medications may further diminish libido in both sexes and cause impotence in males. Depression, disrupted family roles, and the psychological impact of losing urination exacerbate sexual difficulties. Sexual performance may start as stable or normal predialysis but decline postdialysis and remain impaired. However, deteriorating sexual function that is markedly disproportional to the progression of renal disease suggests factors other than the strictly physiological.

Insomnia, restless legs syndrome, and sleep apnea syndrome occur frequently in ESRD (Sabbatini et al. 2002; Springer 2000). Fractured, nonrestorative sleep contributes to illness intrusiveness and should be given therapeutic priority (see Appendix 13 in this volume, "Commonly Used Drugs With Sedative-Hypnotic Properties").

Informed Consent and Decision Making in ESRD Patients

Several factors make ESRD patients particularly challenging to work with in psychotherapy. The effects of uremia and electrolyte imbalance often profoundly affect energy, mental alertness, and the ability to remember. The regimens required of dialysis patients are time-consuming and complex. When other medical problems such as diabetes coexist, the cognitive demands of attending to medical care could overload anyone. Regular psychotherapy may seem like one more burden rather than a resource.

The cognitive effects of chronic uremia may affect the ability of ESRD patients to make decisions about their medical care. These patients are often candidates for more than one type of medical treatment: hemodialysis, peritoneal dialysis, or kidney transplantation. Informed consent requires information processing that puts the uremic patient at a disadvantage (see Chapter 12 in this volume, "Assessing Decisional Capacity and Informed Consent in Medical Patients: A Short, Practical Guide").

Adherence to Medical Treatment

Adherence to or compliance with medical care affects behaviors as seemingly simple as buckling seat belts and those as complex as ESRD's dietary restrictions. Also termed *behavioral self-regulation,* a patient's relationship to given medical advice is a multifaceted phenomenon (Christensen et al. 2002; Eitel et al. 2000; Kaveh and Kimmel 2001) with practical consequences for health and survival. For example, ESRD patients usually rank compliance with fluid restrictions as most stressful of all. Notably, noncompliance with fluid restrictions is a major cause of death from congestive heart failure in ESRD patients.

The *Health Belief Model* (Becker and Maiman 1975) defines how personal health beliefs interact to affect compliance with medical care. The model identifies five criteria that guide interventions with noncompliant patients:

1. Perceived *susceptibility* to negative health consequences caused by not following medical advice
2. Perceived *seriousness* of these consequences
3. Perceived *costs* versus benefits of performing the prescribed adherence behavior
4. Perceived *barriers* (i.e., relative difficulty of incorporating the adherence behavior into the person's lifestyle)
5. Degree of *concern* about the disease itself and its consequences

Case Example

A nephrologist referred for consultation Mr. B, a 61-year-old unmarried dialysis patient who had developed ESRD secondary to uncontrolled hypertension and was nonadherent to fluid restrictions, despite adequate cognitive understanding. Upon interview, it was revealed that the patient, a highly decorated Vietnam veteran, believed in "getting through" hardship by "making the best of things" and "not getting upset." Although slightly anxious, he reported that he was getting used to dialysis and was feeling more comfortable with the staff. He was concerned about the possibility of renal transplantation, saying that he saw what happened to people in Vietnam and he did not want to be "anyone's guinea pig." Dialysis was working just fine for him, according to the patient. In fact, he fancied himself a bit of a perfectionist, often aggravated by others' incompetence. He admired the efficiency of the dialysis staff, even though there were frightening events that occurred on the unit that reminded him of wartime. Mr. B. stated he "was always thirsty," so he drank water liberally and ate fruit (which he desperately missed) in the evenings and mornings before dialysis, thinking that the extra fluid intake could be "taken off," and was willing to spend "the extra hour or two on the machine." He would never consider missing a dialysis session. The staff reported that he was never late and was otherwise a model patient. There was no drug or alcohol abuse or family history of psychiatric illness.

Intervention: Mr. B. did fear the consequences of untreated renal failure; within the framework of his knowledge, he was reasonably adherent. He coordinated drinking fluid with his dialysis, believing the kidneys operated along a plumbing model of "fluid in, fluid out," and did not understand that he thereby jeopardized his health. An educational intervention clarified how fluid and electrolyte ("chemical") shifts could adversely affect blood pressure and the heart. Helping him devise his own logbook of fluid intake (with provisions for occasional splurges) capitalized on his obsessional style and improved his adherence to the fluid restrictions.

The literature on the psychology of adherence to medical care is extensive; for a review, see DiMatteo et al. (2000).

Psychodynamic Factors in ESRD

Illness is supposed to be the great equalizer, afflicting everyone democratically. However, renal failure often selects for those individuals already least able to comply with medical advice, such as smokers, or diabetic patients who cannot adhere to their medical regimen. Therefore, as Levy (2000) has noted, "renal failure, although universal, is skewed in the direction of the patient who is less likely to be able to cooperate with the arduous medical regimen of dialysis and renal transplantation" (p. 234).

Alcohol and substance abusers are at especially high risk of developing renal failure, often secondary to rhabdomyolysis and myoglobinuria. These individuals are already challenging to care for within the medical system. The complications of following a dialysis protocol may become overwhelming for patient and dialysis staff alike.

Not all dialysis patients cope poorly. *Denial* is an important defense that allows titration of awareness; it is often adaptive in the medical setting. Personality variables, such as the need for independence and the ability to use denial effectively, will affect coping and comfort. Denial is high in these patients as a group (Levy 2000). Renal patients tend to feel very much "overdoctored," and so psychotherapy will have a better chance of succeeding if it is conducted in conjunction with clinic visits or dialysis runs (Levy 2000). In most cases, a supportive and practical approach works best.

The value of positive transference transcends the psychotherapy hour and psychodynamically based treatments: for example, patients' satisfaction with their nephrologists correlates with regular attendance at dialysis sessions, and may correlate with survival in some patients (Kovac et al. 2002).

Although there are no studies systematically applying insight-oriented techniques, there are occasional anecdotal reports on how psychodynamics affect dialysis patients (Fargnoli 1990; Martis et al. 1988), including reports of dialysis as a reexperience of childhood sexual abuse (Krawczyk and Raskin 1990) and the association of dialysis with vampires (Perard 1985).

The subjective experience of patients regarding their illness is not always predictable. For example, in one classic study (House 1987), 80 patients on a renal unit were interviewed to assess their psychiatric status and social functioning, then were reinterviewed 1 year later. An unexpected finding was that 11 patients commented positively on some aspect of their experience:

> Typical comments were: "I feel as if I've grown up…as if I'm more aware of what life's all about." "Every day is a bonus now…I'm always hopeful." Several people commented that they worried less over unimportant things and "noticed life" more. These comments were often made by people who had at some time recovered from a medical crisis, and did not necessarily reflect current mental state….It is clear that individual statements about the value of life on treatment are not related, in a simple direct way, to current levels of social or physical function. (House 1987, p. 449)

One interesting study (Baines and Jindal 2002) found that even after successful kidney transplantation, patients may present with feelings of bereavement, grief, or low mood, despite a much-desired outcome. The authors speculated that feelings of loss are generated as patients contemplate their future and deal with their "imagined past," which has been irretrievably lost to chronic illness. These feelings must be distinguished from those experienced relative to other aspects of care (e.g., feelings for the cadaveric donor or the donor family). Without intervention, the patient may become psychiatrically symptomatic and less likely to adhere to medical care (Baines and Jindal 2002).

- *Bottom line:* Never assume to know the meanings of an illness or procedure for a particular patient and the resulting impact on behavior concerning illness.

Employment, Disability, and the Insurance Trap

Practically, the demands of thrice-weekly dialysis would intrude on most full-time occupations. Neuropsychologically, impaired cognitive functioning also helps to account for the lower employment rates seen among ESRD patients (Bremer et al. 1998). Many hemodialysis patients who were employed before their illness no longer work full-time or retire disabled from full-time work (van Manen et al. 2001). It has been noted that

> return to work remains the Achilles' heel in the overall rehabilitation of the patient with ESRD….Studies have consistently shown that the longer patients have been unemployed, the less likely they are to return to work. This is due to many factors, including economic disincentives associated with the availability of disability benefits and the potential loss of benefits through part-time employment. Second, experienced workers who have been chronically unemployed may not have positions available to them to which they can readily return. (Evans et al. 1990, p. 829)

Disability payments are essential for patients incapacitated by illness, but they may impede psychological and occupational rehabilitation. To work psychiatrically with medical patients is to gain an education about disability insurance. The least restrictive (and most expensive) disability policies 1) are noncancelable as long as the premiums are paid, regardless of the insured person's illness or its duration; 2) have "own occupation" riders, stating that a person is considered "disabled" if unable to perform his or her *specific* occupation; and 3) include partial disability provisions, permitting part-time employment while still providing prorated disability income to supplement earnings. Most policies issued today, however, *are* cancelable and have *no* partial disability or own-occupation benefits. Attempting to earn an income again under these circumstances is a gamble with high stakes: patients risk zero reimbursement if they can perform *any* job for *any* income, however removed from their own occupation or below their standard of living. Sometimes the insurance carrier may drop them—permanently—if they are judged "no longer disabled." Should there be a medical exacerbation, these patients may be left financially stranded, uninsurable, and without income except for the small allowance provided by Social Security.

These practical concerns are discordant with the psychological needs of patients who seek to transform their "sick identity" and recover a sense of productivity even while coping with chronic illness. Unfortunately, many individuals will never qualify for reinsurance by another insurance carrier, even if hired again by a new employer. Sometimes employed spouses stay locked into jobs they do not want in order to keep the patient insured.

The insurance trap exacerbates the psychological morbidity of an already formidable illness. Some patients may conclude that they remain better providers if they stay occupationally disabled and "collect the check." The disincentives to finding meaningful work, even for the patient who can physically accommodate it part-time, create secondary psychological disability, which poses challenges in psychotherapy with these patients.

Rational Treatment Withdrawal and Suicide

Estimates of the suicide rate in dialysis patients have varied, but the rates reported usually are higher than those in the general population or in other chronic illnesses. Patients who are maintained on dialysis because they are not candidates for renal transplantation are considered to be terminally ill. Rational treatment withdrawal now accounts for a segment of all ESRD deaths. It is erroneous, though, to assume that "most" dialysis patients "want to commit suicide" because of the stressors they endure. Rational treatment withdrawal is not synonymous with the active desire to kill oneself by suicide. Suicide is motivated specifically by the wish to die, and it accounts for only a fraction of deaths following rational treatment withdrawal.

> The large majority of people with ESRD do not articulate terminal care wishes, do not speak directly to their families about death, do not discuss this subject with medical staff, and do not complete the legal options available to them. Denial is a powerful coping mechanism for individuals with ESRD, and it is the rare patient who considers discontinuing dialysis or seriously contemplates death. People who receive dialysis are preoccupied not with death but with the ordinary activities of life. (Cohen 2002, p. 560)

Patients who choose treatment withdrawal are a heterogeneous group, including nondepressed individuals who wish to live but who have made a rational decision to terminate medical intervention, as well as those who are depressed and actively want to die (i.e., commit suicide). Psychiatrists may be asked to distinguish between these two groups.

Comment: At what point does denial become "too much," prolonging suffering by fruitless medical interventions? Conversely, when is "too little" denial present, short-circuiting hope before a fair fight has even begun? It is impossible to generalize. Personal comfort of the patient is probably a good benchmark. Reasonableness of expected outcome would be another. An ESRD patient who is expressing the wish to stop treatment may be seeking reassurance or support or may have a treatable psychiatric illness such as depression. It is a clinical pearl of palliative care that many patients feel more optimistic about any medical treatment after their psychiatric illness has been treated and their concerns have been heard. Most suicides among terminally ill patients occur in the setting of clinical depression or impaired judgment. That said, none of the patients who decided to terminate dialysis in a multicenter study at eight dialysis facilities in Canada and the United States were suicidal or irrational (Cohen et al. 2000a, 2000b, 2000c). "Patients had decided that progressive deterioration left them unable to enjoy life further and that dialysis was prolonging suffering rather than prolonging life" (Cohen 2002, p. 560). One operational principle may be helpful: although everyone has to die, and has the right to be sad about dying, no one has to die depressed.

A clinical practice guideline to assist with specific dialysis-related ethics consultations has been issued by the Association of Renal Physicians (Moss et al. 2001). See also the section on advance directives in Chapter 12 of this volume.

■ REFERENCES

Aminoff M: Neurological complications of systemic disease, in Neurology in Clinical Practice, 3rd Edition. Edited by Bradley W, Daroff R, Fenichel G, et al. Boston, MA, Butterworth-Heinemann, 2000, pp 1009–1044

Aronoff G, Berns J, Brier M, et al: Drug Prescribing in Renal Failure: Dosing Guidelines for Adults, 4th Edition. Philadelphia, PA, American College of Physicians, 1999

Asconape J: Some common issues in the use of antiepileptic drugs. Semin Nephrol 22:27–39, 2002

Baines L, Jindal R: Loss of the imagined past: an emotional obstacle to medical compliance in kidney transplant recipients. Prog Transplant 12:305–308, 2002

Becker M, Maiman L: Sociobehavioral determinants of compliance with health and medical care recommendations. Med Care 13:10–24, 1975

Bendz H, Aurell M, Lanke J: A historical cohort study of kidney damage in long-term lithium patients: continued surveillance needed. Eur Psychiatry 16:199–206, 2001

Bremer BA, Wert KM, Durica AL, et al: Neuropsychological, physical, and psychosocial functioning of individuals with end-stage renal disease. Ann Behav Med 19:348–352, 1998

Camsari T, Cavdar C, Yemez B, et al: Psychosexual function in CAPD and hemodialysis patients. Perit Dial Int 19:585–588, 1999

Christensen A, Moran P, Wiebe J, et al: Effect of a behavioral self-regulation intervention on patient adherence in hemodialysis. Health Psychol 21:393–397, 2002

Cohen L: Renal disease, in The American Psychiatric Publishing Textbook of Consultation-Liaison Psychiatry: Psychiatry in the Medically Ill, 2nd Edition. Edited by Wise MG, Rundell JR. Washington, DC, American Psychiatric Publishing, 2002, pp 557–562

Cohen L, Germain M, Poppel D, et al: Dialysis discontinuation and palliative care. Am J Kidney Dis 36:140–144, 2000a

Cohen L, Germain M, Poppel D, et al: Dying well after discontinuing the life-support treatment of dialysis. Arch Intern Med 160:2513–2518, 2000b

Cohen L, Steinberg M, Hails K, et al: The psychiatric evaluation of death-hastening requests: lessons from dialysis-discontinuation. Psychosomatics 41:195–203 (commentary: pp 193–194), 2000c

Cohen L, Tessier E, Germain M, et al: Update on psychotropic medication use in renal disease. Psychosomatics 45:34-48, 2004

Daneker B, Kimmel PL, Ranich T, et al: Depression and marital dissatisfaction in patients with end-stage renal disease and in their spouses. Am J Kidney Dis 38:839–846, 2001

DasGupta K, Jefferson J: Treatment of mania in the medically ill, in Psychotropic Drug Use in the Medically Ill (Advances in Psychosomatic Medicine, Vol 21). Edited by Silver P. New York, Karger, 1994, pp 138–162

Devins G, Mandin H, Hons R, et al: Illness intrusiveness and quality of life in end-stage renal disease: comparison and stability across treatment modalities. Health Psychol 9:117–142, 1990

DiMatteo MR, Lepper HS, Croghan TW: Depression is a risk factor for noncompliance with medical treatment: meta-analysis of the effects of anxiety and depression on patient adherence. Arch Intern Med 160:2101–2107, 2000

Eitel P, Friend R, Griffin K, et al: Cognitive control and consistency in compliance. Psychol Health 13:953–973, 2000

Evans R, Rader B, Manninen D, et al: The quality of life of hemodialysis recipients treated with recombinant human erythropoietin. JAMA 263:825–830, 1990

Fargnoli D: Symbolic equations and impotence in uremia, in Psychological and Physiological Aspects of Chronic Renal Failure (Contributions to Nephrology, Vol 77). Edited by D'Amico G, Colasanti G. Basel, Switzerland, Karger, 1990, pp 56–64

Fujisawa M, Ichikawa Y, Yoshiya K, et al: Assessment of health-related quality of life in renal transplant and hemodialysis patients using the SF-36 health survey. Urology 56:201–206, 2000

Gitlin M: Lithium and the kidney: an updated review. Drug Saf 20:231–243, 1999

House A: Psychosocial problems of patients on the renal unit and their relation to treatment outcome. J Psychosom Res 31:441–452, 1987

Johnson G: Lithium: early development, toxicity, and renal function. Neuropsychopharmacology 19:200–205, 1998

Kaveh K, Kimmel PL: Compliance in hemodialysis patients: multidimensional measures in search of a gold standard. Am J Kidney Dis 37:244–266, 2001

Kimmel PL: Psychosocial factors in adult end-stage renal disease patients treated with hemodialysis: correlates and outcomes. Am J Kidney Dis 35:S132–140, 2000

Kimmel PL: Psychosocial factors in dialysis patients. Kidney Int 59:1599–1613, 2001

Kimmel PL, Peterson RA, Weihs KL, et al: Psychosocial factors, behavioral compliance and survival in urban hemodialysis patients. Kidney Int 54:245–254, 1998a

Kimmel PL, Thamer M, Richard CM, et al: Psychiatric illness in patients with end-stage renal disease. Am J Med 105:214–221, 1998b

Kimmel PL, Peterson RA, Weihs KL, et al: Multiple measurements of depression predict mortality in a longitudinal study of chronic hemodialysis outpatients. Kidney Int 57:2093–2098, 2000

Kovac JA, Patel SS, Peterson RA, et al: Patient satisfaction with care and behavioral compliance in end-stage renal disease patients treated with hemodialysis. Am J Kidney Dis 39:1236–1244, 2002

Krawczyk J, Raskin V: Psychological distress related to sexual abuse in a patient undergoing hemodialysis. Am J Psychiatry 147:673–674, 1990

Levy NB: Psychiatric considerations in the primary medical care of the patient with renal failure. Adv Ren Replace Ther 7:231–238, 2000

Levy NB, Cohen L: End-stage renal disease and its treatment, in Psychiatric Care of the Medical Patient. Edited by Stoudemire A, Fogel B, Greenberg D. New York, Oxford University Press, 2000, pp 791–799

Lockwood A: Toxic and metabolic encephalopathies, in Neurology in Clinical Practice, 3rd Edition. Edited by Bradley W, Daroff R, Fenichel G, et al. Boston, MA, Butterworth-Heinemann, 2000, pp 1475–1493

Martis C, et al: Que peut espérer la nephrologie de la psycha-nalyse? ou La rencontre "du discours médical" et "du discours psychanalytique" [What can nephrology hope from psychoanalysis? or The meeting of medical language with psychoanalytic language] (French). Psychologie-Médicale 20:1835–1838, 1988

McMahon LP, Mason K, Skinner SL, et al: Effects of haemoglobin normalization on quality of life and cardiovascular parameters in end-stage renal failure. Nephrol Dial Transplant 15:1425–1430, 2000

Moss A, Association of Renal Physicians, The American Society of Nephrology Working Group: Shared Decision Making in dialysis: a new clinical practice guideline to assist with dialysis-related ethics consultations. J Clin Ethics 12:406–414, 2001

Perard D: La grand-mère machine-vampire de Marie-Sophie [Marie-Sophie's machine-vampire grandmother]. Perspectives-Psychiatriques 23:386–397, 1985

Perlis RH, Sachs GS, Lafer B, et al: Effect of abrupt change from standard to low serum levels of lithium: a reanalysis of double-blind lithium maintenance data. Am J Psychiatry 159:1155–1159, 2002

Sabbatini M, Minale B, Crispo A, et al: Insomnia in maintenance haemodialysis patients. Nephrol Dial Transplant 17:852–856, 2002

Schou M: Lithium treatment at 52. J Affect Disord 67:21–32, 2001

Shidler NR, Peterson RA, Kimmel PL: Quality of life and psychosocial relationships in patients with chronic renal insufficiency. Am J Kidney Dis 32:557–566, 1998

Springer J: Restless legs syndrome: a common disorder in dialysis patients. Journal of Visual Impairment and Blindness 95:491–493, 2000

van Manen JG, Korevaar JC, Dekker FW, et al: Changes in employment status in end-stage renal disease patients during their first year of dialysis. Perit Dial Int 21:595–601, 2001

Wilson K: Mania associated with dialysis: a literature review and new patient report. Psychosomatics 39:543–546, 2000

Wuerth D, Finkelstein SH, Ciarcia J, et al: Identification and treatment of depression in a cohort of patients maintained on chronic peritoneal dialysis. Am J Kidney Dis 37:1011–1017, 2001

Wyszynski A, Wyszynski B: A Case Approach to Medical-Psychiatric Practice. Washington, DC, American Psychiatric Press, 1996

The Patient With Pulmonary Disease

Antoinette Ambrosino Wyszynski, M.D.
Elyse D. Weiner, M.D.

Asthma is defined as a disease of airways that is characterized by increased tracheobronchial responsivity to many stimuli, causing widespread narrowing of the air passages. *Chronic obstructive pulmonary disease* (COPD) is a condition in which there is chronic obstruction of airflow, despite periods of improvement, due to chronic bronchitis and/or emphysema. Both illnesses are increasing in prevalence, creating a population of chronically ill, often psychiatrically distressed individuals. The treatment of the psychiatric issues that arise in both conditions is relatively uncomplicated: avoid benzodiazepines, use selective serotonin reuptake inhibitors (SSRIs) for depressive and anxiety states, and try atypical antipsychotics carefully because there are not yet enough accumulated data on their use. Brief medical updates on asthma and COPD precede the discussion of psychiatric issues.

■ MEDICAL UPDATE ON ASTHMA

As many as 10–15 million individuals in the United States have asthma. The prevalence, morbidity, and mortality of asthma in the United States and other Western countries have dramatically increased during the past two decades (Gathchel and Oordt 2003). More than 5,000 people die from asthma each year. Asthma ranks as the most common chronic disease among children, and it is one of the leading causes of admission to pediatric hospitals. Many primary care physicians now view asthma from a biopsychosocial perspective and develop multidisciplinary treatment plans that attend to psychological factors (such as anxiety and depression) and environmental factors (such as smoking or living in an inner-city environment).

Asthma is characterized by increased tracheobronchial responsivity that causes widespread narrowing of the air passages. The patient experiences paroxysms of dyspnea, coughing, and wheezing. It is an episodic disease, with acute exacerbations interspersed with symptom-free periods. The pathophysiology of asthma involves narrowing of airway diameter caused by smooth muscle contraction, vascular congestion, bronchial wall edema, and thick, tenacious secretions. The net result is an increase in the work of breathing as airway resistance increases, causing decreased forced

Wyszynski AA, Wyszynski B (eds.): *Manual of Psychiatric Care for the Medically Ill.* Washington, D.C., American Psychiatric Publishing, Inc., 2005

expiratory volume (FEV) and flow rate, hyperinflation of the lungs and thorax, and numerous other changes. Although asthma is defined as an "airways disease," an asthmatic attack compromises almost all aspects of pulmonary function. In persons severely ill with asthma, there frequently is electrocardiographic evidence of right ventricular hypertrophy and pulmonary hypertension.

The mortality rate from asthma is relatively low: fewer than 5,000 deaths per year out of a population of approximately 10 million patients at risk. Inner-city death rates appear to be rising, perhaps because of limited availability of health care. There is generally a good prognosis, particularly for individuals with asthma whose disease is mild and develops in childhood. (Exceptions include patients with comorbid problems, such as cigarette smoking.)

Asthma is a disease characterized by exacerbations and remissions, rather than by a progressive downhill course. Spontaneous remissions occur in approximately 20% of adult-onset asthma cases, and about 40% of patients experience improvement, with less frequent and severe attacks, as they grow older (McFadden 2003).

There are two main types of asthma: allergic asthma and idiosyncratic asthma. The following are their key features.

Allergic Asthma

- The most common type of asthma; atopy is the largest risk factor for its development.
- Occurs most often in children and young adults.
- Patients have a personal and/or family history of allergic diseases such as rhinitis, urticaria, and eczema.
- Intradermal injection of extracts from airborne antigens produces positive wheal-and-flare skin reactions. Levels of serum immunoglobulin E (IgE) are increased. Provocation tests involving the inhalation of specific antigen are positive.
- Physical precipitants include environmental irritants or allergens, exercise, and infection. There is often a seasonal pattern.
- A nonseasonal form may result from allergy to feathers, animal danders, dust mites, molds, and other environmental antigens.

Idiosyncratic Asthma

- No personal or family history of allergy.
- Negative skin tests.

- Normal serum levels of IgE, so the disease cannot be classified on the basis of defined immunological mechanisms.
- Precipitants for the cycle may be as benign as the common cold, causing paroxysms of wheezing and dyspnea.
- Episodes may persist for several months.

Emotional Precipitants of Asthmatic Attacks

Individuals with asthma have a higher incidence of anxiety and depressive disorders compared to the general population. In addition, psychological and emotional issues strongly affect the course of life-threatening asthma. Stress, anxiety, depression, and suggestion affect asthmatic episodes; emotional precipitants of asthmatic attacks rival allergic factors and infection. Psychological stimuli, such as suggestion, induce asthmatic attacks *independently* of age, gender, asthma severity, atopy, or method of pulmonary assessment. Anxiety may precipitate dyspnea, and dyspnea in turn induces more anxiety, creating a cycle that potentially interferes with medical and psychiatric interventions.

Vagal efferent activity, and perhaps endorphins, seem to mediate changes in airway caliber. Suggestion has been the most frequently studied psychological variable. When vulnerable individuals are given the appropriate suggestion, they can actually induce variations in the pharmacological effects of adrenergic and cholinergic stimuli on their airways. The medical illness and the psychological state mutually potentiate each other. Behavioral factors also may produce differences in outcome, such as variable adherence to the medical regimen, changeable exposure to asthma triggers, and variable accuracy of asthma symptom perception (Lehrer et al. 2002).

Treatment of Asthma

The most successful treatment for allergic asthma is to *eliminate the causative agent* from the environment. Medication management of asthma is complicated, with many potential drug-drug interactions. Certain medications used in treating asthma—catecholamines, anticholinergics, and steroids—have known neuropsychiatric side effects. There are two general categories of medications (see Box 5–1): bronchodilators, which inhibit smooth muscle contraction for rapid relief of symptoms, and anti-inflammatory agents, which prevent and/or reverse inflammation for long-term control of asthma.

Box 5–1. Medications used to treat asthma and chronic obstructive pulmonary disease

Bronchodilators (drugs that inhibit smooth muscle contraction)
- Theophylline: associated with *anxiety,* especially at blood levels >20 μg/mL
- Catecholamines (epinephrine, isoproterenol, and isoetharine)
- Anticholinergics (atropine methylnitrate, ipratropium bromide)
- Other β-adrenergic agonists (metaproterenol, terbutaline, fenoterol, albuterol): linked with tachycardia-associated *anxiety*

Anti-inflammatory agents
- Steroids, systemic (prednisone): associated with *anxiety, depression, mania, delirium*
- Steroids, inhaled (beclomethasone, budesonide, flunisolide, fluticasone propionate, and triamcinolone acetonide): psychiatric side effects uncommon
- Mast cell–stabilizing agents (cromolyn sodium and nedocromil sodium)
- Leukotriene modifiers (e.g., zileuton): inhibit synthesis of enzymes involved in the production of the cysteinyl leukotrienes, which induce asthma

---

Patient education includes basic medical facts, information about medicines relevant to asthma, and techniques for using inhalers and avoiding allergens. Patients are encouraged to devise a daily self-management plan that includes an asthma diary to encourage self-monitoring.

Psychological interventions for asthma include education, psychotherapy, hypnosis, yoga, written emotional-expression exercises, relaxation training, and biofeedback techniques. A comprehensive review in 2003 found that differences in efficacy among psychological treatment modalities were ambiguous (Schmaling et al. 2003).

■ MEDICAL UPDATE ON COPD

Chronic obstructive pulmonary disease is characterized by reduced maximal expiratory flow during forced exhalation. COPD includes two distinct processes, emphysema and chronic bronchitis, although most often they present in combination. COPD may coexist with asthma, and sometimes the two are difficult to distinguish from each other. In COPD, unlike asthma, the clinical course is progressive.

COPD develops from an inflammatory process in the airways and distal airspaces. Oxidative stress is thought to produce the inflammation of COPD. The term refers to the increased activity of oxidants combined with decreased activity of antioxidants. For example, cigarette smoke produces high concentrations of oxygen free radicals. Experimental evidence suggests that prolonged cigarette smoking impairs respiratory epithelial ciliary movement, inhibits function of alveolar macrophages, and leads to hypertrophy and hyperplasia of mucus-secreting glands. COPD rarely occurs in nonsmokers. Usually patients are in their 50s, have been smoking one pack of cigarettes per day for at least 20 years, and have presented to their internist with a productive cough or acute chest illness. Exertional dyspnea does not usually occur until the patient is 60–70 years of age (Honig and Ingram 2002).

Although 90% of all COPD patients are current or former tobacco smokers, only 15%–20% of smokers lose FEV_1 (forced expiratory volume in 1 second) at a rate fast enough to manifest COPD. Familial clustering of COPD cases strongly suggests a genetic susceptibility to the effects of tobacco smoke. Twin studies show that even after controlling for active and passive smoking, FEV_1 correlates more closely in monozygotic than dizygotic twins (Honig and Ingram 2003).

In normal individuals, FEV_1 normally reaches a lifetime peak at age 25 and then undergoes a linear decline. Annual loss of FEV_1 is accelerated among susceptible individuals who develop COPD, and the loss is hastened by mucus hypersecretion. Acute exacerbations of COPD do not alter the rate of decline.

"Smoker's cough" occurs frequently early in the disease and becomes purulent only during exacerbations. As COPD progresses, exacerbations become both more frequent and more severe. The patient experiences progressive dyspnea and decreased exercise tolerance. As hypoxemia worsens, erythrocytosis and cyanosis may occur. *Morning headache often signals the onset of significant CO_2 retention.* Weight loss occurs in advanced disease and correlates with an adverse prognosis. Cor pulmonale occurs with severe blood gas derangements and is accompanied by peripheral edema and water retention. Anxiety, depression, and sleep disturbances are frequent psychiatric complications.

■ MOOD, SUBJECTIVE DYSPNEA, AND OBJECTIVE PULMONARY FUNCTION

Breathlessness may seem like an inappropriate reason for a psychiatric consultation in an asthmatic or COPD patient. However, research has shown dyspnea to be highly subjective and to be influenced by a variety of physical and psychological factors, including mood disorders. For example, there is wide variation among individuals in subjective dyspnea corresponding to any given FEV_1.

Several explanations may account for this variability. One is methodological: assessed dyspnea levels will vary within a single patient according to the method of assessment. In addition, emotional and psychiatric factors such as depression are particularly likely to complicate the perception of dyspnea (Rushford et al. 1998). Finally, respiratory and anxiety disorders share dyspnea as a primary symptom, often coexist, and are mutually exacerbating.

The mechanism by which airflow perception is affected by psychiatric disorders remains speculative. Several explanations are possible (Rietveld 1998): psychiatric disorders may create distractibility and disabling emotional symptoms, making concentration difficult and affecting perception; or the overlap between airway symptoms (e.g., shortness of breath) and symptoms of certain psychiatric disorders may obscure the cause.

- *Bottom line:* These data have practical consequences for the psychiatric evaluation of asthmatic and COPD patients. Illness-related disability closely correlates with the *subjective* perception of dyspnea—sometimes more closely than with *objectively* measured pulmonary function. When complaints of dyspnea disproportionately exceed objective measures of respiratory disease, they may indicate a psychiatric condition. Asthma and COPD patients with comorbid mood or anxiety disorders should be assessed for their accuracy in reporting their pulmonary status.

■ THE NEUROPSYCHIATRY OF HYPOXIA

Be sure to *check oxygen saturation* in the workup of mental status changes in COPD patients. Do not assume that it can be surmised from level of consciousness. Clinical myth has flagged alertness as a sensitive indicator of oxygenation, but it has been found that alertness is preserved even in the setting of moderate hypoxemia (Grant et al. 1987). Only extreme hypoxia causes alertness to suffer in an obvious way. Using state of consciousness to estimate a patient's level of oxygenation is of limited value—*hypoxic, cognitively impaired patients may appear perfectly awake.*

The *rate* at which hypoxia develops—rather than the absolute *level* of oxygen saturation—determines the acute neuropsychiatric consequences of hypoxemia (Griggs and Arieff 1992; Lipowski 1990). In the setting of chronic hypoxia, for example, oxygen saturations as low as 60 mm Hg may produce few mental status changes, whereas abrupt declines from higher baselines usually result in delirium (Lipowski 1990).

Nonetheless, even mild hypoxemia produces cognitive changes, such as problems in abstraction, perceptual motor integration, and language function (Fix et al. 1982; Prigatano et al. 1983). One classic study (Grant et al. 1987) revealed that the effects of progressive hypoxemia became most apparent in *perceptual learning* and problem solving (the neuropsychological tests that are most sensitive to cerebral dysfunction). Surprisingly, other measures of disease severity, such as pulmonary function tests, did not closely predict the levels of neuropsychological deficits. At the same time, the degree of hypoxemia was not always congruent with the extent of lung disease as measured by pulmonary function tests; for example, some patients showed advanced lung disease who were only mildly hypoxemic.

These data suggest that neuropsychological abilities decline differentially in chronic lung disease. Elderly patients with chronic respiratory disease are particularly susceptible.

■ HYPERCAPNIA

The changes produced by CO_2 retention resemble barbiturate intoxication. *Acute* increases of PCO_2 to 70 mm Hg usually produce confusional states; in *chronic* hypercapnia, however, alertness is preserved (Lipowski 1990).

■ DELIRIUM

Risk factors for delirium in COPD and asthma include hypoxia, hypercapnia, and medications (particularly antibiotics, systemic steroids, and antiviral medications). Sudden changes in mental status examination ratings should trigger a workup for etiology (see Appendix 4, "'VINDICTIVE MADS,'" and Chapter 1, "The Delirious Patient," in this volume).

ANXIETY DISORDERS IN PATIENTS WITH LUNG DISEASE

There is a well-documented relationship between respiratory disease and anxiety disorders. Recent studies have supported the high incidence of anxiety disorders, particularly panic/agoraphobic spectrum disorders, in asthma patients compared with the general population (Goodwin et al. 2003; Nascimento et al. 2002). There is symptomatic overlap between acute asthmatic episodes and those panic/agoraphobic spectrum disorders having prominent respiratory symptoms (i.e., breathlessness, choking, smothering sensations, chest pain). Distinguishing between asthma and anxiety is crucial. When a panic attack is confused with an asthmatic crisis, antiasthmatic drugs may be inappropriately prescribed. These medications are known to worsen anxiety and potentially induce more panic attacks (Pohl et al. 1990); they include theophylline (especially at blood levels >20 µg/mL), bronchodilators, and systemic steroids.

Several hypotheses may explain the high comorbidity between respiratory disease and anxiety disorders (Carr 1998; Perna et al. 1997; Verburg et al. 1995). First, there may be a subset of vulnerable asthmatic patients with a neurophysiologic or neuroanatomic diathesis to panic attacks. Respiratory dysfunction may trigger panic attacks in predisposed individuals by stimulating the locus coeruleus and/or central chemoreceptors hypersensitive to PCO_2. For example, hyperventilation and hypersensitivity to carbon dioxide occur in patients with respiratory disease and in those with panic disorder (Gorman et al. 1988). CO_2 rebreathing, lactic acid infusion, or hyperventilation can induce panic attacks. A similar mechanism might operate in patients with chronic airway obstruction, in which hyperventilation occurs in response to a chronically elevated PCO_2 level.

A second hypothesis is that medications used to treat respiratory illnesses (e.g., theophylline, anticholinergics, β_2-agonist bronchodilators, and steroids either in administration or withdrawal) may induce anxiety symptoms that are indistinguishable from primary anxiety disorders.

A third possibility is that the somatic symptoms associated with respiratory disease could exacerbate catastrophic cognitions and panic attacks in patients vulnerable to anxiety (Clark 1986); the cognitive-

behavioral model of panic disorder would support this hypothesis.

Fourth, patients with advanced lung disease have high rates of functional disability, poorer quality of life, and lower self-esteem. Life domains such as work, social interaction, and sexual intimacy are affected (Wingate and Hansen-Flaschen 1997). These stressors would plausibly place the patient at risk for anxiety and depressive disorders.

Treatment of Anxiety Disorders

Benzodiazepines

Because of their respiratory depressant properties, benzodiazepines are the psychotropics that pose the most problems for patients with pulmonary disease.

Increased PCO_2 normally drives breathing. Many COPD patients are chronically hypercapnic and lose their sensitivity to increased PCO_2. As a result, their drive to breathe becomes more dependent on low oxygen saturation (hypoxia) than on PCO_2. Benzodiazepines can blunt the ventilatory response to hypoxia, thereby inducing more hypercapnia. Thus, these medications may initiate a dangerous cycle: chronically increased PCO_2 leads to further *dependence* on hypoxia to drive breathing; but in the setting of benzodiazepine-induced diminished *sensitivity* to hypoxia, there results further CO_2 retention. If this process occurs in a patient with marginal respiratory reserve, respiratory failure can follow. Patients with moderate to severe COPD are particularly at risk for CO_2 retention with long-acting benzodiazepines such as diazepam (Valium) and chlordiazepoxide (Librium), even at relatively low doses. Respiratory depression gradually worsens as active metabolites accumulate, with the potential for significant benzodiazepine-induced CO_2 retention.

Many patients with chronic respiratory disease suffer sleep apnea—a relative contraindication to benzodiazepines.

For short-term treatment of acute anxiety in the setting of COPD, lorazepam is the benzodiazepine of choice (Fait et al. 2002; Greenberg and Kradin 2002; Thompson 2000). It may be administered orally, intramuscularly, or intravenously, and it has no active metabolites. Medical clearance should be obtained prior to prescribing it, however.

Alternatives to Benzodiazepines

The SSRI antidepressants or buspirone (BuSpar) are preferred over lorazepam for patients with chronic anxiety and lung disease.

The antihistamines, such as hydroxyzine (Vistaril, Atarax) and diphenhydramine (Benadryl), do not cause respiratory depression, but they may not be sufficiently effective for the severely anxious, dyspneic patient. β-Blockers like propranolol are contraindicated for anxiolysis because they cause bronchoconstriction. Sedative-hypnotics and barbiturates (e.g., amobarbital sodium) have significant respiratory depressant effects and should be avoided.

Antipsychotics.   There are times when pulmonary patients are incapacitated by panic about suffocating, and at such times dyspnea and psychological state reciprocally worsen. Although a benzodiazepine may be the most effective psychotropic, concerns about respiratory depression may supervene. In these situations, the anxiolytic effects of a sedating neuroleptic may be helpful. None causes respiratory depression.

Among the conventional antipsychotics, haloperidol (Haldol) has a long safety record in medical patients. Dystonic effects on respiration are rare. The phenothiazines have anticholinergic properties, so they may adversely affect the respiratory system by drying secretions. Tardive dyskinesia constitutes a risk in long-term treatment with all traditional neuroleptics, so these agents should be used only as a brief intervention.

Atypical antipsychotics that possess novel receptor binding profiles may prove to be useful alternatives to anxiolytics for patients with COPD. Generally, olanzapine (Zyprexa) is considered a safe drug in pulmonary patients, and it has sedative properties. It should be used with caution in patients with risk factors for diabetes or cardiovascular disease (see Chapter 3 in this volume, "The Patient With Cardiovascular Disease," pp. 61–62). There is one case report of an elderly patient with chronic lung disease who developed CO_2 narcosis and respiratory failure after treatment with olanzapine and rechallenge (Mouallem and Wolf 2001). It was unclear how olanzapine's general sedative effects could have translated into respiratory depression in this patient.

- Recent data suggest that ziprasidone (Geodon) may have antianxiety efficacy, as it is both a serotonin 5-HT_{1A} agonist and a norepinephrine antagonist. This concept was studied by comparing a 20-mg oral dose of ziprasidone versus 10 mg of diazepam versus placebo in nonpsychotic volunteers undergoing minor dental surgery. The investigators found that ziprasidone had a peak anxiolytic effect comparable to that of diazepam but had a later on-

set of action, approximately at 3 hours (compared with 1–1.5 hours for diazepam). The only adverse event related to treatment was nausea and vomiting in one subject (Wilner et al. 2002).

- Clozapine (Clozaril) has been associated with allergic asthma as well as respiratory arrest. This medication should be used with careful respiratory monitoring.

- Although no reports were available on risperidone (Risperdal) or quetiapine (Seroquel) specifically in this setting, these medications are generally well tolerated in medical patients. There are not enough data to comment on the safety of aripiprazole (Abilify) for patients with lung disease.

An unexpected possible consequence of a neuroleptic prescription is that the medical staff may infer that the patient has been psychotic. Therefore, the rationale for starting an antipsychotic for anxiolysis should be documented clearly in the patient's chart.

■ A WORD ON ALLERGIES AND PSYCHOTROPICS

In certain individuals with high associated morbidity, medications may induce bronchial narrowing and acute asthmatic episodes. The most common offenders are aspirin, coloring agents such as tartrazine, β-adrenergic antagonists, and sulfiting agents. Tartrazine (FD&C Yellow #5), a dye contained in several psychotropic drugs, can provoke severe bronchospasm for up to several hours after ingestion. Susceptible individuals may have a history of sensitivity to aspirin and bronchospasm from foods colored yellow or orange, such as soft drinks or candy. Fortunately, only a small percentage of asthmatic patients respond with severe exacerbations, and pharmaceutical companies have been phasing out tartrazine.

■ COMPLICATIONS OF END-STAGE PULMONARY DISEASE THAT HAVE RELEVANCE FOR PSYCHOPHARMACOLOGY

- *Renal dysfunction.* Chronic hypoxemia and hypercapnia have been shown to cause increased circulating levels of norepinephrine, renin, and aldosterone and decreased levels of antidiuretic hormone. This effect results in defective excretion of salt and water loads. Dose adjustments are necessary for renally metabolized psychotropics such as lithium or gabapentin (Neurontin).

- *Congestive heart failure* secondary to right ventricular dysfunction. In patients with advanced COPD, use caution if administering psychotropic medications that are known to have cardiovascular side effects (e.g., tricyclic antidepressants or phenothiazines).
- *Cachexia and muscle wasting* in advanced COPD. These patients are medically fragile; "start low, go slow."
- *Osteoporosis,* particularly in patients receiving chronic steroid therapy. These patients are prone to fractures. Be cautious about sedating them; sedation predisposes to falls.

Patients with chronic respiratory disease often have several specialists who participate in their care. Box 5–2 lists suggestions on how to coordinate the care of COPD patients who develop psychiatric comorbidity.

■ MAJOR DEPRESSION IN PATIENTS WITH LUNG DISEASE

Depression is common among lung disease patients; the estimated comorbidity of COPD and depression exceeds 20% (Borson et al. 1992). There are challenges in diagnosing depression in this population:

- Medication side effects, such as fluctuations in exogenous corticosteroid levels, create secondary mood problems.
- Symptoms of chronic respiratory disease overlap with symptoms of depression, such as fatigue, lethargy, and loss of interest in activities. For assessing depression, vegetative symptoms are less useful than quality of mood and thought content.

Appendix 15 discusses strategies useful for diagnosing depression in medically ill patients.

Treatment of Major Depression

Many pulmonary patients are elderly and have multisystem disease. For this reason, it is important to choose an antidepressant that minimizes side effects like hypotension and cardiotoxicity. Any medication with anticholinergic effects may promote drying of bronchial secretions, making them more tenacious and promoting bronchial plugging. SSRIs remain the primary treatment for depression in pulmonary disease, as in most medical illnesses. Except for occasional reports of idiosyncratic reactions (de Kerviler et al. 1996; Fleisch et al. 2000; Gonzalez-Rothi et al. 1995), these medications are safe to use in the setting of lung disease.

Box 5–2. **Psychiatric comorbidities and COPD: keys to coordinating care**

Communication with other care team members is crucial to psychiatric treatment of patients with COPD. To ensure the proper coordination of care:

- **Medication history:**
  Report changes in psychiatric medication to all doctors.
  Obtain from the primary care physician a complete list of the patient's medications and medical problems to prevent drug-drug interactions.

- **Onset of depression, anxiety:**
  Report warning signs of depression and anxiety to other care team members, and urge doctors to refer patients who exhibit these signs. Primary care physicians often miss these potential warning signs:

  - Weight loss
  - Nonadherence with treatment
  - Irritability, hostility

  - Declining hygiene
  - Talk about death, hopelessness
  - Increased benzodiazepine use

- **Suicidality:**
  Alert other doctors to the warning signs of suicidality. Patients older than 65 and those with depression or chronic health problems are at increased risk of suicide. Risk factors:

  - Talk about being a burden to one's family
  - Severe hopelessness and worthlessness

  - Guns in the home
  - Giving away one's possessions

Note. COPD=chronic obstructive pulmonary disease.
Source. Reprinted from Cantor L, Jacobson R: "COPD: How to Manage Comorbid Depression and Anxiety." *Current Psychiatry* 2:45–54, 2003. Used with permission of the publisher, Dowden Health Media.

Before SSRIs came into use, many studies established the efficacy and safety in COPD patients of the tricyclic antidepressants (TCAs), particularly nortriptyline (Pamelor, Aventyl). Nortriptyline tends to produce fewer problems with hypotension and anticholinergic side effects than other TCAs. It should be started at low doses and carefully titrated upward. Note that the TCAs have more adverse drug-drug interactions than the SSRIs. For example, TCAs potentiate the anticholinergic effects of the bronchodilator atropine, as well as the pressor effects of epinephrine. It is usually safe to use TCAs with the more selective β_2-agonist bronchodilators, such as metaproterenol and albuterol.

Monoamine oxidase inhibitors (MAOIs) should be avoided because they intensify and prolong the effects of agents such as epinephrine, antihistamines, and anticholinergic agents. MAOIs are contraindicated with numerous agents, including sympathomimetic medications.

Electroconvulsive Therapy (ECT)

There are case reports of patients who received theophylline for pulmonary conditions and experienced status epilepticus during ECT. In contrast, in seven patients on theophylline, Rasmussen and Zorumski (1993) reported safe and effective administration of ECT. However, it is prudent to taper theophylline whenever possible before ECT, withhold the morning dose, and closely monitor blood levels (Datto et al. 2002).

Drug-Drug Interactions

Certain drug-drug interactions are particularly relevant to combinations of COPD/asthma and psychiatric medications (Cozza et al. 2003), as displayed in Table 5–1.

- *Theophylline* is primarily metabolized by the 1A2 system; therefore, potent inhibitors of this enzyme system can potentially cause elevations in theophylline levels and psychiatric symptomatology. Fluvoxamine (Luvox) has been shown to be a "potent inhibitor" of the 1A2 system in human liver microsomes, and there are several reports of its causing toxic theophylline serum concentrations (Diot et al. 1991; Rasmussen et al. 1995; van den Brekel and Harrington 1994).
- *Prednisone*, often used in asthma exacerbations, is an inducer of the P450 cytochrome 3A4 subtype. This subtype is involved in the metabolism of many psychiatric medications, including a host of antidepressants, antipsychotics, benzodiazepines, mood stabilizers, and methadone, potentially lowering levels or effective doses of these drugs (Cozza et al. 2003). Clinical relevance may be limited, however, as no reports of this interaction were found.

Table 5–1. Drug-drug interactions: selected psychotropics and COPD medications

Psychotropic	Potential interactions
Alprazolam (Xanax)	Itraconazole (Sporanox), fluconazole (Diflucan), cimetidine (Tagamet): increase alprazolam levels
Bupropion (Wellbutrin, Zyban)	Lowers seizure threshold, so use cautiously with other drugs having similar potential (e.g., theophylline) May increase adverse effects of levodopa, amantadine (Symmetrel)
Buspirone (BuSpar)	Erythromycin, itraconazole: increase buspirone levels
Diazepam (Valium), lorazepam (Ativan)	Theophylline may decrease serum levels of these drugs
Fluoxetine (Prozac)	May increase prothrombin time and INR if taken with warfarin (Coumadin)
Nefazodone (Serzone)	Could increase atorvastatin, simvastatin levels
Paroxetine (Paxil)	May interact with warfarin Cimetidine increases paroxetine levels Reports of increased theophylline levels
Risperidone (Risperdal)	Metabolized by 2D6 enzyme; potential exists for interactions, but none reported
Valproic acid (Depakote, Depakene)	May increase prothrombin time and INR in patients taking warfarin

Note. COPD=chronic obstructive pulmonary disease; INR=international normalized ratio (a standardized measurement of warfarin therapy effectiveness).
Source. Adapted from Cantor L, Jacobson R: "COPD: How to Manage Comorbid Depression and Anxiety." *Current Psychiatry* 2:45–54, 2003. Used with permission of the publisher, Dowden Health Media.

- *Chronic smoking,* often an active problem in COPD patients, induces the 1A2 subtype. Theophylline clearance is increased, and its half-life decreased, almost twofold in this interaction (Zevin and Benowitz 1999). When smokers on theophylline are admitted to the hospital, the theophylline dose should be adjusted, because once they stop smoking as inpatients, theophylline clearance will fall by 35% within a week.

In addition to Cozza et al. (2003), useful Web sites for help with P450 interactions can be found at http://www.Drug-Interactions.com and http://mhc.com/Cytochromes (accessed June 2004).

■ MEDICAL UPDATE ON SLEEP PROBLEMS IN COPD

Sleep produces the following respiratory changes, even in those without lung disease (McNicholas 2002):

- Diminished responsiveness of the respiratory center to chemical, mechanical, and cortical inputs, particularly during rapid eye movement (REM) sleep
- Diminished responsiveness of the respiratory muscles (accessory muscles more affected than diaphragm) to respiratory center outputs, particularly during REM sleep
- Ventilatory decrements during non-REM sleep and greater decrements during REM sleep, mainly because of reduced tidal volume
- Circadian changes in airway caliber, with mild nocturnal bronchoconstriction—an effect that is exaggerated among asthmatic patients

Normal subjects do not experience clinically significant deterioration in pulmonary function. In those with COPD and other types of chronic lung disease, these changes can be dangerous, producing episodes of hypoxemia, particularly during REM sleep (Braghiroli and Alvarez-Sala 2002; Krahn and Richardson 2000). COPD patients are burdened by two additional changes:

- Sleep quality disturbances (↓ slow wave and REM sleep, as well as ↑ arousals). These disruptions contribute to the chronic fatigue and lethargy that further undermine quality of life in COPD patients.
- Sleep-related hypoxemia and hypercapnia (see left column, "Primary Events," in Figure 5–1). Normal sleep-related hypoventilation, particularly during REM sleep, produces nocturnal hypoxemia in COPD. Patients with COPD are particularly likely to die at night, especially if they are hypoxemic at baseline.

People with asthma often experience episodes of nocturnal and early-morning awakening, difficulty in maintaining sleep, and daytime sleepiness (Bohadana et al. 2002). Asthma tends to destabilize and worsen at night, probably because of a nocturnal increase in airway inflammation and bronchial responsiveness. Sleep fragmentation with frequent nighttime awakenings may arise secondary to nocturnal asthma attacks, anti-asthma medications, and diurnal variation of airway flow rates (usually, valleys occur at 4:00 P.M. and 4:00 A.M.) (Weilburg and Winkelman 2002).

For reviews of sleep disorders in the medically ill, see Weilburg and Winkelman (2002) and Krahn and Richardson (2000). More general discussions are by Kryger et al. (2000) and Reite et al. (2002).

Managing Insomnia

COPD patients are more predisposed than healthy individuals to the respiratory depressant effects of even short-acting benzodiazepines. For example, one study found that midazolam (Versed) produced respiratory depression more quickly in COPD patients compared with healthy control subjects (2 and 3.5 minutes, respectively); moreover, COPD patients required twice as long to return to baseline-level pulmonary function (Saidman 1985).

Although there are optimistic case reports on using benzodiazepines in COPD patients, a 2003 comprehensive analysis warned that the duration of most trials using benzodiazepines as hypnotics in COPD was too short to assess impact with long-term use (George and Bayliff 2003). At least two risk factors increase the likelihood of adverse outcome with benzodiazepines: 1) more advanced pulmonary disease and 2) the presence of hypercapnia. Reports on using alternatives such as zolpidem (Ambien) (Girault et al. 1996; Murciano et al. 1993; Steens et al. 1993) and zaleplon (Sonata) (George et al. 1999) show that they are safe and effective in the setting of COPD.

Appendix 13 lists commonly used drugs with sedative-hypnotic properties. See also Box 5–3 for recommendations for managing insomnia in COPD patients.

■ SLEEP APNEA SYNDROME AND COPD: A REVIEW

Sleep apnea is defined as an intermittent cessation of airflow at the nose and mouth during sleep. *Sleep apnea syndrome* refers to a clinical disorder that arises from recurrent apneas during sleep. Patients com-

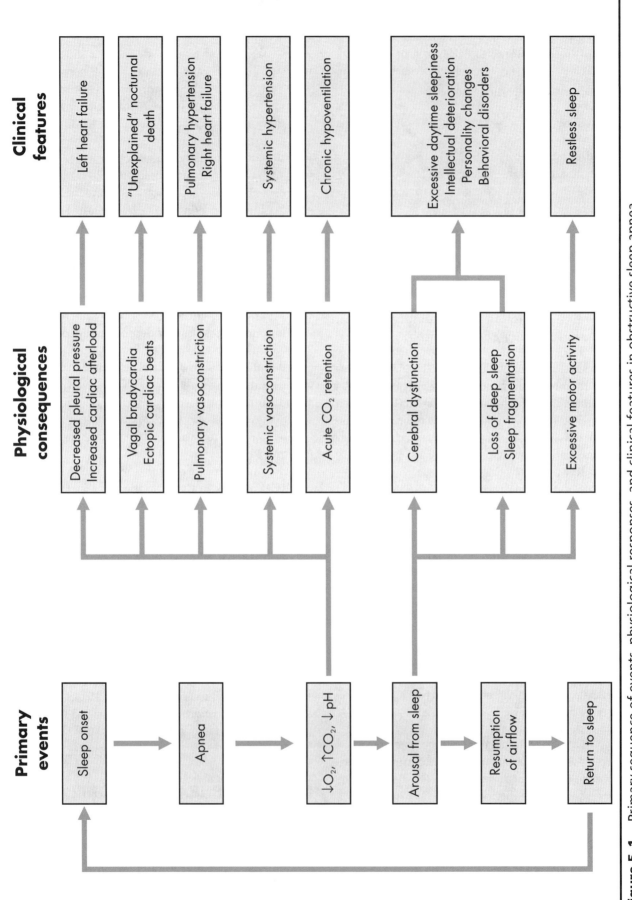

Figure 5–1.   Primary sequence of events, physiological responses, and clinical features in obstructive sleep apnea.

Source.   Phillipson EA: "Sleep Apnea," in *Harrison's Principles of Internal Medicine*, 15th Edition, Chapter 264, p. 1521. New York, McGraw-Hill Medical Publishhing, 2001. Used with permission.

Box 5–3.   **Recommendations for managing insomnia in COPD patients**

1. Identify the specific cause of insomnia.

2. Consult with the pulmonologist to optimize pulmonary health.

3. Screen for drugs known to aggravate insomnia (e.g., theophylline, systemic steroids).

4. Use medications with limited systemic effects (e.g., inhalers).

5. Make behavioral interventions to improve sleep hygiene (e.g., avoid caffeine-containing drinks in the evening, avoid daytime catnaps).

6. Assess baseline pulmonary function and arterial blood gases before prescribing hypnotics.

7. For problems with sleep maintenance, use zolpidem (Ambien) or zaleplon (Sonata). Zaleplon's shorter half-life allows administration within 4 hours of morning awakening without daytime somnolence.

8. Patients with hypercapnia are at heightened risk for respiratory failure with respiratory depressant medications. Options include low-dose tricyclic antidepressants (Hajak et al. 2001; Lin 1993), the cyclic antidepressant trazodone, buspirone (Reite et al. 2002), and sedating atypical antipsychotics (see Appendix 13).

9. Medicate with caution during periods of disease exacerbation. (For patients who have used a benzodiazepine regularly, small, continued doses of the hypnotic may be necessary to avoid withdrawal.)

10. Monitor medicated patients for *confusion, morning somnolence,* or *morning headache* (a possible symptom of CO_2 retention). Monitor for increased dyspnea or increased mucus secretion. Check oxygen saturation. Encourage intermittent use (2–3 times weekly) rather than nightly use of insomnia medications.

Note.   COPD=chronic obstructive pulmonary disease.
Source.   Adapted from data in George and Bayliff 2003.

monly complain of poor sleeping, morning headache, and daytime fatigue and sleepiness. If they are elderly, are in the intensive care unit, or suffer a serious medical illness, the sleep disorder may go unrecognized because it is misattributed to a secondary etiology, such as advanced age, noise, or anxiety (Krahn and Richardson 2000).

Sleep apnea is one of the leading causes of excessive daytime sleepiness. It is estimated to occur in at least 2% of middle-aged women and 4% of middle-aged men (Phillipson 2002). Sleep apnea occurs in a minority of COPD patients (about 10%–15%) (McNicholas 2002). Although higher than would be expected in a normal population, the prevalence of sleep apnea is much lower than other causes of sleep disturbance in COPD patients.

Impaired respiratory drive seems to predispose to sleep apnea. Sleep apnea patients with normal pulmonary function resaturate to normal PO_2 levels in between apneic periods. Sleep apnea patients with COPD typically develop more severe nocturnal hypoxemia; they begin each apneic period already hypoxic. These individuals develop complications of chronic hypoxemia, such as cor pulmonale and polycythemia.

There are two general types of sleep apnea: *obstructive sleep apnea* (OSA) and *central sleep apnea* (CSA).

Obstructive Sleep Apnea

In OSA, respiratory drive remains intact, but airflow is interrupted by occlusion of the oropharyngeal airway. A brief arousal from sleep results, causing a restoration of airway patency and airflow and subsequent return to sleep. This sequence is repeated up to 400–500 times per night, resulting in marked sleep fragmentation. Obesity predisposes to structural compromise of the airway because fat masses in the neck or in soft pharyngeal tissue compress the pharynx (Phillipson 2002). Alcohol exacerbates breathing difficulties by 1) selectively depressing the upper airway muscles and 2) inhibiting the arousal response that terminates each apnea.

Narrowing of the upper airways during sleep predisposes to OSA and results in snoring. Usually, snoring predates the development of OSA. However, most people who snore neither have nor develop OSA. Although snoring alone does not warrant an investigation for OSA, people who snore may benefit from preventive counseling, especially regarding weight gain and alcohol consumption (Phillipson 2002). Figure 5–1 shows the primary sequence of events, physiological responses, and clinical features of obstructive sleep apnea.

Central Sleep Apnea

In CSA, an abnormality in the central drive for respiration, rather than a mechanical obstruction in the upper airway, causes apnea and a sequence of events similar to those of OSA. There are two etiological categories for CSA: 1) defects in the metabolic respiratory control system or respiratory neuromuscular apparatus and 2) transient abnormalities in the central respiratory drive.

Some types of CSA are more easily flagged because they lead to obvious medical complications such as respiratory failure, polycythemia, pulmonary hypertension, and/or right-sided heart failure. Other types of CSA produce mainly sleep-related symptoms: nocturnal awakenings, morning fatigue, and daytime sleepiness. When lung disease and CSA coexist, CSA may be overlooked as a cause of daytime sleepiness and fatigue because the symptoms are attributed to COPD alone. Cardiovascular, central nervous system, and pulmonary pathology are the most common underlying etiologies of CSA.

Diagnosis

Routine sleep studies are not indicated for most COPD patients; the PO_2 level while awake can be used as an index of nocturnal hypoxia. Sleep studies are ordered only if the clinician suspects the sleep apnea syndrome on the basis of medical complications, such as cardiopulmonary failure, neuropsychiatric changes, or systemic hypertension (McNicholas 2002).

The two types of sleep apnea syndrome are associated with similar medical complications. Both are diagnosed and distinguishable on polysomnography, which is an overnight sleep study that includes recording of 1) electrographic variables (electroencephalogram, electrooculogram, and submental electromyogram) that permit the identification of sleep and its various stages, 2) ventilatory variables that identify apneas and classify them as central or obstructive, 3) arterial O_2 saturation by ear or finger oximetry, and 4) heart rate (Phillipson 2002). Continuous measurement of transcutaneous PCO_2 (which reflects arterial PCO_2) also assists in the differential diagnosis of patients with CSA.

The key diagnostic findings in OSA are recurrent apneas (episodes of airflow cessation occurring at the nose and mouth) despite evidence of continuing respiratory effort. The key diagnostic findings in CSA are recurrent apneas that are not accompanied by respiratory effort.

Additional workup may include direct or endoscopic evaluation of the upper airway.

Treatment

There are several approaches to treating OSA and CSA. See Box 5–4 for treatment strategies for sleep apnea syndrome. Benzodiazepines and sedative-hypnotics have been implicated in worsening or precipitating sleep apnea in patients with COPD (Cohn et al. 1992; Guilleminault 1990). These agents should be used with caution.

Box 5–4. **Treatment strategies for sleep apnea syndrome**

Mild to moderate sleep apnea
1. Modest weight reduction (with referral to a nutritionist, when appropriate)
2. Avoidance of nocturnal alcohol (because it reduces activity of the upper airway musculature)
3. Avoidance of the supine position when sleeping
4. Intraoral appliances designed to keep the mandible and tongue forward

Severe sleep apnea
1. Nasal continuous positive airway pressure (CPAP) during sleep
2. Resection of nasal polyps, hypertrophied adenoids, and tonsils
3. Surgery: uvulopalatopharyngoplasty (increases pharyngeal diameter by resecting redundant soft tissue; reserved for CPAP treatment failures); mandibular advancement and hyoid osteotomy; tracheostomy (rarely performed; reserved for treatment failures)

Central sleep apnea
Treatment depends on the underlying etiology.

Source. Adapted from data in Phillipson 2002.

■ **REFERENCES**

Bohadana AB, Hannhart B, Teculescu DB: Nocturnal worsening of asthma and sleep-disordered breathing. J Asthma 39:85–100, 2002

Borson S, McDonald G, Gayle T, et al: Improvement in mood, physical symptoms, and functions with nortriptyline for depression in patients with chronic obstructive pulmonary disease. Psychosomatics 33:190–201, 1992

Braghiroli A, Alvarez-Sala R: Sleep disordered breathing and COPD. Sleep Breath 6:1–2, 2002

Carr RE: Panic disorder and asthma: causes, effects and research implications. J Psychosom Res 44:43–52, 1998

Clark D: A cognitive approach to panic. Behav Res Ther 24:461–470, 1986

Cohn M, Morris D, Juan D, et al: Effects of estazolam and flurazepam on cardiopulmonary function in patients with chronic obstructive pulmonary disease. Drug Saf 7:152–158, 1992

Cozza KL, Armstrong SC, Oesterheld JR: Concise Guide to Drug Interaction Principles for Medical Practice: Cytochrome P450s, UGTs, P-Glycoproteins, 2nd Edition. Washington, DC, American Psychiatric Publishing, 2003

Datto C, Rai AK, Ilivicky HJ, et al: Augmentation of seizure induction in electroconvulsive therapy: a clinical reappraisal. J ECT 18:118–125, 2002

de Kerviler E, Tredaniel J, Revlon G, et al: Fluoxetine-induced pulmonary granulomatosis. Eur Respir J 9:615–617, 1996

Diot P, Jonville AP, Gerard F, et al: Interaction possible entre théophylline et fluvoxamine (letter; French). Thérapie 46:170–171, 1991

Fait M, Wise M, Jachna J, et al: Psychopharmacology, in The American Psychiatric Publishing Textbook of Consultation-Liaison Psychiatry: Psychiatry in the Medically Ill, 2nd Edition. Edited by Wise MG, Rundell JR. Washington, DC, American Psychiatric Publishing, 2002, pp 939–987

Fix A, Golden C, Daughton D, et al: Neuropsychological deficits among patients with COPD. Int J Neurosci 16:99–105, 1982

Fleisch M, Blauer F, Gubler J, et al: Eosinophilic pneumonia and respiratory failure associated with venlafaxine treatment. Eur Respir J 15:205–208, 2000

Gathchel R, Oordt M: Asthma, in Clinical Health Psychology and Primary Care: Practical Advice and Clinical Guidance for Successful Collaboration. Edited by Gathchel R, Oordt M. Washington, DC, American Psychological Association, 2003, pp 103–115

George CF, Bayliff CD: Management of insomnia in patients with chronic obstructive pulmonary disease. Drugs 63:379–387, 2003

George CF, Series F, Kryger MH, et al: Efficacy and safety of zaleplon vs zolpidem in chronic obstructive pulmonary disease (COPD) and insomnia (abstract). Sleep 22:S320, 1999

Mouallem M, Wolf I: Olanzapine-induced respiratory fail-

Girault C, Muir JF, Mihaltan F, et al: Effects of repeated administration of zolpidem on sleep, diurnal and nocturnal respiratory function, vigilance, and physical performance in patients with COPD. Chest 110:1203–1211, 1996

Gonzalez-Rothi R, Zander D, Ros P: Fluoxetine hydrochloride (Prozac)-induced pulmonary disease. Chest 107:1763–1765, 1995

Goodwin R, Jacobi F, Thefeld W: Mental disorders and asthma in the community. Arch Gen Psychiatry 60:1125–1130, 2003

Gorman J, Fyer M, Goetz R, et al: Ventilatory physiology of patients with panic disorder. Arch Gen Psychiatry 45:31–39, 1988

Grant I, Prigatano G, Heaton R, et al: Progressive neuropsychologic impairment and hypoxemia. Arch Gen Psychiatry 44:999–1006, 1987

Greenberg D, Kradin R: Lung disease, in The American Psychiatric Publishing Textbook of Consultation-Liaison Psychiatry: Psychiatry in the Medically Ill, 2nd Edition. Edited by Wise MG, Rundell JR. Washington, DC, American Psychiatric Publishing, 2002, pp 546–551

Griggs R, Arieff A: Hypoxia and the central nervous system, in Metabolic Brain Dysfunction in Systemic Disorders. Edited by Arieff A, Griggs R. Boston, MA, Little, Brown, 1992, pp 39–54

Guilleminault C: Benzodiazepines, breathing, and sleep. Am J Med 88 (suppl 3A):25–28, 1990

Hajak G, Rodenbeck A, Voderholzer U, et al: Doxepin in the treatment of primary insomnia: a placebo-controlled, double-blind, polysomnographic study. J Clin Psychiatry 62:453–463, 2001

Honig E, Ingram R Jr: Chronic bronchitis, emphysema, and airways obstruction, in Harrison's Online, DOI 101036/ 1096–7133ch258. New York, McGraw-Hill, 2002

Krahn L, Richardson J: Sleep disorders in the medically ill, in Psychiatric Care of the Medical Patient. Edited by Stoudemire A, Fogel B, Greenberg D. New York, Oxford University Press, 2000, pp 683–697

Kryger M, Roth T, Dement W: Principles and Practice of Sleep Medicine, 3rd Edition. Philadelphia, PA, WB Saunders, 2000

Lehrer P, Feldman J, Giardino N, et al: Psychological aspects of asthma. J Consult Clin Psychol 70:691–711, 2002

Lin CC: Effects of protriptyline on day and night time oxygenation in patients with chronic obstructive pulmonary disease (Chinese). J Formos Med Assoc 92 (suppl 4):S232–S236, 1993

Lipowski Z: Delirium: Acute Confusional States. New York, Oxford University Press, 1990

McFadden E Jr: Asthma, in Harrison's Online DOI 101036/ 1096-7133ch252. New York, McGraw-Hill, 2003

McNicholas W: Impact of sleep on COPD, in Harrison's Online, DOI 101036/1096–7133edl2379. New York, McGraw-Hill, 2002

ure. Am J Geriatr Psychiatry 9:304–305, 2001

Murciano D, Armengaud MH, Cramer PH, et al: Acute effects of zolpidem, triazolam and flunitrazepam on arterial blood gases and control of breathing in severe COPD. Eur Respir J 6:625–629, 1993

Nascimento I, Nardi AE, Valenca AM, et al: Psychiatric disorders in asthmatic outpatients. Psychiatry Res 110:73–80, 2002

Perna G, Bertani A, Politi E, et al: Asthma and panic attacks. Biol Psychiatry 42:625–630, 1997

Phillipson EA: Sleep apnea, in Harrison's Online, DOI 101036/1096-7133ch264. New York, McGraw-Hill, 2002

Pohl R, Yeragani VK, Balon R: Effects of isoproterenol in panic disorder patients after antidepressant treatment. Biol Psychiatry 28:203–214, 1990

Prigatano G, Parsons O, Wright E, et al: Neuropsychological test performance in mildly hypoxemic patients with COPD. J Consult Clin Psychol 51:108–116, 1983

Rasmussen BB, Maenpaa J, Pelkonen O, et al: Selective serotonin reuptake inhibitors and theophylline metabolism in human liver microsomes: potent inhibition by fluvoxamine. Br J Clin Pharmacol 39:151–159, 1995

Rasmussen KG, Zorumski CF: Electroconvulsive therapy in patients taking theophylline. J Clin Psychiatry 54:427–431, 1993

Reite M, Ruddy J, Nagel K: Evaluation and Management of Sleep Disorders, 3rd Edition. Washington, DC, American Psychiatric Publishing, 2002

Rietveld S: Symptom perception in asthma: a multidisciplinary review. J Asthma 35:137–146, 1998

Rushford N, Tiller JW, Pain MC: Perception of natural fluctuations in peak flow in asthma: clinical severity and psychological correlates. J Asthma 35:251–259, 1998

Saidman L: Midazolam: pharmacology and uses. Anesthesiology 62:310–324, 1985

Schmaling KB, Lehrer PM, Feldman JM, et al: Asthma, in Handbook of Psychology, Vol 9: Health Psychology. Edited by Nezu AM, Nezu CM, Geller PA. New York, Wiley, 2003, pp 99–120

Steens RD, Pouliot Z, Millar TW, et al: Effects of zolpidem and triazolam on sleep and respiration in mild to moderate chronic obstructive pulmonary disease. Sleep 16:318–326, 1993

Thompson W: Pulmonary disease, in Psychiatric Care of the Medical Patient. Edited by Stoudemire A, Fogel B, Greenberg D. New York, Oxford University Press, 2000, pp 757–774

van den Brekel AL, Harrington L: Toxic effects of theophylline caused by fluvoxamine. CMAJ 151:1289–1290, 1994

Verburg K, Griez E, Meijer J, et al: Respiratory disorders as a possible predisposing factor for panic disorder. J Affect Disord 33:129–134, 1995

Weilburg J, Winkelman J: Sleep disorders, in The American Psychiatric Publishing Textbook of Consultation-Liaison Psychiatry: Psychiatry in the Medically Ill, 2nd Edition. Edited by Wise MG, Rundell JR. Washington, DC, American Psychiatric Publishing, 2002, pp 495–518

Wilner K, Anziano R, Johnson A, et al: The anxiolytic effect of the novel antipsychotic ziprasidone compared with diazepam in subjects anxious before dental surgery. J Clin Psychopharmacol 22:206–210, 2002

Wingate BJ, Hansen-Flaschen J: Anxiety and depression in advanced lung disease. Clin Chest Med 18:495–505, 1997

Zevin S, Benowitz N: Drug interactions with tobacco smoking: an update. Clin Pharmacokinet 36:425–438, 1999

99

The Patient With GI Symptoms and Psychiatric Distress

Antoinette Ambrosino Wyszynski, M.D.
Brian D. Bronson, M.D.
Khleber Chapman Attwell, M.D., M.P.H.

Patients with gastrointestinal (GI) complaints and psychiatric symptoms are encountered often in clinical practice. Irritable bowel syndrome (IBS), the main focus of this chapter, is the most frequently occurring functional GI disorder (the others include globus hystericus, pseudodysphagia, and nonulcer dyspepsia). Up to 50% of outpatients referred to gastroenterologists ultimately receive a diagnosis of IBS. Terms that have been used synonymously with IBS include *spastic colon/colitis, colonic neurosis, dyskinesia of the colon, functional diarrhea/enterocolonopathy, nervous diarrhea,* and *unhappy colon.*

This chapter will focus on conditions with GI complaints that often masquerade as primary psychiatric illness. Knowing the differential diagnosis of psychological and GI complaints helps to distinguish in triage between patients requiring additional workup and those who would benefit from a primarily psychiatric intervention. Medical conditions of this type include acute intermittent porphyria (which may present in the emergency room as psychiatric symp-

tomatology occurring with an "acute abdomen" but no surgical findings), B12 (cobalamin) deficiency (overlooked because of its psychiatric presentation), and pancreatic cancer (whose initial presentation may be atypical, treatment-resistant depressive or anxiety states). Table 6–1 summarizes the conditions discussed in this chapter.

■ IRRITABLE BOWEL SYNDROME

The nature of IBS is elusive; the illness presents with symptoms ranging from constipation to diarrhea to abdominal pain. Irritable bowel pain often varies in intensity and location, occurring in atypical abdominal areas as well as in extra-abdominal sites. The pain is either crampy or a generalized ache with superimposed periods of abdominal cramps. Sharp, dull, gaslike, or nondescript pains are also consistent with IBS. Pain can be so severe that it interferes with daily activities, causing patients to avoid situations where no

Table 6–1. Differential diagnosis of gastrointestinal and psychiatric symptoms

	Pancreatic cancer	Acute intermittent porphyria	B_{12} deficiency	Irritable bowel syndrome
Presentation	Atypical depressive or anxiety states, with vague GI symptoms Vague, intermittent epigastric pain that sounds consistent with a somatizing disorder	Initially: delusions, hallucinations, behavioral changes, abdominal pain ("Madness of King George") May correlate with the *menstrual cycle* or present postpartum	Variable presentation, including mood disorders, schizophreniform or paranoid psychoses, or dementia Can be mistaken for chronic alcohol-induced pathology	Constipation or diarrhea, but without systemic progression or pathology Anxiety disorders frequent
Pathology	Theories: paraneoplastic process with "false neurotransmitters" or neuroendocrine abnormalities; tumor-released antibodies affecting serotonin	Porphobilinogen deaminase (hydroxymethylbilane synthase) deficiency. Autosomal dominant inheritance with incomplete penetrance, heterozygotes asymptomatic until precipitant exposure	Defects in intestinal absorption of B_{12} Most common cause: nonautoimmune atrophic gastritis in the elderly (see also Table 6–6)	Theories: abnormal visceral perception; altered gut motility; autonomic nervous system abnormalities; diet; infection; psychological factors
Diagnosis	Clinical suspicion; most common in males ages 60–80. Risk factors: cigarette smoking; chronic pancreatitis; diabetes mellitus; chemical exposure	Occurrence of symptoms on exposure to precipitants: low-calorie diet, infection, or medications undergoing oxidation During acute attacks: excess urine porphobilinogen and 5-aminolevulinate	Clinical suspicion, especially in elderly patients High serum methylmalonic acid (MMA) and homocysteine levels	Abdominal pain relieved by defecation and associated with changed stool frequency or consistency (See Rome II criteria, Table 6–3) Rule out fever, blood in stools, nocturnal pain, weight loss or anorexia, anemia
Treatment	Chemotherapy; prognosis poor	Avoid precipitants of intravenous heme. Use narcotic analgesics and psychotropics with caution (see Table 6–5).	Intramuscular B_{12} Prophylaxis (for patients over 65): 0.1 mg oral crystalline cobalamin daily	Bulking agents, antispasmotics, antidepressants, psychotherapy

bathroom is readily available. Unlike inflammatory bowel disease, such as Crohn's disease or ulcerative colitis, IBS pain does not undermine the patient's nutritional status or normal sleep pattern. The "red flags" listed in Table 6–2 should raise the alarm that a process other than IBS is operating, prompting further investigation.

Table 6–2. "Red flag" conditions in irritable bowel syndrome

Presence of any of the following calls for further investigation to rule out other disease processes:

Fever	Weight loss or anorexia
Blood in stools	Anemia
Nocturnal pain	Abnormal blood studies
Abnormal physical findings	Family history of inflammatory bowel
Onset in patients >50 years of age	disease or malignancy

Abdominal pain with changes in bowel habits is part of the Rome II criteria for IBS (Thompson et al. 2000), which are listed in Table 6–3. Patients may present with a confusing array of bowel symptoms, such as loose stools, usually after meals and in the morning, alternating with episodes of constipation, or constipation alternating with diarrhea. Those with diarrhea may experience fecal urgency during periods of stress; stools are characteristically loose and frequent but of normal total daily volume. Patients with constipation may have a sense of incomplete fecal evacuation leading to repeated, uncomfortable attempts at stool passage.

Many patients report mucus in their stools, but this does not indicate structural or "inflammatory" bowel disease; IBS patients have histologically normal colons, unlike patients with ulcerative colitis or Crohn's disease. Rather, IBS is a disorder of intestinal *motility*. Results of sigmoidoscopy and routine blood testing are normal. Colonoscopy usually reveals hypermotility. Studies of pathogenesis and treatment have yielded ambiguous results because no clear diagnostic markers for IBS exist. In addition, symptoms may show wide variation among individuals.

The American Gastroenterological Association (AGA) currently recommends a complete physical examination, a fecal occult blood test and complete blood count for screening purposes, sigmoidoscopy, and additional testing when indicated (American Gastroenterological Association 2002). A sedimentation rate (particularly in younger patients), serum chemis-

Table 6–3. Rome II diagnostic criteria for irritable bowel syndrome

Abdominal discomfort or pain of at least 12 weeks' duration (which need not be consecutive), occurring in the preceding 12 months, that has 2 of 3 features:
    Relieved by defecation; and/or
    Onset associated with a change in frequency of stool; and/or
    Onset associated with a change in form (appearance) of stool.
Symptoms that cumulatively support the diagnosis of irritable bowel syndrome:
    Abnormal stool frequency (for research purposes, "abnormal" defined as >3 bowel movements/day or <3 bowel movements/week)
    Abnormal stool form (lumpy/hard or loose/watery stool)
    Abnormal stool habits (straining, urgency, or feeling of incomplete evacuation)
    Passage of mucus
    Bloating or feeling of abdominal distention
The diagnosis of a functional bowel disorder always presumes the absence of a structural or biochemical explanation for the symptoms.

Source. Thompson et al. 2000.

tries and albumin, and stool test for ova and parasites are recommended, with test selection based on symptom pattern, geographic area, and clinical features (e.g., predominant diarrhea, areas of endemic infection). The AGA recommends colonoscopy for patients over age 50 years because of a higher pretest probability of colon cancer. In younger patients, colonoscopy or sigmoidoscopy is advised only if there are clinical features suggestive of more serious disease, such as diarrhea accompanied by weight loss.

Symptoms of gastroesophageal reflux are reported by one-third of patients with IBS (Talley 2003). Other frequent complaints include headache, backache, fatigue, sexual dysfunction, and genitourinary symptoms (such as urinary frequency).

Epidemiology

Many people with IBS learn to live with their symptoms and never seek medical care for them. The worldwide prevalence of IBS has been estimated at the relatively stable rate of 10%–20%. IBS is more commonly reported in lower socioeconomic groups. Although the GI symptoms tend to be chronic and recurrent, up to 30% of patients become asymptomatic over time. In Western nations, women are more likely to receive a diagnosis of IBS; this gender pattern may be culture-specific (e.g., in India the pattern is men>women). The prevalence of IBS diagnoses declines with advancing age.

Pathophysiology

The medical workup can be more of a frustration than a relief to IBS patients, who may infer that they are thought to be "imagining" or "giving themselves" symptoms when the test results are within normal limits. Aggravated family members often feel ruled by the patient's GI complaints and bathroom routines, so they frequently support this formulation. Interpersonal and self-esteem issues arise, engendering more anxiety, which feeds back to the sensitized gut to produce more GI distress. Even though anxiety affects colonic function in everyone, the increased colonic sensitivity in IBS cannot be explained solely by psychological factors or emotional states like anxiety. It is helpful to explain to patients that there are *objective* findings producing a *different*—albeit not diseased— physiology. However, note that none of the abnormalities discussed below is specific enough to be used as a criterion for diagnosis. Moreover, there is not yet a disease model that plausibly unifies all of the known abnormalities. Instead, the physiological changes documented in IBS probably interact with genetics and environment to contribute to symptom development.

Abnormal Visceral Perception

Increased rectal resistance and sensitivity to experimental stretch or balloon distention has been found in the majority of IBS patients. Sensitivity to distention has also been found in the colon and/or small intestine in a subset of IBS patients. It is not known whether increased gut sensitivity results from an end-organ abnormality, an increased relay of afferent inputs, or altered central processing of visceral sensation. Studies have shown that visceral hypersensitivity in IBS is not explained by a low general pain threshold but rather appears to be specific for gut distention.

Altered Gut Motility

Although there are many abnormalities in IBS, it is unclear whether they are clinically relevant or perhaps represent artifact or epiphenomena (Talley 2003). Although the colon in IBS does appear to be hyperresponsive to stress, cholinergic drugs, or hormonal factors (e.g., cholecystokinin), basal colonic motility is not altered in IBS. Among the abnormalities reported

to occur in parallel with IBS pain are disturbed small-bowel and colonic transit, certain types of small intestinal motor patterns (such as ileal propulsive waves), and jejunal pressure waves occurring during periods of fasting. Hypotheses about pathogenesis speculate that abnormalities in sensory perception cause alterations in local neural reflexes that in turn change motor function in IBS patients. Extraintestinal motor dysfunction has been recognized in the lung, urinary bladder, and gallbladder of IBS patients, suggesting a generalized abnormality of either smooth muscle or the nervous system.

Autonomic Nervous System Abnormalities

A minority of IBS patients have vagal dysfunction and sympathetic adrenergic dysfunction.

Diet

Diet exacerbates symptoms in many patients. For example, sorbitol, fructose, and bile acids have been shown to induce symptoms such as diarrhea and bloating in susceptible individuals. Variations in fiber intake also may play a role in precipitating certain IBS episodes. Dietary exclusions followed by gradual, sequential reinstitution of foods can induce symptomatic improvement in many patients with functional diarrhea, providing some support for food sensitivity as a trigger.

Infection

Experts believe that an acute, self-limited gastrointestinal infection may "prime" the gut, resulting in functional disturbances such as IBS. A small percentage of IBS patients (10%–25%) experienced a viral illness or traveler's diarrhea prior to the onset of their symptoms, an association that was confirmed in prospective studies of acute bacterial gastroenteritis. Chronic inflammatory cells and enteroendocrine cells in the rectum increase significantly in "postinfectious IBS." Some IBS patients have an excess of mast cells and mast cell degranulation in the terminal ileum and colon. Hypothetically, acute inflammation could permanently sensitize gut afferent receptors, thus sustaining symptoms in predisposed individuals even after the initial stimulus remits and inflammation resolves.

IBS and Psychological Factors

The relationship between the brain and the gut remains "both complex and profound" (Lydiard 2001).

Although fewer than one-half of persons with IBS seek treatment, the literature shows that those who do tend to display high levels of neuroticism, more illness behavior, ineffective coping styles, and an increased incidence of psychiatric disorders and physical/sexual abuse (Lydiard 2001). The most common psychiatric diagnoses in the community-based IBS population are major depression, panic disorder, social phobia, generalized anxiety disorder, posttraumatic stress disorder, and somatization disorder. Psychiatric diagnoses occur at a much higher rate in the IBS population than in population-based controls (63% and 24.8%, respectively). These findings prove critical because they demonstrate the independent association between IBS and psychiatric disorders, eliminating the treatment-seeking status from its prior role in selection bias.

Psychological stress clearly worsens irritable bowel symptoms, regardless of the original pathophysiology. The enteric nervous system has been called the "third division" of the autonomic nervous system. For individuals with IBS, it is puzzling why there is so high a prevalence of preexisting anxiety disorders. A recent hypothesis links autonomic dysregulation, anxiety, and abnormal gut motility, positing a self-reinforcing cycle that reciprocally worsens all three (Lydiard 2001; Lydiard et al. 1993). Specifically, increased CNS arousal in this model stimulates GI distress and increased motility via the CNS-mediated sympathetic outflow, in turn causing the afferent vagal neurons of the distal colon to stimulate the locus coeruleus, which mediates fear and arousal states. Perturbations of the bladder, bowel, or stomach also send afferent input into this nucleus, causing increased neuronal firing. Whatever the mechanism, it seems as though a potentially uncontrollable feedback loop sets itself in motion between the gut (GI symptoms) and the brain (anxiety). Perhaps the autonomic symptoms suffered by patients with combined IBS and anxiety symptoms share some common pathophysiology, mediated by the locus coeruleus, thus linking the two conditions. Many studies have suggested that corticotropin-releasing factor may serve as a common limbic-GI neuropeptide/enteric neurotransmitter; if so, this would have important research implications for treatment (Lydiard 2001; Lydiard et al. 1993).

Compared with other chronic GI disorders, such as Crohn's disease and ulcerative colitis, the course and treatment of IBS are relatively benign. Therapy for IBS is not stressful; there is no risk of undergoing surgery, colostomy, steroid use, disfigurement, or malnutrition. Nonetheless, the reported prevalence of psychi-

atric comorbidity for IBS is *far greater* than for either Crohn's disease or ulcerative colitis, with estimates often exceeding 50%.

Although there are few data to support IBS as a precursor to psychiatric illness, emotional factors in the patient's history, including childhood parental loss, somatization, and sexual or physical abuse, may predate IBS symptoms. The first case-control study in this area challenged the association between functional bowel disorders (FBDs) and previous abuse experiences. Patients with idiopathic constipation ($n=53$) were compared with matched control groups of 50 IBS patients, 51 Crohn's disease patients, and 53 nonpatient control subjects (Hobbis et al. 2002). Measures of previous abuse experiences were a self-report questionnaire and a semistructured interview. No significant differences were found among all four groups for measures of abuse or for psychological stress. Those individuals with a history of abuse were more psychologically distressed, irrespective of their FBD status. These findings challenge the practice among gastroenterologists of questioning IBS patients about abuse experiences (Ilnyckyj and Bernstein 2002).

Methodological Problems

Although the interaction between brain and bowel is undisputed, methodological problems affect many studies that report on the concurrence of IBS symptoms and psychopathology. Problems include sample bias, sample heterogeneity, and sampling error. For example, psychosocial factors determine treatment-seeking behavior, creating a self-selected population that comes to medical attention and enters the researched world of "patienthood." Although 15%–20% of the general population have symptoms consistent with IBS, only a minority actually seek medical help (Talley 2003). Notably, the "nonpatient" subgroup has no greater prevalence of psychological distress than do symptom-free control subjects (Whitehead et al. 1988).

Sample heterogeneity confounded studies conducted prior to the adoption of the Rome II diagnostic criteria. Subjects were included who reported "abdominal pain" and "altered bowel habits" *without any other evidence for IBS*, potentially adding patients with somatization disorder and inflating associations between psychopathology and IBS. In addition, most of the early research on the prevalence of psychiatric disorders in IBS was based on clinic populations, not general community samples. IBS clinic attendees may be a distinct subgroup and cannot be extrapolated to represent people with IBS in general.

- *Bottom line:* These conclusions can be drawn about IBS and psychological factors: 1) Psychotherapeutic and psychopharmacologic interventions depend on better understanding of the chemical mediation of memory, stress, and emotions on the enteric nervous system (Ringel 2002). 2) The causal relationship between IBS and psychiatric morbidity remains poorly understood. 3) The two conditions appear to interact, but without a clear path of one clearly precipitating the other. 4) Individuals with IBS who do seek medical attention are often, but not always, psychologically distressed people who may benefit from psychiatric intervention.

Psychiatric Management of IBS Patients

Psychological Management

Once the medical workup establishes that the symptoms are consistent with IBS, the goal of psychological management is to frame the irritable bowel as *different*, not *diseased*. In practice, this is harder to achieve than it sounds; people with IBS talk *with* the gut, rather than *from* the gut. Their language of distress is somatization: diarrhea, constipation, straining, burping, odor, pain. It takes patience and tact to help them translate bowel language into words, particularly when they are riveted into positions of intense shame and despair—hiding out in restrooms, sitting on toilets until it is "safe," usually too embarrassed to go into detail in psychotherapy about their "bathroom stuff."

Like detectives, IBS patients have usually scouted out and created mental maps of public restrooms, particularly for their morning route to work. Few people are willing or able to leave their homes without having first fully evacuated. If the bowel has not "behaved," that is, fully evacuated or ceased spasming, the patient may be regularly late for appointments or work. When pressed, IBS patients imagine dire consequences of limited toilet access—usually, that they will soil themselves in full public view and become smelly, humiliated outcasts. It is rare to encounter an IBS patient who has not had at least one episode of stained underwear, whether from diarrhea or the overly vigorous treatment of constipation gone awry. Some patients evolve "bowel-induced agoraphobia," fearing that the urge to defecate will unpredictably strike if they leave home, particularly after breakfast. (The gastrocolic reflex, the peristaltic movement of the colon that often occurs 15 to 20 minutes after food enters the stomach, is intense after the first meal of the day.) Some IBS patients are so unnerved by having to get somewhere on time in the morning that they refuse to make appointments altogether. Many individuals feel shame about going into public bathrooms, especially at work, where stalls provide minimal privacy. The anticipated helpless exposure of the noises and smells coming from their "messy" bowel movements often heightens anxiety. There may result avoidance of social situations where the patient anticipates there will be minimal bathroom privacy. (Unlike the patient with social phobia, the IBS patient specifically fears that anxiety will cause the bowel to become overly active at the wrong time and cause a *realistically* embarrassing situation. Unlike the hypochondriac, the typical IBS patient is relieved that there is nothing seriously wrong, and is eager to "fix" the errant bowel.)

Family members often become exasperated rather than empathic, feeling that the patient has become an in-house dictator (e.g., requiring aisle seats at the movies or theater for easy access to the restroom, or needing frequent "rest stops" on excursions). Airplane trips may be particularly challenging; in a situation where anxiety peaks, the patient must synchronize the departure from home for the airport to coincide with being "finished" with the inevitable bowel spasms. The prospect of confinement to an airplane seat at intervals, prohibited from using the restroom, often brings anticipatory misery for the patient. Patients whose work keeps them outdoors or on the road (e.g., in sales, making deliveries) have no regular bathroom to count on, making daily life challenging.

Techniques of Management

Emphasizing that IBS "does not mean you are sick" is well-intentioned but will meet with skepticism. The therapist soon learns that this is one unhappy way to live. The approach requires walking a tightrope between overmedicalizing the condition (implying that the patient is sicker than anyone is saying) and overpsychologizing (minimizing the medical and calling attention to emotional factors before the patient is ready to acknowledge them). Avoid jargon and "psycholingo" or risk dropout by the patient. Individuals with IBS see psychiatrists for "stress management" and because it "might" improve their medical illness, not necessarily because of "issues" other than managing a wild bowel. Often, the psychiatric referral feels like one more shameful happening in a life filled with shameful events. For example, the question "Does IBS bring up control issues?" might result in the incredulous, angry response: "Picture your bowels having a mind of their own, with the doctors telling you there is no definite cause and so no clear-cut treatment. Then they suggest I see a shrink. My bowels may be out of control, but *I'm* not. And I'm not crazy, either." Interventions that start with the patient's practical problems, such as specifics of managing a bowel regimen and the impact on daily life, have better likelihood of succeeding.

Similarly, given that some individuals have traumatic backgrounds, be cautious about appearing "overinterested" in the psychological history, particularly if there is a history of sexual or physical abuse. People with such backgrounds may be sensitive to the crossing of boundaries and may leave treatment if they feel it to be psychologically intrusive. For those ready to explore connections between their emotional and enteric lives, regular meetings may be welcomed and quite helpful. Psychological treatment will be easier for individuals who already connect exacerbations (especially diarrhea) to emotional precipitants or environmental stressors. Most psychotherapy techniques have been shown to be helpful (Hasler 2002; Spanier et al. 2003), and psychotherapy appears to be cost-effective (Creed et al. 2003). Currently, no one type of psychotherapy is recommended over any other because controlled studies have shown clinical improvement with just about all of them, even when administered over relatively *brief* periods of time. Among the helpful behavioral techniques have been relaxation therapy, hypnosis (which may reduce visceral gut perception and in controlled trials is beneficial in IBS), and biofeedback (most valuable in constipation with pelvic floor dysfunction). It is not clear whether improvement relates to actual changes in GI physiology, improved coping strategies, or different interpretation of enteroceptive signals from the gut (American Gastroenterological Association 2002).

A central feature with these patients is the feeling that IBS undermines their dignity and is humiliating to live with. Anyone working with IBS patients must remain sensitive to this fact, regardless of psychotherapeutic model. With highly symptomatic patients, there is the risk of sending mixed messages about the seriousness of the illness, which can exacerbate the patient's anxiety.

It is tempting to recommend a "division of labor" with the gastroenterologist, requesting visits with the specialist for the GI complaints—particularly when a litany of physical complaints seems to invade the psychotherapy sessions. Unfortunately, encouraging trips to the GI specialist reinforces the "sick patient" role and encourages medical testing. A better approach is to sequester a portion of each meeting for a medical update and then use the remaining time for the psychological work, of whatever technique.

The psychiatrist must be convinced that the medical prognosis is benign and that the patient will get better with conservative treatment. This conviction must withstand complaints of persistent abdominal pain, seemingly haphazard changes in bowel habits, and an often-evolving pattern of conditioned avoidance of activities. IBS patients are often alert to "waffling" by their physicians and will react with alarm—and more GI symptoms. Try to ensure that the workup is completed as quickly as possible before engaging the patient in psychiatric treatment so that such treatment can proceed unimpeded by doubts of more serious medical pathology.

- *Bottom line:* The psychiatrist who works with an IBS sufferer must be willing to listen to and elicit details about bowel movements and bathroom visits. It will help the patient to correlate these symptoms to dietary indiscretions, medication noncompliance, and, eventually, emotional and/or cognitive states. For example, lapses in effective diet plans may be reflective of psychological reactions, such as denial or such as anger toward significant others and the use of GI symptoms to punish them. It is usually a relief for IBS patients to find someone who listens without becoming impatient (like their families) or disgusted by their intimate bodily functions. One final observation: clinical trials have demonstrated very large placebo responses for IBS treatments. Although this finding makes it difficult to measure the precise efficacy of any given agent, it also suggests what clinicians have long known: that an ongoing, consistent, supportive relationship with a caring physician may be the most therapeutic strategy of all (Moss and Modlin 2002).

Psychopharmacological Treatment of Depression and Anxiety in IBS

Psychopharmacological agents have been useful in two major subsets of patients with IBS (Wald 2002): 1) those with pain and/or gastrointestinal symptoms refractory to standard medical treatment and 2) patients with IBS and a comorbid psychiatric illness, usually depression and/or one of the anxiety disorders.

Those with refractory symptoms benefit from the neuromodulatory and analgesic properties of antidepressants. Tricyclic antidepressants (TCAs) have played an important role because of their analgesic properties, apparently altering GI physiology (e.g., visceral sensitivity, motility, and secretion) (American

Gastroenterological Association 2002). Benefits occur sooner and at doses lower than those prescribed for major depression, occurring independently of the presence of psychological symptoms (Clouse et al. 1994). Several case reports have suggested the usefulness of serotonergic agents such as paroxetine (Kirsch and Louie 2000; Masand et al. 2002), mirtazapine (Thomas 2000), and fluvoxamine (Emmanuel et al. 1997).

It is difficult to offer evidence-based conclusions about treating coexisting psychiatric disorders in IBS patients, because controlled studies are lacking (Lydiard 2001; Wald 2002). Practical experience has shown that for patients with predominant diarrhea and depression, the constipating side effects of TCAs may be helpful. For depressed patients with predominant constipation, a selective serotonin reuptake inhibitor (SSRI) may be preferable. Most reports find that both classes of antidepressants improve accompanying anxiety as well as depression.

In an algorithm for the initiation of antidepressants for IBS, Clouse (2003) recommended the following procedures in anxious or depressed patients: 1) initiate an SSRI at usual dosage, monitor for symptom response, and add a low-dose TCA for persistent IBS symptoms, *or* 2) initiate a very low dose TCA regimen, monitor for symptom response, and add an SSRI for persistent psychiatric symptoms.

The AGA does not recommend anxiolytics as independent agents for IBS because of weak treatment effects and the potential for physical dependence. To date, no studies have appeared comparing SSRIs and TCAs in IBS.

Medical Update on Treating IBS

According to the AGA (American Gastroenterological Association 2002), the treatment strategy for IBS depends on the nature and severity of the symptoms, the degree of functional impairment, and the presence of psychosocial difficulties affecting the course of the illness. Patients with mild symptoms usually respond to reassurance, education, and treatments not requiring prescription medication. Patients are reassured that their symptoms are not imagined, that they occur commonly in the general population, and that they will not evolve into something life-threatening such as cancer. Individuals with moderate or severe symptoms may require medications that affect gut physiology or psychological treatments. A minority of patients are treatment refractory and need referral to a multidisciplinary pain center.

Correcting Precipitating Factors

Occasionally, dietary and lifestyle modifications are enough to calm an acute exacerbation. These may include 1) eliminating lactose or known gas-producing foods in patients with diarrhea, flatulence, or bloating (e.g., carbonated beverages; cabbage, beans, legumes, and lentils, which are fermented in the colon; and sorbitol, an ingredient of sugar-free chewing gum); 2) avoiding certain known triggers, such as alcohol, caffeine, and spicy or fatty foods; and 3) increasing fiber intake in patients with constipation. (Occasionally, a sudden increase in fiber content, as in adoption of the Heart Smart Diet, may precipitate an IBS flare.)

Diet

A gradual transition to a high-fiber diet has become the goal for IBS patients, although patients with constipation are more likely to benefit. The daily target of 20–30 grams of fiber per day is approximately double the amount in the normal American diet. For some patients, too rapidly increasing dietary fiber may precipitate an IBS flare. Fiber supplements (e.g., methylcellulose, polycarbophil, psyllium) should be started once daily and increased weekly by one dose per day until symptoms improve or until the patient achieves a daily consumption of 5–10 grams three times daily. An anti-gas diet may be helpful for patients with excessive flatus (see preceding section).

Drug Therapy

A number of medications are used for IBS, with the choice of drug being based on the target symptom (e.g., constipation, diarrhea, bloating). The newly released agents for diarrhea-predominant IBS (alosetron; Lotronex) and constipation-predominant IBS (tegaserod; Zelnorm) act at the serotonin 5-HT receptor and appear to offer new relief for the control of symptoms and pain. Medications used for treatment of IBS are listed in Table 6–4.

■ PANCREATIC CANCER

Since the early twentieth century, pancreatic cancer has been known to present *psychiatric symptoms that predate systemic signs,* masquerading as primary psychiatric illness and delaying diagnosis. Timely diagnosis is crucial with this illness; the onset of physical symptoms signals that the disease has spread beyond the pancreas, making it unresectable and resulting in a median survival of less than 6 months (Kedra et al. 2001). It is fatal in more than 98% of the patients it afflicts. The in-

Table 6–4. Medications used to treat irritable bowel syndrome

Symptom	Strategies
Constipation	Tegaserod (Zelnorm); bulking agents (e.g., psyllium, methylcelluose, polycarbophil), lactulose/milk of magnesia, polyethylene glycol, enemas
Diarrhea	Alosetron (Lotronex), loperamide (Imodium), loperamide/simethicone, cholestyramine (Questran)
Bloating	Simethicone (Mylicon), charcoal, lactobacillus
Flatus	α-Galactosidase (Beano) enzyme with vegetable meals
Postprandial pain	Anticholinergics (e.g., dicylomine [Bentyl], hyoscyamine [Levsin, Anaspaz, Cystospaz]; oral, sublingual)
Chronic pain	Tricyclic antidepressants, low-dose (25–75 mg): amitriptyline (Elavil), doxepin (Sinequan), imipramine (Tofranil), nortriptyline (Pamelor)
	Trazodone (Desyrel) 100 mg (divided doses)
	Selective serotonin reuptake inhibitors

Source. Adapted from Talley 2003.

cidence of pancreatic cancer in the United States has increased significantly as the median life expectancy of the American population has been extended. In the year 2000, pancreatic cancer ranked as the fifth most common cause of cancer-related mortality.

The triad of *depression, anxiety,* and *premonition of impending doom* ("*doom anxiety*") was described in many of the early clinical case reports. One study analyzed case reports of pancreatic cancer patients that included enough information to make a retrospective DSM-III-R classification (Green and Austin 1993). Psychiatric diagnoses clustered as follows: 71% depression-related disorder, 48% anxiety-related-disorder, and 29% symptoms of both.

Attention has focused on depression and on the question of whether the link between pancreatic cancer and depression is a true correlation or medical folklore. Holland and colleagues (1986) conducted the largest controlled study, using a large cohort of patients with advanced pancreatic cancer ($n=107$) matched to those with advanced gastric cancer ($n=111$). Both groups were about to undergo chemotherapy on one of two nearly identical chemotherapy protocols. Patient self-ratings of depression, tension-anxiety, fatigue, confusion-bewilderment, and total mood disturbance were significantly higher for the pancreatic cancer group (Holland et al. 1986).

Mechanism

Theories of the substrates of pancreatic cancer have included 1) a tumor-mediated paraneoplastic process that alters mood by producing "false neurotransmitters" or neuroendocrine abnormalities, 2) immunologic interference with the activity of serotonin by an antibody induced against a protein released by the tu-

mor, and 3) metabolic abnormalities due to an increased bicarbonate load coming from obstructed pancreatic ducts (Bernhard and Hürny 1998).

Risk Factors

Demographically, an increased risk for pancreatic cancer exists in patients of advanced age, male gender, black race, or Jewish descent (Mayer 2002). It rarely develops before the age of 50; most patients are between ages 60 and 80 at diagnosis. The causes of pancreatic cancer remain ambiguous. Cigarette smoking is the most consistent risk factor. Heavy smokers have a two to three times greater incidence of pancreatic cancer; it is not yet known whether this is a direct carcinogenic effect of tobacco metabolites on the pancreas or of some other factor that occurs more frequently in cigarette smokers. Other risk factors include chronic pancreatitis, long-standing diabetes mellitus (which has been implicated both as an early manifestation of pancreatic carcinoma and as a predisposing factor), and various dietary factors. Generally, high intakes of fat or meat have been found to increase risk, whereas high intakes of fruits and vegetables reduce risk. However, when these data have been examined in greater detail, the association between pancreatic cancer and diet becomes more complex; for example, the effect may vary by source of fat (meat, nonmeat, dairy, nondairy), total calorie intake, total cholesterol intake, and gender. Alcohol and coffee consumption are not risk factors. Exposures to certain chemicals, usually in farming or manufacturing settings, and certain occupations (e.g., stone miner, cement worker, gardener, textile worker) have also been associated with an increased risk. Two genetic mutations have been identified in association with pancreatic cancer.

Diagnosis

When jaundice does not occur as an obvious warning signal, the initial complaints of fatigue, weight loss, and anorexia are often nonspecific and may prompt psychiatric referral (Wolff et al. 2003). Furthermore, the majority of patients describe abdominal pain as vague, intermittent, epigastric pain that may sound consistent with a somatizing disorder. The physical origin is less likely to be missed when the pain has a gnawing, visceral quality.

- *Bottom line:* Pancreatic cancer should be included in the differential diagnosis of patients who are middle-aged or older and who present with vague abdominal pain that is accompanied by anxiety, agitation, and depression (Bernhard and Hürny 1998).

■ ACUTE INTERMITTENT PORPHYRIA

Acute intermittent porphyria (AIP), one of a group of metabolic diseases called the porphyrias, presents clinically in diverse ways, typically involving the central nervous system. The illness is caused by a genetic deficiency of porphobilinogen deaminase (an enzyme required in the heme biosynthesis pathway, also called hydroxymethylbilane synthase), leading to accumulation of precursors called porphyrins (Gonzalez-Arriaza and Bostwick 2003). AIP is inherited as an autosomal dominant gene with incomplete penetrance. This makes familial expression of the illness variable, potentially disguising the role of family history. Most heterozygotes remain asymptomatic unless exposed to precipitants that increase production of porphyrins.

Precipitants

Precipitants of AIP include drugs oxidized by the cytochrome P450 liver enzymes, such as therapeutic doses of barbiturates, anticonvulsants, estrogens, contraceptives, and alcohol (Croarkin 2002; Desnick 2001; Moore 1999). Also linked to attacks are low-calorie diets, infection, surgery, premenstrual hormonal changes, sun exposure, dehydration, and excessive cigarette smoking (Croarkin 2002; Gonzalez-Arriaza and Bostwick 2003; Grandchamp 1999). The contributions of these precipitants may not be obvious, adding to the often-confusing nature of the illness.

Symptoms

AIP symptoms include acute abdominal pain and/or pain in the limbs or back, often associated with nausea, vomiting, headache, and severe constipation. Tachycardia, hypertension, fever, and urine discoloration also occur commonly (Suarez et al. 1997). Abdominal crises may resemble an acute abdomen and result in laparotomy. Psychiatric symptoms often accompany the attacks and may conceal the metabolic etiology (Lishman 1998). The patient may initially become acutely depressed, agitated, or violent—*symptoms of evolving delirium, the most common neuropsychiatric syndrome.* Marked emotional lability with histrionic behavior is common. Psychotic and paranoid symptoms may resemble schizophrenia, and the patient may be misdiagnosed as having a primary psychiatric condition. Exacerbations may *correlate with the menstrual cycle* in some women, and latent porphyria may first express itself during or shortly after pregnancy—adding to the diagnostic confusion. Complications include the rapid progression to coma.

Course

Acute attacks may last from days to months, varying in frequency and severity. Symptoms may be *completely absent* in periods of remission. In addition to the neuropsychiatric effects, the adverse psychosocial consequences of the illness are considerable, impairing quality of life and producing a high incidence of anxiety and depression in AIP patients (Millward et al. 2001; Wikberg et al. 2000).

Diagnosis

Two variants of AIP, variegate porphyria and hereditary coproporphyria, may be detected both during and between acute attacks through elevated 24-hour stool levels of protoporphyrinogen/protoporphyrin and coproporphyrinogen, respectively (Gonzalez-Arriaza and Bostwick 2003). AIP itself is associated with excess urine porphobilinogen and 5-aminolevulinate—during acute attacks only. When there is clinical suspicion of AIP, genetic testing most reliably identifies carriers (Grandchamp 1999).

Treatment

The primary treatment of all the acute porphyrias requires avoiding precipitants (Gonzalez-Arriaza and Bostwick 2003). Intravenous heme is given in order to reduce porphyrin precursor excretion. Rate of recovery varies depending on the degree of neuronal damage.

Psychotropic medications must be used *selectively and with caution,* as they may precipitate attacks. No controlled studies exist on the use of psychotropics in AIP (Croarkin 2002). Phenothiazines are preferred for medicating nausea, vomiting, psychosis, and restlessness; chloral hydrate for insomnia; and benzodiazepines for anxiety (Desnick 2001). Table 6–5 summarizes anecdotally reported uses of psychotropics in AIP.

- *Bottom line:* Screen patients presenting with unexplained intermittent abdominal pain and psychiatric symptomatology for AIP, particularly in the emergency room setting.

■ B$_{12}$ (COBALAMIN) DEFICIENCY

Vitamin B$_{12}$ (cobalamin) deficiency produces a broad array of psychiatric symptoms, ranging from mood disorders to schizophreniform and paranoid psychoses. In advanced stages, it causes dementia. Gastrointestinal complaints, when they occur, reflect the impact of cobalamin deficiency on the rapidly proliferating gastrointestinal epithelium (Babior and Bunn 2002). Megaloblastosis of the small intestinal epithelium, which results in malabsorption, may cause diarrhea; anorexia with moderate weight loss is an atypical presentation of this condition (Babior and Bunn 2002).

Intestinal absorption of vitamin B$_{12}$ depends on a series of steps, including the liberation of vitamin B$_{12}$ from bound dietary animal proteins by gastric acid, its transfer to intrinsic factor (IF) produced by gastric parietal cells, and ultimately absorption of the B$_{12}$-IF

complex in the small intestine. The causes of B$_{12}$ deficiency are multifold because defects in this complex pathway can occur at any step (Dharmarajan and Norkus 2001). Table 6–6 lists causes of B$_{12}$ deficiency.

Etiology

Nonautoimmune Atrophic Gastritis

Nonautoimmune atrophic gastritis has become the most common cause of B$_{12}$ deficiency in elderly persons. Decreased gastric acid secretion impairs separation of B$_{12}$ from dietary animal protein, leading to malabsorption, whereas intestinal absorption of free vitamin B$_{12}$ (found in supplements) remains intact (Andres 2002; Baik and Russell 1999). B$_{12}$ deficiency increases with advancing age, with a prevalence ranging from 12%–25% in persons 65 and over (van Asselt et al. 2000; Van Goor et al. 1995). Atrophic gastritis accounts for roughly half of the cases of subclinical B$_{12}$ deficiency in elderly individuals (Andres 2002; Lindenbaum et al. 1994; van Asselt et al. 1998, 2000). Some commonly prescribed medications, including acid-lowering agents, will exacerbate malabsorption. Common agents that interfere with absorption are listed in Table 6–7.

Pernicious Anemia

Insufficient IF secondary to antigastric parietal cell and anti-IF antibodies is caused by impaired intestinal B$_{12}$ absorption. There is usually, but not always, a macrocytic anemia. Other symptoms of pernicious anemia include megaloblastic hyperplasia of the bone marrow, gastric achlorhydria, and, frequently, subacute combined degeneration of the spinal cord (see the Neuropsychiatric Syndromes section below). The onset is usually insidious, with gradually increasing weakness, anorexia, soreness of the tongue, and a

Table 6–5. Psychotropics with use anecdotally reported in acute intermittent porphyria

	Reportedly safe	Reportedly unsafe
Antipsychotics	Haloperidol, phenothiazines (chlorpromazine, trifluoperazine), droperidol, olanzapine, risperidone, clozapine	No reports
Antidepressants	Fluoxetine, sertraline, venlafaxine	No reports
Mood stabilizers	Lithium	Carbamazepine Valproic acid
Anxiolytics	Chlordiazepoxide, lorazepam, clonazepam, buspirone	No reports
Hypnotics	Triazolam, temazepam, trazodone, chloral hydrate	
Miscellaneous	Diphenhydramine	Barbiturates

Source. Adapted from data in Croarkin 2002; Desnick 2001; Holroyd and Seward 1999; Ibrahim and Carney 1995; and Moore 1999.

Table 6–6. Causes of B_{12} deficiency

Defective release of B_{12} from food due to...
    Gastric achlorhydria
    Partial gastrectomy
    Drugs that block acid secretion

Inadequate production of intrinsic factor due to...
    Pernicious anemia
    Total gastrectomy

Other causes
    Malabsorption
    Inadequate intake: alcoholics, strict vegans
    Competition for cobalamin (parasites, bacteria)
    Other medications: *p*-aminosalicylic acid, colchicine, neomycin
    Disorders of terminal ileum (sprue, enteritis, intestinal resection, neoplasms)

Source.   Adapted from Babior and Bunn 2002.

Table 6–7. Agents impairing B_{12} absorption

Acid blockers	Other drugs
Lansoprazole (Prevacid)	Metformin (Glucophage)
Omeprazole (Prilosec)	Cholestyramine (Questran)
Cimetidine (Tagamet)	*p*-Aminosalicylate
Famotidine (Pepcid)	Colchicine
Nizatidine (Axid)	Neomycin
Ranitidine (Zantac)	

Source.   Adapted from data in Dharmarajan and Norkus 2001; Herbert 1994; Herbert and Das 1994; and Schenk et al. 1999.

characteristic yellow pallor. The illness affects men and women equally. The average patient presents near age 60. Incidence is highest in individuals of northern European descent and in African Americans; pernicious anemia is much less common in southern Europeans and Asians. It occurs more frequently in patients with other autoimmune-related diseases, including Graves' disease, myxedema, thyroiditis, idiopathic adrenocortical insufficiency, vitiligo, and hypoparathyroidism. Relatives of pernicious anemia patients have an increased incidence of the disease and may be asymptomatic, but with anti-IF antibody in their serum. Treatment involves administration of glucocorticoids, which may produce neuropsychiatric complications. Patients with pernicious anemia are at increased risk for gastric carcinoma.

Poor Intake

Vitamin B_{12} occurs only in meat products, eggs, and dairy products. Alcoholics and strict vegans are at risk for diet-induced deficiency states. Intake/malabsorp-

tion syndromes must be of several years' duration before individuals become symptomatic (Dharmarajan and Norkus 2001).

Neuropsychiatric Symptoms

There is no *prototypical psychiatric presentation* accompanying B_{12} deficiency. Many case reports cite B_{12} deficiency presenting surreptitiously as primary psychiatric syndromes. Psychiatric symptoms may predate and occur independently of neurological and hematological abnormalities. Previous claims have been challenged that neurologic and psychiatric symptoms are *late* manifestations of B_{12} deficiency, occurring in the setting of *anemia or macrocytosis*. It is now known that patients with neurological and psychiatric symptoms may have serum B_{12} levels that are only moderately below normal. *Hallucinations or changes in personality and mood may be the presenting symptoms.*

Neurological symptoms develop in the majority of patients with untreated vitamin B_{12} deficiency and may also predate hematological findings. The neurologic syndrome of B_{12} deficiency has a typical presentation of symmetrical paresthesias in the feet and fingers, the inability to maintain balance when standing with eyes closed and feet together (Romberg's sign), and associated disturbances of vibratory sense and proprioception due to vacuolation in the posterior columns. In later stages there is corticospinal tract involvement, with spastic paresis and ataxia. This combined syndrome is called subacute combined degeneration (SCD) of the spinal cord (i.e., degenerative changes of the dorsal and lateral columns). Administration of *folate* may *precipitate* the onset of SCD if B_{12} deficiency is not treated first.

Diagnosis

Significant macrocytosis in the presence of a megaloblastic anemia is commonly caused by cobalamin deficiency. (Other causes of macrocytosis include folate deficiency, liver disease, alcoholism, hypothyroidism, and aplastic anemia [Babior and Bunn 2002].) The normal range of cobalamin in serum is 200–900 pg/mL; values <100 pg/mL indicate clinically significant deficiency (see Table 6–6).

Tests of serum methylmalonic acid (MMA) and homocysteine levels improve the sensitivity and specificity of B_{12} measurements and are important in the differential diagnosis of megaloblastic anemias (Baik and Russell 1999; Dharmarajan and Norkus 2001). (Table 6–8 compares the uses of these two tests in differential diagnosis.) These tests measure tissue vitamin stores, flagging a deficiency state even when serum B_{12} levels are borderline or even normal. Elevated MMA is a more specific flag for vitamin B_{12} deficiency, except in cases of chronic renal failure, which independently raises MMA (Bjorn et al. 2001; Dharmarajan and Norkus 2001; Savage et al. 1994). In the geriatric population, plasma homocysteine may correlate more closely than plasma MMA with neuropsychiatric dysfunction (Bjorn et al. 2001). The cognitive decline associated with deficiencies of B_{12}, folate, and B_6 is not well understood but may be linked to their direct relationship to elevated homocysteine, an independent risk factor for microvascular disease in the brain (Gonzalez-Gross et al. 2001).

The authors of one review (Dharmarajan and Norkus 2001) recommended yearly B_{12} screening in vulnerable patients, including people over age 65 and those with autoimmune disease, chronic pancreatitis, Crohn's disease, gastric or small-bowel surgery, gastritis, HIV infection, malabsorption syndromes, multiple sclerosis, strict vegan diet, use of histamine H_2 receptor antagonists or proton pump inhibitors, thyroid disease, or unexplained anemia. The recommendation also included screening every 5 years for individuals over 50.

Folate Supplementation and Occult B_{12} Deficiency

Folate and B_{12} deficiencies often occur together. Both cause macrocytic anemia and gastrointestinal symptoms, and folate deficiency is also independently associated with neurological symptoms similar to those seen with vitamin B_{12} deficiency (Skeen 2002). Folate fortification of food (by order of the U.S. Food and Drug Administration in 1998) has had a paradoxical effect. Because the macrocytic anemia resolves along with the folate deficiency, there is greater likelihood that accompanying occult B_{12} deficiency will go undetected (Babior and Bunn 2002). Elderly persons are at greatest risk. Such patients may present with neuropsychiatric abnormalities, including peripheral neuropathy, gait disturbance, memory loss, and psychiatric symptoms, but without macrocytosis or obviously deficient serum B_{12} levels. MMA levels obtained by screening are extremely useful, reflecting B_{12} deficiency at the tissue level. Treatment with cobalamin tends to improve the psychiatric abnormalities, normalizing serum MMA. Unfortunately, neurologic defects do not always reverse with cobalamin supplementation.

Treatment

Early identification and treatment of B_{12} deficiency can greatly reduce patient morbidity, since neuropsychiatric deficits are potentially reversible with early intervention. One prospective study reported improvements on tests of verbal word learning, verbal fluency, and similarities after healthy, nondemented community-dwelling elderly persons with low B_{12} levels on screening received cobalamin supplementation (van Asselt et al. 2001).

Replacement therapy is the mainstay of treatment for cobalamin deficiency. Historically, monthly parenteral therapy was recommended, particularly in cases of pernicious anemia where insufficient IF presumably prevented the efficacy of oral replacement

Table 6–8. Differential diagnosis using serum methylmalonic acid (MMA) and homocysteine levels

| | Serum level | | |
	In B_{12} deficiency	In folate deficiency	Notes
MMA	↑	Normal	Specific marker for B_{12} deficiency except in renal failure
Homocysteine	↑	↑	Elevated in folate deficiency, B_6 deficiency, renal failure, hypothyroidism, aging

with free vitamin B$_{12}$. More recent evidence suggests that high-dose (1,000–2,000 mg/day) daily oral replacement therapy may be as effective as parenteral treatment (Oh and Brown 2003). The response to treatment is usually quick, beginning hematologically as bone marrow morphology reverts toward normal. The patient should experience increased strength and improved sense of well-being. Most patients require only replacement therapy. Some patients develop severe anemia, requiring transfusions. If treatment continues, the complications of the deficiency state do not progress or return, although some neurologic symptoms may not resolve even with optimal therapy. Pernicious anemia patients are at risk for gastric carcinoma and require careful follow-up.

Prophylaxis

Some experts have recommended the use of 0.1 mg oral crystalline cobalamin prophylaxis daily in people over age 65 years. This recommendation has been made because defective cobalamin absorption occurs so commonly in older people and may present covertly, as neurologic illness, rather than with hematologic symptoms.

■ REFERENCES

American Gastroenterological Association: Medical position statement: irritable bowel syndrome. Gastroenterology 123:2105–2107, 2002

Andres E: Food-cobalamin malabsorption in the elderly. Am J Med 113:351–352, 2002

Babior BM, Bunn HF: Megaloblastic anemias, in Harrison's Online, DOI 101036/1096–7133ch107. Edited by Braunwald E, Fauci A, Isselbacher K, et al. McGraw-Hill, 2002. Available at: http://harrisons.accessmedicine.com. Accessed June 12, 2003.

Baik H, Russell R: Vitamin B$_{12}$ deficiency in the elderly. Annu Rev Nutr 19:357–377, 1999

Bernhard J, Hürny C: Gastrointestinal cancer, in Psychooncology. Edited by Holland J, Breitbart W. New York, Oxford University Press, 1998, pp 324–339

Bjorn H, Anders I, Nilson K, et al: Markers for the functional availability of cobalamin/folate and their association with neuropsychiatric symptoms in the elderly. Int J Geriatr Psychiatry 16:873–878, 2001

Clouse R: Antidepressants for irritable bowel syndrome. Gut 52:598–599, 2003

Clouse R, Lustman P, Geisman R, et al: Antidepressant therapy in 138 patients with irritable bowel syndrome: a five-year clinical experience. Aliment Pharmacol Ther 8:409–416, 1994

Creed F, Fernandes L, Guthrie E, et al: The cost-effectiveness of psychotherapy and paroxetine for severe irritable bowel syndrome. Gastroenterology 124:303–317, 2003

Croarkin P: From King George to neuroglobin: the psychiatric aspects of acute intermittent porphyria. J Psychiatr Pract 8:398–405, 2002

Desnick R: The Porphyrias, in Harrison's Principles of Internal Medicine, 15th Edition. Edited by Braunwald E, Fauci A, Kasper D, et al. New York, McGraw-Hill Medical, 2001, pp 2261–2267

Dharmarajan T, Norkus E: Approaches to vitamin B$_{12}$ deficiency: early treatment may prevent devastating complications. Postgrad Med 110:99–105, 2001

Emmanuel N, Lydiard R, Crawford M: Treatment of irritable bowel syndrome with fluvoxamine (letter). Am J Psychiatry 154:711–712, 1997

Gonzalez-Arriaza H, Bostwick J: Acute porphyrias: a case report and review. Am J Psychiatry 160:450–458, 2003

Gonzalez-Gross M, Marcos A, Pietrzik K: Nutrition and cognitive impairment in the elderly. Br J Nutr 86:313–321, 2001

Grandchamp B: Acute intermittent porphyria. Semin Liver Dis 18:17–24, 1999

Green A, Austin C: Psychopathology of pancreatic cancer: a psychobiologic probe. Psychosomatics 34:208–221, 1993

Hasler W: The irritable bowel syndrome. Med Clin North Am 86:1525–1551, 2002

Herbert V: Staging vitamin B-12 (cobalamin) status in vegetarians. Am J Clin Nutrition 59:1213S–1222S, 1994

Herbert V, Das K: Folic acid and vitamin B$_{12}$, in Modern Nutrition in Health and Disease, 8th Edition. Edited by Shils M, Olson J, Shikie M. Philadelphia, PA, Lea & Febiger, 1994, pp 402–405

Holland J, Hughes A, Tross S, et al: Comparative psychological disturbance in patients with pancreatic and gastric cancer. Am J Psychiatry 143:982–986, 1986

Holroyd S, Seward R: Psychotropic drugs in acute intermittent porphyria. Clin Pharmacol Ther 66:323–325, 1999

Ibrahim Z, Carney M: Safe use of haloperidol in acute intermittent porphyria (letter). Ann Pharmacother 29:200, 1995

Ilnyckyj A, Bernstein C: Sexual abuse in irritable bowel syndrome: to ask or not to ask—that is the question. Can J Gastroenterol 16:801–805, 2002

Kedra B, Popiela T, Sierzega M, et al: Prognostic factors of long-term survival after resective procedures for pancreatic cancer. Hepatogastroenterology 48:1762–1766, 2001

Kirsch M, Louie A: Paroxetine and irritable bowel syndrome. Am J Psychiatry 157:1523–1524, 2000

Lindenbaum J, Rosenberg I, Wilson P, et al: Prevalence of cobalamin deficiency in the Framingham elderly population. Am J Clin Nutr 60:2–11, 1994

Lishman W: Organic Psychiatry, 3rd Edition. London, Blackwell Scientific, 1998

Lydiard R: Irritable bowel syndrome, anxiety, and depression: what are the links? J Clin Psychiatry 62 (suppl 8):38–45, 2001

Lydiard R, Fossey M, Marsh W, et al: Prevalence of psychiatric disorders in patients with irritable bowel syndrome. Psychosomatics 34:229–234, 1993

Masand P, Gupta S, Schwartz T, et al: Paroxetine in patients with irritable bowel syndrome: a pilot open-label study. Prim Care Companion J Clin Psychiatry 4:12–16, 2002

Mayer R: Pancreatic Cancer, in Harrison's Online, DOI 101036/1096–7133ch92. Edited by Braunwald E, Fauci A, Isselbacher K, et al. McGraw-Hill, 2002. Available at: http://harrisons.accessmedicine.com. Accessed May 23, 2003.

Millward LM, Kelly P, Deacon A, et al: Self-rated psychosocial consequences and quality of life in the acute porphyrias. J Inherit Metab Dis 24:733–747, 2001

Moore M: Porphyria: A Patient's Guide. Porphyria Research Unit, The University of Queensland, Department of Medicine. 1999. Available at: http://www.uq.edu.au/porphyria/safedrug.htm. Accessed May 23, 2003.

Moss S, Modlin I: Summation: irritable bowel and the irritable physician. J Clin Gastroenterol 35 (suppl):S68–S70, 2002

Oh R, Brown DL: Vitamin B_{12} deficiency. Am Fam Physician 67:979–986 [summary for patients 67:993–994], 2003

Ringel Y: Brain research in functional gastrointestinal disorders. J Clin Gastroenterol 35 (suppl):S23–S25, 2002

Savage D, Lindenbaum J, Stabler S, et al: Sensitivity of serum methylmalonic acid and total homocysteine determinations for diagnosing cobalamin and folate deficiencies. Am J Med 96:239–246, 1994

Schenk BE, Kuipers EJ, Klinkenberg-Knol EC, et al: Atrophic gastritis during long-term omeprazole therapy affects serum vitamin B_{12} levels. Aliment Pharmacol Ther 13:1343–1346, 1999

Skeen MB: Neurologic manifestations of gastrointestinal disease. Neurol Clin 20:195–225, vii, 2002

Spanier AJ, Howden CW, Jones MP: A systematic review of alternative therapies in the irritable bowel syndrome. Arch Intern Med 163:265–274, 2003

Suarez J, Cohen M, Larkin J, et al: Acute intermittent porphyria: clinical pathological correlation: report of a case and review of the literature. Neurology 48:1678–1683, 1997

Talley N: Functional gastrointestinal disorders, in Current Diagnosis and Treatment in Gastroenterology, 2nd Edition. Edited by Friedman S, McQuaid K, Grendell J. Lange Medical/McGraw-Hill, 2003. Available at: http://online.statref.com/document.aspx?fxid=23&docid=55. Accessed May 23, 2003.

Thomas S: Irritable bowel syndrome and mirtazapine. Am J Psychiatry 157:1341–1342, 2000

Thompson W, Longstretch G, Drossman D, et al: Section C, Functional Bowel Disorders, and Section D, Functional Abdominal Pain, in Rome II: Functional Gastrointestinal Disorders: Diagnosis, Pathophysiology, and Treatment, 2nd Edition. Edited by Drossman D, Talley N, Thompson W, et al. McLean, VA, Degnon Associates, 2000, pp 351–432

van Asselt DZ, de Groot LC, Van Staveren WA, et al: Role of cobalamin intake and atrophic gastritis in mild cobalamin deficiency in older Dutch subjects. Am J Clin Nutr 68:328–334, 1998

van Asselt DZ, Blom HJ, Zuiderent R, et al: Clinical significance of low cobalamin levels in older hospital patients. Neth J Med 57:41–49, 2000

van Asselt DZ, Pasman JW, van Lier HJ, et al: Cobalamin supplementation improves cognitive and cerebral function in older, cobalamin-deficient persons. J Gerontol A Biol Sci Med Sci 56:M775–M779, 2001

Van Goor L, Woisky M, Lagaay A, et al: Review: cobalamin deficiency and mental impairment in elderly people. Age Ageing 24:536–542, 1995

Wald A: Psychotropic agents in irritable bowel syndrome. J Clin Gastroenterol 35 (suppl):S53–S57, 2002

Whitehead W, Bosmajian L, Zorderman A, et al: Symptoms of psychologic distress associated with irritable bowel syndrome: comparison of community and medical clinic samples. Gastroenterology 95:709–714, 1988

Wikberg A, Jansson L, Lithner F: Women's experience of suffering repeated severe attacks of acute intermittent porphyria. J Adv Nurs 32:1348–1355, 2000

Wolff RA, Abbruzzese J, Evans DB: Neoplasms of the exocrine pancreas, in Holland-Frei Cancer Medicine 6, 6th Edition. Edited by Kufe D, Pollock R, Weichselbaum R, et al. Hamilton, ON, BC Decker, 2003, pp 1585–1614

The Obstetrics Patient

Antoinette Ambrosino Wyszynski, M.D.
Shari I. Lusskin, M.D.

The selective serotonin reuptake inhibitors (SSRIs) have replaced benzodiazepines, sedatives, and tricyclic antidepressants as first-line medications for anxiety and depressive disorders in pregnant women. Before their arrival, the emphasis was on "making do" until the infant was delivered, because of worries about teratogenicity.

The SSRIs have streamlined, but not eliminated, clinical decision making. The risks to the fetus shift over time, creating uncertainty about intervention. Pregnancy dysregulates occult and established psychiatric illness, particularly in the postpartum period. Several management problems arise when treating women of childbearing age:

1. How should a patient be managed while she attempts to conceive?
2. How should a single depressive episode, versus more than two episodes, be factored into treatment planning?
3. If a woman is euthymic and already pregnant when she arrives for evaluation, should one continue medication during the first trimester? Would the same medications be OK for the second and the third trimester?
4. What would the treatment recommendations be if a patient wanted to breastfeed? Would the recommendations change if a patient had already suffered from postpartum depression after a prior pregnancy?
5. How does a history of bipolar disorder change the clinical decision making?
6. How should psychosis be handled if it occurs?
7. Should one ever advise electroconvulsive therapy (ECT) in pregnancy? Is it safe?

The permutations of these treatment decisions can be dizzying. For the depressed patient, the path to treatment has been made easier by the Consensus Guideline Project for the treatment of depression. (Altshuler et al. 2001) (see the sections in this chapter on depression occurring in the conception, pregnancy, and postpartum periods). For the patient with bipolar disorder, a consensus guideline for the management of bipolar disorder in pregnant and postpartum women is also available (Yonkers et al. 2004).

Unfortunately, parallel consensus studies do not exist for managing schizophrenia and anxiety disorders in pregnancy. As an alternative, we have gathered the recommendations from the current literature for these patients, organizing the data according to four stages of the reproductive cycle: Phase I, Conception; Phase II, Pregnancy; Phase III, Postpartum; and Phase IV, Breastfeeding.

Box 7–1 highlights the numerous resources available to assist the clinician in assessing the safety of various medications during pregnancy and lactation. Table 7–1 lists the differential diagnosis of psychiatric problems encountered in pregnancy and the postpartum period.

Box 7–1. **Clinician resources for safety data on medications in pregnancy and lactation**

The UpToDate series in Obstetrics, Gynecology, and Women's Health (http://www.uptodate.com; accessed June 2004). Provides material that is periodically revised by psychiatrists who specialize in the care of pregnant patients.

Briggs G, Freeman R, Yaffe S: *Drugs in Pregnancy and Lactation,* 6th Edition. Philadelphia, PA, Lippincott Williams & Wilkins, 2002. Revised every 4 years.

Friedman J, Polifka JE: *Teratogenic Effects of Drugs: A Resource for Clinicians (TERIS),* 2nd Edition. Baltimore, MD, Johns Hopkins University Press, 2000.

TERIS (206-43-2465; http://www.depts.washington.edu/~terisweb; accessed June 2004).

ReproTox (202-293-5237; http://www.reprotox.org; accessed June 2004).

Physician Assistance Department of the drug manufacturer (numbers obtainable in the *Physicians' Desk Reference*) often provides medication-specific literature searches, recent articles, or summaries.

The U.S. Food and Drug Administration (FDA) "ABC" rating system: not considered accurate and currently in the process of revision (Yonkers et al. 2004). Sometimes the FDA rating designations can lead to erroneous conclusions that certain medications are safer to use in pregnancy than others. Of limited usefulness in clinical decision making. It is more accurate to do a quick literature search to update drug safety summaries.

Table 7–1. DSM-IV-TR differential diagnosis of psychiatric problems encountered in pregnancy and the postpartum period

Category	Differential Diagnosis
Mood disorders	Major depressive disorder[a] Bipolar I or II disorder[a] Mood disorder due to [general medical condition][b] Substance-induced mood disorder
Psychotic disorders (usually affective)	Major depressive disorder with psychotic features Bipolar I disorder Psychotic disorder due to [general medical condition][b] Substance-induced psychotic disorder Schizophrenia and schizoaffective disorder Brief psychotic disorder[a]
Anxiety disorders	Generalized anxiety disorder Panic disorder Obsessive-compulsive disorder Anxiety disorder due to [general medical condition][b] Substance-induced anxiety disorder
Eating disorders	Anorexia nervosa (AN) Bulimia nervosa (BN) Eating disorder not otherwise specified (and subtypes of AN and BN: e.g., restricting, bingeing)

[a]Specify with postpartum onset, within 4 weeks of giving birth (but clinically may present later).
[b]Especially new-onset conditions, such as thyroid disorders, lupus, or HIV infection.

It is important to note that substance-induced disorders should be included in the differential diagnosis of pregnant and lactating women (see Table 7–1). Most clinicians know about the complications of heavy substance abuse during pregnancy, such as fetal alcohol syndrome. However, cigarette smoking and heavy caffeine use also pose risks to the mother and fetus (Ness et al. 1999). One study found that up to one-third of a sample of 186 obstetrics clinic patients were at risk for psychiatric disorders and/or substance abuse, as identified by screening questionnaires (Kelly et al. 2001). Of those identified, only a minority (23%) received specific treatment. Although clinic attendees may not represent the general population, these findings highlight the importance of careful diagnostic workup, including obtaining a urine toxicology screen for all patients.

Limitations of space make it inevitable that psychotherapy will get short shrift in our review, despite its primacy in treating the pregnant patient. The techniques of psychotherapy form volumes unto themselves. Methodologies that have been specifically studied in pregnancy and/or postpartum include interpersonal psychotherapy (O'Hara et al. 2000; Spinelli and Endicott 2003; Zlotnick et al. 2001), cognitive-behavioral therapy (Appleby et al. 1997), marital therapy, group psychotherapy, and family therapy.

■ PHASE I: CONCEPTION

Always note the date of the last menstrual period and the patient's method of birth control. About 50% of all pregnancies are unplanned, so this will help the clinician track pregnancy and early exposure to psychotropic medications. Ideally, decisions regarding medications will be made prior to conception.

Given poor compliance with birth control methods and the inherent failure rate of each method, many women will conceive inadvertently while taking medications. Among those who are making a considered choice, however, many are reluctant to conceive a baby while on medications. Understandably, most prospective mothers-to-be wish to remain medication-free for as long as possible. The danger of recurrence of the psychiatric disorder is often overlooked in the desire for a "natural" or "chemical-free" pregnancy. Responsible counseling is essential. This requires discussions about the genetics of mental illness and its natural history with and without treatment. The clinician must discuss the relative risks and benefits of us-

ing medication during pregnancy. Some women may once again mourn the fact that they have an illness, reacting with grief, anger, and often anxiety for their future offspring. The clinician should try not to short-circuit these reactions, but to help the patient process them.

Sometimes these discussions alone may bring relief; many women assume that they cannot bear a child because they are taking medication, or make erroneous assumptions about the risks of transmitting their illness to their children. Frank conversations about the genetics of the illness and the treatment options in pregnancy may bring a welcome surprise.

Whenever possible, the clinician should try to include the other prospective parent in these discussions and to proceed along the model of informed consent. Informed consent is likely to be more reliably obtained when the couple has engaged in responsible decision making together. We discuss informed consent further in the section Phase II: Pregnancy, below. Table 7–2, which summarizes what is known about the natural history of depression, psychosis, and bipolar disorder associated with pregnancy, may assist in these discussions.

Try to outline a relapse prevention and management strategy, preferably *before* the patient attempts conception. Such an approach allows for advance planning—alerting the obstetrician, preparing for the impact on job or finances should the patient become disabled, and enlisting family or friends for assistance at home or if the patient requires hospitalization. Some patients might also find it reassuring to pursue a second opinion with a psychiatrist experienced in treating psychiatric syndromes in pregnant women.

Although this approach potentially burdens an already upset individual with too much information, most families respond favorably to having a safety net—a "game plan just in case" of a recurrence. Reassurances that the patient will not become symptomatic again, or statements like "We'll cross that bridge when we come to it," are well-meaning but not useful. During a recurrence, it is easier to call on a strategy formed together as a team, when the patient felt well, than to scramble to put one together during a crisis. Generally, the more informed the patient and family, the better the clinical course.

Medication changes are best effected before the patient becomes pregnant. This procedure will help to minimize the number of medications to which the fetus will be exposed. It is also a strategy to buy time with the patient so that she is more likely to be euthymic at conception and remain so throughout the pregnancy.

Table 7–2. Natural history of psychiatric illness associated with pregnancy and the postpartum period

Type	Characteristics	Studies
Depression	1st and 3rd trimesters are the time of peak depressive symptoms.	Evans et al. 2001; Kumar and Robson 1984; Steiner and Yonkers 1998
	Risk factors for antenatal and postpartum depression: personal[a] or family history of depression before, during,[b] after, or unassociated with pregnancy.	Beck 1996; Kumar and Robson 1984; Llewellyn et al. 1997
Psychotic disorders	Schizophrenic and schizoaffective disorders: high risk of relapse off medication.	Cohler et al. 1975; Davidson and Robertson 1985; McNeil et al. 1984; Protheroe 1969
	The postpartum period is a time of highest vulnerability to new-onset psychotic illness in the life cycle of a woman.	Agrawal et al. 1997; Kendell et al. 1987; Terp and Mortensen 1998; Videbech and Gouliaev 1995
Bipolar disorder	Natural course unknown; bipolar patients off lithium are at high risk for relapse during pregnancy and the postpartum period.	Viguera et al. 2000
	High risk of manic or depressive psychosis off medication, particularly if medication is not slowly tapered.	Viguera et al. 2002
	Risk factors for bipolar symptomatology for patients not taking medication: personal or family history of affective illness, particularly bipolar disorder.	

[a]It is estimated that 50%–62% of women with a prior history of postpartum depression will develop it again.
[b]Depression during pregnancy strongly predicts postpartum depression.

Unipolar Depression

In 2001, a panel of 36 national experts in the field of women's mental health completed a written survey covering a total of 858 treatment options in 117 specific clinical situations pertaining to depressive disorders across the reproductive cycle (Altshuler et al. 2001). Depression severity (mild to severe) was specified for most clinical situations. Treatment options included a range of pharmacological, psychosocial, and alternative medicine approaches. Categorical rank was assigned statistically to each option. Guideline tables indicating preferred treatment strategies were then developed for key clinical situations.

We have tried to abstract the principles of treatment that were detailed in that guideline, to allow for changes in the research literature that occur over time. Figure 7–1 and Figure 7–2 are algorithms for treating depression during conception and pregnancy. A few points are important to consider when using these algorithms:

1. We have used the terms *least-risk antidepressant* (LRAD) and *unknown-risk antidepressant* (URAD) to capture the principle of "risk management" relative to treating depression across the reproductive cycle. Risk is relative; as new studies are published,

the safety of a particular medication is established or undermined. It is up to the clinician to remain up to date about safety data on medications in pregnancy and lactation (see Box 7–1 for a list of clinician resources).

2. Patients may tolerate an unacceptable level of psychopathology in order to have a medication-free pregnancy. The concept of "what the patient can tolerate" relative to untreated psychopathology must be replaced by "what is clinically appropriate," given a careful discussion of risks and benefits. Women who choose to delay intervention because their depressive symptoms are minimal or mild should be educated about the signs or symptoms of a deepening depression and should be followed closely.

3. Regardless of what a woman says early on, she may in the end decide to breastfeed. Antidepressants should be chosen with this possible outcome in mind.

4. As noted in the preceding section, if medication changes are to be made (e.g., the switch from an unknown-risk antidepressant to a least-risk antidepressant), they are best made before conception.

Figure 7–1 provides an algorithm based on the principles of treatment recommended by the Consensus Guideline Project for the treatment of unipolar depression in women who are trying to conceive (Altshuler et al. 2001). Strategies for women trying to conceive are shown for 1) those who become depressed but are not taking medication and 2) those who are already taking antidepressants and have been in remission.

Depression Complicated by Psychosis

If psychosis complicates depression, it is usually in the form of paranoid delusions of persecution or about the fetus, often superimposed on a primary mood disorder (Misri and Lusskin 2004c). Hallucinations are relatively uncommon. Treatment involves adding small doses of antipsychotic medication to the antidepressant regimen. Once the psychotic symptoms remit and the mood has improved, the antipsychotic may be tapered, with caution, but the antidepressant should be continued throughout pregnancy and into the postpartum period. Patients with this complication, especially if untreated, are also at risk for postpartum psychosis. See also the discussion in this chapter on treating psychosis in pregnancy.

- *Warning!* "Unipolar" depression may really be bipolar disorder in dysphoric disguise, which will be unmasked and dysregulated by antidepressant treatment. Once mania occurs, the patient is obligated to undergo treatment with mood stabilizers, which all have teratogenic potential in the first trimester. Appendix 16, "Screening Worksheet for Bipolar Spectrum Disorders," helps identify women at risk for this illness.

Bipolar Disorder

The new expert consensus guidelines summarize much of the literature on the natural history of bipolar disorder in pregnancy and the various treatment options (Yonkers et al. 2004).

A woman with a bipolar history faces difficult choices. Reproductive events increase her risk of affective dysregulation, and many patients will require combination therapy to manage their illness, thus exposing a fetus to multiple medications. Although the odds are that the baby will have no malformations attributable to medication, one must note that all first-trimester antimanic agents have teratogenic potential. Some of these malformations may not be detectable until late in the second trimester (weeks 16–20), leaving the choice for therapeutic abortion until late in the

pregnancy. Some malformations may not be detectable at all during prenatal testing, making the choices even harder. Emotional bonding may start as soon as the pregnancy is diagnosed, so a termination or miscarriage at any stage can be emotionally devastating. We also know that discontinuing lithium, in particular, places a woman with bipolar disorder at grave risk for relapse, both during and (especially) after the pregnancy (Viguera et al. 2000). Specific relapse statistics in pregnancy for alternative mood stabilizers, such as valproic acid (Depakote, Depakene), carbamazepine (Tegretol), and olanzapine (Zyprexa), are not available. It is well established that bipolar patients who have discontinued these medications are at risk for relapse as well. Information on the teratogenicity of these agents is provided at the end of this chapter in Appendix 7–A, "Psychotropics in Pregnancy and Lactation."

Ideally, the treatment plan for every woman of reproductive age with bipolar disorder will take into consideration the potential for pregnancy. Given the variable teratogenic potential of all mood stabilizers, changes to relatively safer medications are best accomplished prior to conception; for example, lithium has less teratogenic potential than valproic acid. During an established pregnancy, the risk of switching medications or treatment modalities has to be balanced against the risks of continuing treatment. Careful decision making will minimize the risks to both the mother and the fetus (Yonkers et al. 2004)

The following strategies are helpful for bipolar patients on lithium who are planning to conceive (Cohen et al. 1994a; Viguera et al. 2002):

- *Minimal risk of relapse:* Try to taper lithium slowly, before pregnancy, over the course of 6 weeks, to minimize rebound relapses. Use high-potency neuroleptics as substitute maintenance, but without using mood stabilizers until the second trimester.
- *Moderate risk of relapse:* Do not discontinue medication until documentation of pregnancy. Slowly taper and discontinue lithium during organogenesis, 4–12 weeks after the last menstrual period. Achieving conception may take several months, and this approach minimizes the lithium-free period, thus lowering the risk of affective disorder recurrence. Also, in the setting of early pregnancy (i.e., after one missed menstrual period, or at approximately 2 weeks postconception), the window of lithium exposure is small.
- *Severe risk of relapse:* Continue lithium throughout the period of conception and early pregnancy. Conduct necessary tests of fetal development at weeks 16–20.

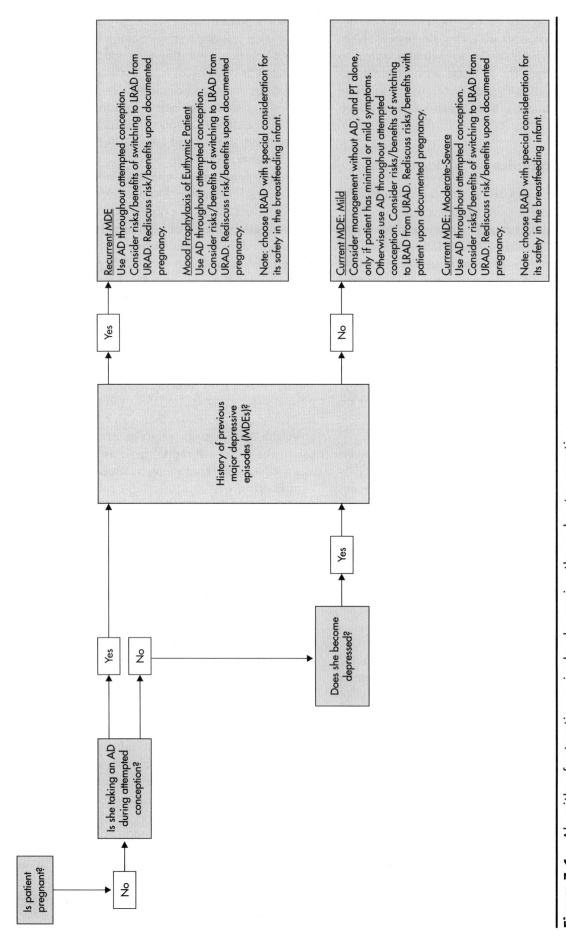

Figure 7–1. Algorithm for treating unipolar depression throughout conception.

Abbreviations: AD=antidepressant; LRAD=least-risk antidepressant; PT=psychotherapy; T=trimester; URAD=unknown-risk antidepressant.

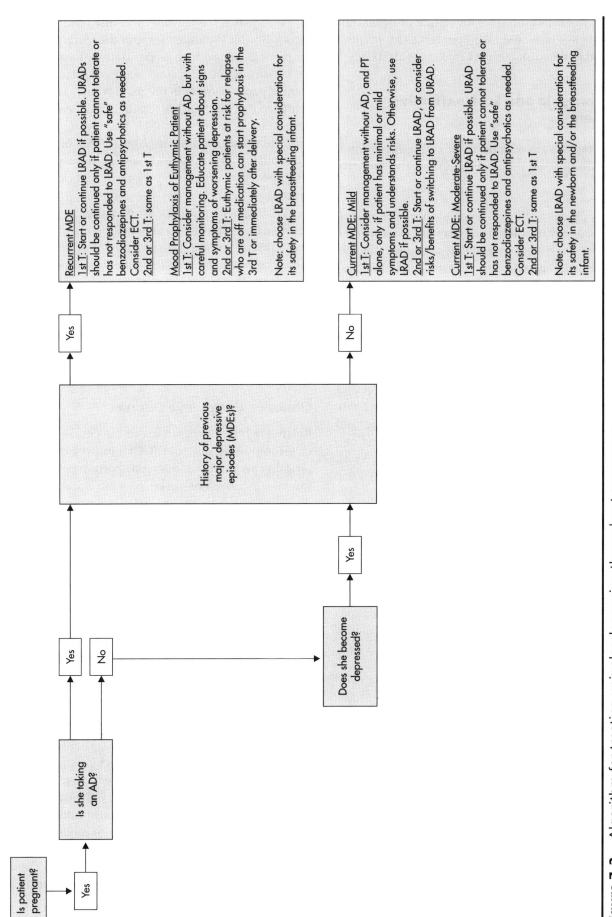

Figure 7–2. Algorithm for treating unipolar depression throughout pregnancy.

Abbreviations: AD=antidepressant; ECT=electroconvulsive therapy; LRAD=least-risk antidepressant; PT=psychotherapy; T=trimester; URAD=unknown-risk antidepressant.

The consensus guidelines for bipolar disorder during pregnancy outline similar approaches for patients taking other mood stabilizers (Yonkers et al. 2004).

Schizophrenia and Schizoaffective Disorders

Several factors are of concern in caring for women with schizophrenia (Miller 1997; Miller and Finnerty 1998):

- Schizophrenic women tend to have more unplanned and unwanted pregnancies than women without this diagnosis, and they are more often victims of violence during pregnancy (Miller and Finnerty 1996). They may not have the benefit of preconception counseling and may present already in the first trimester, when prenatal care becomes the top priority.
- Unmedicated schizophrenic patients have a much higher risk of decompensating both during and after pregnancy (Cohler et al. 1975; Davidson and Robertson 1985; McNeil et al. 1984; Protheroe 1969).
- The high rate of relapse for schizophrenic and schizoaffective patients is diminished with maintenance antipsychotic treatment (Robinson et al. 1999).

It is usually advisable to continue antipsychotic treatment for a pregnant patient with schizophrenia or schizoaffective disorder. More difficult, however, are questions of informed consent for the patient whose psychotic process has impaired her ability to think clearly about risk and benefit. As noted, it is advisable to include the partner and family in the informed consent discussion, to document clearly the rationale for pharmacotherapy, and to proceed with involuntary treatment if necessary.

Anxiety Disorders

Panic Disorder

There are inconsistent findings about the impact of pregnancy on panic disorder. Some authors have suggested that pregnancy provides a protective effect, diminishing the intensity and number of symptoms (Cowley and Roy-Burne 1989; George et al. 1987). Others have documented persistent panic attacks during pregnancy and in the postpartum period (Cohen et al. 1994b, 1996), rendering advice about the predicted course of panic disorder off medication unreliable.

The SSRIs have become first-line treatments for panic disorder. Although some of the SSRIs approved for panic disorder, such as paroxetine (Paxil), do not yet have a large accumulated safety record in the treatment of panic disorder in pregnant women, there is no evidence that any SSRI is teratogenic when used for depression. Alternatively, their therapeutic predecessors, the tricyclic antidepressants (TCAs) imipramine (Tofranil) and nortriptyline (Pamelor, Aventyl), have a long history of safe use in pregnancy and can be used as backup.

A patient with mild disease may attempt a medication-free first trimester by slowly tapering off medication but reinstituting it if symptoms reappear, before they become disabling. If the patient has severe panic disorder with a history of relapsing when off medications, pharmacotherapy should be continued throughout the pregnancy. A structured form of psychotherapy, such as cognitive-behavioral therapy, may allow for regular monitoring, serve to support the patient, and teach her strategies for managing anxiety.

Obsessive-Compulsive Disorder

Relatively little is known about the course of obsessive-compulsive disorder (OCD) in pregnancy. Empirically, pregnancy and the postpartum period seem to confer increased risk of onset or exacerbation of this disorder (Abramowitz et al. 2003; Chelmow and Halfin 1997; Hertzberg et al. 1997; Maina et al. 1999; Neziroglu et al. 1992; Sichel et al. 1993). Although generalizations are limited by scanty research in the area of OCD in pregnancy, clinical observations suggest that earlier onset and moderate to severe symptoms before pregnancy predict a more severe disease course in pregnancy (Misri and Lusskin 2004c).

Misri and Lusskin (2004c) described a subtype of OCD, with onset often in the third trimester, in which ego-dystonic obsessional symptoms develop, often without compulsive rituals. Obsessional thoughts are about harming the baby, without the compulsion to act, but careful evaluation is nonetheless warranted. Compulsive behaviors that can have significant psychosocial ramifications, such as checking the baby excessively or avoiding knives, may develop in response to the obsessional thoughts. Severe OCD can overlap with psychosis in both pregnant and nonpregnant women. Obsessional thoughts require careful evaluation to rule out psychosis.

Under the best of circumstances, OCD is a therapeutic challenge. In pregnancy and postpartum, the illness becomes even more complex because of concerns about fetal safety and exacerbation in the postpartum period. One study reported that women with OCD may be at increased risk for postpartum depression, underscoring the importance of careful postpartum evaluation of women with OCD (Williams and Koran 1997). Symptoms may also interfere with adherence to prenatal care and proper care of the infant.

Eating Disorders From Conception to Postpartum

Anorexia nervosa (both restricting type and bulimic type) and bulimia nervosa often do not come to medical attention until pregnancy, even though the woman may have been symptomatic since adolescence or throughout young adulthood. Typically, the psychiatrist is asked to evaluate such a patient when she develops hyperemesis gravidarum (excessive nausea and vomiting) or a mood disorder. It is the exception, rather than the rule, that an eating disorder has already been identified before referral.

The prevalence of eating disorders among women of childbearing potential has been reported to be 4% (King 1989). Although not well studied, the prevalence during pregnancy has been estimated to be closer to 1%, due to symptom remission in some pregnant women and impaired fertility associated with eating disorders (Turton et al. 1999).

Although active eating disorders may impair fertility, the associated amenorrhea or oligomenorrhea does not necessarily stop ovulation, and women with these disorders may become pregnant unexpectedly (Mitchell-Gieleghem et al. 2002). Women with eating disorders who are underweight and require infertility treatments in order to become pregnant are more likely to miscarry. Eating disorders should ideally be in full remission before any assisted reproductive technology is offered to the patient (Norre et al. 2001). Anorexia nervosa is easily suspected when the patient presents with below-normal body weight. Bulimia nervosa, in contrast, has been called the "invisible eating disorder" because the patient may have a normal or above-normal weight (Mitchell-Gieleghem et al. 2002).

Obstetricians do not typically ask about a history of eating disorders or current symptomatology (Abraham 2001). Moreover, women with anorexia or bulimia tend to conceal their abnormal eating patterns and use of compensatory behaviors (fasting, laxative abuse, diuretic abuse, purging, and excessive exercise) because of denial, shame, and/or guilt (Abraham 2001).

Warning signs of an eating disorder during pregnancy include the following (Franko and Spurrell 2000):

- Hyperemesis gravidarum
- Lack of weight gain in two consecutive prenatal visits in the second trimester
- A history of an eating disorder

Risk factors for active disease in pregnancy include a prior history of disease (eating disorders may be "reactivated" in pregnancy, and current symptoms may be concealed), younger age, unemployment, lower educational level, and poorer housing (Mitchell-Gieleghem et al. 2002; Turton et al. 1999). Eating disorders can, however, occur in all socioeconomic groups (Mitchell-Gieleghem et al. 2002).

A higher risk of fetal and maternal complications is conferred by the presence of eating disorders in the mother. Studies have shown a greater incidence of hyperemesis gravidarum, miscarriage, intrauterine growth retardation, prematurity, cesarean section, and postpartum depression (Abraham 1998; Bulik et al. 1999; Conti et al. 1998; Franko and Spurrell 2000; Franko et al. 2001; Morgan et al. 1999). As an example, a large prospective study comparing the pregnancy outcome of 302 women hospitalized with an eating disorder before pregnancy and 900 control subjects found that women with eating disorders had significantly higher rates of preterm birth (7.0% vs. 4.3%) and of infants small for gestational age (19.6% vs. 12.0%) (Sollid et al. 2004).

Eating disorder symptoms may improve in pregnancy, often because the woman has made a commitment to caring for the fetus (Mitchell-Gieleghem et al. 2002). One recent prospective study reported that both anorexia and bulimia symptoms improved during pregnancy, with symptom remission persisting in the patients with bulimia nervosa up to 9 months postpartum. Patients with anorexia nervosa were more likely than patients with bulimia nervosa to return to their pre-pregnancy baseline symptom levels within 6 months of delivery (Blais et al. 2000). In the same group of patients, a subsequent study showed that women with active disease during pregnancy were more likely to have a cesarean section and to develop postpartum depression compared with women in remission. Although most of the pregnancies yielded healthy babies born at term, there was a higher incidence of congenital defects compared with the general population (Franko et al. 2001).

Disordered eating and its associated compensatory behaviors pose risks for both mother and fetus. Anorexia nervosa predisposes to intrauterine growth retardation, as well as malnutrition in the mother. Bulimia nervosa may lead to excessive weight gain as the woman's ability to compensate for binge eating becomes limited; for example, she may decide to stop purging or be unable to exercise excessively.

Pregnant women with eating disorders require careful evaluation for comorbid psychiatric disorders such as antenatal depression. Pharmacotherapy with adjunctive psychotherapy is often necessary. Team management is essential, combining the expertise of an internist, a nutritionist, the obstetrician or family practitioner, and the psychiatrist. This approach must continue into the postpartum period and should include a pediatrician; women with either anorexia nervosa or bulimia nervosa are more likely to underfeed their babies than are women without eating disorders (Lacey and Smith 1987; Russell et al. 1998). The high incidence of relapse of eating disorders after delivery, as well as the comorbidity with postpartum depression, mandates careful long-term follow-up of those patients identified in pregnancy.

Comment on Oral Contraceptives

Oral contraceptives can cause mood changes, particularly depression. In the nongravid woman, discontinuing oral contraceptives or changing the preparation may alleviate the mood symptoms. Progesterone is usually the causative factor, although some women develop mood symptoms in response to estrogen alone. Preparations containing lower progestin-to-estrogen ratios have fewer depressive effects (Lawrie et al. 1998). The same principles will apply later in life—such that perimenopausal women given oral contraceptives or postmenopausal women given hormone replacement therapy may suffer a relapse of depression when given estrogen replacement therapy.

■ PHASE II: PREGNANCY

The goal of management is to minimize the use of medication in the first trimester, when fetal organ formation (organogenesis) is at its height. The brain develops through all three trimesters and beyond, so the risks of medication for neurological development persist beyond the first trimester.

Nonpharmacological interventions can buy time. They include psychotherapy and environmental manipulation (e.g., getting adequate sleep, avoiding caffeine, reducing one's work schedule, receiving help with chores and childcare). If the condition worsens, homecare by family or friends may be an option. Somatic treatments (pharmacotherapy and/or ECT)

usually are warranted when the condition progresses to the point of needing homecare or hospitalization.

Other strategies for minimizing exposure include the following (Misri and Lusskin 2004d):

- Slowly reducing rather than abruptly stopping medications, to lessen withdrawal symptoms. This strategy permits better monitoring for relapse, allowing for prompt intervention.
- Using the lowest possible therapeutic dose
- Choosing medications known to have the lowest fetal toxicity if use of medications is unavoidable
- Minimizing the number of medications used whenever possible (e.g., many women with bipolar disorder will require combination therapy)
- Preventing psychiatric complications by careful history taking. Depressed women with undiagnosed bipolar disorder who are given antidepressants may become manic, forcing the addition of mood stabilizers, which are all potential teratogens (see Appendix 16 in this volume, "Screening Worksheet for Bipolar Spectrum Disorders").
- Choosing a medication with minimal effects on the fetus and newborn. As noted above, the choice of medication in pregnancy will also reflect whether or not a woman plans to breastfeed. This strategy spares the patient the risks of medication changes during the postpartum period, the time of greatest vulnerability to relapse.
- Avoiding the temptation to try a newly released medication. Until enough data demonstrate its safety in human pregnancy, stick with a tried-and-true drug unless there is a compelling reason to switch (e.g., if the woman has been unresponsive to all other treatments, has conceived while taking the newer medication, and runs a high risk of relapse if it is discontinued). The clinician should stay up to date and access a current database of medications before using them in pregnant or lactating women.

Comment: Although it is important to minimize exposure to medications, do not undertreat the mother in the hope of reducing risks to the fetus; to do so exposes the fetus to the risks of untreated illness as well as to the risks of medications.

Risks, Benefits, and Informed Consent

Medicating a pregnant woman requires informed consent. As with any patient, a reassuring, compassionate manner should not preempt her right to know the potential risks and benefits. The clinician must be knowledgeable about the existing data and their limitations. It is up to the clinician to remain informed about the current findings for a particular drug in pregnant and lactating woman. In addition to conducting a search of a medical database, several other sources will be helpful. They are listed in Box 7–1.

A Word About the FDA "ABC" Rating System

Although the teratogenicity rating system used by the U.S. Food and Drug Administration (FDA) is a point of reference, we feel it is of limited usefulness in clinical decision making. The ratings (A, B, C, D, or X) can be misleading. For example: bupropion (Wellbutrin) is rated category B; nortriptyline (Pamelor, Aventyl) is rated category D. Does this reflect bupropion's superior teratogenic profile compared with nortriptyline? Is it a safer choice than nortriptyline? In fact, bupropion's rating derives entirely from animal studies. On the other hand, there has been a large body of data supporting the safety of nortriptyline in human pregnancy. Certainly during 30 years of use there have been safety concerns about nortriptyline in pregnancy, as with all tricyclics. The result is that nortriptyline has been assigned a higher risk category than a medication like bupropion, which is a relative newcomer and has fewer documented safety concerns. A simplistic interpretation of the FDA rating system could lead to the erroneous conclusion that bupropion is safer to use in pregnancy than nortriptyline. Instead, we feel it is best to do a quick literature search to update drug safety summaries such as those listed in Box 7–1. The FDA rating system is currently undergoing revision (Yonkers et al. 2004).

Risk-Benefit Discussions

The clinician should try to provide *written* information to the expectant couple. Anxiety or the psychiatric condition itself may interfere with processing what is heard. Printed patient education material allows the couple to review at home and return with questions. Information sheets and consent forms are no substitute, however, for an actual discussion of risks and benefits with the prescribing physician. Consent and doctor-patient discussions must be documented in writing for medicolegal reasons. Whenever possible, consent should be obtained from the other expectant parent as well.

- An example of such documentation might be: "The risks, benefits, and alternatives to treatment with [name of medication], including but not limited to

teratogenicity, neurobehavioral teratogenicity, and neonatal intoxication and withdrawal syndromes, were discussed with the patient and her partner, who agree with the plan."

Factors That Affect the Fetus and Newborn

Most individuals imagine structural (morphological) teratogenicity, such as the limb deformities of the thalidomide catastrophe, when they think of the risk of in utero exposure to medications. However, there are other problems that must enter into informed clinical decision making and informed consent. Table 7–3 lists factors that affect the fetus and newborn, and Table 7–4 lists factors that determine the teratogenic risks of a drug. As in the titration of a drug dosage, such information must be disclosed in a manner that is sensitive to a patient's capacity to process the data. The decision to use medications may evolve over time (see also Chapter 12 in this volume, "Assessing Decisional Capacity and Informed Consent in Medical Patients").

Table 7–3. Factors affecting the fetus and newborn

Factor	Type of effect
Teratogenicity	Structural (morphological; e.g., limb deformity)
	Neurobehavioral (long-term effects of exposure on neurobehavioral development after birth; e.g., effects on early developmental milestones)
Intoxication	Fetal
	Neonatal (at delivery; during breastfeeding)
Withdrawal	Fetal
	Neonatal and infant (at delivery; during breastfeeding)

Unipolar Depression

Pharmacotherapy

A detailed discussion of specific antidepressants is included in this chapter in Appendix 7–A, "Psychotropics in Pregnancy and Lactation." It may be used with Figures 7–1 and 7–2, the algorithms for treating depression during conception and pregnancy. Alternatives to medication include ECT, light therapy, and psychotherapy (for mild disease).

The tricyclic antidepressants have been used for more than 50 years, but the SSRIs are actually better

Table 7–4.   Factors determining the teratogenic risks of a drug

1. **Drug-related factors**
    Dosage
    Regularity of drug use
    Stage of drug exposure
2. **Environmental factors**
    Illicit drugs
    Alcohol
    Tobacco
    Other toxins
3. **Genetic factors**
    Genetic constitution of the fetus

Guidelines for organogenesis:
Central nervous system: gestational days 10–25
Limb development: gestational days 24–26
Cardiovascular system: gestational days 20–40

studied. Neither class of antidepressants appears to increase the risk for teratogenicity or miscarriage. There are limited reports of neonatal complications such as preterm delivery or poor neonatal adaptation, which are discussed in Appendix 7–A in this chapter. Venlafaxine, trazodone, and nefazodone also appear to be relatively safe. There are very few data on mirtazapine and on bupropion, and these drugs should only be used if better-studied drugs are not an option. Monoamine oxidase inhibitors are generally contraindicated. When depression is complicated by psychosis, antidepressants must be used in combination with antipsychotics. Treatment involves adding small doses of antipsychotic medication to the antidepressant regimen. Once the psychotic symptoms remit and the mood has improved, the antipsychotic may be tapered, with caution, but the antidepressant should be continued throughout pregnancy and into the postpartum period. Patients with depression and psychosis during pregnancy, especially if untreated, are also at risk for postpartum psychosis. For severe depression, and mania, electroconvulsive therapy offers another treatment option (see section on ECT below). For mild disease, light therapy holds promise but is still in the experimental stages.

Light Therapy

The first pilot study (*N*=16) for light treatment in pregnant women showed improvement in mean depression ratings by 49% after 3 weeks of treatment, without adverse effects (Oren et al. 2002). Note that there is a very high placebo response rate in light ther-

apy studies for pregnancy, postpartum, and premenstrual dysphoric disorders.

Electroconvulsive Therapy

ECT is an accepted technique for the treatment of a number of conditions in pregnancy, including depression, mania, and psychosis. No direct evidence of teratogenicity was found in one review of more than 300 cases of ECT used in pregnancy (Miller 1994a). Complications were few (*n*=28) and included benign fetal cardiac arrhythmias, abdominal pain, mild vaginal bleeding, self-limited uterine contractions, and premature labor (which appeared to be caused by factors other than ECT). There were three stillbirths/neonatal deaths, but these were not attributed to ECT. The author concluded that modifications in technique could further reduce the risk of complications by preventing maternal aspiration, respiratory alkalosis, and aortocaval compression.

Two studies have described ECT-induced premature labor, which was managed with tocolytic therapy. In both reports, the babies were born healthy and close to full term (Bhatia et al. 1999; Polster and Wisner 1999).

- *Bottom line:* ECT offers a safe and effective alternative to drugs and may be combined with medications as needed. Box 7–2 summarizes recommendations on use of ECT during pregnancy and the postpartum period from the American Psychiatric Association's Task Force Report on the practice of electroconvulsive therapy.

A Special Consideration: Physical Restraint During Pregnancy

Although this prospect is disagreeable to everyone, sometimes it is impossible to guarantee the safety of an agitated, pregnant patient without physical restraint.

- A second- or third-trimester patient should be positioned in the *left lateral position* (i.e., on her left side), so that the uterus is displaced to the left (i.e., toward the spleen and away from the inferior vena cava). Frequent positional changes will minimize patient discomfort.
- The usual supine (face up) position is contraindicated for extended periods of time during the second half of pregnancy. Compression of the aorta and vena cava by the gravid uterus in supine position may obstruct the venous return to the heart

---

Box 7–2. **Electroconvulsive therapy (ECT) in pregnancy and the puerperium** (see also p. 317)

In pregnancy

a. ECT may be used in all three trimesters of pregnancy and during the puerperium.

b. In pregnant patients, obstetric consultation should be obtained prior to ECT.

c. The risks of ECT anesthetic agents to the fetus are likely to be less than the risks of alternative pharmacologic treatments for psychiatric disorders and also less than the risks of untreated mental illness. Nonetheless, potential teratogenic effects and neonatal toxicities should be discussed in the informed consent process.

d. Pregnant patients should be well oxygenated but not hyperventilated during ECT.

e. The risk of aspiration is increased in pregnant patients and should be assessed on an individual basis. Modifications in ECT procedure should be considered in order to diminish this risk and may include withholding anticholinergic agents; administering nonparticulate antacids, gastrointestinal motility enhancing agents, or histamine-2 blockers; or endotracheal intubation.

f. Medications used to minimize the risk of aspiration or for symptomatic treatment of nausea, headache, or muscle soreness should be appropriate for use during pregnancy.

g. Intravenous hydration with a non-glucose-containing solution is suggested before each ECT treatment.

h. When gestational age is more than 14–16 weeks, noninvasive monitoring of fetal heart rate should be done before and after each ECT treatment.

i. After 20 weeks of pregnancy, uterine blood flow should be optimized by placing a wedge under the patient's right hip to displace the uterus from the aorta and vena cava.

j. If the pregnancy is high risk or close to term, additional monitoring may be indicated at the time of ECT.

k. At facilities administering ECT to pregnant women, resources for managing obstetric and neonatal emergencies should be readily accessible.

In the puerperium (the period after childbirth)

a. Breastfeeding does not usually need to be interrupted during an index or continuation/maintenance course of ECT. However, the informed consent process should include a discussion of the potential risks to the infant of breastfeeding during the ECT course.

b. Anesthetic agents administered with ECT generally pose little risk to the nursing infant.

c. Because other medications given during ECT may be excreted into breast milk, the indications for such medications and their potential effects on the nursing infant should be evaluated before they are administered.

d. Infant medication exposure from breastfeeding immediately after an ECT treatment may be lessened by delaying feeding for several hours or by collecting and storing breast milk for administration by bottle.

Source. American Psychiatric Association: *The Practice of Electroconvulsive Therapy: Recommendations for Treatment, Training, and Privileging.* Task Force Report of the American Psychiatric Association. Washington, DC, American Psychiatric Association, 2001, p. 57. Copyright 2001 American Psychiatric Association. Used with permission.

and produce a vasovagal-like syndrome termed the *supine hypotensive syndrome of pregnancy* (Landon 2001). The accompanying symptoms of hypotension and bradycardia are usually relieved by placing the patient in the left lateral position.

Physical restraint is not without psychological side effects, such as damaged rapport with the patient and intensified paranoia. In some cases, antipsychotic medication may be less traumatic psychologically. Although there is no formula for intervention, women requiring physical restraints also require definitive

somatic treatment such as pharmacotherapy and/or ECT.

Bipolar Disorder

Diagnostic Issues

Often the diagnosis of mania is difficult to make in pregnancy, particularly in the hypomanic phase:

> In the pregnant manic patient, an increase in goal-directed activity (e.g., shopping, cleaning, traveling, redecorating the house) may at first be perceived as

productive and useful signs of "nesting," until people around her realize that these activities are inappropriate and excessive....A manic woman with preeclampsia [for example] may be advised to remain at bedrest, but will not be able to rest because she feels compelled to be excessively active. (Misri and Lusskin 2004d)

The consequences of missing the early declaration of a manic illness, or misattributing it to psychosocial factors, are grave; the patient's judgment will deteriorate, compromising the safety of mother and fetus alike. Appendix 16 in this volume, "Screening Worksheet for Bipolar Spectrum Disorders," helps identify women at risk for this illness.

Buying Time

For the first-trimester patient who is hypomanic, it may be possible to buy time, and avoid mood stabilizers with their potential for teratogenicity, by the following methods (Misri and Lusskin 2004d):

- Environmental manipulation, such as promoting adequate sleep and reducing stress (e.g., giving the patient time off from work, reducing household and childcare responsibilities)
- Benzodiazepines on an as-needed basis (but do not undermedicate!)

With luck, these strategies may avert or attenuate a manic episode. However, if symptoms do not remit, or if the patient is not sleeping or has become agitated, treatment must become more aggressive.

Recommendations for the Treatment of Bipolar Disorder in Pregnancy

1. A trial of lithium prior to conception should be considered. The risk of birth defects from lithium is less than from the anticonvulsants. The anticonvulsant drugs should be used in pregnancy only if better-studied drugs, such as lithium, are ineffective (Yonkers et al. 2004) (see Appendix 7–B, "A Primer on Using Lithium in Pregnancy and Lactation").
2. Clinicians who have pregnant patients taking antiepileptic drugs are encouraged to contact the Antiepileptic Drug Pregnancy Registry (http://www.aedpregnancyregistry.org; toll free: 888-233-2334; accessed June 2004) as early in the pregnancy as possible to include their patients for prospective monitoring.
3. The incidence of neural tube defects for patients taking anticonvulsants *may* be reduced by the fol-

lowing strategies (American Academy of Pediatrics Committee on Drugs 2000; Holmes 2002; Iqbal et al. 2001; Kennedy and Koren 1998; L.B. Holmes, personal communication, June 2003; see also http://search.marchofdimes.com/pnhec/887.asp, accessed June 2004):

- Folic acid (vitamin B$_9$) treatment, using up to 4 mg/day, from periconception through the end of the first trimester. Preconception consultation with the obstetrician is recommended.
- Monotherapy if possible
- Lowest possible dose of drug

4. α-Fetoprotein screening for neural tube defects
5. Ultrasonography between 16 and 20 weeks of pregnancy to detect cardiac abnormalities (associated with lithium; see Appendix 7–B in this chapter) and neural tube defects (associated with antiepileptic drugs)
6. ECT is indicated for the treatment of both mania and severe depression, especially if there is severe agitation or an acute risk of suicide, or if pharmacotherapy is refused or not tolerated. Refer to ECT guidelines in Box 7–2 and in the Unipolar Depression section above.

Schizophrenia and Schizoaffective Disorders

Schizophrenic women are probably among the most vulnerable to the psychiatric complications of pregnancy. These patients are at high risk of psychotic relapse while not taking their medication, placing prenatal care as well as their own medical-psychiatric well-being in jeopardy. For example, a diagnosis of schizophrenia was among several significant predictors of poorer prenatal care and more complicated births (Goodman and Emory 1992; Miller et al. 1990, 1992; Spielvogel and Wile 1992). The misperceptions and bizarre behavior of women with chronic mental illness interfered with their making use of available services (Miller et al. 1990). Schizophrenic women have a higher incidence of fetal growth retardation, preterm birth, and perinatal death (Bennedsen 1998; Bennedsen et al. 1999).

Comprehensive psychosocial management before and after delivery is crucial in helping a patient with a chronic mental illness to deliver and raise a healthy infant (Patton et al. 2002). Although we could find no specific guidelines, years of research have accrued to support using maintenance antipsychotics for the pregnant schizophrenic patient.

The goal of pharmacological management in pregnancy is to reduce symptoms while using the lowest doses and numbers of agents. Consider the following indications for neuroleptics during pregnancy:

- Inability to care for oneself or to cooperate with prenatal care
- Impairment of reality testing, inducing potential danger to self or others
- Disorganized thought, behavior, and perception

Treatment

Note that schizophrenia itself has been found to double statistically the risks of malformations and fetal demise, independently of medication exposure (Altshuler et al. 1996). High-potency, conventional antipsychotics such as haloperidol (Haldol), perphenazine (Trilafon), trifluoperazine (Stelazine), and thiothixene (Navane), when used in nonpsychotic women, were shown to be less teratogenic than low-potency conventional antipsychotics such as chlorpromazine (Thorazine). In psychotic women, high-potency conventional antipsychotics are generally preferred over the low-potency conventional antipsychotics, despite the risk of extrapyramidal effects (Patton et al. 2002).

There is evidence of neurobehavioral teratogenicity in animal studies following fetal exposure to conventional high- and low-potency antipsychotics (Altshuler et al. 1996; American Academy of Pediatrics Committee on Drugs 2000). No effects on behavioral, emotional, or cognitive development have been found in human studies, although prospective, developmental studies have yet to be launched (Altshuler et al. 1996; American Academy of Pediatrics Committee on Drugs 2000).

The novel or atypical antipsychotics have only limited data for use in pregnancy. Currently, recommendations are that they be used in pregnancy only if the patient has a history of nonresponse to the better-studied, conventional antipsychotic medications or is at significant risk for relapse if the drug is discontinued (Patton et al. 2002). *It is generally not prudent to switch drugs when the patient is already pregnant, because this exposes the fetus to the twin risks of maternal relapse and exposure to a second medication.* Medication changes from a novel to a typical antipsychotic should be accomplished prior to conception (see Appendix 7–A in this chapter, "Psychotropics in Pregnancy and Lactation," for specific medications; see also the section above regarding physical restraint in pregnancy).

Extrapyramidal Side Effects

Diphenhydramine (Benadryl) is considered to be the treatment of choice for extrapyramidal side effects caused by the conventional antipsychotics in pregnant women. Limited data suggest that benztropine (Cogentin) is also safe, although there is a report of paralytic ileus in two newborns exposed in utero (ReproTox 2004). There are not enough data to comment on the safety of trihexyphenidyl (Artane) or amantadine (Symmetrel) in human pregnancy or lactation.

Anxiety Disorders

Benzodiazepines have become subordinated to SSRIs and to the serotonin-norepinephrine reuptake inhibitor venlafaxine (Effexor) in the treatment of most anxiety disorders. They are usually added at the beginning of treatment and then withdrawn gradually once the SSRI has taken full effect. This is a fortuitous development; regular benzodiazepine use in pregnancy has been controversial. Thirty years of studies have variously linked, exonerated, reconvicted, and then cleared the prototypical benzodiazepine, diazepam (Valium), from an association with congenital defects. Methodological problems have confounded this literature, making meaningful analysis a challenge. Of course, there will be many women who have to remain on a benzodiazepine long-term, adding the further complications of polypharmacy with the antidepressants.

Two teratology reviews have concluded that benzodiazepines pose little teratogenic risk, but the data are insufficient to conclude that there is no risk (Briggs et al. 2002; Friedman and Polifka 2000). Details and exceptions are noted in Appendix 7–A in this chapter, "Psychotropics in Pregnancy and Lactation."

Obsessive-Compulsive Disorder

Somatic treatments for OCD include the SSRIs, clomipramine, venlafaxine, benzodiazepines, and antipsychotics. Cognitive-behavioral therapy has been the most efficacious nonsomatic treatment for OCD. See Appendix 7–A for details on specific medications.

Insomnia

Environmental manipulation, such as avoiding caffeine and alcohol and promoting good sleep hygiene, are the first line of treatment for insomnia. For women requiring medications, diphenhydramine, benzodiazepines, and low-dose TCAs are options.

Although not typically the hypnotic of choice, diphenhydramine has a long history of use in human pregnancy. Experience suggests that it is a safe (but not entirely effective) hypnotic for pregnant women (Briggs et al. 2002). It is most useful for transient mild insomnia. For more persistent insomnia, low-dose amitriptyline (Elavil) or imipramine (Tofranil) (10–20 mg po qhs) may be tried. Because of the potential for drug-drug interactions, avoid the combination of TCAs and SSRIs in pregnancy unless the patient was taking such a combination before becoming pregnant. When these drugs are ineffective or not an option, and for patients with insomnia secondary to depression, low-dose benzodiazepines such as clonazepam (Klonopin) or lorazepam (Ativan) can be useful.

The data on zolpidem (Ambien) and zaleplon (Sonata) are too limited at this writing to assess their safety in humans (Briggs et al. 2002). We recommend switching to diphenhydramine, or to clonazepam if the former is ineffective.

Temazepam (Restoril) and triazolam (Halcion) are *contraindicated* during pregnancy (Briggs et al. 2002). The mechanism for this interaction is unknown. It is unclear why triazolam is also contraindicated, since we could locate no data that support its association with congenital defects.

Eating Disorders

See the section Eating Disorders From Conception to Postpartum, earlier in this chapter under Phase I: Conception.

■ PHASE III: POSTPARTUM

The tragedy of Andrea Yates highlighted the malignancy of postpartum illness when she killed all five of her small children in 2001 while suffering from postpartum psychosis (Denno 2003). Postpartum states span a range of problems, involving sometimes the recurrence of a preexisting condition, at other times the onset of a new disorder. The most benign of the postpartum syndromes is "postpartum blues," also known as the "baby blues." The most potentially lethal is postpartum psychosis, which carries the risks of suicide and infanticide.

Table 7–1 lists the differential diagnosis of psychiatric problems encountered in pregnancy and the postpartum period. Table 7–2 shows the natural history of psychiatric illness associated with pregnancy and the postpartum period.

Postpartum Blues

Postpartum blues (PPB) is a common syndrome typically experienced by women within the first 2 weeks after delivery, with peak symptoms occurring between the third and seventh day after delivering the baby. New mothers report "feeling very emotional," with characteristic symptoms including "moodiness" ranging from euphoria to tearful sadness, anxiety, insomnia, poor appetite, and irritability.

Diagnosis

There are no well-established criteria for the diagnosis, and DSM-IV-TR (American Psychiatric Association 2000) offers no specific designation for this condition. Psychosis and suicidal ideation do not occur as symptoms of PPB but signal a graver condition, such as a major affective disorder.

Etiology

There is speculation about a hormonal cause of PPB. For example, one prospective study of 191 women found weak support for an association between PPB and estrogen withdrawal (O'Hara et al. 1991). Risk factors for PPB include a history of the following: depression, premenstrual mood changes, depressive symptoms during pregnancy, depression in family, and a variety of psychosocial stressors.

Sequelae

Although recovery is usually complete with conservative treatment, women who develop PPB are at greater risk for developing postpartum depression (O'Hara et al. 1991). If symptoms persist beyond 2 weeks or worsen, the woman should seek evaluation for postpartum depression. A self-assessment checklist may be printed out for patient use at http://www.pndsa.co.za/ms-fc.htm (accessed June 2004).

Treatment

The blues are usually transitory and rarely require pharmacological treatment. The key therapeutic interventions are reassurance and support. Low-dose benzodiazepines may be used for insomnia and anxiety.

Comment: It is difficult for nonparents to imagine the unremitting pressure of a newborn's demands, the household work an infant generates, and the practical strain of keeping up with it all. Unlike the rigors of medical or surgical training, the new mother is on call

24 hours a day, 7 days a week, without days off, without a night float, ancillary staff, call rotation, lunch break, or scheduled vacation. If there are other children at home, and the family is already stretched by limited financial or social resources, the job becomes overwhelming. Add sleep deprivation, the blues, and guilt about not being happy, and the result may be enough to uncover psychiatric vulnerabilities. Adequate sleep and periodic rest breaks are essential to a "blue" mother's mental health treatment plan. Experienced clinicians have recommended short-term use of low-dose benzodiazepines, such as clonazepam (0.5–1 mg po qhs) or lorazepam (0.5–1 mg po qhs), to help control insomnia (Misri and Lusskin 2004a). This strategy is certainly preferable to using alcohol for inducing sleep, because doing so may exacerbate the mood swings of PPB. However, benzodiazepines may affect the breastfeeding infant. It may be possible to use formula or frozen, medication-free breast milk for a night or two while the exhausted mother catches up on her sleep.

Postpartum Depression

The onset of postpartum depression (PPD) varies. In fact, many "postpartum" episodes actually begin during pregnancy, but patients might not come to diagnostic attention until after delivery (Cooper et al. 1999; Evans et al. 2001; Lee et al. 2001; O'Hara et al. 1990; Yonkers et al. 2001). These data have practical implications:

- Screening women for depression *while they are pregnant* may identify those at risk for PPD.

The approximate incidence of postpartum depression in the United States is usually quoted at about 10% (O'Hara et al. 1990). The publication of the 1984 landmark study detailing correlates with PPD (Kumar and Robson 1984) has been followed by many others. Methodological problems have included flawed correlation attributions, however. Most clinically relevant are these specific aspects of patient history (Wisner et al. 2002):

- Occurrence of depression during the index pregnancy. (*Note:* A woman who is depressed during pregnancy is likely to remain so after delivery.)
- Previous postpartum depression
- History of depression unassociated with pregnancy
- Family psychiatric history
- Pregnancy loss within the past 12 months, whether through miscarriage, stillbirth, or abortion for un-

planned pregnancy (Janssen et al. 1996; Major et al. 2000; Neugebauer et al. 1997). Women who conceive less than 1 year after a stillbirth appear to be at higher risk for depression in the third trimester of the next pregnancy and at 1 year postpartum compared with those who waited 12 months or more to conceive (Hughes et al. 1999).
- Abrupt or premature discontinuation of antidepressants

Patients with these risk factors should be carefully monitored for PPD. It should be remembered that most postpartum visits occur in the obstetrician's office, without psychiatric involvement. Screening instruments like the Edinburgh Postnatal Depression Scale (Figure 7–3) have been shown to improve detection of PPD compared with simple clinical interview by the obstetrician (Evins et al. 2000). The scale is a 10-item self-report questionnaire validated specifically for the detection of depression in the postpartum period (Cox et al. 1987). Responses are scored 0, 1, 2, or 3, with a maximum score of 30; scores ≥12 or 13 identify most women with PPD. Women who are symptomatic but not suicidal or functionally impaired should be evaluated again, at least within 1 month, or referred for psychiatric follow-up (Wisner et al. 2002).

Etiology and Pathogenesis

The peak symptoms of postpartum mood changes occur during a rapid flux of gonadotropins and hormones, which has led to the study of biochemical variables. It is not surprising that investigators have had difficulty controlling for the interaction of genetic predisposition with the simultaneous covariance of multifold hormonal shifts, key life events, and multifaceted environmental changes. There have been many studies, varied methodologies, and no one emergent biological factor to account for the problem of PPD. Since 1996 alone, investigators have studied estrogen (Ahokas et al. 2001; Bloch et al. 2000; Gregoire et al. 1996; Hendrick et al. 1998), progesterone (Harris et al. 1996; Lawrie et al. 1998), testosterone (Hohlagschwandtner et al. 2001), thyroid hormone (Harris et al. 1996; Kent et al. 1999; Pedersen 1999), corticotropin-releasing hormone (Schmeelk et al. 1999), cortisol (Harris et al. 1996), and even cholesterol (van Dam et al. 1999).

Diagnosis

DSM-IV-TR does not consider PPD to be a separate class of affective disorder, but adds to major depressive disorder a "postpartum onset" specifier, (i.e., oc-

Edinburgh Postnatal Depression Scale

Name: _____   Baby's age:_____   Date: _____

As you have recently had a baby, we would like to know how you are feeling. Please UNDERLINE the answer which comes closest to how you have felt IN THE PAST 7 DAYS, not just how you feel today.

Here is an example, already completed.
    I have felt happy:
        Yes, all the time
        <u>Yes, most of the time</u>
        No, not very often
        No, not at all

This would mean: "I have felt happy most of the time" during the past week. Please complete the other questions in the same way.

1. I have been able to laugh and see the funny side of things:
    As much as I always could
    Not quite so much now
    Definitely not so much now
    Not at all

2. I have looked forward to things:
    As much as I ever did
    Rather less than I used to
    Definitely less than I used to
    Hardly at all

*3. I have blamed myself unnecessarily when things went wrong:
    Yes, most of the time
    Yes, some of the time
    Not very often
    No, never

4. I have been anxious or worried for no good reason:
    No, not at all
    Hardly ever
    Yes, sometimes
    Yes, very often

*5. I have felt scared or panicky for no very good reason:
    Yes, quite a lot
    Yes, sometimes
    No, not much
    No, not at all

*6. Things have been getting overwhelming:
    Yes, most of the time I have not been able to cope at all
    Yes, sometimes I haven't been coping as well as usual
    No, most of the time I have coped quite well
    No, I have been coping as well as ever

*7. I have been so unhappy that I have had difficulty sleeping:
    Yes, most of the time
    Yes, sometimes
    Not very often
    No, not at all

*8. I have felt sad or miserable:
    Yes, most of the time
    Yes, quite often
    Not very often
    No, not at all

*9. I have been so unhappy that I have been crying:
    Yes, most of the time
    Yes, quite often
    Only occasionally
    No, never

*10. The thought of harming myself has occurred to me:
    Yes, quite often
    Sometimes
    Hardly ever
    Never

RESPONSE SCORING AND NOTES:
Response categories are scored 0, 1, 2, and 3 according to increased severity of the symptoms. (e.g., #4, "No, not at all" = 0 points)
Items marked with an asterisk are reverse scored (i.e., 3, 2, 1, 0). (e.g., #5, "Yes, quite a lot" = 3 points)
The total score is calculated by adding together the scores for each of the ten items.
The validation study showed that mothers who score above a threshold 12/13 were likely to be suffering from a depressive illness of varying severity. Nevertheless, the EPDS score should not override clinical judgment. A careful clinical assessment should be carried out to confirm the diagnosis. The scale indicates how the mother has felt during the previous week, and in doubtful cases it may be usefully repeated after 2 weeks. The scale will not detect mothers with anxiety disorders, phobias, or personality disorders (Cox et al. 1987, p. 786).
A high score on the EPDS indicates the likelihood of postpartum depression being present in the mother. It is meant to be administered and interpreted under the supervision of a physician (J.L. Cox, personal communication, 2003).

Figure 7–3. Edinburgh Postnatal Depression Scale.

Source. From Cox J, Holden J, Sagovsky R: "Detection of Postnatal Depression: Development of the 10-Item Edinburgh Postnatal Depression Scale. *British Journal of Psychiatry* 150:82–786, 1987. Used with permission.

curring *within 4 weeks* after delivery). The same designation is also used for other affective disorders, such as mania or mixed states, occurring after pregnancy. Certainly the vulnerability to PPD has been established for up to 1 year after delivery, but DSM has yet to account for this phenomenon.

Vegetative disturbances lose value for diagnosing depression in people with other physical conditions, and women who have just given birth are no exception. Sleep and appetite disturbance, lack of energy, and disturbances of libido normally occur postpartum. One should look instead for exaggerated disturbances in these domains; for example, the mother is unable to sleep even when the baby sleeps, or she finds that food has no appeal. Pay particular attention to the quality of mood and the presence of guilt. Experts have described the following population-specific symptoms (Misri and Lusskin 2004a):

- Obsessional thoughts about harming herself or the baby. Fortunately, such thoughts are not necessarily indicative of the desire to take action and are usually ego-dystonic to the woman. They must be pursued, however, because they may be symptomatic of a psychotic process. When psychosis occurs, it raises the risk of suicide or infanticide. Interviews of depressed new mothers must include questions about suicidal or infanticidal ideation. Direct questioning may not be effective; if the mother has not volunteered this information, another way to elicit it is to inquire whether she has had any "scary" thoughts, specifically about harming herself or the baby.
- Significant anxiety, often with panic attacks
- Intense irritability and anger
- Feelings of guilt, especially about real or imagined inadequacies relative to the baby
- A sense of being overwhelmed or unable to care for the baby
- Feeling like a failure as a mother

If she has not bonded adequately with her infant, the mother may become overwhelmed with self-blame and guilt. Unfortunately, remorse and shame may interfere with her seeking appropriate help.

Prognosis and Outcome

Although the American Academy of Pediatrics has concluded that "antidepressants' effects on infants are unknown but possibly of concern," the verdict on *untreated* maternal depression is unanimous: it can be devastating.

Study after study has documented problems in the behavioral, intellectual, social, and interpersonal development of infants with depressed mothers. The family system also becomes "ill." For example, in one study of 54 first-time mothers and 42 fathers who were their husbands or partners, 28% of the fathers became depressed in the first postpartum year (Areias et al. 1996). Predictably, the father's personal history of depression was a significant risk factor (odds ratio 20.95). However, another risk factor for paternal depression was development of depression in the mother beginning during or shortly after pregnancy (odds ratio 42.3). This fascinating research, which is beyond the scope of this chapter, has been summarized by other authors (Jacobsen 1999; Meersand and Turchin 2003; Spinelli 2003b).

PPD unfortunately predicts future depressive episodes, both associated and unassociated with pregnancy (Nonacs and Cohen 1998). Among the most serious complications of untreated PPD are the progression to delusional depression (which is a type of postpartum psychosis), suicide, and, rarely, infanticide (see the section Postpartum Psychosis below for further details).

Differential Diagnosis

The differential diagnosis for postpartum depressive mood disorders should include the following:

- Postpartum blues (PPB; no DSM-IV-TR diagnosis) (*Note:* Any depressive syndrome accompanied by psychosis or lasting beyond 2 weeks postpartum ceases qualifying for PPB.)
- Postpartum depression (PPD) without psychotic features
- Postpartum depression with psychotic features (consider bipolar disorder, depressed)
- Bipolar I or II disorder, depressed phase. In a sample of 30 women with occult bipolar disorder, 20 (67%) experienced a postpartum mood episode, almost exclusively depressive, as the initial presentation of their bipolar disorder (Chaudron and Pies 2003; Freeman et al. 2002).
- Mood disorder due to a general medical condition with major depressive-like episode or with depressive features. Depressive symptoms have been reported as the presenting feature in hypothyroidism (Gunnarsson et al. 2001), infection with HIV, and systemic lupus erythematosus (SLE). The differential diagnoses of these conditions are discussed below in the section on postpartum psychosis.
- Substance-induced depressive disorder. Effects of prescription drugs, illicit drugs, alcohol, and over-

the-counter and herbal remedies may mimic and precipitate psychiatric disorders in pregnancy and the postpartum period.

Treatment

Psychotherapy. The recent literature on psychotherapy in the postpartum period contains reports on the usefulness of a variety of psychotherapies, including cognitive therapy (Appleby et al. 1997), interpersonal psychotherapy (Klier et al. 2001; O'Hara et al. 2000; Zlotnick et al. 2001), group therapy (Meager and Milgrom 1996; Morgan et al. 1997), and marital therapy (Misri et al. 2000b). Psychotherapy should be considered as the first-line treatment option for mild postpartum depression, especially if the woman has no prior history of depression. It is also useful for moderate to severe episodes of PPD as an adjunct to pharmacotherapy.

Pharmacotherapy. Breastfeeding guides the choice of medication. Specific medications are discussed in Appendix 7–A in this chapter. If the woman does not breastfeed, the selection criteria for antidepressants are the same as for depression unassociated with pregnancy. On the other hand, the choice of medication may not be so straightforward. If the postpartum depression is the first presentation of an affective illness, especially if the patient has mood-congruent psychotic symptoms, then bipolar disorder may be the primary diagnosis. In that case, treatment with mood stabilizers should be considered early in the course (Chaudron and Pies 2003).

Electroconvulsive therapy. ECT has a long history of efficacy in pregnant and postpartum patients (Miller 1994a; Reed et al. 1999), particularly when a treatment team is available that includes a psychiatrist, an obstetrician, and an anesthesiologist. Particular indications for ECT are as follows:

- Severe depression with psychotic features
- Acute mania
- Patient at risk for suicide or infanticide

See Box 7–2 for information on the use of ECT in pregnancy and the puerperium. Although there are no reports of adverse effects on nursing infants from the ECT anesthetics, it has been suggested that exposure can be minimized by storing breast milk the day before (Rabheru 2001).

Light therapy. There is a paucity of data on the use of light therapy in pregnancy and the postpartum period. There is one case report of its potential value in

treating PPD (Corral et al. 2000). See the section above on light therapy in pregnancy.

Hormonal therapy. A small study showed improvement in PPD after treatment with transdermal estradiol, but there were several methodological limitations to the study, the most significant of which was that more than one-half of the women in the treatment and control groups were already taking antidepressants (Gregoire et al. 1996). Kumar et al. (2003) demonstrated, in a well-designed open study of 29 women, that transdermal estradiol, begun within 48 hours of delivery, did not reduce the risk of recurrence of postpartum psychosis in 29 women; 12 patients relapsed, most within 1–2 weeks of delivery. This study found no evidence to support the hypothesis that postpartum psychosis results from the rapid fall in circulating estrogens after delivery.

Estrogen is not recommended as a primary treatment for either postpartum depression or postpartum psychosis, but it may eventually prove useful as an adjunct in some cases. The administration of a long-acting progestogen for contraception, given within 48 hours of delivery, increased the risk of PPD in a study of 180 women (Lawrie et al. 1998).

Patient Self-Help Resources

Postpartum Support International (http://www.postpartum.net; accessed June 2004) offers support groups, with meetings at local, state, national, and international levels, and provides useful information for women, families, and clinicians.

Postpartum Psychosis
Problems With Definition

There has been great debate about whether postpartum psychosis (PPP) comprises a separate illness from other psychotic states or lies along a continuum with them, particularly with bipolar disorder. Part of the problem has been methodological; the criteria for PPP have been vague, with early studies calling many different postpartum states "postpartum psychosis": major depression with psychotic features, bipolar disorder with manic episode, schizophrenia, schizophreniform disorder, and brief reactive psychosis. Even more confusing are the variable definitions of the postpartum period—anywhere from 0–3 weeks to 12 months after delivery. Hospital admission records often are the only source of epidemiological data, but they frequently lack diagnostic specifics (e.g., psychotic depression vs. schizophrenia). This confusion has complicated evaluating the pre-DSM-IV literature in a clinically meaningful way.

- At this time, DSM-IV-TR does not have "postpartum psychosis" as a diagnosis. Instead, use the standard criteria for psychosis (e.g., depressed, mixed, or manic episode, schizoaffective disorder or schizophrenia) with the "postpartum-onset" specifier if symptoms develop within 4 weeks of birth.
- For those psychotic states that develop a few months after birth, DSM-IV-TR has no postpartum specifier.

Features

Postpartum psychosis occurs infrequently: 1–2 per 1,000 births (0.1%–0.2%) (Terp and Mortensen 1998). The major risk factors for its occurrence are as follows (Nonacs and Cohen 1998):

- *Bipolar disorder.* Women with bipolar disorder are at greater risk for postpartum psychosis than are those with unipolar depression; PPP may be the first episode of a bipolar disorder (Chaudron and Pies 2003; Yonkers et al. 2004). Those who remained well during pregnancy but had discontinued lithium prior to pregnancy are still at significantly increased risk of relapse, which may take the form of a manic psychosis or a major depressive episode, within the first month postpartum (Viguera et al. 2000).
- *Schizophrenia.* Although clinical lore has it that schizophreniform illness precipitated by an acute stressor augurs a good prognosis, this is not true for schizophreniform presentations associated with pregnancy. One 25-year follow-up study tracked 82 patients who had been treated for postpartum illness (Davidson and Robertson 1985). *The risk of nonpuerperal recurrence for schizophrenic illness was 100%,* followed closely by bipolar disorder (66%) and recurrent unipolar depression (43%).
- *Postpartum psychosis, personal history.* Recurrence rates are as high as 70% (Nonacs and Cohen 1998).
- *Postpartum psychosis, family history* (Jones and Craddock 2001)

Mothers with these risk factors require careful monitoring and prophylactic management.

Vulnerability Over Time

The relative risk of hospital admission for psychosis varies according to time from delivery (Kendell et al. 1987; Lier et al. 1989; Terp and Mortensen 1998). The following data (Kendell et al. 1987) suggest that pregnancy and childbirth precipitate mental illness in biologically vulnerable individuals and that the higher risk of hospitalization continues for up to 2 years postpartum: postpartum month 1 >postpartum month 3 >postpartum year 2 >antepartum.

Clinical Features

Postpartum psychotic states usually present within 2 weeks of delivery. They have been described as follows (Attia et al. 1999; Kendell et al. 1987; Misri and Lusskin 2004b; Terp and Mortensen 1998; Videbech and Gouliaev 1995):

- Usually affective in nature, either manic or depressive, but with lability and mixed mood states common. Only a minority are schizophreniform (i.e., presenting in the absence of clear mood disturbance).
- Delirium-like presentation: disorientation, "perplexity," sleep dysregulation, and a subjective experience of confusion (workup for delirium usually negative); these features not always present (Chaudron and Pies 2003)
- Psychomotor restlessness
- Hallucinations and delusions are prominent (and tend to be mood-congruent rather than bizarre or schizophreniform).
- Suicidal and infanticidal ideation may present initially, or rapidly evolve.
- Rapid, malignant course may follow. Treatment should not be delayed while the general medical workup is under way.
- Late-onset postpartum psychosis often is associated with delusional depression and has resulted from an untreated or incompletely treated postpartum depression.

Prognosis

Women who suffer pregnancy-related psychotic episodes often want to know their risk for recurrence if they do (or do not) become pregnant again. The following trends have been distilled from the literature, which can be reviewed in detail elsewhere (Attia et al. 1999; Chaudron and Pies 2003; Misri and Lusskin 2004b; Wyszynski and Wyszynski 1996; Yonkers et al. 2004):

- Postpartum psychotic illness predisposes to additional psychotic episodes unrelated to pregnancy.

- After postpartum psychosis, which is usually accompanied by affective symptoms, the risk of future affective episodes stays higher than for the general population, whether the woman becomes pregnant again or not.
- Puerperal (pregnancy-related) illness may serve to activate nonpuerperal psychiatric illness, with each episode increasing the likelihood of developing a chronic, relapsing affective disorder.
- Mothers without psychiatric history prior to their index postpartum psychotic episode seem to have the most benign course, relative to frequency and severity of lifetime psychiatric symptomatology.
- Suicide is a complication of recurrent psychotic episodes.

Suicide

Fortunately, women during pregnancy and in the first year after childbirth have a suicide rate that is lower than expected in the general female population (Appleby 1991; Marzuk et al. 1997). Warnings still remain in force for certain members of the pregnant population who are vulnerable because of the following factors:

- *Psychiatric admission:* Postpartum psychiatric admission serves as a marker for increased suicide risk: by 70-fold in the first year postpartum and 17-fold across a woman's life span (Appleby et al. 1998). An earlier epidemiological study found that postpartum women who committed suicide tended to use violent methods (self-incineration, jumping from a height, jumping in front of a train), suggesting that these individuals may have been psychotic (Appleby 1991).
- *Teen age:* Although pregnant teens were at less risk than nonpregnant teens, they carried a suicide risk five times greater than that for pregnant women as a group (Appleby 1991).
- *Stillbirth:* Women after stillbirth have a suicide rate approaching that of the general female population and therefore are more vulnerable than their pregnant counterparts and other postpartum women (Appleby 1991).

Comment: When conducting screening evaluations, consider the secondary finding that pregnant women are vulnerable to domestic violence (Guth and Pachter 2000). Homicide exceeded suicide as the leading cause of pregnancy-associated deaths in a study that reviewed death records in Maryland from 1993 to 1998 (Horon and Cheng 2001).

Infanticide

The absolute risk of infanticide is difficult to determine. Some children whose cause of death was diagnosed as sudden infant death syndrome (SIDS), for example, may have been victims of fatal child abuse (Overpeck et al. 1998). In one series, the perpetrator of infant homicide in the first week of life tended to be the mother, while after the first week it was a male (the father or stepfather) (Overpeck et al. 1998). Maternal age under 17 years, a mother 17–19 years old having a second or subsequent child, and a first birth to a mother less than 15 years old with little education and little or no prenatal care were risk factors for death in the first 4 months of life.

A 2003 volume on infanticide summarizes some of the psychiatric, legal, and treatment issues pertaining to this tragic complication of mental illness (Spinelli 2003a). Denial of pregnancy may precede neonaticide (defined as infant murder occurring on the day of birth) and may serve as a risk factor for it (Miller 2003). Postpartum psychosis is a risk factor for infanticide. Women with ego-dystonic ruminations about harming their babies are thought to be at lower risk but merit careful evaluation for the presence of psychosis.

Comment: In some other countries, including England and Canada, the criminal justice system considers neonaticide and infanticide to be symptoms of mental illness. In the United States, they are considered murder or manslaughter.

Differential Diagnosis

Postpartum psychosis implies a primary psychiatric disorder, but other conditions may present as or coexist with PPP. See Appendix 4 in this volume, "'VINDICTIVE MADS': Differential Diagnosis of Mental Status Changes."

A few conditions deserve particular attention in postpartum patients:

- *Substance-induced psychotic disorder:* Recreational drugs, some herbal medications, sympathomimetic over-the-counter diet drugs used to lose excess pregnancy weight, and prescription drugs (e.g., high-dose metronidazole, an antifungal used in obstetric and gynecologic practice) may induce psychosis, complicating the postpartum diagnostic picture.
- *Psychotic disorder due to thyroid disease:* Thyroiditis occurs relatively commonly postpartum, often due to autoimmunity. Psychosis may result from either the hyperthyroid phase or subsequent hypothy-

roidism. "Myxedema madness," often a paranoid psychosis with features of delirium, may be the only sign of hypothyroidism (Heinrich and Grahm 2003; Lehrmann and Jain 2002).

If onset occurs in the postpartum period, psychosis may be misattributed to PPP. Patients with bipolar disorder who have been maintained on lithium throughout pregnancy run the dual risk of postpartum breakthrough mania or depression and hypothyroidism as a complication of chronic lithium therapy. Be sure to consider both diagnoses in the workup of postpartum psychosis in these patients.

- *Psychotic disorder due to systemic lupus erythematosus (SLE).* This autoimmune illness has a peak incidence in women of childbearing age and may flare as a result of pregnancy, particularly during the first 6 weeks postpartum (Hahn 2001). If lupus cerebritis were first to occur after pregnancy, it could present as postpartum psychosis. The test for serum antinuclear antibodies remains the best way to screen for SLE (Hahn 2001).
- *Psychotic disorder due to HIV.* Infection with the human immunodeficiency virus should be suspected in a patient with postpartum mental status changes if she has risk factors for HIV other than pregnancy (see Chapter 9, "The HIV-Infected Patient," in this volume). Psychiatric symptomatology, such as affective psychosis accompanied by confusional states, may be the presenting feature of infection with HIV, even in the absence of systemic signs (de Ronchi et al. 2000).

Workup

Routine tests should include baseline complete blood count, liver function tests, serum electrolyte levels, thyroid function including a thyroid-stimulating hormone level (TSH), renal function tests, and a urine drug screen. Recommendations for a more complete workup of mental status changes can be found in Appendix 1 in this volume, "American Psychiatric Association Guidelines for Assessing the Delirious Patient."

A note on thyroid function: Several changes in thyroid physiology accompany normal pregnancy (Gabbe et al. 2002). These changes include alterations in thyroxine-binding globulin and decreases in circulating extrathyroidal iodide. Total thyroxine (T_4) and total triiodothyronine (T_3) levels begin to increase in the first trimester and peak at midgestation. The free T_4 levels rise slightly in the first trimester and then decrease so that by delivery, the free T_4 levels are 10%–15% lower than in nonpregnant women. However, these changes are small, and in most pregnant women serum free T_4 concentrations remain within the normal nonpregnant range. Free T_3 levels follow a parallel pattern. TSH concentrations decrease transiently in the first trimester and then rise to prepregnant levels by the end of the first trimester. TSH levels then remain stable throughout the remainder of gestation. Thus, despite alterations in thyroid morphology, histology, and laboratory indices, *the pregnant woman should remain euthyroid clinically and by laboratory evaluation.*

Treatment

Postpartum psychosis is a medical emergency requiring the mother's hospitalization for her protection and that of the infant. General principles of treatment of postpartum psychosis (Misri and Lusskin 2004b) involve the following:

- Early identification
- Rapid evaluation
- Hospitalization
- Coordinated care of mother and infant
- Involvement of family and other supports

Most women with this condition are too ill to breastfeed their infants. A positive consequence, however, is that the atypical antipsychotics may be used without worrying about a nursing infant's ingestion of them. These medications offer advantages over conventional agents: not only do they reduce psychotic symptoms, but they also have mood-stabilizing properties, fewer extrapyramidal side effects, and less risk of tardive dyskinesia. When oral administration is not possible because of agitation, high-potency antipsychotics, such as haloperidol (Haldol) or ziprasidone (Geodon), are initially administered parenterally and then withdrawn when the patient can take the oral medication. Medications are then titrated according to symptoms. Lorazepam is often coadministered with antipsychotics to potentiate their sedative effect and reduce the total required antipsychotic dose. Mood stabilizers and/or antidepressants are added according to clinical indication.

ECT is indicated for acute agitation, when the woman is at high risk for suicide or infanticide, and when she has refused or not responded to medications (see Box 7–2 on ECT).

Insomnia should be a target symptom for treatment, so providing for a bedtime dose of medication has therapeutic importance.

After the psychotic symptoms have resolved, psychosocial intervention is crucial for reestablishing the patient in her role as mother. Careful follow-up, supervised mother-infant interaction, and community involvement are essential to making psychiatric rehabilitation work for the mother and child.

Prophylaxis

It has been estimated that up to 50% of women with bipolar disorder experience recurrence of a mood disorder (depression or mania) in the postpartum period (Nonacs and Cohen 1998). Prophylactic treatment with lithium decreased the rate of recurrence to 10% in one study; no similar studies have been done with other mood stabilizers (Austin and Mitchell 1998; Cohen et al. 1995). Women with a history of postpartum psychosis have a 70% relapse rate (Nonacs and Cohen 1998).

Maintenance therapy with lithium reduces relapse in patients with bipolar disorder and has the advantage of being potentially effective on the depressive phase of bipolar disorder. Anticonvulsants are useful alternatives to lithium as mood-stabilizing agents in postpartum psychosis (manic type) and, unlike lithium, are approved by the American College of Pediatrics for use by breastfeeding mothers (Briggs et al. 2002). (See Appendix 7–B in this chapter on the use of lithium.)

■ PHASE IV: BREASTFEEDING

It can be agonizing for a patient to agree to take medication while breastfeeding. A new mother must weigh the uncertainty of exposing her baby to drugs against the risks of withholding the benefits of breast milk. This ambiguity can be unnerving to a woman deeply committed to breastfeeding her child; she may feel that continuing her medication creates a conflict of interest, placing her own welfare above that of the baby. As a result, she may decide to stop medication "temporarily" against medical advice until the newborn has benefited from breast milk, at least for a few months. The clinician's role is crucial in highlighting the risks of relapse even when medication is withdrawn even temporarily.

The following questions may help the patient give informed consent:

- Does the new mother believe that the psychiatric medication is crucial to her health, with complications resulting from nonadherence? Is there wishful thinking that her medication is "something op-

tional," a lifestyle choice that can be made electively, according to convenience or desire?
- Does the woman recognize that avoiding medications, whether or not she is breastfeeding, puts her at risk for relapse, decompensation, and hospitalization (with the attendant separation from her baby and other children)? Such a complication risks disruption of mother-infant bonding during the time of greatest vulnerability for recurrence, the postpartum period.
- Has the mother considered the unambiguous, clearly documented impact of untreated psychiatric illness on the cognitive, behavioral, and social development of infants (Jacobsen 1999)?

Until the new mother has factored these risks against the potential impact of medication in breast milk and considered the option of substituting formula for breast milk, she has not made a fully informed decision. In the spirit of comprehensive management and a team approach to postpartum disorders, the treating clinician should discuss the diagnosis and treatment recommendations with the pediatrician, especially when the mother is breastfeeding. This will also help to avoid conflicting recommendations.

- *Recommendations:* The following is a summary of the data available at the time of this writing on the use of psychotropic medications during breastfeeding. Details for specific medications can be found in Appendix 7–A, "Psychotropics in Pregnancy and Lactation," in this chapter. It is best to perform a search of the current literature before finalizing a treatment plan for the woman who plans to breastfeed.

Antidepressants

The American Academy of Pediatrics classifies the antidepressants as "drugs whose effect on the nursing infant is unknown but may be of concern" (American Academy of Pediatrics Committee on Drugs 2001). The contrast between the growing database on SSRI exposure through breastfeeding and the rare adverse report is encouraging. Long-term data are still pending on the developmental effects of SSRI exposure through breast milk, but the little evidence that we have is reassuring (see Appendix 7–A in this chapter).

Mood Stabilizers

Lithium is generally considered *incompatible* with breastfeeding because it accumulates in both maternal breast milk and infant serum, leading to potential toxicity in the nursing infant (American Academy of Pediatrics Committee on Drugs 2001; Llewellyn et al. 1998). Note also that newborns generally are vulnerable to dehydration, which would heighten their risk for lithium toxicity.

Despite these potential hazards, a recent literature review (Misri and Lusskin 2004e) confirmed that case reports of adverse effects of lithium on breastfeeding infants have been rare. Very careful monitoring of the mother and the infant is advised during breastfeeding (see Appendix 7–B in this chapter, "A Primer on Using Lithium in Pregnancy and Lactation").

The anticonvulsants valproic acid (Depakote, Depakene) and carbamazepine (Tegretol) have won their place among mood stabilizers. The American Academy of Pediatrics Committee on Drugs and the American Academy of Neurology consider both valproic acid and carbamazepine to be compatible with breastfeeding because of consistent, although limited, reports of low to unquantifiable concentrations of these medications in breast milk; levels have been reported to be higher in infants who were also exposed during pregnancy (American Academy of Pediatrics Committee on Drugs 2001; Yonkers et al. 2004). The relative safety of these agents in breastfeeding stands in contrast to their teratogenic potential in pregnancy.

Infants exposed to either of these anticonvulsants during breastfeeding should be monitored for possible hepatic complications, with maternal and infant serum drug levels and liver function tests every 2–4 weeks or as indicated by the clinical situation (Misri and Lusskin 2004e).

Gabapentin (Neurontin), topiramate (Topamax), and lamotrigine (Lamictal) have also been used for the treatment of bipolar disorder, but data on breastfeeding are quite limited (see Appendix 7–A).

Antipsychotics

Breastfeeding on antipsychotics is not recommended due to a lack of information (Misri and Lusskin 2004e), particularly because medication-free alternatives, such as formula, are available to the baby. However, some women will still breastfeed while taking these medications. It is hoped that women with chronic psychotic illnesses like schizophrenia will receive assistance and be monitored closely, because their ability to parent may be compromised by their disorder. When antipsychotic medications are continued, it is best to avoid polypharmacy, use the lowest doses possible, and monitor the infant carefully, using standard-

ized developmental screening tools if available. See Appendix 7–A for specific studies and medications.

Anxiolytics

Benzodiazepines are not contraindicated during breastfeeding but should be used cautiously (and are not a substitute for antidepressants or antipsychotics). The main concern is sedation in the newborn. For this reason, low doses of medications with no active metabolites, such as clonazepam or lorazepam, are preferred (Misri and Lusskin 2004e).

■ REFERENCES

Abraham S: Sexuality and reproduction in bulimia nervosa patients over 10 years. J Psychosom Res 44:491–502, 1998

Abraham S: Obstetricians and maternal body weight and eating disorders during pregnancy. J Psychosom Obstet Gynaecol 22:159–163, 2001

Abramowitz J, Schwartz S, Moore K, et al: Obsessive-compulsive symptoms in pregnancy and the puerperium: a review of the literature. J Anxiety Disord 17:461–478, 2003

Agrawal P, Bhatia MS, Malik SC: Post partum psychosis: a clinical study. Int J Soc Psychiatry 43:217–222, 1997

Ahokas A, Kaukoranta J, Wahlbeck K, et al: Estrogen deficiency in severe postpartum depression: successful treatment with sublingual physiologic 17beta-estradiol: a preliminary study. J Clin Psychiatry 62:332–336, 2001

Altshuler LL, Cohen L, Szuba MP, et al: Pharmacologic management of psychiatric illness during pregnancy: dilemmas and guidelines. Am J Psychiatry 153:592–606, 1996

Altshuler LL, Cohen LS, Moline ML, et al: The Expert Consensus Guideline Series: treatment of depression in women. Postgrad Med (spec no):1–107, 2001

American Academy of Pediatrics Committee on Drugs: Use of psychoactive medication during pregnancy and possible effects on the fetus and newborn. Pediatrics 105:880–887, 2000

American Academy of Pediatrics Committee on Drugs: The transfer of drugs and other chemicals into human milk. Pediatrics 108:776–789, 2001

American Psychiatric Association: Diagnostic and Statistical Manual of Mental Disorders, 4th Edition, Text Revision. Washington, DC, American Psychiatric Association, 2000

Antiepileptic Drug Pregnancy Registry. Available at: http://www.aedpregnancyregistry.org. Toll-free telephone: 888-233-2334. Accessed June 2004.

Appleby L: Suicide during pregnancy and in the first postnatal year. BMJ 302:137–140, 1991

Appleby L, Warner R, Whitton A, et al: A controlled study of fluoxetine and cognitive-behavioural counselling in the treatment of postnatal depression. BMJ 314:932–936, 1997

Appleby L, Mortensen PB, Faragher EB: Suicide and other causes of mortality after post-partum psychiatric admission. Br J Psychiatry 173:209–211, 1998

Areias ME, Kumar R, Barros H, et al: Correlates of postnatal depression in mothers and fathers. Br J Psychiatry 169:36–41, 1996

Arnold L, Suckow R, Lichtenstein P: Fluvoxamine concentrations in breast milk and in maternal and infant sera (letter). J Clin Psychopharmacol 20:491–493, 2000

Attia E, Downey J, Oberman M: Effects of postpartum disorders on parenting and on offspring, in Postpartum Mood Disorders. Edited by Miller L. Washington, DC, American Psychiatric Press, 1999, pp 99–117

Austin MP, Mitchell PB: Psychotropic medications in pregnant women: treatment dilemmas. Med J Aust 169:428–431, 1998

Baab SW, Peindl KS, Piontek CM, et al: Serum bupropion levels in 2 breastfeeding mother-infant pairs. J Clin Psychiatry 63:910–911, 2002

Bader TF, Newman K: Amitriptyline in human breast milk and the nursing infant's serum. Am J Psychiatry 137:855–856, 1980

Barnas C, Bergant A, Hummer M, et al: Clozapine concentrations in maternal and fetal plasma, amniotic fluid, and breast milk (letter). Am J Psychiatry 151:945, 1994

Beck CT: A meta-analysis of predictors of postpartum depression. Nurs Res 45:297–303, 1996

Begg EJ, Duffull SB, Saunders DA, et al: Paroxetine in human milk. Br J Clin Pharmacol 48:142–147, 1999

Bennedsen BE: Adverse pregnancy outcome in schizophrenic women: occurrence and risk factors. Schizophr Res 33:1–26, 1998

Bennedsen BE, Mortensen PB, Olesen AV, et al: Preterm birth and intra-uterine growth retardation among children of women with schizophrenia. Br J Psychiatry 175:239–245, 1999

Bhatia SC, Baldwin SA, Bhatia SK: Electroconvulsive therapy during the third trimester of pregnancy. J ECT 15:270–274, 1999

Birnbaum CS, Cohen LS, Bailey JW, et al: Serum concentrations of antidepressants and benzodiazepines in nursing infants: a case series. Pediatrics 104:e11, 1999

Biswas P, Wilton L, Shakir S: The pharmacovigilance of mirtazapine: results of a prescription event monitoring study on 13554 patients in England. J Psychopharmacol 17:121–126, 2003

Blacker KH, Weinstein BJ, Ellman GL: Mother's milk and chlorpromazine. Am J Psychiatry 119:178–179, 1962

Blais MA, Becker AE, Burwell RA, et al: Pregnancy: outcome and impact on symptomatology in a cohort of eating-disordered women. Int J Eat Disord 27:140–149, 2000

Bloch M, Schmidt PJ, Danaceau M, et al: Effects of gonadal steroids in women with a history of postpartum depression. Am J Psychiatry 157:924–930, 2000

Bonnot O, Vollset S, Godet P, et al: Maternal exposure to lorazepam and anal atresia in newborns? Results from a hypothesis generating study of benzodiazepines and malformations (abstract). Teratology 59:439–440, 1999

Brent NB, Wisner KL: Fluoxetine and carbamazepine concentrations in a nursing mother/infant pair. Clin Pediatr (Phila) 37:41–44, 1998

Breyer-Pfaff U, Nill K, Entenmann KN, et al: Secretion of amitriptyline and metabolites into breast milk (letter). Am J Psychiatry 152:812–813, 1995

Briggs G, Freeman R, Yaffe S: Drugs in Pregnancy and Lactation, 6th Edition. Philadelphia, PA, Lippincott Williams & Wilkins, 2002

Bulik CM, Sullivan PF, Fear JL, et al: Fertility and reproduction in women with anorexia nervosa: a controlled study. J Clin Psychiatry 60:130–135, 1999

Burch KJ, Wells BG: Fluoxetine/norfluoxetine concentrations in human milk. Pediatrics 89:676–677, 1992

Burt VK, Suri R, Altshuler L, et al: The use of psychotropic medications during breast-feeding. Am J Psychiatry 158:1001–1009, 2001

Celermajer DS, Bull C, Till JA, et al: Ebstein's anomaly: presentation and outcome from fetus to adult. J Am Coll Cardiol 23:170–176, 1994

Chambers CD, Johnson KA, Dick LM, et al: Birth outcomes in pregnant women taking fluoxetine. N Engl J Med 335:1010–1015, 1996

Chambers CD, Anderson PO, Thomas RG, et al: Weight gain in infants breastfed by mothers who take fluoxetine. Pediatrics 104:e61, 1999

Chaudron LH, Jefferson JW: Mood stabilizers during breast-feeding: a review. J Clin Psychiatry 61:79–90, 2000

Chaudron LH, Pies RW: The relationship between postpartum psychosis and bipolar disorder: a review. J Clin Psychiatry 64:1284–1292, 2003

Chelmow D, Halfin VP: Pregnancy complicated by obsessive-compulsive disorder. J Matern Fetal Med 6:31–34, 1997

Cohen LS, Rosenbaum JF: Psychotropic drug use during pregnancy: weighing the risks. J Clin Psychiatry 59:18–28, 1998

Cohen LS, Friedman JM, Jefferson JW, et al: A reevaluation of risk of in utero exposure to lithium. JAMA 271:146–150 [erratum 271:1485], 1994a

Cohen LS, Sichel DA, Dimmock JA, et al: Impact of pregnancy on panic disorder: a case series. J Clin Psychiatry 55:284–288, 1994b

Cohen LS, Sichel DA, Robertson LM, et al: Postpartum prophylaxis for women with bipolar disorder. Am J Psychiatry 152:1641–1645, 1995

Cohen LS, Sichel DA, Faraone SV, et al: Course of panic disorder during pregnancy and the puerperium: a preliminary study. Biol Psychiatry 39:950–954, 1996

Cohler BJ, Gallant DH, Grunebaum HU, et al: Pregnancy and birth complications among mentally ill and well mothers and their children. Soc Biol 22:269–278, 1975

Conti J, Abraham S, Taylor A: Eating behavior and pregnancy outcome. J Psychosom Res 44:465–477, 1998

Cooper PJ, Tomlinson M, Swartz L, et al: Post-partum depression and the mother-infant relationship in a South African peri-urban settlement. Br J Psychiatry 175:554–558, 1999

Cornelissen M, Steegers-Theunissen R, Kollee L, et al: Supplementation of vitamin K in pregnant women receiving anticonvulsant therapy prevents neonatal vitamin K deficiency. Am J Obstet Gynecol 168:884–888, 1993

Corral M, Kuan A, Kostaras D: Bright light therapy's effect on postpartum depression (letter). Am J Psychiatry 157:303–304, 2000

Costei AM, Kozer E, Ho T, et al: Perinatal outcome following third trimester exposure to paroxetine. Arch Pediatr Adolesc Med 156:1129–1132, 2002

Cowe L, Lloyd DJ, Dawling S: Neonatal convulsions caused by withdrawal from maternal clomipramine. Br Med J (Clin Res Ed) 284:1837–1838, 1982

Cowley D, Roy-Burne P: Panic disorder during pregnancy. J Psychosom Obstet Gynaecol 10:193–210, 1989

Cox JL, Holden JM, Sagovsky R: Detection of postnatal depression: development of the 10-item Edinburgh Postnatal Depression Scale. Br J Psychiatry 150:782–786, 1987

Croke S, Buist A, Hackett LP, et al: Olanzapine excretion in human breast milk: estimation of infant exposure. Int J Neuropsychopharmacol 5:243–247, 2002

Dahl ML, Olhager E, Ahlner J: Paroxetine withdrawal in a neonate (letter). Br J Psychiatry 171:391–392, 1997

Davidson J, Robertson E: A follow-up study of postpartum illness, 1946–1978. Acta Psychiatr Scand 71:451–457, 1985

Denno D: Who is Andrea Yates? A short story about insanity. Duke Journal of Gender Law & Policy 10:1–139, 2003

de Ronchi D, Faranca I, Forti P, et al: Development of acute psychotic disorders and HIV-1 infection. Int J Psychiatry Med 30:173–183, 2000

Diav-Citrin O, Shechtman S, Arnon J, et al: Is carbamazepine teratogenic? A prospective controlled study of 210 pregnancies. Neurology 57:321–324, 2001

Dickson RA, Hogg L: Pregnancy of a patient treated with clozapine. Psychiatr Serv 49:1081–1083, 1998

Dickson RA, Dawson DT: Olanzapine and pregnancy. Can J Psychiatry 43:196–197, 1998

Einarson A, Fatoye B, Sarkar M, et al: Pregnancy outcome following gestational exposure to venlafaxine: a multicenter prospective controlled study. Am J Psychiatry 158:1728–1730, 2001

Einarson A, Bonari L, Voyer-Lavigne S, et al: A multicentre prospective controlled study to determine the safety of trazodone and nefazodone use during pregnancy. Can J Psychiatry 48:106–110, 2003

Epperson CN, Anderson GM, McDougle CJ: Sertraline and breast-feeding (letter). N Engl J Med 336:1189–1190, 1997

Epperson [C]N, Czarkowski KA, Ward-O'Brien D, et al: Maternal sertraline treatment and serotonin transport in breast-feeding mother-infant pairs. Am J Psychiatry 158:1631–1637, 2001

Ericson A, Kallen B, Wiholm B: Delivery outcome after the use of antidepressants in early pregnancy. Eur J Clin Pharmacol 55:503–508, 1999

Evans J, Heron J, Francomb H, et al: Cohort study of depressed mood during pregnancy and after childbirth. BMJ 323:257–260, 2001

Evins G, Theofrastous J, Galvin S: Postpartum depression: a comparison of screening and routine clinical evaluation. Am J Obstet Gynecol 182:1080–1082, 2000

Franko DL, Spurrell EB: Detection and management of eating disorders during pregnancy. Obstet Gynecol 95:942–946, 2000

Franko DL, Blais MA, Becker AE, et al: Pregnancy complications and neonatal outcomes in women with eating disorders. Am J Psychiatry 158:1461–1466, 2001

Freeman MP, Smith KW, Freeman SA, et al: The impact of reproductive events on the course of bipolar disorder in women. J Clin Psychiatry 63:284–287, 2002

Frey B, Schubiger G, Musy JP: Transient cholestatic hepatitis in a neonate associated with carbamazepine exposure during pregnancy and breast-feeding. Eur J Pediatr 150:136–138, 1990

Friedman J, Polifka J: Teratogenic Effects of Drugs: A Resource for Clinicians (TERIS), 2nd Edition. Baltimore, MD, Johns Hopkins University Press, 2000

Fries H: Lithium in pregnancy. Lancet 1:1233, 1970

Gabbe SG, Niebyl JR, Simpson JL (eds): Obstetrics: Normal and Problem Pregnancies, 4th Edition. New York, Churchill Livingstone, 2002

George DT, Ladenheim JA, Nutt DJ: Effect of pregnancy on panic attacks. Am J Psychiatry 144:1078–1079, 1987

Gillen-Goldstein J, Young B: An overview of fetal heart rate assessment, in UpToDate (http://www.uptodate.com). Edited by Rose BD. Wellesley, MA, UpToDate, 2004

Glaxo SmithKline Bupropion Pregnancy Registry: Interim Report 9/1/97–2/28/03. Issued June 2003. Research Triangle Park, NC, PharmaResearch Corp, 2003, pp 1–22

Goldstein DJ, Corbin LA, Sundell KL: Effects of first-trimester fluoxetine exposure on the newborn. Obstet Gynecol 89:713–718, 1997

Goldstein DJ, Corbin LA, Fung MC: Olanzapine-exposed pregnancies and lactation: early experience. J Clin Psychopharmacol 20:399–403, 2000

Goodman SH, Emory EK: Perinatal complications in births to low socioeconomic status schizophrenic and depressed women. J Abnorm Psychol 101:225–229, 1992

Gracious BL, Wisner KL: Phenelzine use throughout pregnancy and the puerperium: case report, review of the literature, and management recommendations. Depress Anxiety 6:124–128, 1997

Gregoire AJ, Kumar R, Everitt B, et al: Transdermal oestrogen for treatment of severe postnatal depression. Lancet 347:930–933, 1996

Guberman AH, Besag FM, Brodie MJ, et al: Lamotrigine-associated rash: risk/benefit considerations in adults and children. Epilepsia 40:985–991, 1999

Gunnarsson T, Sjoberg S, Eriksson M, et al: Depressive symptoms in hypothyroid disorder with some observations on biochemical correlates. Neuropsychobiology 43:70–74, 2001

Guth AA, Pachter L: Domestic violence and the trauma surgeon. Am J Surg 179:134–140, 2000

Hagg S, Granberg K, Carleborg L: Excretion of fluvoxamine into breast milk (letter). Br J Clin Pharmacol 49:286–288, 2000

Hahn B: Systemic lupus erythematosus, in Harrison's Principles of Internal Medicine, 15th Edition. Edited by Braunwald E, Fauci A, Kasper D. New York, McGraw-Hill Medical, 2001, pp 1922–1928

Harris B, Lovett L, Smith J, et al: Cardiff puerperal mood and hormone study, III: postnatal depression at 5 to 6 weeks postpartum, and its hormonal correlates across the peripartum period. Br J Psychiatry 168:739–744, 1996

Heikkinen T, Ekblad U, Kero P, et al: Citalopram in pregnancy and lactation. Clin Pharmacol Ther 72:184–191, 2002

Heinrich TW, Grahm G: Hypothyroidism presenting as psychosis: myxedema madness revisited. Prim Care Companion J Clin Psychiatry 5:260–266, 2003

Hendrick V, Altshuler LL, Suri R: Hormonal changes in the postpartum and implications for postpartum depression. Psychosomatics 39:93–101, 1998

Hendrick V, Altshuler L, Wertheimer A, et al: Venlafaxine and breast-feeding (letter). Am J Psychiatry 158:2089–2090, 2001a

Hendrick V, Fukuchi A, Altshuler L, et al: Use of sertraline, paroxetine and fluvoxamine by nursing women. Br J Psychiatry 179:163–166, 2001b

Hendrick V, Smith LM, Hwang S, et al: Weight gain in breastfed infants of mothers taking antidepressant medications. J Clin Psychiatry 64:410–412, 2003a

Hendrick V, Smith LM, Suri R, et al: Birth outcomes after prenatal exposure to antidepressant medication. Am J Obstet Gynecol 188:812–815, 2003b

Hertzberg T, Leo RJ, Kim KY: Recurrent obsessive-compulsive disorder associated with pregnancy and childbirth. Psychosomatics 38:386–388, 1997

Hill RC, McIvor RJ, Wojnar-Horton RE, et al: Risperidone distribution and excretion into human milk: case report and estimated infant exposure during breast-feeding (letter). J Clin Psychopharmacol 20:285–286, 2000

Hohlagschwandtner M, Husslein P, Klier C, et al: Correlation between serum testosterone levels and peripartal mood states. Acta Obstet Gynecol Scand 80:326–330, 2001

Holmes LB: The teratogenicity of anticonvulsant drugs: a progress report. J Med Genet 39:245–247, 2002

Horon IL, Cheng D: Enhanced surveillance for pregnancy-associated mortality—Maryland, 1993–1998. JAMA 285:1455–1459, 2001

Hughes PM, Turton P, Evans CD: Stillbirth as risk factor for depression and anxiety in the subsequent pregnancy: cohort study. BMJ 318:1721–1724, 1999

Ilett KF, Hackett LP, Dusci LJ, et al: Distribution and excretion of venlafaxine and O-desmethylvenlafaxine in human milk. Br J Clin Pharmacol 45:459–462, 1998

Ilett KF, Kristensen JH, Hackett LP, et al: Distribution of venlafaxine and its O-desmethyl metabolite in human milk and their effects in breastfed infants. Br J Clin Pharmacol 53:17–22, 2002

Ilett KF, Hackett LP, Kristensen JH, et al: Transfer of risperidone and 9-hydroxyrisperidone into human milk. Ann Pharmacother 38:273–276, 2004

Iqbal MM, Gundlapalli SP, Ryan WG, et al: Effects of antimanic mood-stabilizing drugs on fetuses, neonates, and nursing infants. South Med J 94:304–322, 2001

Iqbal MM, Sobhan T, Ryals T: Effects of commonly used benzodiazepines on the fetus, the neonate, and the nursing infant. Psychiatr Serv 53:39–49, 2002

Isenberg K: Excretion of fluoxetine in human breast milk (letter). J Clin Psychiatry 51:169, 1990

Jacobsen T: Effects of postpartum disorders on parenting and on offspring, in Postpartum Mood Disorders. Edited by Miller L. Washington, DC, American Psychiatric Press, 1999, pp 119–139

Janssen HJ, Cuisinier MC, Hoogduin KA, et al: Controlled prospective study on the mental health of women following pregnancy loss. Am J Psychiatry 153:226–230, 1996

Jensen PN, Olesen OV, Bertelsen A, et al: Citalopram and desmethylcitalopram concentrations in breast milk and in serum of mother and infant. Ther Drug Monit 19:236–239, 1997

Jones I, Craddock N: Familiality of the puerperal trigger in bipolar disorder: results of a family study. Am J Psychiatry 158:913–917, 2001

Kaplan B, Modai I, Stoler M, et al: Clozapine treatment and risk of unplanned pregnancy. J Am Board Fam Pract 8:239–241, 1995

Kelly R, Zatzick D, Anders T: The detection and treatment of psychiatric disorders and substance use among pregnant women cared for in obstetrics. Am J Psychiatry 158:213–219, 2001

Kemp J, Ilett KF, Booth J, et al: Excretion of doxepin and N-desmethyldoxepin in human milk. Br J Clin Pharmacol 20:497–499, 1985

Kendell RE, Chalmers JC, Platz C: Epidemiology of puerperal psychoses. Br J Psychiatry 150:662–673 [erratum 151:135], 1987

Kennedy D, Koren G: Valproic acid use in psychiatry: issues in treating women of reproductive age. J Psychiatry Neurosci 23:223–228, 1998

Kent GN, Stuckey BG, Allen JR, et al: Postpartum thyroid dysfunction: clinical assessment and relationship to psychiatric affective morbidity. Clin Endocrinol (Oxf) 51:429–438, 1999

Kesim M, Yaris F, Kadioglu M, et al: Mirtazapine use in two pregnant women: is it safe? (letter) Teratology 66:204, 2002

King MB: Eating disorders in a general practice population: prevalence, characteristics and follow-up at 12 to 18 months. Psychol Med Monogr Suppl 14:1–34, 1989

Kirchheiner J, Berghofer A, Bolk-Weischedel D: Healthy outcome under olanzapine treatment in a pregnant woman. Pharmacopsychiatry 33:78–80, 2000

Klier CM, Muzik M, Rosenblum KL, et al: Interpersonal psychotherapy adapted for the group setting in the treatment of postpartum depression. J Psychother Pract Res 10:124–131, 2001

Knott C, Reynolds F: Therapeutic drug monitoring in pregnancy: rationale and current status. Clin Pharmacokinet 19:425–433, 1990

Kris EB, Carmichael DM: Chlorpromazine maintenance therapy during pregnancy and confinement. Psychiatr Q 31:690–695, 1957

Kristensen JH, Ilett KF, Hackett LP, et al: Distribution and excretion of fluoxetine and norfluoxetine in human milk. Br J Clin Pharmacol 48:521–527, 1999

Kristensen JH, Hackett LP, Kohan R, et al: The amount of fluvoxamine in milk is unlikely to be a cause of adverse effects in breastfed infants. J Hum Lact 18:139–143, 2002

Kulin NA, Pastuszak A, Sage SR, et al: Pregnancy outcome following maternal use of the new selective serotonin reuptake inhibitors: a prospective controlled multicenter study. JAMA 279:609–610, 1998

Kumar C, McIvor RJ, Davies T, et al: Estrogen administration does not reduce the rate of recurrence of affective psychosis after childbirth. J Clin Psychiatry 64:112–118, 2003

Kumar R, Robson KM: A prospective study of emotional disorders in childbearing women. Br J Psychiatry 144:35–47, 1984

Lacey JH, Smith G: Bulimia nervosa: the impact of pregnancy on mother and baby. Br J Psychiatry 150:777–781, 1987

Laine K, Heikkinen T, Ekblad U, et al: Effects of exposure to selective serotonin reuptake inhibitors during pregnancy on serotonergic symptoms in newborns and cord blood monoamine and prolactin concentrations. Arch Gen Psychiatry 60:720–726, 2003

Landon M: Medical complications of pregnancy: cardiac disease, in Obstetrics and Gynecology Principles for Practice. Edited by Ling F, Duff P. New York, McGraw-Hill Medical, 2001, pp 134–145

Lawrie TA, Hofmeyr GJ, De Jager M, et al: A double-blind randomised placebo controlled trial of postnatal norethisterone enanthate: the effect on postnatal depression and serum hormones. Br J Obstet Gynaecol 105:1082–1090, 1998

Lee D, Yip A, Chiu H, et al: A psychiatric epidemiological study of postpartum Chinese women. Am J Psychiatry 158:220–226, 2001

Lehrmann JA, Jain S: Myxedema psychosis with grade II hypothyroidism. Gen Hosp Psychiatry 24:275–277, 2002

Lester BM, Cucca J, Andreozzi L, et al: Possible association between fluoxetine hydrochloride and colic in an infant. J Am Acad Child Adolesc Psychiatry 32:1253–1255, 1993

Lier L, Kastrup M, Rafaelsen O: Psychiatric illness in relation to pregnancy and childbirth, II: diagnostic profiles, psychosocial and perinatal aspects. Nordisk Psykiatrisk Tidsskrift 43:535–542, 1989

Littrell KH, Johnson CG, Peabody CD, et al: Antipsychotics during pregnancy (letter). Am J Psychiatry 157:1342, 2000

Llewellyn AM, Stowe ZN, Nemeroff CB: Depression during pregnancy and the puerperium. J Clin Psychiatry 58 (suppl)15:26–32, 1997

Llewellyn A[M], Stowe ZN, Strader JR Jr: The use of lithium and management of women with bipolar disorder during pregnancy and lactation. J Clin Psychiatry 59 (suppl 6):57–64, 1998

Maina G, Albert U, Bogetto F, et al: Recent life events and obsessive-compulsive disorder (OCD): the role of pregnancy/delivery. Psychiatry Res 89:49–58, 1999

Major B, Cozzarelli C, Cooper ML, et al: Psychological responses of women after first-trimester abortion. Arch Gen Psychiatry 57:777–784, 2000

Mammen OK, Perel JM, Rudolph G, et al: Sertraline and norsertraline levels in three breastfed infants. J Clin Psychiatry 58:100–103, 1997

Marzuk PM, Tardiff K, Leon AC, et al: Lower risk of suicide during pregnancy. Am J Psychiatry 154:122–123, 1997

Matalon S, Schechtman S, Goldzweig G, et al: The teratogenetic effect of carbamazepine: a meta-analysis of 1255 exposures. Reprod Toxicol 16:9–17, 2002

Matheson I, Skjaeraasen J: Milk concentrations of flupenthixol, nortriptyline and zuclopenthixol and between-breast differences in two patients. Eur J Clin Pharmacol 35:217–220, 1988

Matheson I, Evang A, Overo KF, et al: Presence of chlorprothixene and its metabolites in breast milk. Eur J Clin Pharmacol 27:611–613, 1984

Matheson I, Pande H, Alertsen AR: Respiratory depression caused by N-desmethyldoxepin in breast milk (letter). Lancet 2:1124, 1985

McElhatton PR, Garbis HM, Elefant E, et al: The outcome of pregnancy in 689 women exposed to therapeutic doses of antidepressants: a collaborative study of the European Network of Teratology Information Services (ENTIS). Reprod Toxicol 10:285–294, 1996

McNeil TF, Kaij L, Malmquist-Larsson A: Women with nonorganic psychosis: pregnancy's effect on mental health during pregnancy. Acta Psychiatr Scand 70:140–148, 1984

Meager I, Milgrom J: Group treatment for postpartum depression: a pilot study. Aust N Z J Psychiatry 30:852–860, 1996

Mee R, Drummond-Webb J: Congenital heart disease, in Sabiston Textbook of Surgery, 16th Edition. Edited by Townsend C, Beauchamp R, Evers B, et al. Philadelphia, PA, WB Saunders, 2001, pp 1262–1263

Meersand P, Turchin W: The mother-infant relationship: from normality to pathology, in Infanticide: Psychosocial and Legal Perspectives on Mothers Who Kill. Edited by Spinelli M. Washington, DC, American Psychiatric Publishing, 2003, pp 209–233

Merlob P, Mor N, Litwin A: Transient hepatic dysfunction in an infant of an epileptic mother treated with carbamazepine during pregnancy and breastfeeding. Ann Pharmacother 26:1563–1565, 1992

Miller LJ: Psychiatric medication during pregnancy: understanding and minimizing risks. Psychiatric Annals 24:69–75, 1994a

Miller LJ: Use of electroconvulsive therapy during pregnancy. Hosp Community Psychiatry 45:444–450, 1994b

Miller LJ: Sexuality, reproduction, and family planning in women with schizophrenia. Schizophr Bull 23:623–635, 1997

Miller LJ: Denial of pregnancy, in Infanticide: Psychosocial and Legal Perspectives on Mothers Who Kill. Edited by Spinelli MG. Washington, DC, American Psychiatric Publishing, 2003, pp 81–104

Miller LJ, Finnerty M: Sexuality, pregnancy, and childrearing among women with schizophrenia-spectrum disorders. Psychiatr Serv 47:502–506, 1996

Miller LJ, Finnerty M: Family planning knowledge, attitudes and practices in women with schizophrenic spectrum disorders. J Psychosom Obstet Gynaecol 19:210–217, 1998

Miller WH {Jr}, Resnick MP, Williams MH, et al: The pregnant psychiatric inpatient: a missed opportunity. Gen Hosp Psychiatry 12:373–378, 1990

Miller WH Jr, Bloom JD, Resnick MP: Chronic mental illnesses and perinatal outcome. Gen Hosp Psychiatry 14:171–176, 1992

Misri S, Lusskin SI: Postpartum Blues and Depression, in UpToDate (http://www.uptodate.com). Edited by Rose BD. Wellesley, MA, UpToDate, 2004a

Misri S, Lusskin SI: Postpartum Psychosis, in UpToDate (http://www.uptodate.com). Edited by Rose BD. Wellesley, MA, UpToDate, 2004b

Misri S, Lusskin SI: Psychiatric Disorders in Pregnancy, in UpToDate (http://www.uptodate.com). Edited by Rose BD. Wellesley, MA, UpToDate, 2004c

Misri S, Lusskin SI: Treatment of Psychiatric Disorders in Pregnancy, in UpToDate (http://www.uptodate.com). Edited by Rose BD. Wellesley, MA, UpToDate, 2004d

Misri S, Lusskin SI: Use of Psychotropic Medications in Breastfeeding Women, in UpToDate (http://www.uptodate.com). Edited by Rose BD. Wellesley, MA, UpToDate, 2004e

Misri S, Sivertz K: Tricyclic drugs in pregnancy and lactation: a preliminary report. Int J Psychiatry Med 21:157–171, 1991

Misri S, Kim J, Riggs KW, et al: Paroxetine levels in postpartum depressed women, breast milk, and infant serum. J Clin Psychiatry 61:828–832, 2000a

Misri S, Kostaras X, Fox D, et al: The impact of partner support in the treatment of postpartum depression. Can J Psychiatry 45:554–558, 2000b

Mitchell-Gieleghem A, Mittelstaedt ME, Bulik CM: Eating disorders and childbearing: concealment and consequences. Birth 29:182–191, 2002

Morgan JF, Lacey JH, Sedgwick PM: Impact of pregnancy on bulimia nervosa. Br J Psychiatry 174:135–140 [erratum 174:278], 1999

Morgan M, Matthey S, Barnett B, et al: A group programme for postnatally distressed women and their partners. J Adv Nurs 26:913–920, 1997

National Toxicology Program (NTP) and Center for the Evaluation of Risks to Human Reproduction (CERHR): Expert panel report on the reproductive and developmental toxicity of fluoxetine. NTP-CERHR-Fluoxetine-04. April 2004. Available at: http://cerhr.niehs.nih.gov/news/fluoxetine/fluoxetine_final.pdf. Accessed July 2004.

Ness RB, Grisso JA, Hirschinger N, et al: Cocaine and tobacco use and the risk of spontaneous abortion. N Engl J Med 340:333–339, 1999

Neugebauer R, Kline J, Shrout P, et al: Major depressive disorder in the 6 months after miscarriage. JAMA 277:383–388, 1997

Neziroglu F, Anemone R, Yaryura-Tobias JA: Onset of obsessive-compulsive disorder in pregnancy. Am J Psychiatry 149:947–950, 1992

Nonacs R, Cohen LS: Postpartum mood disorders: diagnosis and treatment guidelines. J Clin Psychiatry 59 (suppl 2): 34–40, 1998

Nordeng H, Lindemann R, Perminov KV, et al: Neonatal withdrawal syndrome after in utero exposure to selective serotonin reuptake inhibitors. Acta Paediatr 90:288–291, 2001

Norre J, Vandereycken W, Gordts S: The management of eating disorders in a fertility clinic: clinical guidelines. J Psychosom Obstet Gynaecol 22:77–81, 2001

Nulman I, Koren G: The safety of fluoxetine during pregnancy and lactation. Teratology 53:304–308, 1996

Nulman I, Rovet J, Stewart DE, et al: Neurodevelopment of children exposed in utero to antidepressant drugs. N Engl J Med 336:258–262, 1997

Nulman I, Rovet J, Stewart DE, et al: Child development following exposure to tricyclic antidepressants or fluoxetine throughout fetal life: a prospective, controlled study. Am J Psychiatry 159:1889–1895, 2002

Oana Y: Epileptic seizures and pseudoseizures from the viewpoint of the hierarchy of consciousness. Epilepsia 39 (suppl 5):21–25, 1998

Oca MJ, Donn SM: Association of maternal sertraline (Zoloft) therapy and transient neonatal nystagmus. J Perinatol 19:460–461, 1999

O'Hara MW, Zekoski EM, Philipps LH, et al: Controlled prospective study of postpartum mood disorders: comparison of childbearing and nonchildbearing women. J Abnorm Psychol 99:3–15, 1990

O'Hara MW, Schlechte JA, Lewis DA, et al: Prospective study of postpartum blues: biologic and psychosocial factors. Arch Gen Psychiatry 48:801–806, 1991

O'Hara MW, Stuart S, Gorman LL, et al: Efficacy of interpersonal psychotherapy for postpartum depression. Arch Gen Psychiatry 57:1039–1045, 2000

Ohman I, Vitols S, Tomson T: Lamotrigine in pregnancy: pharmacokinetics during delivery, in the neonate, and during lactation. Epilepsia 41:709–713, 2000

Ohman I, Vitols S, Luef G, et al: Topiramate kinetics during delivery, lactation, and in the neonate: preliminary observations. Epilepsia 43:1157–1160, 2002

Öhman R, Hägg S, Carleborg L, et al: Excretion of paroxetine into breast milk. J Clin Psychiatry 60:519–523, 1999

Olesen OV, Bartels U, Poulsen JH: Perphenazine in breast milk and serum (letter). Am J Psychiatry 147:1378–1379, 1990

Omtzigt JG, Los FJ, Grobbee DE, et al: The risk of spina bifida aperta after first-trimester exposure to valproate in a prenatal cohort. Neurology 42:119–125, 1992

Oren DA, Wisner KL, Spinelli M, et al: An open trial of morning light therapy for treatment of antepartum depression. Am J Psychiatry 159:666–669, 2002

Ornoy A, Arnon J, Shechtman S, et al: Is benzodiazepine use during pregnancy really teratogenic? Reprod Toxicol 12:511–515, 1998

Overpeck MD, Brenner RA, Trumble AC, et al: Risk factors for infant homicide in the United States. N Engl J Med 339:1211–1216, 1998

Patton SW, Misri S, Corral MR, et al: Antipsychotic medication during pregnancy and lactation in women with schizophrenia: evaluating the risk. Can J Psychiatry 47:959–965, 2002

Pedersen CA: Postpartum mood and anxiety disorders: a guide for the nonpsychiatric clinician with an aside on thyroid associations with postpartum mood. Thyroid 9:691–697, 1999

Perlis RH, Sachs GS, Lafer B, et al: Effect of abrupt change from standard to low serum levels of lithium: a reanalysis of double-blind lithium maintenance data. Am J Psychiatry 159:1155–1159, 2002

Pinelli JM, Symington AJ, Cunningham KA, et al: Case report and review of the perinatal implications of maternal lithium use. Am J Obstet Gynecol 187:245–249, 2002

Piontek CM, Wisner KL, Perel JM, et al: Serum fluvoxamine levels in breastfed infants. J Clin Psychiatry 62:111–113, 2001

Pittard WB 3rd, O'Neal W Jr: Amitriptyline excretion in human milk (letter). J Clin Psychopharmacol 6:383–384, 1986

Polster DS, Wisner KL: ECT-induced premature labor: a case report (letter). J Clin Psychiatry 60:53–54, 1999

Protheroe C: Puerperal psychoses: a long-term study, 1927–1961. Br J Psychiatry 115:9–30, 1969

Rabheru K: The use of electroconvulsive therapy in special patient populations. Can J Psychiatry 46:710–719, 2001

Rambeck B, Kurlemann G, Stodieck SR, et al: Concentrations of lamotrigine in a mother on lamotrigine treatment and her newborn child. Eur J Clin Pharmacol 51:481–484, 1997

Rampono J, Kristensen JH, Hackett LP, et al: Citalopram and demethylcitalopram in human milk; distribution, excretion and effects in breast fed infants. Br J Clin Pharmacol 50:263–268, 2000

Ratnayake T, Libretto SE: No complications with risperidone treatment before and throughout pregnancy and during the nursing period (letter). J Clin Psychiatry 63:76–77, 2002

Reed P, Sermin N, Appleby L, et al: A comparison of clinical response to electroconvulsive therapy in puerperal and non-puerperal psychoses. J Affect Disord 54:255–260, 1999

ReproTox. An Information System on Environmental Hazards to Human Reproduction and Development. Available at: http://www.reprotox.org. Accessed June 2004.

Robinson D, Woerner MG, Alvir JM, et al: Predictors of relapse following response from a first episode of schizophrenia or schizoaffective disorder. Arch Gen Psychiatry 56:241–247, 1999

Rosa FW: Spina bifida in infants of women treated with carbamazepine during pregnancy. N Engl J Med 324:674–677, 1991

Russell GF, Treasure J, Eisler I: Mothers with anorexia nervosa who underfeed their children: their recognition and management. Psychol Med 28:93–108, 1998

Saks B: Mirtazapine: treatment of depression, anxiety, and hyperemesis gravidarum in the pregnant patient—a report of 7 cases. Arch Women Ment Health 3:165–170, 2001

Schimmell MS, Katz EZ, Shaag Y, et al: Toxic neonatal effects following maternal clomipramine therapy. J Toxicol Clin Toxicol 29:479–484, 1991

Schmeelk KH, Granger DA, Susman EJ, et al: Maternal depression and risk for postpartum complications: role of prenatal corticotropin-releasing hormone and interleukin-1 receptor antagonist. Behav Med 25:88–94, 1999

Schmidt K, Olesen OV, Jensen PN: Citalopram and breast-feeding: serum concentration and side effects in the infant. Biol Psychiatry 47:164–165, 2000

Schou M, Amdisen A: Lithium and pregnancy, 3: lithium ingestion by children breast-fed by women on lithium treatment. Br Med J 2:138, 1973

Schou M, Weinstein MR: Problems of lithium maintenance treatment during pregnancy, delivery and lactation. Agressologie 21(A):7–9, 1980

Schou M, Goldfield MD, Weinstein MR, et al: Lithium and pregnancy, I: report from the Register of Lithium Babies. Br Med J 2:135–136, 1973

Sichel DA, Cohen LS, Dimmock JA, et al: Postpartum obsessive compulsive disorder: a case series. J Clin Psychiatry 54:156–159, 1993

Simhandl C, Zhoglami A, Pinder R: Pregnancy during use of mirtazapine (abstract PM02098). Abstracts of the 21st CINP Congress. Glasgow, Scotland, 1998

Skausig OB, Schou M: [Breast feeding during lithium therapy] (Danish). Ugeskr Laeger 139:400–401, 1977

Sollid CP, Wisborg K, Hjort J, et al: Eating disorder that was diagnosed before pregnancy and pregnancy outcome. Am J Obstet Gynecol 190:206–210, 2004

Sovner R, Orsulak P: Excretion of imipramine and desipramine in human breast milk. Am J Psychiatry 136:451–452, 1979

Spielvogel A, Wile J: Treatment and outcomes of psychotic patients during pregnancy and childbirth. Birth 19:131–137, 1992

Spigset O, Carieborg L, Öhman R, et al: Excretion of citalopram in breast milk. Br J Clin Pharmacol 44:295–298, 1997

Spinelli MG (ed): Infanticide: Psychosocial and Legal Perspectives on Mothers Who Kill. Washington, DC, American Psychiatric Publishing, 2003a

Spinelli MG: The promise of saved lives: recognition, prevention, and rehabilitation, in Infanticide: Psychosocial and Legal Perspectives on Mothers Who Kill. Edited by Spinelli MG. Washington, DC, American Psychiatric Publishing, 2003b, pp 235–255

Spinelli MG, Endicott J: Controlled clinical trial of interpersonal psychotherapy versus parenting education program for depressed pregnant women. Am J Psychiatry 160:555–562, 2003

Stahl MM, Neiderud J, Vinge E: Thrombocytopenic purpura and anemia in a breast-fed infant whose mother was treated with valproic acid. J Pediatr 130:1001–1003, 1997

Stancer HC, Reed KL: Desipramine and 2-hydroxydesipramine in human breast milk and the nursing infant's serum. Am J Psychiatry 143:1597–1600, 1986

Steiner M, Yonkers K: Depression in Women. London, Martin Dunitz, 1998

Stewart RB, Karas B, Springer PK: Haloperidol excretion in human milk. Am J Psychiatry 137:849–850, 1980

Stiskal JA, Kulin N, Koren G, et al: Neonatal paroxetine withdrawal syndrome. Arch Dis Child Fetal Neonatal Ed 84:F134–F135, 2001

Stoner SC, Sommi RW Jr, Marken PA, et al: Clozapine use in two full-term pregnancies (letter). J Clin Psychiatry 58:364–365, 1997

Stowe ZN, Owens MJ, Landry JC, et al: Sertraline and desmethylsertraline in human breast milk and nursing infants. Am J Psychiatry 154:1255–1260, 1997

Stowe ZN, Cohen LS, Hostetter A, et al: Paroxetine in human breast milk and nursing infants. Am J Psychiatry 157:185–189, 2000

Sykes PA, Quarrie J, Alexander FW: Lithium carbonate and breast-feeding. Br Med J 2:1299, 1976

Taddio A, Ito S, Koren G: Excretion of fluoxetine and its metabolite, norfluoxetine, in human breast milk. J Clin Pharmacol 36:42–47, 1996

Taylor TM, O'Toole MS, Ohlsen RI, et al: Safety of quetiapine during pregnancy. Am J Psychiatry 160:588–589, 2003

Tede N, Foster E: Congenital heart disease in adults, in Current Diagnosis and Treatment in Cardiology, 2nd Edition. Edited by Crawford MH. New York, Lange Medical/McGraw-Hill Medical, 2003

Tennis P, Eldridge RR, International Lamotrigine Pregnancy Registry Scientific Advisory Committee: Preliminary results on pregnancy outcomes in women using lamotrigine. Epilepsia 43:1161–1167, 2002

Tenyi T, Trixler M, Keresztes Z: Quetiapine and pregnancy (letter). Am J Psychiatry 159:674, 2002

TERIS [Teratogen Information System] Clinical Teratology Web. Available at: http://www.depts.washington.edu/~terisweb. Accessed June 2004.

Terp IM, Mortensen PB: Post-partum psychoses: clinical diagnoses and relative risk of admission after parturition. Br J Psychiatry 172:521–526, 1998

Tomson T, Ohman I, Vitols S: Lamotrigine in pregnancy and lactation: a case report. Epilepsia 38:1039–1041, 1997

Tunnessen WW Jr, Hertz CG: Toxic effects of lithium in newborn infants: a commentary. J Pediatr 81:804–807, 1972

Turton P, Hughes P, Bolton H, et al: Incidence and demographic correlates of eating disorder symptoms in a pregnant population. Int J Eat Disord 26:448–452, 1999

van Dam RM, Schuit AJ, Schouten EG, et al: Serum cholesterol decline and depression in the postpartum period. J Psychosom Res 46:385–390, 1999

Videbech P, Gouliaev G: First admission with puerperal psychosis: 7–14 years of follow-up. Acta Psychiatr Scand 91:167–173, 1995

Viguera AC, Nonacs R, Cohen LS, et al: Risk of recurrence of bipolar disorder in pregnant and nonpregnant women after discontinuing lithium maintenance. Am J Psychiatry 157:179–184, 2000

Viguera AC, Cohen LS, Baldessarini RJ, et al: Managing bipolar disorder during pregnancy: weighing the risks and benefits. Can J Psychiatry 47:426–436, 2002

Waldman MD, Safferman AZ: Pregnancy and clozapine (letter). Am J Psychiatry 150:168–169, 1993

Warner JP: Evidence-based psychopharmacology, 3: assessing evidence of harm: what are the teratogenic effects of lithium carbonate? J Psychopharmacol 14:77–80, 2000

Weinstein MR, Goldfield M: Lithium carbonate treatment during pregnancy; report of a case. Dis Nerv Syst 30:828–832, 1969

Weinstock L, Cohen LS, Bailey JW, et al: Obstetrical and neonatal outcome following clonazepam use during pregnancy: a case series. Psychother Psychosom 70:158–162, 2001

Whalley LJ, Blain PG, Prime JK: Haloperidol secreted in breast milk. Br Med J (Clin Res Ed) 282:1746–1747, 1981

Wiles DH, Orr MW, Kolakowska T: Chlorpromazine levels in plasma and milk of nursing mothers (letter). Br J Clin Pharmacol 5:272–273, 1978

Williams KE, Koran LM: Obsessive-compulsive disorder in pregnancy, the puerperium, and the premenstruum. J Clin Psychiatry 58:330–334 [quiz 335–336], 1997

Wisner KL, Perel JM: Serum nortriptyline levels in nursing mothers and their infants. Am J Psychiatry 148:1234–1236, 1991

Wisner KL, Perel JM: Nortriptyline treatment of breast-feeding women (letter). Am J Psychiatry 153:295, 1996

Wisner KL, Perel JM, Wheeler S: Tricyclic dose requirements across pregnancy. Am J Psychiatry 150:1541–1542, 1993

Wisner KL, Perel JM, Foglia JP: Serum clomipramine and metabolite levels in four nursing mother-infant pairs. J Clin Psychiatry 56:17–20, 1995

Wisner KL, Perel JM, Blumer J: Serum sertraline and *N*-desmethylsertraline levels in breast-feeding mother-infant pairs. Am J Psychiatry 155:690–692, 1998

Wisner KL, Parry BL, Piontek CM: Postpartum depression. N Engl J Med 347:194–199, 2002

Wright S, Dawling S, Ashford JJ: Excretion of fluvoxamine in breast milk (letter). Br J Clin Pharmacol 31:209, 1991

Wyszynski A, Wyszynski B: A Case Approach to Medical-Psychiatric Practice. Washington, DC, American Psychiatric Press, 1996

Yapp P, Ilett KF, Kristensen JH, et al: Drowsiness and poor feeding in a breast-fed infant: association with nefazodone and its metabolites. Ann Pharmacother 34:1269–1272, 2000

Yogev Y, Ben-Haroush A, Kaplan B: Maternal clozapine treatment and decreased fetal heart rate variability. Int J Gynaecol Obstet 79:259–260, 2002

Yonkers KA, Ramin SM, Rush AJ, et al: Onset and persistence of postpartum depression in an inner-city maternal health clinic system. Am J Psychiatry 158:1856–1863, 2001

Yonkers KA, Wisner KL, Stowe Z, et al: Management of bipolar disorder during pregnancy and the postpartum period [consensus guidelines]. Am J Psychiatry 161: 608–620, 2004

Yoshida K, Smith B, Craggs M, et al: Investigation of pharmacokinetics and of possible adverse effects in infants exposed to tricyclic antidepressants in breast-milk. J Affect Disord 43:225–237, 1997

Yoshida K, Smith B, Craggs M, et al: Fluoxetine in breast-milk and developmental outcome of breast-fed infants. Br J Psychiatry 172:175–178, 1998a

Yoshida K, Smith B, Craggs M, et al: Neuroleptic drugs in breast-milk: a study of pharmacokinetics and of possible adverse effects in breast-fed infants. Psychol Med 28:81–91, 1998b

Zlotnick C, Johnson SL, Miller IW, et al: Postpartum depression in women receiving public assistance: pilot study of an interpersonal-therapy-oriented group intervention. Am J Psychiatry 158:638–640, 2001

Appendix 7–A

Psychotropics in Pregnancy and Lactation

■ SELECTIVE SEROTONIN REUPTAKE INHIBITORS (SSRIs)

Fluoxetine (Prozac) in Pregnancy

As the antidepressant with the most data in pregnancy and lactation, fluoxetine has also been subjected to the most rigorous analysis of any antidepressant to date. Data collected over the years (e.g., Goldstein et al. 1997; McElhatton et al. 1996) suggest no increased risk of miscarriage, major anatomical malformations, or stillbirths. There is some controversy over whether exposure, especially in the third trimester, increases the risk of premature birth or low birth weight (see p. 150).

The data on long-term effects of in utero exposure are reassuring, both for fluoxetine and the tricyclic antidepressants. Absence of neurobehavioral teratogenicity was shown in two studies. In the first, 55 infants exposed to fluoxetine in utero were compared with a group exposed to tricyclic antidepressants and with an unexposed control group. They were followed for 16 to 86 months after birth. No differences were found among the three groups in global IQ scores, language development, or behavioral development, or in birth weight or perinatal complications (Nulman et al. 1997). Another study compared 40 infants exposed to fluoxetine throughout pregnancy with 46 exposed to tricyclics and 36 nonexposed infants with nondepressed mothers. No adverse effects were found on global IQ, language development, or temperament at up to 71 months postpartum. More important, however, was the correlation (via multiple regression analysis) of lower cognitive and language achievement by the children with the duration and number of maternal postpartum depressive episodes (Nulman et al. 2002).

Sertraline (Zoloft), Paroxetine (Paxil), Fluvoxamine (Luvox), and Citalopram (Celexa) in Pregnancy

Although there are fewer data available for these medications than for fluoxetine, there have been no reports of increased rates of major malformations, stillbirths,

miscarriages, prematurity, or negative effects on birth weight. A large study from the Swedish Medical Birth Registry and the Lundbeck Safety Database evaluated women using SSRIs other than fluoxetine and found no increase in the rate of congenital malformations in infants exposed solely to citalopram ($n=364$), paroxetine ($n=118$), or sertraline ($n=32$) (Ericson et al. 1999). *Note:* At this writing, no data are available yet on escitalopram (Lexapro) in either pregnancy or lactation, although it is expected to be similar to citalopram in terms of reproductive toxicity risks.

In a series from nine Teratology Information Centers in Canada and the United States, outcomes were examined in 147 pregnancies exposed to sertraline, 97 to paroxetine, and 26 to fluvoxamine (Kulin et al. 1998). No increased risks were found for major malformations, miscarriage, stillbirth, or prematurity, and there were no significant differences in birth weight or gestational age compared with a control group exposed only to nonteratogenic agents. An additional study of 11 infants exposed to citalopram throughout pregnancy offers some information on long-term effects. The study found no complications at birth (Heikkinen et al. 2002). On delivery, infant plasma concentrations of citalopram and its metabolite were detected at two-thirds of maternal concentration but by age 2 months had declined to very low or undetectable levels, even in breastfed infants. Neurological development was normal for both exposed and control infants at age 12 months, and the two groups did not differ in weight.

Neonatal Complications and SSRIs

Fluoxetine

Two studies illustrate the complexity of determining whether or not there are neonatal complications with fluoxetine. One study reported an increased risk of perinatal complications, such as transient respiratory distress, feeding difficulties, jitteriness, and decreased birth weight, with third-trimester fluoxetine exposure compared with exposure limited to the first and second trimesters (Chambers et al. 1996). In contrast, a study of 138 women taking SSRIs during pregnancy, including 73 taking fluoxetine at the time of delivery, found no increase in the risk of neonatal complications compared with population norms (Hendrick et al. 2003b). As in many studies, the conclusions were limited by the lack of a control group of depressed mothers who were not on medications.

An expert panel from the Center for the Evaluation of Risks to Human Reproduction (CERHR), which is part of the National Toxicology Program of the U.S. Department of Health and Human Services, reviewed all of the data available as of March 2004 on fluoxetine use in pregnancy and breastfeeding to assess its reproductive and developmental toxicity (National Toxicology Program and Center for the Evaluation of Risks to Human Reproduction 2004). Although the panel highlighted the limitations of the data and stressed the importance of balancing the risks of untreated maternal mental illness against the risks of treatment, it nonetheless concluded that

> sufficient evidence exists for the Panel to conclude that fluoxetine exhibits developmental toxicity as characterized by an increased rate of poor neonatal adaptation (e.g., jitteriness, tachypnea, hypoglycemia, hypothermia, poor tone, respiratory distress, weak or absent cry, diminished pain reactivity, or desaturation with feeding) at typical maternal therapeutic doses (20–80 mg/day orally). These effects appear to result more readily from in utero exposure late in gestation. The observed toxicity may be reversible, although long-term follow-up studies have not been conducted to look for residual effects. The evidence suggests that developmental toxicity can also occur in the form of shortened gestational duration and reduced birth weight at term. (National Toxicology Program and Center for the Evaluation of Risks to Human Reproduction 2004, p. 144)

Other SSRIs

A small number of case reports and case series describe transient neonatal withdrawal syndromes with SSRIs other than fluoxetine (Costei et al. 2002; Dahl et al. 1997; Kent et al. 1999; Nordeng et al. 2001; Oca and Donn 1999; Stiskal et al. 2001). One study found that third-trimester paroxetine was associated with a significantly higher rate of complications in newborns compared with 1) a control group with no medication exposure and 2) those whose exposure was limited to the first or second trimester (Costei et al. 2002). Pregnant women were enrolled prospectively, but outcome data were collected by telephone interviews with the mothers rather than by chart reviews, thus predisposing to recall bias. Twelve of 55 infants experienced complications ($P=0.03$), which included respiratory distress ($n=9$), hypoglycemia ($n=3$), and jaundice ($n=1$). The infants were hospitalized for up to 2 weeks after delivery but had no long-term adverse effects. Although these complications were described as withdrawal symptoms, both jaundice and hypoglycemia are common neonatal complications.

A 2003 study compared the infants of 20 mothers exposed to fluoxetine or citalopram (20–40 mg/day) with 20 unmedicated matched control subjects (Laine et al. 2003). SSRI-exposed infants, evaluated at 4 days of age, had a fourfold increase in the rate of serotonergic symptom scores (e.g., tremor, restlessness, and rigidity) compared with nonexposed control subjects. There were no differences between the groups at 2 weeks and 2 months of age. The authors concluded that symptoms reflected high CNS serotonergic activity rather that SSRI withdrawal, but methodological limitations, including the small sample size, limit the validity of this conclusion.

Comment: Other authors caution about revising management recommendations for treatment with SSRIs until larger and better studies have been conducted. Transient neonatal symptoms are still poorly understood and await further elucidation. The risks of untreated maternal mental illness should not be underestimated (Misri and Lusskin 2004d). It is a relatively consistent finding that frequency and intensity of maternal depression correlate more strongly with behavioral teratogenicity for early-childhood development than does fetal exposure to SSRI medication.

Breastfeeding and SSRIs

The contrast between the growing database on SSRI breastfeeding and the rare adverse report gives cause for optimism. Long-term data are still pending on the developmental effects of SSRI exposure through breast milk, but the little that we have is also reassuring.

Fluoxetine (Prozac)

Fluoxetine remains the most frequently studied SSRI (Brent and Wisner 1998; Burch and Wells 1992; Isenberg 1990; Kristensen et al. 1999; Nulman and Koren 1996; Taddio et al. 1996; Yoshida et al. 1998a). The active metabolite (norfluoxetine) is predisposed to accumulate in infants. No adverse events were noted in 180 out of 190 cases of infants whose mothers took fluoxetine during lactation (Burt et al. 2001). Fluoxetine was found to be above adult therapeutic levels in one

3-week-old baby of a nursing mother who was taking 20 mg/day (Lester et al. 1993). The baby suffered colic (constant crying, sleep disturbance, frequent vomiting, watery stools) while breastfeeding, which resolved when switched to a bottle. It could not be determined if other constituents of the breast milk caused the colic.

Reduced weight gain was noted in some infants who were breastfed by mothers taking fluoxetine, although the weights reported were not statistically lower than the national mean (Chambers et al. 1999). In contrast, a study of 78 breastfeeding mother-infant pairs who were exposed to various SSRIs or venlafaxine found that the babies gained significantly less weight if the mothers were depressed for 2 months or more postpartum. There was no correlation between weight gain and drug exposure, highlighting once again the negative impact of maternal depression on the infant (Hendrick et al. 2003a). On the other hand, the CERHR Expert Panel highlighted the complexities facing the clinician by concluding that

> exposure to fluoxetine through breast milk may result in reduced postnatal growth during early infancy. However, the possibility that this diminished growth may be related to prenatal rather than postnatal exposure could not be excluded. The long-term implications of these findings cannot be evaluated without further longitudinal data. (National Toxicology Program and Center for the Evaluation of Risks to Human Reproduction 2004, p. 144)

Better-designed and larger studies are clearly needed before a definitive conclusion can be reached.

Sertraline (Zoloft)

Low or undetectable serum levels of sertraline and its metabolite desmethylsertraline have been reported in infant serum in more than 70 infants (Burt et al. 2001; Epperson et al. 1997; Hendrick et al. 2001b; Mammen et al. 1997; Stowe et al. 1997; Wisner et al. 1998). Platelet serotonin uptake (an assay of central serotonergic activity) was unchanged in 19 breastfeeding infants exposed to sertraline, despite the presence of low serum levels of sertraline and its metabolite (Epperson et al. 2001).

Paroxetine (Paxil)

Although paroxetine does find its way into breast milk, there is the advantage to infants of no active metabolites. No adverse neonatal effects have been reported in more than 70 cases, with infant levels very low or undetectable (Begg et al. 1999; Hendrick et al.

2001b; Misri et al. 2000a; Öhman et al. 1999; Stowe et al. 2000).

Fluvoxamine (Luvox)

In 10 cases of fluvoxamine exposure, there were no adverse effects, and low concentrations in breast milk and infant serum were found (Arnold et al. 2000; Hagg et al. 2000; Hendrick et al. 2001b; Kristensen et al. 2002; Piontek et al. 2001; Wright et al. 1991).

Citalopram (Celexa)

There have been at least 20 case studies examining infants exposed to citalopram while breastfeeding (Heikkinen et al. 2002; Jensen et al. 1997; Rampono et al. 2000; Schmidt et al. 2000; Spigset et al. 1997). Short-lasting symptoms of sleep problems correlated to high serum concentration of citalopram in one study, improving when the dose was decreased (Schmidt et al. 2000). Whereas concentrations of citalopram and its metabolite were two to three times higher in breast milk than in maternal plasma in nine mother-infant pairs, serum concentrations in infants remained low or undetectable (Heikkinen et al. 2002). One-year neurodevelopmental outcomes were reported as normal.

■ OTHER ANTIDEPRESSANTS

Venlafaxine (Effexor)

Venlafaxine is a reuptake inhibitor for both serotonin and norepinephrine. There are fewer data on venlafaxine than on the SSRI or TCA classes of antidepressants. A multicenter prospective study reported venlafaxine's safety (at average dose 75 mg/day, range 37.5–300 mg/day) in 150 women who were exposed during pregnancy and followed for 6–12 months postpartum (Einarson et al. 2001). Venlafaxine was taken by 34 patients through the entire pregnancy. The control groups consisted of women treated with SSRIs (fluoxetine, sertraline, paroxetine, and fluvoxamine) for depression and women taking other nonteratogenic agents. The rate of major malformations for women taking venlafaxine was comparable to that in the other two groups and was no higher than the baseline rate of birth defects in the general population (i.e., 1%–3%). Premature births did not differ among groups. Additional data in support of safety in pregnancy come from the study by Hendrick et al. (2003a) described in the above section on fluoxetine. There are no reports of neonatal complications thus far.

- *Note:* It is not advisable to taper venlafaxine close to term with the goal of reducing the potential for neonatal intoxication or withdrawal syndromes. Such a strategy risks exposing the mother to the fairly common venlafaxine-associated withdrawal symptoms, as well as to the risks of relapse of depression. More data are needed to determine the ideal management strategy through labor and delivery.

Breastfeeding

No adverse events have been found in the eight published cases of infants who breastfed while their mothers took venlafaxine. Infant serum levels of the medication and its active metabolite were variable but generally low (Hendrick et al. 2001a; Ilett et al. 1998, 2002).

Nefazodone (Serzone) and Trazodone (Desyrel)

A multicenter prospective controlled study compared 147 women with first-trimester exposure to trazodone (*n*=58) or nefazodone (*n*=89) with women exposed to other nonteratogenic antidepressants or to other nonteratogenic drugs. In the study group, 35% of the women took nefazodone or trazodone throughout pregnancy (Einarson et al. 2003). There were no statistically significant differences between the three groups in the rates of spontaneous abortions, premature labor, or malformations (no difference from expected rate of 1%–3%), or in birth weight.

Breastfeeding

There is one case report only, in which a premature infant who breastfed while the mother was taking nefazodone 300 mg/day developed sedation and poor feeding, which resolved within 72 hours of stopping breastfeeding. Other causes had been excluded. The very low calculated infant dose through breast milk (0.45% of the maternal dose) stands in contrast to the putative side effects of exposure (Yapp et al. 2000). No data are available for trazodone.

Mirtazapine (Remeron)

A prescription event monitoring study in England reported on 41 cases of first-trimester exposure to mirtazapine (Biswas et al. 2003). The study is limited by the lack of complete information about the mothers' diagnoses, doses, and duration of treatment and by

the lack of control groups. Of the 41 babies, 20 were apparently healthy and delivered at term. Of the remaining 21, there were four premature births at 26–36 weeks, with one case of patent ductus arteriosus; there were eight therapeutic terminations; and there were eight spontaneous miscarriages. One outcome was not known.

In another case series, six women were treated through seven pregnancies with mirtazapine, beginning at 10–17 weeks of pregnancy, for anxiety and depression comorbid with hyperemesis gravidarum (Saks 2001). All seven babies were healthy and delivered at term, although one required treatment for mild pulmonary hypertension and persistent fetal circulation. In the case of two pregnant women exposed briefly to mirtazapine and trifluoperazine (Stelazine) between the first and fifth weeks of pregnancy, both babies were healthy and born at term (Kesim et al. 2002). Although one developed transient gastroesophageal reflux, there was no evidence of congenital anomalies up to 6 months in age. There is also one case report, available as an abstract, of the delivery at term of a healthy infant following exposure to mirtazapine during the first 26 days of pregnancy (Simhandl et al. 1998).

- *Recommendation:* Mirtazapine should be used during pregnancy and breastfeeding only if safer alternatives are not an option.

Breastfeeding

No data are available on the use of mirtazapine during breastfeeding.

Bupropion (Wellbutrin, Zyban)

Although there are no published case reports on the use of bupropion during pregnancy, the manufacturer released preliminary findings from the manufacturer's registry (Glaxo SmithKline Bupropion Pregnancy Registry 2003). Definitive conclusions regarding the risk of particular birth defects could not be drawn because of the small sample size. There were 322 cases of first-trimester exposure. Nine babies were born with birth defects, and there was one therapeutic termination for a congenital anomaly. There were 11 additional terminations and 40 spontaneous miscarriages. A total of 261 babies were born without birth defects. The manufacturer is continuing to enroll patients in the registry; for more information, contact the Bupropion Pregnancy Registry at 1-800-336-2176 (toll-free) or 910-256-0549 (collect).

- *Recommendation:* Bupropion should be used only if safer alternatives are not an option.

Breastfeeding

No quantifiable levels of bupropion or its metabolite and no adverse effects were reported in the infants of two breastfeeding mothers (Baab et al. 2002).

Tricyclic Antidepressants (TCAs)

TCAs in Pregnancy

Most tricyclic antidepressants have received FDA risk designations of C or D, implying that risk is unknown or that there is evidence of substantial risk. Early reports from chart reviews and case studies linked tricyclics with congenital defects, such as limb anomalies. However, reexamination of the data has shown no increased risk of congenital defects compared with the general population for TCA exposure in utero (Altshuler et al. 1996). There is a general consensus, based on 30 years of experience gleaned from more than 400 case reports, that TCAs are relatively safe in pregnancy, particularly when used in modified doses, with plasma concentration monitoring, and in collaboration with an obstetrician (Altshuler et al. 1996; Cohen and Rosenbaum 1998). Long-term follow-up data on TCA exposure have been reassuring as well (Nulman et al. 2002). There is also no apparent increase in the risk of miscarriage or stillbirth.

Neonatal Complications

One study reported that infants born to mothers who received more than 150 mg of tricyclics per day showed jaundice and severe withdrawal symptoms, perhaps due to the relative immaturity of the neonatal liver (Misri and Sivertz 1991). All symptoms resolved in 3–6 days. Infants born to mothers whose tricyclics had been discontinued 4–7 days prior to delivery showed *negligible withdrawal symptoms.* Reducing the tricyclic dosage before delivery may lessen the risk of neonatal withdrawal (e.g., jitteriness, irritability, seizures, hypotonia, and tachypnea) after the baby is born. However, lowering the TCA dose may predispose the mother to withdrawal symptoms and relapse of depression just when she is most vulnerable in the postpartum period; thus this technique should only be tried if the mother can be monitored frequently. If a severe neonatal withdrawal syndrome develops, the infant can be given a low dose of antidepressant and gradually tapered off the drug (Miller 1994b).

Long-Term Effects

The two studies done on long-term effects of fluoxetine followed children who had been exposed to TCAs in utero as control subjects. No effects were found on language development or IQ in the TCA-exposed children. As noted above in the section on fluoxetine, there was a negative correlation of adverse effects with the degree of maternal depression, but not with the degree of medication exposure (Nulman et al. 1997, 2002).

Use: Despite these encouraging data, the TCAs have been moved aside by the SSRIs as first line-treatments because of their side effect profile for orthostatic hypotension and dizziness (the latter both secondary to and independent of orthostatic hypotension), and antihistaminic and anticholinergic side effects (sedation; constipation, urinary retention). Nortriptyline (Pamelor, Aventyl) and desipramine are the preferred tricyclics for depressed pregnant patients because they have the fewest side effects. The more sedating medications, imipramine and amitriptyline, may be useful especially in low doses of 10–20 mg at night for treatment of sleep disturbances, whether alone or adjunctively to other antidepressants (Misri and Lusskin 2004d).

Dosing: The progressive physiological changes of pregnancy require dose *increases;* pregnancy reduces protein-binding capacity, enhances hepatic metabolism, causes progesterone-induced decline in gastrointestinal motility (reducing absorption), and increases the volume of distribution (Knott and Reynolds 1990). Tricyclic dose requirements have been shown to increase during the second half of pregnancy; during the final trimester, the mean required dose was 1.6 times higher than that needed during the nonpregnant state (Wisner et al. 1993).

Breastfeeding

Approximately 10% of the maternal TCA concentration crosses to breast milk (Misri and Sivertz 1991), resulting in infant serum levels that are variable. No adverse effects have been documented for exposure to amitriptyline (Elavil), nortriptyline (Pamelor, Aventyl), imipramine (Tofranil), desipramine (Norpramin), or clomipramine (Anafranil) (Bader and Newman 1980; Birnbaum et al. 1999; Breyer-Pfaff et al. 1995; Matheson and Skjaeraasen 1988; Pittard and O'Neal 1986; Schimmell et al. 1991; Sovner and Orsulak 1979; Stancer and Reed 1986; Wisner and Perel 1991, 1996; Wisner et al. 1995; Yoshida et al. 1997). Doxepin (Sinequan) and its metabolite have been reported, in one case (Matheson et al. 1985), to accumulate in a nursing infant, causing sedation and respiratory distress. The active metabolite can accumulate in nursing infants because of its long half-life (37 hours) (Matheson et al. 1985). However, another case study did not report any adverse effects (Kemp et al. 1985).

Clomipramine (Anafranil)

Clomipramine is frequently used for the treatment of obsessive-compulsive disorder. Few studies exist specifically on clomipramine. The two that have been published focused on neonatal toxicity. In one of these studies (Schimmell et al. 1991), three of six infants who were exposed in utero to clomipramine had symptoms of mild toxicity. Mild respiratory distress, mild hypotonia, tremors, and jitteriness were noted in one newborn; all symptoms resolved spontaneously by age 6 days. Another infant suffered mild hypotonia, which lasted several weeks. The third infant required oxygen therapy for transient tachypnea. No other signs of toxicity were noted. In the other study (Cowe et al. 1982), seizures were experienced in two infants withdrawing from clomipramine.

Given these data, managing maternal clomipramine like any other TCA (i.e., tapering high doses very close to delivery if possible) may help minimize neonatal withdrawal and toxicity, without precipitating relapse in the mother. Long-term follow-up studies for children exposed to clomipramine in utero are not yet available.

Monoamine Oxidase Inhibitors

Monoamine oxidase inhibitors should be avoided in pregnancy; not only are there few data on their use in pregnancy, but animal studies have shown that they are associated with fetal growth restriction (Altshuler et al. 1996). Drug-drug interactions and drug-food interactions increase the risk of hypertensive crisis, making treatment with these agents cumbersome. A case report on the use of phenelzine (Nardil) in pregnancy also reviewed the literature through 1997 (Gracious and Wisner 1997).

■ ANTIPSYCHOTICS

Conventional (Typical) Antipsychotic Medications in Pregnancy and Lactation

Teratogenicity

Teratogenicity data on phenothiazines are drawn from their use as antiemetics in women with hyper-

emesis gravidarum. In a meta-analysis of 74,337 live births, there were 2,591 mother-infant pairs with first-trimester phenothiazine exposure (Altshuler et al. 1996). Data showed that there was an additional risk of 0.4% (4 in 1,000) over baseline risk (2%–4% of live births) in the relative risk of malformations. Thus, phenothiazines confer a relatively small increase in the absolute risk of congenital birth defects.

The meta-analysis also demonstrated that high-potency, conventional antipsychotics (e.g., haloperidol [Haldol], perphenazine [Trilafon], trifluoperazine [Stelazine], and thiothixene [Navane]) were less teratogenic than low-potency conventional antipsychotics (e.g., chlorpromazine) in nonpsychotic women. In psychotic women, high-potency conventional antipsychotics are generally preferred over the low-potency conventional antipsychotics, despite the risk of extrapyramidal effects and tardive dyskinesia (Patton et al. 2002).

- *Note:* Schizophrenia itself has been found to double statistically the risks of malformations and fetal demise, independent of medication exposure (Altshuler et al. 1996).

Long-Term Effects

There *is* evidence of neurobehavioral teratogenicity in animal studies following fetal exposure to conventional high- and low-potency antipsychotics (Altshuler et al. 1996; American Academy of Pediatrics Committee on Drugs 2000). However, no effects on behavioral, emotional, or cognitive development have been found in human studies, although prospective, developmental studies have yet to be launched (Altshuler et al. 1996; American Academy of Pediatrics Committee on Drugs 2000).

Neonatal Side Effects

The incidence of side effects in newborns is unknown, but transient neonatal symptoms have been described subsequent to in utero exposure, particularly with the low-potency antipsychotics. Sedation, hypotension, tachycardia, gastrointestinal effects (functional bowel obstruction and neonatal jaundice), tremor, motor restlessness, hypertonicity, abnormal movements (dystonic and parkinsonian effects), and feeding problems have been reported in newborns (Altshuler et al. 1996; American Academy of Pediatrics Committee on Drugs 2000; Cohen and Rosenbaum 1998).

Extrapyramidal Side Effects

Diphenhydramine (Benadryl) is considered to be the treatment of choice for avoiding extrapyramidal side effects caused by the conventional antipsychotics in pregnant women (Altshuler et al. 1996). Limited data suggest benztropine (Cogentin) is also safe, although there is a case report of paralytic ileus in two newborns exposed in utero (ReproTox 2004). There are not enough data to comment on the safety of trihexyphenidyl (Artane) or amantadine (Symmetrel) in human pregnancy or lactation.

Breastfeeding

Patton et al. (2002) have reviewed the data available on antipsychotics in pregnancy and lactation. As of 2002, fewer than 35 cases had been published on the use of typical antipsychotics in lactating women, and the long-term neurobehavioral effects on the infants had not been documented. Those that were published included reports on the exposure of newborns to the typical antipsychotics chlorpromazine (Thorazine), trifluoperazine (Stelazine), perphenazine (Trilafon), and haloperidol (Haldol) through breast milk (Blacker et al. 1962; Croke et al. 2002; Kris and Carmichael 1957; Matheson and Skjaeraasen 1988; Matheson et al. 1984; Olesen et al. 1990; Stewart et al. 1980; Whalley et al. 1981; Wiles et al. 1978; Yoshida et al. 1998b).

Drowsiness and lethargy in one breastfeeding infant were reported in association with chlorpromazine (Wiles et al. 1978). A prospective controlled trial of typical antipsychotic medications described three infants, exposed to a combination of chlorpromazine and haloperidol through breast milk, who showed developmental delays at age 12–18 months (Yoshida et al. 1998b). However, only one of these three infants had detectable serum concentrations of the medications.

It is relevant that many typical antipsychotic medications, particularly chlorpromazine (Thorazine) and fluphenazine (Prolixin), have long half-lives, predisposing to accumulation and sedation in the nursing infant. Infants should be monitored closely for sedation and other adverse effects.

Novel (Atypical) Antipsychotic Medications in Pregnancy and Lactation

The novel or atypical antipsychotics have only limited data for use in pregnancy. Currently, recommenda-tions are that they be used in pregnancy only if the patient is at risk for relapse or has a history of nonresponse with the better-studied conventional antipsychotic medications (Patton et al. 2002).

Clozapine (Clozaril)

The risk of clozapine-associated agranulocytosis requires monitoring the white blood cell count in the infant; in addition, a case of neonatal seizure has been reported (Stoner et al. 1997). Several case reports have appeared of previously infertile schizophrenic women becoming pregnant when clozapine was substituted for a conventional antipsychotic; this effect was thought to be secondary to normalization of prolactin levels (Dickson and Hogg 1998; Kaplan et al. 1995; Stoner et al. 1997; Waldman and Safferman 1993). Unlike the conventional antipsychotics, which block dopamine and raise prolactin levels, clozapine does not affect prolactin levels, nor does it cause extrapyramidal symptoms or tardive dyskinesia.

There are six published case reports on clozapine use throughout pregnancy. All patients had received a diagnosis of schizophrenia and had been started on clozapine prior to pregnancy (Barnas et al. 1994; Dickson and Hogg 1998; Stoner et al. 1997; Waldman and Safferman 1993; Yogev et al. 2002). There were no congenital anomalies. One woman developed gestational diabetes without any prior history (Waldman and Safferman 1993). Another patient had hyperglycemia prior to treatment with clozapine, which worsened after the medication was started and progressed to gestational diabetes (Dickson and Hogg 1998). These two deliveries were complicated by shoulder dystocia. Both babies were otherwise healthy, with the latter followed to age 3 years. One infant had a seizure at age 8 days, which the authors theorized might reflect clozapine accumulation or clozapine withdrawal. The baby was followed until age 2 years without any evidence of seizure disorder or neurodevelopmental abnormalities (Barnas et al. 1994). Clozapine levels were determined in amniotic fluid at delivery, in maternal and infant serum, and in breast milk (the infant was not breastfed), demonstrating accumulation in infant serum and breast milk.

Neonatal complications: A case report described decreased fetal heart rate variability during labor and delivery in a healthy infant born at 37 weeks (Yogev et al. 2002). Decreased fetal heart rate variability can be a marker for fetal compromise (Gillen-Goldstein and Young 2004). The authors suspected that the decreased fetal heart rate variability represented a transient effect of clozapine on the fetal central nervous system and recommended further studies to determine the broader implications (Yogev et al. 2002). The original manufacturer of clozapine (Clozaril; Novartis Pharmaceuticals) investigated 48 pregnancies. There were 29 babies born to 28 patients who had completed pregnancies with varying degrees of exposure. Of the 29 babies born, 25 were healthy; four of the 29 had complications, including three congenital anomalies. Subsequent analysis in 1997 led to the conclusion that these anomalies were unlikely to be causally related to clozapine treatment and that the drug is not likely to be teratogenic (Novartis Pharmaceuticals, personal communication, July 10, 2003).

Risperidone (Risperdal)

Cases have been reported of risperidone exposure throughout pregnancy in two women with schizophrenia (Ratnayake and Libretto 2002). No maternal or neonatal complications were found in the infants, who were delivered by elective cesarean birth at term. No developmental abnormalities were evident at follow-up at age 9 months for one infant and age 12 months for the other. It is not clear from the case reports whether the infants nursed or not.

Breastfeeding. There is one report in which levels of risperidone were assayed in the breast milk and potential infant exposure was estimated, but the infant was bottle fed (Hill et al. 2000). Two breastfed infants had undetectable plasma concentrations of risperidone and 9-hydroxyrisperidone and had no adverse effects (Ilett et al. 2004).

Olanzapine (Zyprexa)

Like clozapine, olanzapine is less likely to raise prolactin levels and so may reverse antipsychotic-associated infertility (Dickson and Dawson 1998). The manufacturer's safety database reported on 23 prospectively identified exposures to olanzapine (Goldstein et al. 2000). Three of 23 women spontaneously miscarried, for a rate within the expected range (13%). First-trimester exposure occurred for 15 of the remaining 19 pregnancies, without increased incidence of major malformation, stillbirth, prematurity, miscarriage, or perinatal complications. One infant was exposed from the 18th week to delivery, and then during 2 months of breastfeeding (Kirchheiner et al. 2000). Follow-up for 11 months showed no evidence of complications or developmental abnormalities. One woman taking olanzapine experienced a pregnancy that was compli-

cated by excessive weight gain, gestational diabetes, and preeclampsia. The baby was delivered at 30 weeks by elective cesarean section and weighed 4 lb 11 oz with normal Apgar scores; no other information was reported (Littrell et al. 2000). The manufacturer's registry of 96 reports showed one major malformation and seven cases of transient perinatal complications. These were considered within the normal range compared with control subjects (Viguera et al. 2002).

Breastfeeding. The manufacturer's safety database (Goldstein et al. 2000) and a small case series (Croke et al. 2002) provide what we know of olanzapine exposure during breastfeeding. One of three database infants exposed to olanzapine had cardiomegaly, jaundice, and sedation (Goldstein et al. 2000). However, it was not possible to determine the contribution of accumulation in breast milk because this child had been exposed to olanzapine both in utero and during breastfeeding. In the case series, five mother-infant pairs were studied on an inpatient mother-baby unit. All babies appeared to tolerate exposure to olanzapine without side effects (Croke et al. 2002). The serum level was measured in only one infant and was found to be undetectable.

Quetiapine (Seroquel)

The first case report of quetiapine exposure throughout pregnancy reported that a health baby boy was born who showed no adverse effects up to age 6 months (Tenyi et al. 2002). The second case published was of a baby girl exposed in utero to risperidone for the first 2 weeks and then to quetiapine until delivery. She was healthy at delivery at 39 weeks and up to 1 month postpartum (Taylor et al. 2003). The baby was breastfed, but the mother was off medication. There are no published data on quetiapine use during breastfeeding.

Ziprasidone (Geodon) and Aripiprazole (Abilify)

Ziprasidone and aripiprazole have been recently introduced in the United States. There is no information on their use in humans during pregnancy or lactation.

■ ANXIOLYTICS

Diazepam (Valium)

Diazepam is the best-studied benzodiazepine, with major reviews concluding that there is minimal risk of teratogenicity (Briggs et al. 2002; Friedman and Polifka 2000; Iqbal et al. 2002; ReproTox 2004; TERIS 2004);

Transient neonatal syndromes such as the "floppy infant" syndrome, characterized by neonatal hypotonia, apnea, hypothermia, and feeding difficulties, reflect intoxication. Hypertonia, tremors, and irritability, which reflect withdrawal, have been reported (Briggs et al. 2002; Friedman and Polifka 2000; Iqbal et al. 2002).

Alprazolam (Xanax)

Alprazolam was evaluated in a meta-analysis of several studies (Altshuler et al. 1996), and it was found that first-trimester exposure was associated with a statistically significant increase in the rate of cleft palate, from 0.0006 to 0.007; however, the absolute risk for this anomaly remained small (Altshuler et al. 1996). The later Israeli Teratogen Information Service study cited below found no increase in the frequency of any congenital anomalies among infants exposed in 149 pregnancies (Ornoy et al. 1998). Transient neonatal withdrawal syndromes have been reported (Friedman and Polifka 2000; ReproTox 2004; TERIS 2004).

Clonazepam (Klonopin)

Clonazepam is used as an anticonvulsant and as an anxiolytic. Limited data are available for clonazepam, with most coming from studies of women with epilepsy who took other anticonvulsants as well, thus confounding interpretation of the effects of clonazepam alone (Briggs et al. 2002; Friedman and Polifka 2000) (see Anticonvulsants section below). In the Israeli Teratogen Information Service study, there were 69 exposed pregnancies, with no increase in the rate of malformations (Ornoy et al. 1998). This finding was consistent with previous scattered reports that clonazepam as monotherapy for epilepsy did not appear to be teratogenic (Briggs et al. 2002; Friedman and Polifka 2000). A case series of 27 infants exposed to clonazepam during pregnancy for treatment of maternal psychiatric disorders, in doses up to 3 mg/ day, found no increase in the rate of congenital malformations or perinatal problems (Weinstock et al. 2001). Transient neonatal apnea, hypotonia, and cyanosis have been reported (Friedman and Polifka 2000).

Lorazepam (Ativan)

Lorazepam is used orally for anxiety, and parenterally for treatment of anxiety and status epilepticus and as a preanesthetic sedative. Data for this drug are also limited. A Teratogen Information Center study followed 112 patients exposed to lorazepam during pregnancy and found no increase in the rate of malformations (Bonnot et al. 1999; Friedman and Polifka 2000; Ornoy et al. 1998 ; ReproTox 2004; TERIS 2004). There are reports of neonatal sedation (floppy infant syndrome), especially following intravenous use during labor (Friedman and Polifka 2000; ReproTox 2004; TERIS 2004).

Neonatal Complications and Benzodiazepines

Exposure to benzodiazepines, especially at the end of the third trimester, close to delivery, may produce neonatal toxicity, which has been dubbed "floppy infant" syndrome (hypotonia, lethargy, sucking difficulties) (Briggs et al. 2002; Friedman and Polifka 2000; ReproTox 2004; TERIS 2004). Neonatal withdrawal symptoms from benzodiazepines include irritability, restlessness, hypertonicity, diarrhea, and vomiting (Briggs et al. 2002). These complications may be minimized by slowly tapering the mother's anxiolytic to the lowest dose tolerable in terms of symptom control, so that the baby is born with minimal blood levels.

Conclusion: The benzodiazepines appear to be relatively safe in pregnancy and lactation. Clonazepam and lorazepam are generally preferred over alprazolam in pregnancy (Misri and Lusskin 2004d). The short half-life of alprazolam and the risk of interdose withdrawal may result in the pregnant woman needing higher doses. Clonazepam and lorazepam have longer half-lives, allowing more therapeutic hours per dose, as well as smoother tapering with little of the rebound associated with shorter-acting medications. Their lack of active metabolites also lessens the risk of sedation in the newborn, making them the preferred benzodiazepines in breastfeeding women (Misri and Lusskin 2004e).

The very long half-life of diazepam and its long-acting active metabolites predispose to cumulative sedation in the mother and the fetus, making it a less attractive first-choice medication. On the other hand, it is not absolutely necessary to switch from diazepam to a different benzodiazepine for women on long-term diazepam therapy; instead, the aim should be to reduce the dose as much as possible.

Breastfeeding and Benzodiazepines

Benzodiazepines are not contraindicated during breastfeeding but should be used cautiously (and are not a substitute for antidepressants or antipsychotics). The main concern is sedation in the newborn. For this reason, low doses of medications with no active metabolites, such as clonazepam or lorazepam, are preferred (Misri and Lusskin 2004e).

■ ANTICONVULSANTS

Women of reproductive age who take anticonvulsants ideally will take folic acid (1–4 mg/day), regardless of whether or not they plan to become pregnant, to reduce the risks of birth defects should they become pregnant.

Although the anticonvulsants valproic acid and carbamazepine might appear to offer advantages over lithium in pregnancy (because neither drug requires the same careful attention to fluid and electrolyte alterations over the course of pregnancy, and because both are considered by the American Academy of Pediatrics to be compatible with breastfeeding), nonetheless, both are human teratogens. Distinct patterns of anomalies are associated with the use of anticonvulsant drugs for any indication during pregnancy (Holmes 2002). It is important to keep in mind that data regarding the teratogenicity of anticonvulsant drugs have been obtained primarily from exposures in women with epilepsy and that epilepsy itself may confer an increased risk of congenital anomalies (Holmes 2002). Carbamazepine and valproic acid in particular have been associated with cardiac and neural tube defects (Altshuler et al. 1996; American Academy of Pediatrics Committee on Drugs 2000; Holmes 2002; Iqbal et al. 2001).

Carbamazepine (Tegretol)

First-trimester exposure to anticonvulsants increases the risk of neural tube defects, such as spina bifida, from 0.03% in the general population to 1% in women taking carbamazepine (Rosa 1991). Cardiac anomalies and low birth weight have been associated with first-trimester exposure to carbamazepine. One group of investigators reported that the relative risk for major congenital anomalies was 2.4 and the prevalence of heart defects was 2.9%, compared with 0.7% in nonexposed control subjects (Diav-Citrin et al. 2001). A meta-analysis of 1,255 exposed babies showed a 2.89-fold increased risk of major congenital anomalies with carbamazepine exposure compared with control subjects (Matalon et al. 2002). Polypharmacy with other

antiepileptic medications showed a twofold increased risk for teratogenicity.

Carbamazepine and valproic acid have been associated with characteristic craniofacial abnormalities, microcephaly, growth retardation, cleft lip and palate, limb defects, and genital anomalies (Holmes 2002; Viguera et al. 2002). Second- and third-trimester carbamazepine use has been associated with coagulopathy in the newborn, which brings with it an increase in risk of other serious complications, such as neonatal intracerebral hemorrhage. Maternal oral vitamin K_1 (10–20 mg/day) in the last month of pregnancy may reduce the incidence of coagulopathy (Cornelissen et al. 1993).

Valproic Acid (Depakote, Depakene)

Valproic acid has been associated with an even higher risk of neural tube defects than carbamazepine. A prospective cohort study of 261 women with 297 pregnancies exposed to valproic acid yielded a 5.4% risk of neural tube defects (Omtzigt et al. 1992). Preliminary findings from the Antiepileptic Drug Pregnancy Registry (2004) were released in 2002, showing the following: of 123 babies exposed to valproic acid alone, 8.9% had major birth defects, including neural tube defects and cardiac defects, compared with 2.8% of babies exposed to other monotherapies and 1.6% of unexposed control subjects. An increased incidence of multiple anomalies was also found, but these anomalies were not always detectable on prenatal ultrasound. The generalizability of these findings has not been established (Holmes 2002; L.B. Holmes, personal communication, June 2003). Studies are currently under way to determine whether in utero exposure to valproic acid confers an increased risk of long-term neurodevelopmental disorders such as autism (Holmes 2002; L.B. Holmes, personal communication, June 2003).

As noted in the preceding section on carbamazepine, valproic acid has been associated with characteristic craniofacial abnormalities, microcephaly, growth retardation, cleft lip/palate, limb defects, and genital anomalies (Holmes 2002; Viguera et al. 2002).

Lamotrigine (Lamictal), Gabapentin (Neurontin), and Topiramate (Topamax)

A pregnancy registry in the United States established by the manufacturer of lamotrigine reported the following: first-trimester exposure to lamotrigine monotherapy resulted in three major birth defects in 168 babies, yielding a rate of 1.8% that was within the population-based norms. The risk was higher with lamotrigine polytherapy: 10% with valproic acid (5/50 exposures) and 4.3% (5/116 exposures) with anticonvulsants other than valproic acid. The generalizability of the findings is limited by small sample sizes. No specific pattern of congenital malformations emerged in any of the subgroups. A second registry, based in the United Kingdom, which followed women treated with any anticonvulsant drug during pregnancy, found a rate of 4% (95% confidence interval 0.6%–7.6%) for women with epilepsy using lamotrigine monotherapy. This result was consistent with other data on women with epilepsy on monotherapy (Tennis et al. 2002).

We await data on topiramate. To date, little empirical evidence supports the use of gabapentin as a mood stabilizer.

Breastfeeding

The American Academy of Pediatrics Committee on Drugs and the American Academy of Neurology consider valproic acid and carbamazepine compatible with breastfeeding because of consistent, though limited, reports of low to unquantifiable concentrations of these medications in breast milk; levels have been reported to be higher in infants who were also exposed to them during pregnancy (American Academy of Pediatrics Committee on Drugs 2001; Yonkers et al. 2004).

Although valproic acid and carbamazepine appear to be safe for breastfeeding babies, infants should be monitored for possible hepatic complications. Maternal and infant serum drug levels and liver function should be monitored every 2–4 weeks, or more frequently as indicated by the clinical situation (Misri and Lusskin 2004e).

Valproic Acid (Depakote, Depakene)

To date, only one published report has described adverse effects in an infant exposed to valproic acid through breastfeeding (Stahl et al. 1997). A 3-month-old infant developed thrombocytopenia and anemia while the mother was being treated with valproic acid monotherapy. The authors conducted an extensive investigation as to other possible causes, but none were

discovered. The abnormalities resolved 12 to 35 days after breastfeeding was discontinued.

Carbamazepine (Tegretol)

The use of carbamazepine during breastfeeding has been associated with infant hepatic toxicity in two case reports (Frey et al. 1990; Merlob et al. 1992). However, the infants in both cases were exposed to carbamazepine both during pregnancy and through breast milk; therefore, it is unclear whether the adverse effects were the result of in utero or breast milk exposure.

Gabapentin (Neurontin)

No published cases of gabapentin exposure through breast milk yet exist. One unpublished report from the drug manufacturer analyzed blood, urine, and milk samples from six women treated with 400 mg of gabapentin (Chaudron and Jefferson 2000). Plasma concentrations were approximately equal to breast milk concentrations in five of the six. The sixth woman was unable to produce milk.

Lamotrigine (Lamictal)

Lamotrigine is excreted in considerable quantities into human breast milk (Oana 1998; Ohman et al. 2000; Rambeck et al. 1997; Tomson et al. 1997). Infant serum levels average about one-third of maternal levels. This series of case reports reported no adverse events in breastfeeding infants exposed to lamotrigine. However, children who were directly treated with this medication have developed life-threatening rashes (Guberman et al. 1999), so clinicians should remain concerned about infants who are exposed to this medication indirectly through breastfeeding and should monitor them closely for side effects.

Topiramate (Topamax)

Topiramate levels in three mother-infant pairs were looked at during pregnancy and in the postpartum period. Infant levels were found to be 10%–20% of maternal levels, and there were no adverse effects observed in the infants (Ohman et al. 2002).

Appendix 7–B

A Primer on Using Lithium in Pregnancy and Lactation: Why? When? How?

Of the mood stabilizers, by far the most clinical experience is with lithium, which freely crosses the placenta, equilibrating between maternal and cord serum. The Register of Lithium Babies project (Schou and Weinstein 1980; Schou et al. 1973) in the 1970s pooled information about 225 babies who had been exposed to lithium in utero and implicated first-trimester lithium in causing the rare Ebstein's anomaly, which occurs in the general population at a rate of 1 in 20,000 births (0.005%). It affects the cardiovascular system, which is formed during the 3rd through 9th week after conception (corresponding to the 5th through the 11th week of pregnancy).

Thirty years after the initial warnings and many publications later, the high incidence for Ebstein's anomaly associated with lithium has been revised downward from the original 3/100 births (3%) to 1/1,000 births (0.01%) (Altshuler et al. 1996; American Academy of Pediatrics Committee on Drugs 2000; Cohen and Rosenbaum 1998; Iqbal et al. 2001; Warner 2000).

■ EBSTEIN'S ANOMALY

Ebstein's anomaly is characterized by deformity of the tricuspid valve, resulting in variable degrees of tricuspid regurgitation. Atrial septal defect is the most common associated anomaly. The portion of the right ventricle proximal to the tricuspid leaflets is atrialized (thinned), and if the remaining right ventricle is small in size, pump function may be inadequate (Tede and Foster 2003). Cyanosis results from right-to-left shunting across an atrial septal defect or patent foramen ovale in the presence of significant tricuspid regurgitation or elevated right atrial pressures. Although the clinical features are variable, patients experience pro-

gressive cyanosis from right-to-left atrial shunting, symptoms due to tricuspid regurgitation and right ventricular dysfunction, and/or paroxysmal atrial tachyarrhythmias (Celermajer et al. 1994). Without surgical intervention, the patient's chance of surviving to age 50 is about 50%, with survival dependent on the degree of the anatomical and physiological abnormalities (Tede and Foster 2003). Surgical interventions include tricuspid annuloplasty, tricuspid valve reconstruction with creation of a monocuspid valve, and tricuspid valve replacement (Mee and Drummond-Webb 2001).

Comment: Although the risk of Ebstein's anomaly in a lithium-exposed infant is 20 times that in the general population, the chances remain minute in comparison to the mother's odds of a recurrence—almost a sure bet for many patients who discontinue medication.

■ LITHIUM MANAGEMENT DURING PREGNANCY

Pregnancy unbalances previously stable lithium regimens, because of the physiological shifts that occur as the pregnancy progresses. The goals of lithium management are to achieve optimal efficacy at the lowest possible concentration, to avoid episodes of lithium toxicity, and to minimize rapid fluctuations in lithium levels. Management should include the following:

- *Test baseline serum electrolytes, thyroid function, and renal function.* Monitor thyroid-stimulating hormone every 3–6 months during pregnancy because secondary maternal hypothyroidism is a common complication of lithium treatment (Misri and Lusskin 2004d).

Table 7–5.   Lithium dose adjustments in the third trimester and in preeclampsia

Clinical situation	Effect of pregnancy on GFR	Lithium dose adjustment	Comment
Trimester 3			
Early	↑	↑	Dose adjustment maintains steady serum levels.
Late	↓	↓ by 30%–50%	Dose adjustment avoids maternal and neonatal toxicity as maternal GFR and volume of distribution decline. Note prolonged Li$^+$ half-life in neonates (68–96 hours).
Preeclampsia	↓	↓	Sodium-restricted diet promotes salt (Na$^+$, Li$^+$) retention, predisposing to lithium toxicity. Lowered lithium dose decreases the risk of toxicity.

Note.   GFR=glomerular filtration rate.

- *Check serum electrolytes and lithium levels during titration.* Once stable, serum lithium levels, electrolytes, and renal function should be monitored monthly early in pregnancy and weekly in the third trimester, as glomerular filtration rate (GFR) declines (see Table 7–5). Therapeutic lithium levels range from 0.6 to 1.1 mEq/L, with levels of 0.8 or above offering greater protection against relapse. Try to protect the mother against rapid changes in serum lithium level (Perlis et al. 2002).
- *Monitor for nephrogenic diabetes insipidus (NDI).* Polyuria and nocturia are relatively sensitive indicators of renal concentrating capacity for patients taking lithium. However, these symptoms lose much of their discriminatory value because they occur so frequently in pregnancy anyway. As discussed in Chapter 4, "The Patient With Kidney Disease," lithium-induced polyuria is a frequent, reversible side effect that can occur at any time during lithium administration. It occurs as a consequence of the collecting tubules' diminished sensitivity to antidiuretic hormone (ADH), interfering with the production of concentrated urine. When lithium accumulates in collecting tubule cells, blocking ADH, it causes NDI, with true polyuria (24-hour urine volume >3,000 mL). This effect is usually temporary, but is irreversible in 5%–10% of patients. Although this is a rare complication, lithium is the most common cause of NDI. If there is the suspicion of NDI, it is reasonable to assess 24-hour urine volume and consult with a nephrologist.
- *Obtain fetal cardiac ultrasound at weeks 16–20* for patients who have been exposed to lithium prior to week 12 of pregnancy.
- *Adjust lithium dose in the third trimester* and/or in the setting of preeclampsia, to compensate for changes in renal function (see Table 7–5).

- *Closely monitor serum lithium concentrations in the last week of pregnancy* to minimize the risk of maternal and neonatal toxicity. Use intravenous hydration during labor and delivery whenever possible. The lithium dose may be reduced by 30%–50% shortly before delivery in anticipation of the rapid decline in volume of distribution and GFR at delivery.

■ BREASTFEEDING: RISKS AND BENEFITS

Breast milk concentrations are approximately half of the maternal serum concentrations (Fries 1970; Schou and Amdisen 1973; Skausig and Schou 1977; Sykes et al. 1976; Tunnessen and Hertz 1972; Weinstein and Goldfield 1969). Lithium concentrations in the sera of infants are approximately equal to or slightly less than that in breast milk but can range from 5% to 200% of the maternal serum concentrations. Lithium is considered contraindicated in breastfeeding by the American Academy of Pediatrics because of the risk of toxicity in the infant (Briggs et al. 2002).

■ LITHIUM TOXICITY AND MANAGEMENT IN NEWBORNS

- The serum half-life of lithium in newborns is prolonged, averaging 68–96 hours, as compared with the adult's 10–20 hours (Briggs et al. 2002).
- Because the kidneys are immature, the newborn is at risk for high serum levels and for lithium toxicity, even if the mother's serum lithium level was within the therapeutic range.
- Lithium toxicity in babies differs from the clinical picture seen in adults. Symptoms include lethargy

and "floppy infant" syndrome, which is characterized by respiratory difficulties, cyanosis, and hypotonicity (Altshuler et al. 1996; Viguera et al. 2002).

- The infant's lithium level should be monitored closely, although the symptoms of lithium toxicity are usually mild and are self-limiting, disappearing as lithium is eliminated by the newborn (Briggs et al. 2002).

- There are no known long-term neurobehavioral sequelae of neonatal lithium toxicity (American Academy of Pediatrics Committee on Drugs 2000; Iqbal et al. 2001; Pinelli et al. 2002; Viguera et al. 2002).

- Exposure to lithium during the second and third trimesters can also cause fetal thyroid goiter (American Academy of Pediatrics Committee on Drugs 2000; Iqbal et al. 2001).

Chapter

8

The Patient Using Steroids

Antoinette Ambrosino Wyszynski, M.D.
Van Yu, M.D.

Corticosteroids behave like neuropsychiatric wild cards, inducing a spectrum of states as varied as mood disorders, psychotic states, and dementia-like syndromes. They make the detective work of figuring out changes in mental status quite challenging as they stage unpredictable, hit-and-run assaults on mood, cognition, and perception.

It is often tempting to blame steroids for mental status changes, but the odds are that some other etiology is causing the mental status change. A weighted incidence of only 5.7% has been calculated for steroid psychosis (Lewis and Smith 1983). Moreover, corticosteroids are given to patients who may have other causes for mental status derangements, such as CNS lupus, HIV infection, chronic obstructive pulmonary disorder, or brain trauma.

Nonetheless, the unpredictability of steroid-induced neuropsychiatric side effects raises the temptation to blame them automatically. It is better clinical practice to consider the differential diagnosis of mental status changes discussed in Chapter 1 (see also Appendix 4 in this volume, "'VINDICTIVE MADS': Differential Diagnosis of Mental Status Changes.") Note that individuals who experience mental status changes while taking steroids may withhold this in-

formation from their physicians out of embarrassment or fear of being labeled "insane."

Unfortunately, the literature can be as confusing to track as the medications themselves. In this chapter, we will present selected highlights of relevance to clinical practice, focusing on steroid psychosis. The reader should consult the critical review of extant studies from 1950 to 2002 by Sirois (2003).

■ PHENOMENOLOGY OF CORTICOSTEROID-RELATED PSYCHIATRIC SYNDROMES

Our discussion will cover the most psychiatrically relevant steroid-induced reactions. These are usually accompanied by psychosis, typically in the setting of mania.

The *initial response* to corticosteroids is often a sense of well-being, mild euphoria, and improved appetite, which may be misleading in determining etiology retrospectively. Severe steroid-related psychiatric syndromes are relatively rare. The majority of mental changes are mild to moderate and *do not* herald the development of a full-blown psychosis or affective syndrome.

Wyszynski AA, Wyszynski B (eds.): *Manual of Psychiatric Care for the Medically Ill.* Washington, D.C., American Psychiatric Publishing, Inc., 2005

When more severe reactions occur, their onset is unpredictable, and symptoms can shift radically during the course of illness. There is no consistent, predictable presentation of steroid-induced psychiatric syndromes, even in a particular patient (e.g., the patient who presents with depression at one point may present with mania in the future). Many different types of reactions occur, such as steroid-induced obsessive-compulsive behavior and panic attacks. With this in mind, however, some general statements about steroid-induced phenomenology may guide the evaluation.

Most patients should recover fully without residua from steroid psychosis and improve within 2 to 6 weeks (Hall et al. 1979; Lewis and Smith 1983). Persistence of psychiatric symptoms for weeks or months after steroid exposure strongly suggests either another medical etiology (e.g., lupus) or a primary psychiatric syndrome.

■ CLINICAL PROFILE OF CORTICOSTEROID-INDUCED PSYCHIATRIC REACTIONS

Two clinical profiles emerged when 130 cases appearing in the 1974–2001 literature were analyzed (Sirois 2003): an affective profile (75% of cases) and a "toxic-organic" profile (25% of cases). Four types of presentations were described:

1. Steroid-induced affective states, including mania, depression, and mixed states (mania and depression). They were complicated by hallucinations in about half the cases. Mania was more common than depression. *Prodrome:* insomnia and distractibility, often preceding the more obvious mood disturbances by up to 72–96 hours (Shapiro 1993). *Complications:* suicidal or homicidal ideation.
2. Steroid-induced delirium-like presentation, with or without psychotic features. *Prodrome:* confusion, perplexity, and agitation. *Precipitants:* steroid introduction, titration, or withdrawal.
3. Steroid-related cognitive impairment ("steroid dementia"). Decreased attention, concentration, and retention, and slowed mental speed. *Course:* usually reversible, but deficits may last many months, with slow recovery. Steroid-induced etiology is not necessarily flagged by psychosis. *Risk factors:* unclear; may occur with short or long-term exposure, large or small steroid doses. *Clinical relevance:* Subtle cognitive changes may have an impact on the

patient's ability to work responsibly, keep appointments, manage finances, and so forth. Family should be aware of this potential side effect.
4. Steroid withdrawal phenomena: The usual treatment for steroid-associated psychiatric disturbances is to reduce or discontinue the steroids when possible. However, this strategy may paradoxically induce mental disturbances. Steroid withdrawal symptoms are diverse, including depression, mania, depersonalization, fatigue, and delirium. *Diagnostic problems:* The possible exacerbation of the underlying medical illness makes it difficult to distinguish between steroid-induced and steroid-withdrawal mental status disruptions; for example, a decrease in steroid doses may cause a flare of lupus cerebritis with mental status changes.

■ RISK FACTORS FOR STEROID-INDUCED PSYCHOSIS

Psychotic states are the only steroid-related psychiatric syndromes for which enough data are available to permit abstracting risk factors. As shown in Table 8–1, rising steroid dose (especially above 60 mg prednisone or its equivalent) is consistently associated with vulnerability to steroid-induced psychiatric symptoms. Steroid-induced psychiatric symptoms can occur at any time during the course of steroid treatment, although they tend to cluster within the first 2 weeks of steroid exposure (Stiefel et al. 1989). The duration (chronicity) of steroid exposure does not reliably predict the onset, duration, severity, or type of psychiatric sequelae. No single synthetic steroid preparation (e.g., cortisone, dexamethasone, prednisone) appears more likely than any other to cause symptoms.

Prior Psychiatric History

Psychiatrists often screen patients with psychiatric histories before elective procedures requiring corticosteroids, such as transplantation. The assumption is that patients with such histories will be more vulnerable to mental status derangements. Although no controlled data are available, the incidence of steroid-induced psychiatric problems surprisingly does not differ in patients with and without histories of previous psychiatric illness.

Prior Steroid History

An even more unexpected finding is that previous steroid-induced psychiatric complications do not predis-

Table 8–1. Risk factors for steroid-induced psychosis

Potential factor	Effect on steroid-induced syndromes
Dose	>60 mg prednisone or its equivalent increases risk
Onset	Usually within 2 weeks of exposure, but may occur at any time
Duration of steroid treatment (exposure duration)	Not predictive
Type of steroid preparation	Not predictive
Prior steroid exposure	Not predictive
History of psychiatric illness	Not predictive

pose a patient to subsequent episodes (Kershner and Wang-Cheng 1989). The downside is that patients without previous problems may develop steroid-induced psychiatric side effects in the future (Stiefel et al. 1989).

■ TREATMENT OF STEROID-INDUCED PSYCHIATRIC REACTIONS

As with any medication side effect, the first step for steroid-induced psychiatric reactions is to discontinue or taper the steroid. However, this strategy has pitfalls: 1) the patient may be vulnerable to steroid-withdrawal psychiatric symptoms; 2) steroid discontinuation may exacerbate an underlying medical condition that produced mental status changes, such as CNS lupus; and 3) steroid treatment may be the only viable treatment option. Fortunately, other strategies may be helpful when steroids cannot be discontinued.

Antidepressants

There is little to guide the clinician except anecdotal case reports. Most of the literature predates the introduction of selective serotonin reuptake inhibitors (SSRIs) and focuses on tricyclic antidepressants (TCAs). TCAs are ineffective for steroid-induced depression and may even exacerbate corticosteroid-induced psychosis. The reason for this effect is unclear, but it might be due to exacerbation of steroid-induced symptoms by TCAs' anticholinergic properties. One study reported the successful treatment of steroid-withdrawal depression with fluoxetine (Prozac) in a patient with Sjögren's syndrome (Wyszynski and Wyszynski 1993). Another series of four patients who developed major depression on withdrawal of anabolic steroids also responded to fluoxetine (Malone and Dimeff 1992).

- *Bottom line:* SSRIs are a reasonable choice for the first-line treatment of steroid-induced depression, despite the scarcity of clinical reports.

Antipsychotics

Antipsychotics improve and shorten the duration of steroid-induced psychotic syndromes. Various neuroleptics have been described in this context, including thioridazine (Mellaril), chlorpromazine (Thorazine), and haloperidol (Haldol) (Bloch et al. 1994; Shapiro 1993). In the classic study by Hall et al. (1979), phenothiazines (chlorpromazine or thioridazine) produced an excellent response in all 14 patients. Phenothiazines are not optimal because their side effect profile (adverse cardiovascular side effects, particularly for thioridazine; anticholinergic effects) makes them poorly tolerated in medically ill patients. Haloperidol remains the most widely studied neuroleptic because of its efficacy, low anticholinergicity, minimal cardiovascular side effects, and flexibility of administration (oral, intramuscular, or intravenous).

There is a growing literature on using the atypical antipsychotic olanzapine (Zyprexa) for treating steroid-induced psychosis accompanied by features of mania (Brown et al. 1999; Budur and Pozuelo 2003; Goldman and Goveas 2002). Risperidone (Risperdal) also has been reported to be effective (Dasilva et al. 2002; Kramer and Cottingham 1999). However, hyperglycemia leading to ketoacidosis is a potential adverse side effect of olanzapine, and thus glucose levels must be monitored carefully (see also p. 62 in Chapter 3, "The Patient With Cardiovascular Disease").

An informed general strategy may be to apply the principles of managing delirium to these patients, as discussed in Chapter 1 of this volume, "The Delirious Patient."

Mood Stabilizers

Mood stabilizers are helpful in treating steroid-induced affective disorders, with or without accompanying psychotic symptoms. Lithium has been useful for the treatment of steroid-induced mania and depression (Terao et al. 1997). It has been reportedly used as "prophylaxis" against steroid-induced psychosis (Falk et al. 1979; Goggans et al. 1983; Terao et al. 1994). However, steroid-induced vulnerability is unpredictable, so it is difficult to define *prophylaxis* and therefore judge the efficacy of preventive measures.

Because corticosteroids are used to treat diseases that are also complicated by renal dysfunction, such as lupus nephritis, the use of lithium requires careful monitoring or may be contraindicated. Alternative mood stabilizers are reportedly effective and include carbamazepine (Tegretol) (Wada et al. 2001) and valproic acid (Depakote, Depakene) (Abbas and Styra 1994; Kahn et al. 1988; Kline and Jaggers 1999). Note that carbamazepine may decrease serum concentrations of prednisone.

Anxiolytics

Minor episodes of anxiety associated with steroid use are likely to go unreported. Anxiety, emotional lability, and restlessness simulate adjustment disorders; the clinician may miss the medication-induced etiology. Stiefel and colleagues (1989) suggested that the sudden onset of such symptoms during steroid treatment is highly suggestive of a steroid-related etiology. If the symptoms interfere with the patient's quality of life, benzodiazepines may bring symptomatic relief. Lorazepam (Ativan) and oxazepam (Serax) have intermediate half-lives and no active metabolites. They are less likely to produce cumulative CNS or respiratory toxicity, and they are relatively unaffected by parenchymal liver disease because they bypass Phase I oxidation in the liver to directly undergo glucuronidation (Cozza et al. 2003).

Electroconvulsive Therapy

ECT has been effective for severe steroid-induced depression (Allen and Pitts 1978; Douglas and Schwartz 1982; Sutor et al. 1996) and catatonia (Doherty et al. 1991).

Alternate-Day Corticosteroids

Giving corticosteroids on alternate days instead of every day, in an attempt to reduce the incidence of steroid-induced psychiatric complications, appears to be unsuccessful. Joffe and colleagues (1988a, 1988b) assessed mood and cognition on consecutive days in 18 women with systemic lupus erythematosus (SLE) on alternate-day steroid therapy. They demonstrated that substantial alterations in mood, particularly depression and anxiety, occurred between the day-on and the day-off medication in a subgroup of these patients with SLE. Although overall mean scores for the mood and cognitive tests did not differ significantly between on-medication and off-medication days, 10 of the 18 patients had substantial changes in their levels of depression or anxiety. The direction of these alterations was not predictable—some improved on drug-free days, whereas others worsened. These data seem to be consistent with a study of three patients who showed mood cycling when taking 50–60 mg of alternate-day prednisone (Sharfstein et al. 1982). Joffe's patients, however, took a mean alternating daily dose of only 13.9 mg of prednisone, suggesting that even low-dose alternate-day corticosteroids may induce psychiatric morbidity (Joffe et al. 1988a, 1988b).

■ ANABOLIC-ANDROGENIC STEROIDS

Anabolic-androgenic steroids (AAS) are synthetically derived from testosterone. These compounds bind to androgen receptors and have a dual anabolic and androgenic (masculinizing) effect. AAS are medically indicated to treat androgen deficiency syndromes and AIDS-associated wasting (Hengge et al. 2003). An exhaustive review by Brower (2002) showed no cases of abuse or dependence for patients who received therapeutic doses of AAS for medical indications.

However, AAS have also become abused drugs, used to enhance athletic performance and improve appearance by adding muscle bulk in men and women (Gruber and Pope 2000). AAS abusers are more likely also to abuse other drugs and alcohol than nonusers (Irving et al. 2002), a finding confirmed in an animal model (Johansson et al. 2000; Wichstrom and Pedersen 2001). AAS abuse may serve as a "gateway" leading to opioid abuse, as well as causing its own morbidity (Kanayama et al. 2003).

Addition of other drugs to AAS may 1) enhance desired effects (e.g., amphetamines and levothyroxine increase endurance and burn fat); 2) minimize unpleasant side effects (e.g., diuretics counteract AAS-induced edema; opioids, often supplied by dealers of AAS, reduce pain from workouts and injuries); and/or 3) obscure urine detection (e.g., probenecid decreases renal excretion of AAS). These strategies produce myriad adverse medical side effects, such as cardiotoxicity when AAS are combined with amphetamines. Several of the combination drugs, such as androstenedione (the immediate precursor of testosterone), creatine, dehydroepiandrosterone (DHEA), and ephedrine, are available over the counter.

Psychiatric Side Effects

Anabolic-androgenic steroids produce psychiatric effects (mainly mood disorders) both when administered and when withdrawn. The psychiatric effects of AAS span the spectrum. AAS have been used in controlled settings to treat depression (Pope et al. 2003; Yates 2000) but have been associated with mania, depression, psychosis, suicide, and aggression leading to violence and homicide (Bahrke 2000; Midgley et al. 2001; Pope et al. 2000; Thiblin et al. 2000). AAS are ingested both by prescription and in over-the-counter supplements, such as DHEA.

In athletes, AAS are termed *ergogenic* or performance-enhancing drugs, but they may perpetuate mood and body-image problems. A form of body dysmorphic disorder (*muscle dysmorphia*) and a form of eating disturbance (*eating disorder, bodybuilder type*) have been described among AAS abusers (Gruber and Pope 2000; Olivardia et al. 2000). Patients with muscle dysmorphia are chronically dissatisfied and preoccu-

pied with the perception that their musculature is too small. The syndrome was originally termed *reverse anorexia nervosa*. Table 8–2 lists characteristic mental status and physical findings for individuals taking AAS.

Incidence

It has been difficult to determine the incidence of AAS-associated psychiatric disorders because of sampling bias occurring with clinical case reports and convenience samples of AAS users (Brower 2002). A review of four prospective, placebo-controlled trials estimated that manic or hypomanic reactions occur in at least 5% of AAS users and concluded that the effects are dose related (Pope and Brower 2000). Prospective studies have been limited by the ethical constraint on replicating the nonmedical uses of AAS, which would require administering high doses of AAS combined with other drugs. The rates of AAS-induced psychiatric disorders are probably higher than the conserva-

Table 8–2. Physical and mental status findings of patients taking anabolic-androgenic steroids (AAS)

Appearance	Musculature markedly enlarged; neck, shoulders, and chest disproportionately developed. Oversized clothing is often worn, particularly in setting of muscle dysmorphia. Other: facial acne, male pattern baldness, hirsutism, possible needle marks in large muscles.
Behavior	Psychomotor disturbances consistent with manic or depressive states
Attitude	Possibly competitive and aggressive (AAS-induced or characterological)
Speech	Usually normal, although women may have deepened voice
Mood and affect	Variable; range includes irritability, mania or hypomania with elevated mood, dysphoria or depression, anxiety
Thought content	Suicidal, homicidal, or paranoid ideation. Grandiose or persecutory thoughts may progress to delusions. Hallucinations uncommon.
Physical exam	
Men	Gynecomastia, testicular atrophy, and prostatic hypertrophy
Women	Breast tissue atrophy, clitoral hypertrophy
Both	Edema in the extremities due to water retention; possible hepatomegaly and jaundice
Laboratory abnormalities	
ECG	Left ventricular hypertrophy
CBC	Increased RBC, hemoglobin, hematocrit
Liver function tests	Increased ALT, AST, LDH, GGT, and total bilirubin
Urine testing	+/− for AAS or other drugs of abuse
Hormonal levels	Increased testosterone and estradiol (with use of testosterone esters) Decreased testosterone (without use of testosterone esters or during withdrawal) Decreased LH and FSH

Note. ALT=alanine transaminase (formerly SGPT); AST=aspartate transaminase (formerly SGOT); CBC=complete blood count; ECG=electrocardiogram; FSH=follicle-stimulating hormone; GGT=γ-glutamyltransferase; LDH=lactate dehydrogenase; LH=luteinizing hormone; RBC=red blood cells.
Source. Adapted from Brower 2002.

tive estimate of 5%. Even healthy volunteers without prior psychiatric histories develop psychiatric effects following high doses of AAS (Daly et al. 2001, 2003). Vulnerability to psychiatric effects in the AAS-abusing population is increased by prior psychiatric history, comorbid medical conditions, and concurrent drug or alcohol use.

Treatment of Psychiatric Side Effects

No controlled trials of treatment are available for either AAS abuse or AAS dependence. Brower (2000, 2002) noted the following points about treatment of AAS abusers:

1. *Goal:* Abstinence from AAS and other drugs.
2. *Challenges:* Patients often have focused on physical appearance and attractiveness, physical fitness, and success (Kanayama et al. 2001). Physical attributes are a way that AAS users define themselves and compete successfully in a world perceived as populated with winners or losers. Patients must mourn the loss of idealized physical attributes in order to remain abstinent. AAS withdrawal symptoms are typically depressive, which may complicate management. Maintenance of abstinence involves ongoing support and identification of relapse triggers (e.g., *internal triggers:* thinking that one is not big enough, feeling inadequate socially or during workouts, and perceiving one's body as too small; *external triggers:* people or locations associated with using AAS, such as a particular gym).
3. *Techniques:* Supportive psychotherapy is crucial. One approach is for the therapist to use the approach of a coach or teammate—someone on the same side as the patient, knowledgeable about his or her culture and motivations. This technique helps defuse the competitive, aggressive traits that have been advantageous to the patient in other settings but that can undermine treatment. Motivational interviewing techniques may be helpful for AAS users who are treatment averse (Brower and Rootenberg 1999).
4. *Psychopharmacology:* SSRIs are effective for AAS-withdrawal dysphoria and depression. AAS users are at risk for suicide, cardiotoxicity, and prostatic hypertrophy. The SSRIs' low potential for lethal overdose, few adverse cardiac effects, and lack of anticholinergic effects (such as urinary retention) are advantages. SSRIs also may be helpful in treating body dysmorphic disorder (Phillips et al. 2002).

Antipsychotic drugs may be helpful for marked irritability, aggressiveness, or agitation that continues into the withdrawal phase.

■ REFERENCES

Abbas A, Styra R: Valproate prophylaxis against steroid-induced psychosis (letter). Can J Psychiatry 39:188–189, 1994

Allen R, Pitts F: ECT for depressed patients with lupus erythematosus. Am J Psychiatry 135:367–368, 1978

Bahrke M: Psychological effects of endogenous testosterone and anabolic-androgenic steroids, in Anabolic Steroids in Sport and Exercise, 2nd Edition. Edited by Yesalis C. Champaign, IL, Human Kinetics, 2000, pp 247–278

Bloch M, Gur E, Shalev A: Chlorpromazine prophylaxis of steroid-induced psychosis. Gen Hosp Psychiatry 16:42–44, 1994

Brower KJ: Assessment and treatment of anabolic steroid abuse, dependence, and withdrawal, in Anabolic Steroids in Sport and Exercise, 2nd Edition. Edited by Yesalis CE. Champaign, IL, Human Kinetics, 2000, pp 305–332

Brower KJ: Anabolic steroid abuse and dependence. Curr Psychiatry Rep 4:377–387, 2002

Brower KJ, Rootenberg JH: Counseling for substance abuse problems, in Counseling in Sports Medicine. Edited by Ray R, Wiese-Bjornstal DM. Champaign, IL, Human Kinetics, 1999, pp 179–204

Brown E, Khan D, Suppes T: Treatment of corticosteroid-induced mood changes with olanzapine (letter). Am J Psychiatry 156:968, 1999

Budur K, Pozuelo L: Olanzapine for corticosteroid-induced mood disorders (letter). Psychosomatics 44:353, 2003

Cozza KL, Armstrong SC, Oesterheld JR: Concise Guide to Drug Interaction Principles for Medical Practice: Cytochrome P450s, UGTs, P-Glycoproteins, 2nd Edition. Washington, DC, American Psychiatric Publishing, 2003

Daly RC, Su TP, Schmidt PJ, et al: Cerebrospinal fluid and behavioral changes after methyltestosterone administration: preliminary findings. Arch Gen Psychiatry 58:172–177, 2001

Daly RC, Su TP, Schmidt PJ, et al: Neuroendocrine and behavioral effects of high-dose anabolic steroid administration in male normal volunteers. Psychoneuroendocrinology 28:317–331, 2003

Dasilva C, Murse M, Vokey K: Steroid induced psychosis treated with risperidone. Can J Psychiatry 47:388–389, 2002

Doherty M, Garstin I, McClellan R: A steroid stupor in a surgical ward. Br J Psychiatry 158:125–127, 1991

Douglas C, Schwartz H: ECT for depression caused by lupus cerebritis: a case report. Am J Psychiatry 139:1631–1632, 1982

Falk W, Mahnke M, Poskanzer D: Lithium prophylaxis of corticotropin-induced psychosis. JAMA 241:1011–1012, 1979

Goggans F, Weisberg L, Koran L: Lithium prophylaxis of prednisone psychosis: a case report. J Clin Psychiatry 44:111–112, 1983

Goldman L, Goveas J: Olanzapine treatment of corticosteroid-induced mood disorders. Psychosomatics 43:495–497, 2002

Gruber AJ, Pope HG Jr: Psychiatric and medical effects of anabolic-androgenic steroid use in women. Psychother Psychosom 69:19–26, 2000

Hall R, Popkin M, Stickney S, et al: Presentation of the steroid psychoses. J Nerv Ment Dis 167:229–236, 1979

Hengge UR, Stocks K, Wiehler H, et al: Double-blind, randomized, placebo-controlled phase III trial of oxymetholone for the treatment of HIV wasting. AIDS 17:699–710, 2003

Irving L, Wall M, Neumark-Sztainer D, et al: Steroid use among adolescents: findings from Project EAT. J Adolesc Health 30:243–252, 2002

Joffe RT, Denicoff KD, Rubinow DR, et al: Mood effects of alternate-day corticosteroid therapy in patients with systemic lupus erythematosus. Gen Hosp Psychiatry 10:56–60, 1988a

Joffe RT, Wolkowitz OM, Rubinow DR, et al: Alternate-day corticosteroid treatment, mood and plasma HVA in patients with systemic lupus erythematosus. Neuropsychobiology 19:17–19, 1988b

Johansson P, Lindqvist A, Nyberg F, et al: Anabolic androgenic steroids affects alcohol intake, defensive behaviors and brain opioid peptides in the rat. Pharmacol Biochem Behav 67:271–279, 2000

Kahn D, Stevenson E, Douglas C: Effect of sodium valproate in three patients with organic brain syndromes. Am J Psychiatry 145:1010–1011, 1988

Kanayama G, Pope HG Jr, Hudson JI: "Body image" drugs: a growing psychosomatic problem. Psychother Psychosom 70:61–65, 2001

Kanayama G, Cohane GH, Weiss RD, et al: Past anabolic-androgenic steroid use among men admitted for substance abuse treatment: an underrecognized problem? J Clin Psychiatry 64:156–160, 2003

Kershner P, Wang-Cheng R: Psychiatric side effects of steroid therapy. Psychosomatics 30:135–139, 1989

Kline M, Jaggers E: Mania onset while using dehydroepiandrosterone (letter). Am J Psychiatry 156:971, 1999

Kramer J, Cottingham E: Risperidone in the treatment of steroid-induced psychosis (letter). J Child Adolesc Psychopharmacol 9:315–316, 1999

Lewis D, Smith R: Steroid-induced psychiatric syndromes. J Affect Disord 5:319–332, 1983

Malone DJ, Dimeff R: The use of fluoxetine in depression associated with anabolic steroid withdrawal: a case series. J Clin Psychiatry 53:130–132, 1992

Midgley S, Heather N, Davies J: Levels of aggression among a group of anabolic-androgenic steroid users. Med Sci Law 41:309–314, 2001

Olivardia R, Pope HG Jr, Hudson JI: Muscle dysmorphia in male weightlifters: a case-control study. Am J Psychiatry 157:1291–1296, 2000

Phillips K, Albertini R, Rasmussen S: A randomized placebo-controlled trial of fluoxetine in body dysmorphic disorder. Arch Gen Psychiatry 59:381–388, 2002

Pope HG Jr, Brower K: Anabolic-androgenic steroid abuse, in Comprehensive Textbook of Psychiatry, 7th Edition. Edited by Sadock B, Sadock V. Philadelphia, PA, Lippincott Williams & Wilkins, 2000, pp 1085–1095

Pope HG Jr, Kouri E, Hudson J: Effects of supraphysiologic doses of testosterone on mood and aggression in normal men: a randomized controlled trial. Arch Gen Psychiatry 57:133–140, 2000

Pope HG Jr, Cohane GH, Kanayama G, et al: Testosterone gel supplementation for men with refractory depression: a randomized, placebo-controlled trial. Am J Psychiatry 160:105–111, 2003

Shapiro H: Psychopathology in the lupus patient, in Dubois' Lupus Erythematosus, 4th Edition. Edited by Wallace DJ, Hahn BH. Philadelphia, PA, Lea & Febiger, 1993, pp 386–402

Sharfstein S, Sack D, Fauci A: Relationship between alternate-day corticosteroid therapy and behavioral abnormalities. JAMA 248:2987–2989, 1982

Sirois F: Steroid psychosis: a review. Gen Hosp Psychiatry 25:27–33, 2003

Stiefel F, Breitbart W, Holland J: Corticosteroids in cancer: neuropsychiatric complications. Cancer Invest 7:479–491, 1989

Sutor B, Wells L, Rummans T: Steroid-induced depressive psychosis responsive to electroconvulsive therapy. Convuls Ther 12:104–107, 1996

Terao T, Mizuki T, Ohji T, et al: Antidepressant effect of lithium in patients with systemic lupus erythematosus and cerebral infarction, treated with corticosteroid. Br J Psychiatry 164:109–110, 1994

Terao T, Yoshimura R, Shiratuchi T, et al: Effects of lithium on steroid-induced depression. Biol Psychiatry 41:1225–1226, 1997

Thiblin I, Lindquist O, Rajs J: Cause and manner of death among users of anabolic androgenic steroids. J Forensic Sci 45:16–23, 2000

Wada K, Yamada N, Yamauchi, Y, et al: Carbamazepine treatment of corticosteroid-induced mood disorder. J Affect Disord 65:315–317, 2001

Wichstrom L, Pedersen W: Use of anabolic-androgenic steroids in adolescence: winning, looking good or being bad? J Stud Alcohol 62:5–13, 2001

Wyszynski A, Wyszynski B: Treatment of depression with fluoxetine in corticosteroid-dependent central nervous system Sjögren's syndrome. Psychosomatics 34:173–176, 1993

Yates W: Testosterone in psychiatry: risks and benefits. Arch Gen Psychiatry 57:155–156, 2000

Chapter 9

The HIV-Infected Patient

Antoinette Ambrosino Wyszynski, M.D.
Bryan Bruno, M.D.
Patrick Ying, M.D.
Linda Chuang, M.D.
Miriam Friedlander, M.D.
Bruce Rubenstein, M.D.

The relevance of the human immunodeficiency virus (HIV) to clinical practice needs no introduction: this two-decade-old epidemic has affected nearly every country in the world, and the World Health Organization has corrected the "underreported" figure of 1.1 million to a more likely 4.5 million lives affected by the virus. No statistics, however, truly convey the suffering contained within these numbers.

Vulnerable populations. Since first reported in the early 1980s, the demographics of HIV have changed. Women are one of the fastest-growing infected populations, with new cases steadily increasing each year. In the United States, female cases of acquired immunodeficiency syndrome (AIDS) have now been reported in all 50 states and the District of Columbia. African American and Hispanic women are disproportionately affected, with rates 17 times and 6 times higher, respectively, than for Caucasian women (Centers for Disease Control and Prevention 1998). This is

a psychiatrically vulnerable population; low-income and minority women infected with HIV experience greater levels of depression, stress, and anxiety symptoms relative to community norms (Catz et al. 2002).

Women are more medically vulnerable to contract HIV for several reasons. First, male-to-female transmission—the leading risk exposure category for all women—is estimated to be eight times more likely than transmission from female to male. The presence of concurrent sexually transmitted diseases can increase the risk of new HIV infections by two- to fivefold. Second, *a significant vector of disease to women* is represented by the high-risk sexual behaviors among male injection drug users (Centers for Disease Control and Prevention 2002). About one-third of all HIV cases in women are accounted for by either injection drug use or sex with an injection drug user (Centers for Disease Control and Prevention 1998). Injection and noninjection drug use put women at increased risk for HIV infection and are strongly linked to unsafe sex.

Third, men who have sex with both men and women practice riskier sex with *female* than with male partners. For example, one study showed that only a minority engaged in unprotected anal sex with their male partners, *whereas a full two-thirds had unprotected vaginal sex with their female partners* (Ross et al. 1992). These asymmetrical findings reflect a perception of differential risk based on the partner's gender. Fourth, sexual abuse and sexual coercion place certain women at risk (e.g., sex workers) because they are more likely to abuse drugs and engage in high-risk sexual practices.

Substance users also continue to be a vulnerable group for HIV infection. Drugs and alcohol diminish inhibitions and interfere with judgment, adding to HIV risk-taking, such as unprotected sex, methamphetamine use, and needle sharing (Kalichman et al. 2002; Mandell et al. 1999; Semple 2002). It is important to take a careful history and not be misled by stereotypes of substance abusers; whereas heroin or crack cocaine use is well known to place its users at risk, "club drugs" like Ecstasy (MDMA) also disinhibit sexual behavior, heightening risk.

Chronically mentally ill individuals are also predisposed to HIV infection for a number of reasons: high rates of substance use disorders, misunderstandings about HIV transmission, high rates of sexually transmitted diseases, and frequent high-risk behaviors such as "survival sex" (in exchange for food, shelter, or money) (Cournos et al. 2001; McKinnon and Rosner 2000; McKinnon et al. 2001, 2002). Compared with the general population, people with severe mental illness are more likely to have sexual contact with multiple partners. The occurrence of psychosis predisposes people with schizophrenia to high-risk sexual behaviors. Severely mentally ill patients are also vulnerable to not adhering to medical care, causing exacerbations of the underlying condition to be more likely. Preexisting psychiatric disorders will often complicate the recognition of new neuropsychiatric problems, such as HIV-associated dementia complex (HADC), because it becomes difficult to tease apart the mental disorder from the mental status change (as discussed in the next section of this chapter).

Low self-esteem, anxiety, and depression additionally mediate high-risk behavior relative to HIV. For example, a lack of self-acceptance or self-condemnation about being gay (internalized homophobia) correlated with HIV-positive status in a study of men who have sex with men (Ross and Rosser 1996). In another sample, in a study that followed inner-city young people for several years, treatment of depression and anxiety was found to correlate more strongly with reductions

in HIV-related risk behaviors than was knowledge about HIV, access to information, counseling, or knowing someone with AIDS (Stiffman et al. 1995).

Personality variables such as emotional dysregulation, poor impulse control, and hostility have also been associated with high-risk behavior (Trobst 2002). Survivors of sexual or physical abuse sometimes place themselves at risk through behaviors such as sexual compulsivity, revictimization, substance abuse, and chronic depression (Goodman and Fallot 1998; Lenderking et al. 1997). Frequently, these individuals struggle with aspects of posttraumatic stress disorder (PTSD) such as hyperarousal, trauma intrusion phenomena, dissociative phenomena, somatization, and sexual dysfunction. For example, one study (of many) found a relationship between HIV risk behaviors and PTSD among women prisoners (Hutton et al. 2001). A history of emotional, physical, and sexual abuse or other trauma associated with active reexperiencing, hyperarousal, and avoidance increases the risk of engaging in unprotected sex (Bartholow et al. 1994), having difficulty negotiating condom use with partners (Miller 1999), and having higher rates of sexually transmitted diseases, including HIV (Petrak et al. 2000).

■ "PLEASE SEE THIS HIV-POSITIVE PATIENT FOR...": A HIERARCHICAL APPROACH TO THE INITIAL CONSULTATION

One difficulty with this type of HIV/AIDS print summary is that it is outdated as soon as it comes off the press. We have tried to assemble an overview that will remain usable over time, aiming to be pragmatic rather than comprehensive. Box 9–1 lists Internet resources recommended by the American Psychiatric Association Office of HIV Psychiatry. These sites will keep you updated with a quickly changing body of knowledge. Some offer multilingual patient fact sheets and Web materials. The American Psychiatric Association Practice Guideline for the Treatment of the Patients With HIV/AIDS may be found at http://www.psych.org/aids (accessed July 2004).

Central to the understanding of HIV is knowledge of combination antiretroviral therapy, known as highly active antiretroviral therapy (HAART). Since its widespread use in the United States began in 1995, the incidence of AIDS-defining conditions has declined. We quote from the 2003 indications for beginning HAART (Dybul 2002):

Box 9–1. **HIV Internet resources**	
Site	**Web address (accessed July 2004)**

SITES OF CLINICAL INTEREST

Site	Web address
American Psychiatric Association Practice Guideline for the Treatment of Patients With HIV/AIDS	http://www.psych.org/aids
AIDSinfo (combined HIV/AIDS Clinical Trials Information Service [ACTIS] and HIV/AIDS Treatment Information Service [ATIS])	http://www.aidsinfo.nih.gov [Extremely comprehensive site]
Bastyr University AIDS Research Center	http://www.bastyr.edu/research/buarc [Resource links, reports on alternative medicine, evaluation of naturopathic therapies]
CDC Guidelines for Pregnancy and HIV	http://www.cdc.gov/mmwr/preview/mmwrhtml/rr5019a2.htm
CDC Guidelines for Serologic Testing	http://www.cdc.gov/mmwr/preview/mmwrhtml/rr5019a1.htm
Center for AIDS Prevention Studies (CAPS)	http://www.caps.ucsf.edu [Population-specific prevention fact sheets (English, Spanish, French)]
Cytochrome P450 Drug Interaction Table	http://medicine.iupui.edu/flockhart and http://mhc.com/Cytochromes
Johns Hopkins AIDS Service	http://www.hopkins-aids.edu [Full-text online version of the reference book *Medical Management of HIV Disease*]
Medscape HIV/AIDS	http://www.hiv.medscape.com [search: HIV]
National Institute of Allergy and Infectious Diseases (NIAID)	http://www.niaid.nih.gov [Full-text publications on HIV/AIDS]
National Institute on Mental Health Office of AIDS Research	http://www.nimh.nih.gov/oa
Toronto General Hospital University Health Network	http://www.tthhivclinic.com [Medication fact sheets and drug interaction tables]

SITES OF PATIENT INTEREST

Site	Web address
AEGIS (AIDS Education Global Information System)	http://www.aegis.com
The Body	http://www.thebody.com
Critical Path AIDS Project	http://www.critpath.org
Fact Sheets for Patients (English, Spanish, French)	http://hivinsite.ucsf.edu/InSite.jsp?page=li-04-22
The New Mexico AIDS InfoNet	http://www.aidsinfonet.org
Gay Men's Health Crisis	http://www.gmhc.org
International Association of Physicians in AIDS Care	http://www.iapac.org
National Association of People With AIDS	http://www.napwa.org
National Minority AIDS Council	http://www.nmac.org
Project Inform	http://www.projinf.org
San Francisco AIDS Foundation	http://www.sfaf.org
UNAIDS	http://www.unaids.org

Treatment is usually offered to all patients with symptoms ascribed to HIV infection. For asymptomatic patients, the recommendation to treat is based on the readiness of the person to begin therapy; the degree of existing immunodeficiency as determined by the CD4+ T cell count (<350 CD4+ T cells/mm³); the risk for disease progression as determined by the CD4+ T cell count and level of plasma HIV RNA; the potential benefits and risks of initiating therapy in an asymptomatic person; and the likelihood, after counseling and education, of adherence to the prescribed treatment regimen. (p. 381)

Results of therapy are evaluated through plasma HIV RNA levels; these levels should show a logarithmic decrease in viral load at 2–8 weeks, with no detectable virus 4–6 months after treatment initiation. Several factors contribute to treatment failure at 4–6 months: nonadherence; inadequate potency of drugs; suboptimal levels of antiretroviral agents; and viral resistance (Dybul 2002). Patients who adhere carefully to the medication yet still experience treatment failure usually have their regimen changed, guided by the results of their first round and drug-resistance testing. However, the variety of antiretroviral regimens is still limited, and optimal alternatives are not always possible (see Table 9–1). Problems with adherence, toxicity, and resistance further complicate treatment planning, sometimes resulting in the recommendation that patients participate in a clinical trial or use a regimen that might not achieve complete viral suppression. The HIV/AIDS Treatment Information Service Web site (http://www.hivatis.org) provides the most up-to-date information on the current concepts of HIV management.

Comment: HAART has revolutionized the treatment of AIDS, but it has also presented new obstacles. Under the best of circumstances, treatment is psychologically harrowing for patients. There are many unwanted physical side effects, neuropsychiatric complications, and drug-drug interactions. Clinicians sometimes encounter seronegative patients (or seropositive individuals not yet treated) who present after an "unsafe" sexual encounter, panicked by questions about whether to "get HAART." A pragmatic psychiatric approach to these patients would involve reducing anxiety so that the patient pursues expert medical advice.

There is a hierarchy of differential diagnosis for a seropositive patient, regardless of psychiatric chief complaint. The sequence—particularly for hospitalized patients—is as follows: think delirium first, HIV-associated dementia complex second, medical differential diagnosis third, primary psychiatric etiology last. Rationale: *Delirium represents impending brain failure,* analogous in urgency to acute congestive heart failure or acute renal failure. *It is a medical emergency* that may initially present with psychiatric symptoms, such as mood disturbance or psychosis. HIV and AIDS patients are particularly at risk for delirium because

- HIV has a proclivity to attack the brain.
- Polypharmacy is required to mount a full-scale counterattack against HIV.
- AIDS patients are immunocompromised, so they are highly vulnerable to opportunistic infection, malignancies, and other medical complications.

There is another practical concern. HAART is intolerant of mistakes. Brief delays in initiating treatment, or small deviations from the regimen, generate drastic differences in outcome. It would be tragic for the clinician to cause a patient to lose antiretroviral therapeutic time by having assumed, for example,

Table 9–1. A partial list of antiretroviral medications

| | Reverse transcriptase inhibitors | | | |
Protease inhibitors	Nucleoside analogues		Nonnucleoside analogues	Nonnucleotide analogues
Amprenavir (Agenerase)	Abacavir (Ziagen; ABC)	Stavudine (d4T)	Delavirdine (Rescriptor)	Adefovir (Preveon)
Indinavir (Crixivan)	Combivir (AZT+3TC)	Trizivir (AZT+3TC+ABC)	**Efavirenz (Sustiva)**	
Lopinavir and ritonavir (Kaletra)	Didanosine (Videx; ddI)	Zalcitabine (Hivid; ddC)	**Nevirapine (Viramune)**	
Nelfinavir (Viracept)	Lamivudine (Epivir; 3TC)	Zidovudine (Retrovir; ZDV; AZT)		
Ritonavir (Norvir)				
Saquinavir (Invirase, Fortovase)				

Note. Enfuvirtide (Fuzeon) was approved by the U.S. Food and Drug Administration in March 2003. It is the first in a new class of medications, HIV fusion inhibitors. For medications in **boldface type,** drug-drug interactions are particularly problematic.

"depression" or "adjustment disorder" when early-stage encephalopathy was the true etiology. *Recommend serologic testing for HIV for all patients who present with new-onset psychosis, especially if the patient has any risk factors for HIV exposure.* Acute or subacute onset of confusion, memory complaints, affective or mood disturbances, bizarre behavior, abnormal posturing, or symptoms of a medical illness (e.g., fever, weight loss) should raise the possibility of HIV infection.

The following materials may be useful for your consultations:

- Figure 9–1. "The Initial Psychiatric Consultation to an HIV or AIDS Patient"
- Box 9–2. "Assessing HIV Risk Behavior: A Checklist of Behaviors and Attitudes"
- Figure 9–3. "Summary of Psychopharmacology for HIV and AIDS Patients"
- Population-specific fact sheets for patients (organized by gender, by ethnicity, by race, by sexual orientation) available at: http://www.caps.ucsf.edu/FSindex.html (accessed July 2004). Sponsored by the Center for AIDS Prevention Studies at the University of California–San Francisco, all fact sheets are available in English and Spanish, and selected ones are available in Kiswahili.
- Appendix 1. "American Psychiatric Association Guidelines for Assessing the Delirious Patient"
- Appendix 2. "Worksheet for Organizing Medical Chart Information: The Initial Psychiatric Consultation"
- Appendix 4. "'VINDICTIVE MADS': Differential Diagnosis of Mental Status Changes." Frequent causes for delirium in AIDS patients include infection, neoplasms, degenerative disease, intoxication (from medications), endocrine/metabolic abnormalities, and seizures.

■ "THE NEW GREAT IMITATOR"

In the very early years of the AIDS epidemic, the dearth of effective preventive treatments for HIV allowed clinicians to observe the natural history of HIV's effect on mental status (Sewell et al. 1994). HIV was called "the new great imitator" (Sabin 1987). As with neurosyphilis, its impact on the brain could easily be mistaken for primary psychiatric illness. *Psychosis alone* may be its initial presentation (Beckett et al. 1987; Halevie-Goldman et al. 1987; Halstead et al. 1988; Treisman et al. 1994), *sometimes occurring in the absence of either affective changes or detectable cognitive deterioration* (Buhrich et al. 1988). One 1991 chart and literature review found the following characteristics of new-onset HIV-associated psychosis (Harris et al. 1991):

1. Normal initial neurological evaluation (exam, computed tomography [CT] scan, cerebrospinal fluid [CSF])
2. Absence of *an apparent prodromal phase*
3. Persecutory, grandiose, or somatic delusions. When hallucinations also occurred, they were usually auditory in nature.
4. Frequent occurrence of mood and/or affective disturbance (81% of patients), and bizarre behavior (52%)
5. Rapid medical and cognitive deterioration of those psychotic patients who had abnormal CT scans and/or electroencephalograms
6. Neuroleptic-induced improvement of psychotic symptoms, although side effects were frequent

Patients with new-onset HIV-associated psychosis tended to be initially misdiagnosed; admission diagnoses included undifferentiated schizophrenia, schizophreniform disorder, "reactive psychosis," atypical psychosis, depression with psychotic features, and mania. These diagnoses were later revised to AIDS encephalitis, cryptococcal meningitis, or "organic psychosis." It was not possible to determine the incidence of psychosis in this study because of methodological limitations.

Monosymptomatic hypochondriacal psychosis with the delusion of parasitic infestation (Holmes 1989) and catatonia have also been described in AIDS delirium and HIV-associated dementia complex (Scamvougeras and Rosebush 1992; Snyder et al. 1992; Volkow et al. 1987).

The differential diagnosis and treatment of psychosis in HIV are discussed later in this chapter.

■ HIV-ASSOCIATED DEMENTIA COMPLEX

Disease course and pathology are variable in early HIV infection. A mononucleosis-like illness occurs within days to weeks of presumed HIV exposure, with symptoms such as fatigue, fever, lymphadenopathy, and occasionally a rash. These symptoms usually resolve as an immune response to HIV develops and the levels of plasma viremia decrease. Patients who present years later with the clinical syndrome of AIDS do not always recall such a prodrome. For untreated

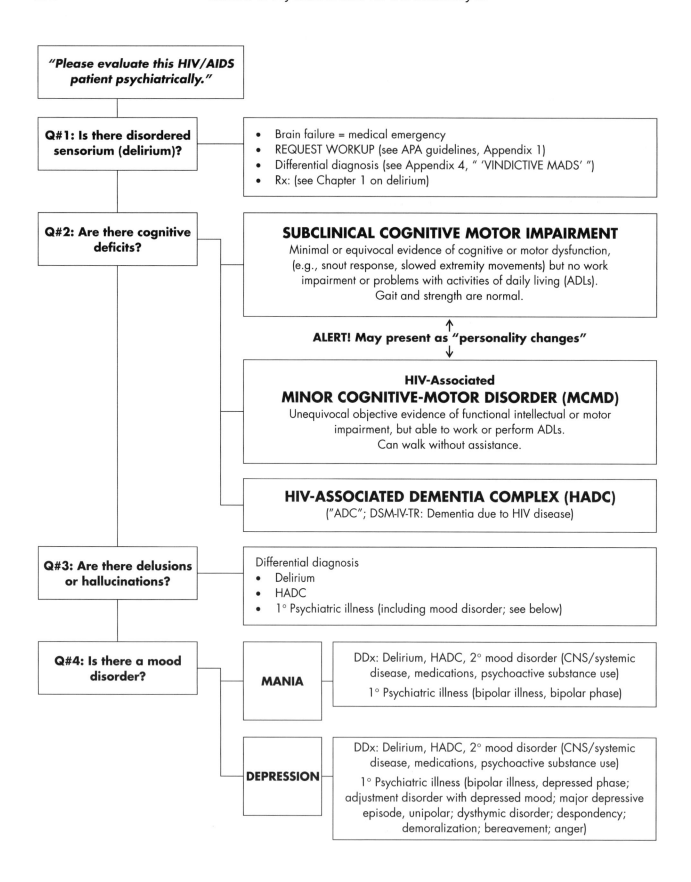

Figure 9–1.   The initial psychiatric consultation to an HIV or AIDS patient: a hierarchical approach.

Abbreviations: 1°=primary; 2°=secondary; APA=American Psychiatric Association; DDx=differential diagnosis; Q=question.

Box 9–2. **Assessing HIV risk behavior: a checklist of behaviors and attitudes**
Take a specific behavioral history: ❑ Frequency of sexual intercourse (vaginal, anal, oral) ❑ Number, gender, and known HIV risk of sex partners ❑ Whether the patient has traded sex (for money, drugs, a place to stay, cigarettes) ❑ Past and current symptoms of sexually transmitted infections ❑ Use of condoms and other contraceptive methods ❑ Use of drugs, particularly those that are injected or sniffed ❑ Sharing of needles, syringes, or other injection equipment Does the person perceive himself/herself to be at risk for HIV infection? (If there is no perception of risk, there will be little motivation for behavioral change.) Does the person believe that changing behavior will have an impact on preventing infection? Does the seropositive person care about infecting others or benefit by avoiding reexposure? Is there an Axis I condition? Would treatment for it improve the ability to cooperate with medical advice (e.g., would adherence improve if depression were treated and resolved)? Assess predisposition to *persistent* high-risk sexual behavior, especially: ❑ Drug or alcohol abuse ❑ Borderline personality disorder ❑ Axis I disorder ❑ History of childhood sexual abuse[a] Is the patient autonomous or fatalistic about the illness? (See Chapter 13.)

[a]Sexual compulsivity, revictimization, substance abuse, and chronic depression enhance the vulnerability to HIV infection of adult survivors of sexual abuse (Goodman and Fallot 1998; Lenderking et al. 1997). Survivor characteristics: trauma intrusion phenomena, dissociative phenomena, somatization, sexual dysfunction (Hutton et al. 2001).

patients, the median time from initial infection to the development of clinical disease is approximately 10 years (Fauci and Lane 2001). The rate of disease progression is directly correlated with HIV RNA levels. Those with high levels of HIV RNA in plasma progress to symptomatic disease faster than do those with low levels.

The virus crosses the blood–CSF barrier early in the infection. Neuropathological findings include cerebral atrophy, myelin pallor, chronic perivascular inflammation, multinucleated giant cells derived from HIV-infected macrophages and microglia, microglial nodules, and reactive gliosis (Jay 2000). Although typically managed by neurologists, HIV-associated dementia complex (HADC) may imitate conditions as varied as neurosyphilis, Alzheimer's disease, depression, anxiety disorders, psychotic disorders, and substance abuse. Furthermore, HADC patients evolve varied neuropsychiatric complications, such as anxiety, depression, mania, and psychosis.

The classification system for HIV infection by the Centers for Disease Control and Prevention emphasizes the clinical importance of the CD4+ T-lymphocyte count in categorizing HIV-related clinical conditions. The American Academy of Neurology categorization of HIV-related central nervous system (CNS) disease has become the standard (see Box 9–3).

HADC is a multifaceted syndrome consisting of cognitive, affective, motor, and behavioral abnormalities in HIV-infected persons (synonyms: AIDS dementia complex, AIDS encephalopathy, HIV encephalopathy). DSM-IV-TR (American Psychiatric Association 2000a) specifically uses the term *dementia due to HIV disease* (code 294.1x). The definitional criteria for HADC according to the American Academy of Neurology AIDS Task Force are listed in Box 9–3. Although it is not as widely used, we have found the Memorial Sloan-Kettering Cancer Center staging system for HADC also useful in the clinical description of HADC and its progression (Table 9–2).

Deficits of HADC

Cognitive deficits of HADC include mental slowing (less verbal, less spontaneous, not as quick); poor concentration and attention (e.g., losing track of conversations);

Box 9–3.   Definitional criteria for HIV-associated dementia complex (HADC) and cognitive impairment (American Academy of Neurology AIDS Task Force)

Probable (must have **each** of the following)
1. a. Acquired abnormality in at least two of the following *cognitive abilities* (present for at least 1 month), verified by reliable history and mental status examination, with history obtained from an informant, supplemented by neuropsychological testing:
   - attention/concentration
   - speed of processing of information
   - visuospatial skills
   - memory/learning
   - speech/language
   - abstraction/reasoning

    b. Cognitive dysfunction causing impairment of work or activities of daily living

2. At least **one** of the following:
    a. Abnormality in *motor function or performance* verified by clinical exam (e.g., slowed rapid movements, abnormal gait, limb incoordination, hyperreflexia, hypertonia, or weakness); neuropsychological tests (e.g., fine motor speed, manual dexterity, perceptual motor skills)

    b. Decline in *motivation or emotional control,* or change in *social behavior* (e.g., change in personality with apathy, inertia, irritability, emotional lability) or new onset of *impaired judgment* (e.g., socially inappropriate behavior or disinhibition)

3. Absence or clouding of consciousness of sufficient interval to establish criterion 1, above

4. Other etiologies ruled out, including active CNS opportunistic infection or malignancy, psychiatric disorders (e.g., depressive disorder), substance use or withdrawal.
    If another potential etiology (e.g., major depression) is present, it cannot be the cause of the above cognitive, motor, or behavioral symptoms and signs in order to diagnose HADC

Possible (must have **one** of the following)
1. Other potential etiology present (must have **each** of the following):
    a. Same as criteria 1, 2, and 3 in **Probable**

    b. Another potential etiology is present, but the cause of criterion 1 above is uncertain.

2. Incomplete clinical evaluation (must have **each** of the following):
    a. Same as criteria 1, 2, and 3 in **Probable**

    b. Etiology cannot be determined (appropriate laboratory or radiologic investigations pending).

Source.   Adapted from Janssen RS, Cornblath DR, Epstein LG, et al.: "Nomenclature and Research Case Definitions for Neurological Manifestations of Human Immunodeficiency Virus–Type 1 (HIV-1) Infection: Report of a Working Group of the American Academy of Neurology AIDS Task Force." *Neurology* 41:778–785, 1991.

Table 9–2.   Adapted Memorial Sloan-Kettering Cancer Center staging system for HIV-associated dementia complex

Stage	Description
0.5 Equivocal	**Subclinical cognitive motor impairment** Either minimal or equivocal symptoms of cognitive or motor dysfunction, or mild signs (snout response, slowed extremity movements) but without impairment of work or capacity to perform activities of daily living (ADLs). Gait and strength are normal.
1 Mild	**Minor cognitive-motor disorder** Unequivocal evidence (symptoms, signs, neuropsychological test performance) of functional intellectual or motor impairment, but able to perform all but the more demanding aspects of work or ADLs. Can walk without assistance.
2–4 Moderate to end stage	**HIV-associated dementia complex** *Stage 2:* Cannot walk or maintain the more demanding ADLs, but can perform basic ADLs of self-care; ambulatory, but may require a single prop *Stage 3:* Major intellectual incapacity or motor disability *Stage 4:* Nearly vegetative

forgetfulness (appointments, names, historical details); confusion (time, place); and difficulties in abstraction, problem solving, or manipulating acquired knowledge.

Behavioral deficits seen in HADC include apathy, social withdrawal; personality changes; and agitated psychosis.

Motor deficits associated with HADC include loss of coordination; fine motor difficulties (e.g., impaired handwriting); eye movement abnormalities; unsteady gait; leg weakness; and tremor.

HIV-Associated Minor Cognitive-Motor Disorder

The diagnosis of HIV-associated minor cognitive-motor disorder (MCMD) is reserved for individuals who demonstrate cognitive or motor dysfunction not severe enough to interfere with activities of daily living or to qualify for a full-blown dementia syndrome. Prevalence estimates made in 1995 (Heaton et al. 1995) are listed in Table 9–3. An important clinical question remains: do MCMD and HADC differ in underlying pathogenesis and clinical course, as well as in severity? Encouragingly, only a minority of patients (about 17%) with MCMD developed HADC in a study by Marder et al. (1998). Trials are under way to determine the impact of HAART on the natural history of both MCMD and HADC.

The symptoms of HADC are often subtle and insidious in onset; slowed decision making is most prominent. This presentation differs from the amnesia, language disturbance, and agnosia typifying the early stages of senile dementia of the Alzheimer type (SDAT). SDAT is a cortical-type dementia. HADC follows a different pattern: it is closer to "subcortical de-

Table 9–3. CDC stage and MCMD

CDC stage	Approximate percentage of patients meeting criteria for MCMD
A	5%
B	27%
C	21%–24%

Note. CDC=Centers for Disease Control and Prevention; MCMD=minor cognitive-motor disorder.
Source. Data from Heaton et al. 1995.

mentia," which has been described in Parkinson's disease, Huntington's disease, Wilson's disease, and other disorders. Although cognitive functioning is eventually globally impaired, insight is often preserved until late in the illness. Depression is common (see Table 9–4). Luckily, dementia is a complication of advanced HIV infection, rarely developing in the early stages of infection (Jay 2000). Table 9–4 compares features of cortical and subcortical dementia.

Assessment

Cognitive slowing appears to be the first cognitive disturbance of HIV infection. Most useful are test batteries that will assess the following: psychomotor speed, information encoding, information retrieval, concentration, and attention. Baseline and longitudinal neuropsychological testing have become the standard for evaluating and tracking cognitive function in seropositive patients. Although the selection of formal neuropsychological test instruments is beyond the scope of this chapter, a few points are worth noting:

Table 9–4. A comparison of subcortical and cortical dementia

Mental status domain	Subcortical dementia (HADC, Parkinson's disease)	Cortical dementia (Alzheimer's disease)
Appearance	Disheveled, ill-appearing	Alert, healthy
Activity	Slow	Normal
Posture	Distorted	Erect
Speech	Abnormal articulation: dysarthria, muteness, etc.	Normal articulation
Language	Normal production	Dysnomia, paraphasia
Cognition	Cannot plan or sequence cognitive operations in problem solving	Unable to manipulate knowledge
Memory	Disorder of retrieval	Disorder of learning
Visuospatial	Sloppy due to movement problems	Constructional disturbance
Emotional state	Apathetic, lacking drive	Unaware, unconcerned

Note. HADC=HIV-associated dementia complex.
Source. From Cummings JL (ed.): *Subcortical Dementia.* Copyright 1990 Jeffrey L. Cummings. Used by permission of Oxford University Press.

Table 9–5.   Clinician-administered tests recommended by the American Psychiatric Association

Mental Alternation Test (MAT)	Patients count to 20, say the alphabet, and then alternate between numbers/letters. Score: correct number/letter alterations in 30 seconds (e.g., 1-A, then 2-B, then 3-C=3). Maximum score: 52 points. Score <15 correlates with HIV-related cognitive impairment. Confounding conditions: subnormal intelligence; delirium; poor concentration (Jones et al. 1993).
HIV Dementia Scale (HDS) (see Figure 9–2)	Four subtests: timed written alphabet, four-item recall in 5 minutes, cube copy time, and antisaccadic task. Score≤10 correlates with HIV-related cognitive impairment (Power et al. 1995).
The Executive Interview (EXIT25)	25 executive cognition tasks in 15 minutes (e.g., abstract thinking; ability to plan, initiate, sequence, monitor, and stop complex behavior). Available from Dr. Donald Royall (royall@uthscsa.edu) (Berghuis et al. 1999; Royall et al. 1992; Schillerstrom et al. 2003).

The Mini-Mental State Examination (MMSE) is not sufficiently sensitive for detecting HIV-associated neurocognitive dysfunction, particularly early MCMD, because it omits assessing response time. Even late in the dementing disease, MMSE scores may underestimate HADC cognitive dysfunction.

The American Psychiatric Association Practice Guideline (American Psychiatric Association 2000b) recommends baseline screening using any one of the three tests listed in Table 9–5. Patients should be reevaluated regularly as part of the treatment plan. If there is evidence of early cognitive impairment, formal neuropsychological testing is useful for documenting areas of cognitive dysfunction as well as areas of relative cognitive strength.

Clinical Course

HADC is a dementia of variable progression and duration. Some HADC patients develop other systemic AIDS manifestations during the course of the dementia. Others have a more indolent, prolonged, and relatively stable course. Some patients may compensate for cognitive loss, whereas others deteriorate rapidly to a severe vegetative dementia over a period of weeks. It is not possible to predict the clinical course for a given patient.

Patients with HADC complain that their thinking is slowed and their concentration diminished. They may report, for example, losing track of the conversation while speaking to people and having to reread a paragraph or page to get it to "sink in." Additionally, they complain of forgetfulness, usually for day-to-day events. In the early stages, individuals may report that they cannot keep up with their personal finances or business activities, describing a state of "puzzlement." Neurobehavioral abnormalities may soon follow, such as motor complaints of clumsiness, sloppy handwriting, tremor, and poor balance, especially with rapid head turns.

- *Caution.* In psychotherapy, the apathy and social withdrawal of insidious-onset HADC may resemble and coincide with psychodynamically motivated phenomena like resistance, denial, and repression.

Case Example of Subtle-Onset HADC

Ms. A was a 38-year-old single mother of two who contracted HIV after a sexual assault by a neighbor at the age of 33, for which she had "no memory." She had been relatively adherent to her medical care, including a recommendation for an antidepressant and supportive psychotherapy. In the past year, however, Ms. A had become more forgetful about her appointments, joking that "it must be the start of menopause," or "I guess I didn't want to talk about something last week." She would forget to bring in her insurance forms so that sessions could be billed, but also began to misplace items unrelated to psychotherapy, such as her children's medical forms and lunch vouchers. Although she initially attributed these reactions to "what was being discussed in psychotherapy," the patient could no longer remember what was discussed from session to session. The patient's sister became concerned that the patient was "acting senile," that is, apathetic, forgetful, easily confused, "not herself." Neurological workup later revealed that the patient was in the early stages of HADC.

Comment: HADC-related cognitive changes are sometimes distinguishable by "forgetfulness" that is not limited to the psychotherapy sessions or psychodynamically valent material. Such memory and problem-solving deficits will adversely affect the patient's ability to follow through and maintain continuity in psychotherapy. Sometimes insight regarding intellectual decline is preserved until late in the illness, and patients may experience reactions of fear, anxiety, and mourning.

Max Score	Score	
4	(__)	MEMORY – REGISTRATION Give four words to recall (dog, hat, green, peach), 1 second to say each. Then ask the patient all 4 after you have said them.
4	(__)	ATTENTION Antisaccadic eye movement task[1]: 20 commands. __ errors in 20 trials (SCORE: ≤ 3 errors=4; 4 errors=3; 5 errors=2; 6 errors=1; >6 errors=0)
6	(__)	PSYCHOMOTOR SPEED Ask patient to write the alphabet in upper case letters horizontally across the page (use back of this record form) and record time: __ seconds (SCORE: ≤ 21 sec=6; 21.1 sec=5; 24.1–27 sec=4; 27.1–30 sec=3; >36 sec=0)
4	(__)	MEMORY – RECALL Ask for 4 words from Registration above. For words not recalled, prompt with "semantic clue," as follows: animal (dog); piece of clothing (hat); color (green); fruit (peach). (SCORE: 1 point for each correct unprompted word, ½ point if correct after prompting.)
2	(__)	CONSTRUCTION Copy the cube below; record time: __ seconds. (SCORE: <25 sec=2; 25–35 sec=1; >35 sec=0)
16 Max	(__) Total Score	(≤10 suggestive of cognitive impairment)

Figure 9–2. HIV Dementia Scale.

[1]Antisaccadic eye movement task: patient focuses on the examiner's (E) nose and looks to and from the E's moving index finger and nose, using alternating hands. E's hands positioned at the patient's shoulder width and eye height. Patient must maintain focus on E's unmoving index finger (i.e., antisaccades). After practice trial, patient is then asked to perform 20 serial anti-saccades. 1 error = looking at moving finger.

Source. Power C, Selnes O, Grim J, et al.: "HIV Dementia Scale: A Rapid Screening Test." *Journal of Acquired Immune Deficiency Syndromes and Human Retrovirology* 8:273–278, 1995. Used with permission from the publisher.

Differential Diagnosis

HADC is in the differential diagnosis of any psychiatric symptom occurring in an HIV-infected individual. Advanced cases are easy to spot and are characterized by global cognitive deterioration, gross impairment of social functioning, disorientation, agitation, mutism, vacant stare, spasticity and myoclonus, bowel and bladder incontinence, and, rarely, coma. The symptoms of early HADC, however, may be easily misdiagnosed as depression, particularly in the initial phases when symptoms coincide with affective changes of depression, including dysphoria, anxiety, irritability, apathy, and social withdrawal. Predominance of dysphoric thought content, such as low self-esteem, irrational guilt, and self-denigration, may help distinguish depressive syndromes from HADC. However, these negative self-perceptions are not pathognomonic and may also reflect patients' awareness of declining cognitive abilities.

Psychotic ideation and inappropriate behavior are relatively uncommon early features of HADC. More typical is the insidious onset of apathy or social withdrawal in a previously healthy seropositive individual. Nonetheless, HADC has also been mistaken for primary psychotic disorders, mania, SDAT, and anxiety and adjustment disorders.

HADC in older patients: Early HADC may be overlooked in the differential diagnosis of dementia in older patients, especially when systemic symptoms or obvious risk factors are absent. Table 9–6 lists factors that should prompt an investigation of serostatus in elderly patients.

Table 9–6. Factors that should prompt serostatus assessment in elderly patients

- Known risk group of patient or sexual partner
- History of surgery or blood transfusion before 1985 (prior to screening of blood supply for HIV)
- Parkinson's-like dementia (with "subcortical" pattern of cognitive deficits)
- Dementia with atypical features (e.g., rapid progression, focal neurological signs)
- Significant systemic symptoms, especially weight loss, opportunistic infections, pneumonia

---

Treatment Considerations in HADC

Nonpharmacological Management Strategies

A spectrum of reactions may occur in caregivers who relate to cognitively impaired patients. One is denial, in which both caregiver and patient minimize the cognitive deficits: "She's always been like this, it's nothing new." Interventions are difficult in this setting because recommendations usually are considered unnecessary. Alternatively, the patient may be treated as incapable of any independent activity, leading the caregiver to "take over" prematurely. This leaves the patient feeling even more powerless and hopeless.

Behavioral abnormalities that result from a dementing illness often challenge the ingenuity and fortitude of the caregivers. The distractibility of mild cognitive impairment may be mistaken for boredom or anxiety, and apathy may be misattributed to depression. Loss of mental flexibility is secondary to dementing illness but may come across as "stubbornness" (Boccellari and Zeifert 1994). If these behaviors are understood to be the result of the dementing process itself, caregivers may be able to make better interventions to help patients modify them.

Suggestions for management strategies for the patient with HADC MCMD appear in Box 9–4. (See also Appendix 5 in this volume for a discussion of general treatment principles for use with dementia patients.)

Pharmacological Treatment

At this writing, the primary treatment for a patient diagnosed with HADC is HAART. Table 9–1 lists the main categories of current antiviral drugs and many of the specific drugs with common brand names. Several of them have potential drug-drug interactions with common psychotropic medications.

Neuropsychiatric side effects. Compiling a comprehensive list of the neuropsychiatric side effects of HIV medications is like trying to hit a moving target. Almost every medication used to treat HIV/AIDS is an offender, particularly in this vulnerable population. We find it more useful to assume that a medication produces psychiatric sequelae until proven otherwise, and to look up what is unfamiliar or unremembered.

Plant-based (herbal) therapy. It is easier to trace drug-drug interactions when the clinician has the patient's complete medication list. However, more than one-quarter of outpatients being treated for HIV in one study reported using herbal medicines (Duggan et al. 2001), yet they did not always report them (Power et al. 2002). Asking about herbal supplements should be a routine part of patient assessments. Appendix 6 in this volume lists commonly used herbal therapies and their potential side effects.

Psychostimulants. The psychostimulants have been used for several years to improve HADC-associated cognitive impairment and fatigue. Their use is symptom-driven (rather than diagnosis-driven), with improvements shown in patients who have the following symptoms: cognitive problems (with or without accompanying depression), fatigue, apathy, social withdrawal, anorexia, suicidal ideation, and deficient self-care. Psychostimulants can also potentiate analgesic effects of narcotic analgesics while minimizing CNS-depressant side effects and lowering the dose required for analgesics to be effective.

A randomized, double-blind, placebo-controlled trial of psychostimulants in ambulatory patients showed that treatment with methylphenidate or with pemoline significantly improved fatigue, decreased levels of depression and psychological distress, and improved quality of life with minimal side effects (Breitbart et al. 2001). There were no significant differences in efficacy between the two medications. Severe side effects were relatively uncommon, with only hyperactivity or jitteriness occurring more often among subjects receiving active medication. *Note:* Because of the risk of unpredictable liver failure resulting in death, pemoline (Cylert) is now available only as a second-line medication, and only if the patient signs a special informed consent form provided by the manufacturer.

Box 9–4: Management strategies for the patient with HIV-associated dementia complex minor cognitive-motor disorder (HADC MCMD)

Advice to patients

1. **Use memory aids** (e.g., write down appointments, important information, or conversations). These reduce the need to ask for help and allow the individual to maintain a sense of control.

2. **Slow down and do one task at a time.** Multitasking produces confusion and frustration.

3. **Use verbal monitoring** (i.e., talk aloud as a task is completed). Problem-solving aloud allows self-cueing that facilitates concentration and maintains focus.

4. **Keep mentally active in nonstressful ways.** Examples: Scrabble, cards, checkers, crossword puzzles, jigsaw puzzles, and video games. Activities should not be overly difficult or frustrating.

5. **Get enough rest and schedule appointments early in the day.** Fatigue worsens cognitive problems, leading to irritability and angry outbursts.

6. **Avoid stressful situations by planning ahead.** For example, shopping, running errands, or dining can be conducted during off-hours, when stimulation and stress are less.

7. **Learn stress-reduction techniques and relaxation exercises** to reduce tension and anxiety.

8. **Get regular exercise.**

9. **Self-manage medications as long as possible.** Devices like watches with an alarm or automated pill boxes that beep when it is time for the next dose are helpful.

10. **Give up tasks that have become too difficult** (e.g., balancing a checkbook). Ask for help.

Advice to caregivers

1. **Maintain orientation** by displaying calendars and clocks. Use an orientation blackboard with the date and the patient's daily schedule, as well as night-lights to minimize "sundowning."

2. **Keep the environment and routine consistent.** Minimize sudden changes, promote familiarity to reduce confusion (e.g., furniture, utensils, personal articles should always be kept in the same place).

3. **Monitor stimulation** to avoid increased confusion, fearfulness, and agitation.

4. **Prepare the patient for change.** Cognitive impairment limits the ability to adjust quickly to change; sudden changes or surprises may increase confusion or cause anxiety.

5. **Avoid challenging demented patients directly** about a particular behavior or trying to convince them of another course of action. Upsetting confrontation may increase frustration and confusion.

6. **Redirect or distract the patient from inappropriate or troublesome behavior** (e.g., by calling the patient's name and shifting to a different focus or activity).

7. **Maintain calm when faced with the demented patient's agitation or confusion.** Displays of emotion on the part of caregivers are likely to escalate the patient's agitation.

Source. Adapted from Boccellari A, Zeifert P: "Management of Neurobehavioral Impairment in HIV-1 Infection." *Psychiatric Clinics of North America* 17:183–203, 1994.

Dosing. A review of psychostimulant preparations appears in Chapter 3, "The Patient With Cardiovascular Disease." In cardiovascularly stable patients, administration should start with a morning dose equivalent to 2.5–5 mg of methylphenidate by mouth, feeding tube, or suppository (Holmes et al. 1994). The dose should be increased by 5 mg every 1–2 days until demonstrable effects are achieved, either improved mood or irritability. Blood pressure and heart rate should be monitored initially, along with adverse effects such as agitation, restlessness, nausea, and psychosis. The medication should be increased gradually, given in divided doses before 1:00 P.M. (so as not to

disturb sleep), until maximum clinical response is achieved. The sustained-release preparation is an alternative if a clinical effect is desired in the afternoon.

Side effects. Patients should be monitored for movement disorders because involuntary dyskinetic movements occur with stimulants, particularly dextroamphetamine or daily doses of methylphenidate above 60 mg. It has been recommended that alternatives to dextroamphetamine be used in HIV patients because of this medication's tendency to produce abnormal involuntary movements and the vulnerability of these patients to side effects (Fernandez and Levy 1994).

Psychosis is a rare side effect of psychostimulants, occurring in patients with a history of psychotic symptoms. Stimulant abuse is rarely a problem in medically ill patients unless there is a previous history of substance abuse.

■ PSYCHOSIS IN HIV

Differential Diagnosis

Psychosis may occur in HADC alone or be symptomatic of delirium in a seropositive patient with or without HADC. (Delirium is discussed at length in Chapter 1 of this volume.) The ages at onset of idiopathic psychosis and HIV infection overlap, so that the differential diagnosis often includes primary psychiatric disorders, such as schizophrenia and bipolar affective disorder. Other causes of psychosis include substance abuse, steroids, and antiretroviral agents such as zidovudine, ganciclovir, abacavir, nevirapine, and efavirenz (Foster et al. 2003). Efavirenz is associated with multiple psychiatric and neurological side effects (Treisman and Kaplin 2002). There have been at least three reported cases in which patients experienced significant psychiatric improvement after discontinuation or reduction of efavirenz (Peyriere et al. 2001). Unfortunately, patients often receive efavirenz after failing other antiretrovirals, so options may be limited.

Isoniazid (INH) is used as a first-line treatment for tuberculosis. It has a number of psychiatric complications, including affective disturbance and psychosis (Gnam et al. 1993; Upadhyaya and Chaturvedi 1989). New-onset psychosis may be a result of opportunistic infections, such as cryptococcosis, herpes encephalitis, or toxoplasmosis, or cancers such as CNS lymphoma. It may also be the manifestation of cytomegalovirus (CMV) retinitis with visual impairment and visual hallucinations (Cohen and Jacobson 2000). There have been cases presenting predominantly with psychotic symptoms that then progressed to HADC, raising the possibility that CNS viral infection may be operative in HIV-related psychosis (Navia et al. 1986).

- *Bottom line:* HIV infection should be considered *in any patient who presents with new-onset psychosis,* especially if the patient has any risk factors for HIV exposure. Acute or subacute onset of confusion, memory complaints, affective or mood disturbances, bizarre behavior, abnormal posturing, or symptoms of a medical illness (e.g., fever, weight loss) should raise the possibility of HIV infection.

Treatment

Most patients respond rapidly to neuroleptics. However, there is a subgroup whose psychosis never completely remits and who show residual cognitive impairment consistent with HADC (Fernandez and Levy 1994). As with any medically fragile group, start with low-dose neuroleptics, cautiously titrating to minimize the risk of side effects. Antipsychotic treatment in the setting of HIV infection follows the same principles as for other medically ill patients. (See Chapter 1 in this volume for an extensive discussion of the workup and management of psychosis secondary to delirium.)

High-potency typical neuroleptics such as haloperidol and depot neuroleptics *should be avoided* because of the heightened vulnerability of HIV patients to side effects such as neuroleptic malignant syndrome and extrapyramidal side effects (Ferrando and Wapenyi 2002). Low-potency antipsychotics such as chlorpromazine (Thorazine) are highly anticholinergic, may contribute to delirium, and predispose to cardiovascular side effects.

Atypical Antipsychotics

Atypical antipsychotics may be particularly helpful in bypassing the problems encountered with typical neuroleptics. Schwartz and Masand (2002), in their review on the use of atypical antipsychotics to treat delirium in the medically ill, recommended the following for risperidone, olanzapine, and quetiapine:

Risperidone (Risperdal).   Recommended dosage for mild to severe agitation is 0.25–0.5 mg twice daily to start, with 0.25–0.5 mg every 4 hours as needed for agitation or increased delirium symptoms. Increase up to 4 mg/day if symptoms initially fail to clear. Numerous reports indicate the effectiveness of risperidone for the treatment of psychosis in the setting of HIV. However, there are reports that coadministration with ritonavir (Norvir), which inhibits its metabolism and raises plasma levels, has led to increases in extrapyramidal symptoms (EPS), neuroleptic malignant syndrome, and reversible coma (Jover et al. 2002; Kelly et al. 2002; Lee et al. 2000).

Olanzapine (Zyprexa).   Recommended dosage for mild to severe agitation is 2.5–5.0 mg at bedtime to start, increasing up to 20 mg/day if symptoms fail to clear. As-needed doses may be added, but daily doses exceeding 20 mg/day have not shown greater efficacy for delirium. Olanzapine has also been used successfully in the HIV population, and the associated weight gain may be beneficial in this population (Cohen and Jacobson 2000; Ferrando and Wapenyi 2002). Ritonavir may decrease the blood levels of olanzapine, ultimately causing higher doses to be needed (Penzak et al. 2001). In addition, atypical antipsychotics (particularly olanzapine) have been associated with hyperglycemia, ketoacidosis, and hypercholesterolemia in several case reports and uncontrolled studies.

Quetiapine (Seroquel). Quetiapine has been used in the setting of delirium in the general medically ill at 25–50 mg twice daily for mild to severe agitation to start, with 25–50 mg every 4 hours as needed for agitation or increased delirium symptoms. Increase up to 600 mg/day. We could find no data on its use in HIV patients.

Clozapine (Clozaril). Clozapine has also been shown to be effective in this setting; however, the risk of agranulocytosis is especially worrisome in patients with HIV. Clozapine is contraindicated for patients taking ritonavir (Ferrando and Wapenyi 2002).

Pimozide (Orap). Pimozide is contraindicated with protease inhibitors because they increase plasma levels and the risk for arrhythmia (McNicholl and Peiperl 2003).

Ziprasidone (Geodon) and Aripiprazole (Abilify). No data are available on use in HIV.

Management

Medications may be discontinued 7–10 days after patients return to baseline with cleared sensorium and alleviation of delirium symptoms, particularly after restoration of the sleep-wake cycle.

Extrapyramidal Side Effects

When antiparkinsonian drugs are required for EPS, amantadine (Symmetrel) is recommended because it is less anticholinergic (and therefore less likely to contribute to delirium) than either benztropine (Cogentin) or trihexyphenidyl (Artane). The starting dose is 50 mg orally bid (up to 100 mg bid). Note, however, that amantadine is a dopamine agonist and has been implicated in causing delusional states in patients with Parkinson's disease and chronic psychosis. If psychosis worsens or does not remit after adding amantadine to a neuroleptic regimen, the drug should be discontinued and the patient reevaluated.

■ MAJOR DEPRESSION IN HIV INFECTION

Prevalence

Prevalence data on major depressive syndromes in the HIV-spectrum population vary. During the early years of the AIDS epidemic, many reports reflected the impression that major depression was an inevitable consequence of living with a stigmatizing and ultimately fatal disease. More recent studies, which are based on self-report measures and standardized diagnostic interviews, have modified that view. Most studies demonstrate that although major depression is more common in HIV-positive individuals than in HIV-negative individuals, depressive disorders seem to be the exception rather than the rule for this population.

In a five-site World Health Organization neuropsychiatric AIDS study, prevalence rates of major depression ranged from 3.0%–10.9% in asymptomatic HIV-positive individuals to 4.0%–18.4% in symptomatic HIV-positive individuals. U.S. national estimates have varied, limited because of their reliance on convenience samples (e.g., clinic patients) and specific subpopulations (e.g., gay men). For example, consistent with prior self-report studies that have yielded prevalence ratings of between 20% and 32%, a study of a representative probability sample of 2,864 adults receiving care for HIV in the United States in 1996 showed that one-third had major depression (Bing et al. 2001). Other studies that rely largely on standardized diagnostic interviews show lower rates of major depression, in the 4%–14% range (Rabkin et al. 1997). A recent meta-analysis of 10 published studies demonstrated that the frequency of major depression was nearly two times higher in HIV-positive subjects than in HIV-negative subjects (Ciesla and Roberts 2001).

- *Bottom line:* These findings support the common-sense practice of assessing depression throughout the course of HIV disease.

Risk Factors

The following factors are associated with a higher risk of HIV-associated depression (Lagana et al. 2002; Lyketsos et al. 1996): history of depression (before contracting HIV), chronic pain, and limited social support. Although some research has shown no consistent association between rates of depression and stage of HIV disease, most suggests that rates of depression increase in the later stages of HIV infection (Kelly et al.

1998; Maj 1996). For example, in a large prospective study using data from 911 HIV-positive men from the Multicenter AIDS Cohort Study, Lyketsos et al. (1996) found that there was a dramatic, sustained rise in depressive symptoms as AIDS developed, beginning as early as 18 months before clinical AIDS was diagnosed. A variety of psychosocial and biological factors could contribute to this rise in depressive symptoms.

Knowledge of positive antibody status is only a relatively weak predictor of profound depression (Hays et al. 1992; Perry et al. 1993). Furthermore, there is no evidence that risk for major depressive disorder correlates with the sexual orientation of HIV-positive individuals (Ciesla and Roberts 2001). In addition, there is no clear association between HADC and depression.

Differential Diagnosis

It is important to distinguish between depression and medical conditions that require emergency intervention. The differential diagnosis of depression should include the following: delirium (brain failure), apathy due to HADC or to substance-induced or withdrawal states; mood disorders (major depressive disorder, unipolar; bipolar disorder, depressed phase; dysthymic disorder; adjustment disorder with depressed mood); bereavement; anger; despondency; and demoralization.

Agitation associated with a depressive syndrome may be difficult to distinguish from dementia-caused agitation. Acute onset, precipitation by a medical or neurological event, mood lability, absence of previous affective history, and nocturnal worsening tend to argue in favor of HADC.

Treatment

The management of major depression in patients with HIV infection should involve a careful assessment of the overall medical status of the patient, including concurrent illnesses and medications. Although psychotherapy is an important component of treatment, this section will focus on psychopharmacological interventions.

Some general guidelines for using psychotropic medications, including antidepressants, in HIV-infected patients include the following:

- Use lower starting doses and slower titration.
- Provide the least complicated dosing schedule possible.

- Consider drug side effect profiles to avoid unnecessary adverse effects.
- Check drug metabolism/clearance pathways to minimize drug interactions and possible end organ damage.

The combination of ritonavir with psychotropics is the most potentially problematic. Although ritonavir inhibits both 3A4 and 2D6, clinically significant drug interactions tend to occur because of its potent 2D6 inhibition.

Clinical trials and efficacy studies demonstrate that antidepressants are generally effective and well tolerated by patients who have symptomatic HIV infection or who are ill with AIDS. A good clinical rule when coprescribing psychotropics and antiretrovirals is to "start low, go slow."

Selective Serotonin Reuptake Inhibitors

The selective serotonin reuptake inhibitors (SSRIs) have replaced the tricyclic antidepressants (TCAs) as first-line medications. Combination with the protease inhibitors (all metabolized by 3A4) is the most potentially problematic. Ritonavir inhibits both 3A4 and 2D6, and clinically significant drug interactions tend to occur because of its potent 2D6 inhibition. Citalopram (Celexa) and escitalopram (Lexapro) retain their advantage in having the least competition for this enzyme system, and hence fewest potential drug-drug interactions with the protease inhibitors

Starting doses of fluoxetine (Prozac), citalopram (Celexa), and paroxetine (Paxil) should be approximately 10 mg/day. Sertraline (Zoloft) should be started at 25 mg/day. Cachectic patients, or those highly sensitive to side effects, may require lower initial doses.

SSRI side effects early in treatment include gastrointestinal upset, dry mouth, headache, and symptoms of anxiety. These generally subside within 7–10 days of a dose change. More enduring are the infamous SSRI sexual side effects, such as decreased libido, anorgasmia, and problems with erection in males.

Despite these problems, clinical experience has shown that SSRIs are effective and have a relatively benign side effect profile in HIV/AIDS patients. For example, one randomized, placebo-controlled trial showed results that were consistent with other double-blind antidepressant studies with HIV-positive patients (Rabkin et al. 1999): 74% of patients with major depression responded to fluoxetine versus 47% with placebo. The SSRIs do not alter CD4 cell counts (Rabkin et al. 1994).

Note that AIDS patients experience heightened vulnerability to side effects such as serotonin syndrome. The use of SSRIs is widespread, so one should not discount this side effect, as discussed in Chapter 1 on delirium. The serotonin syndrome also may be induced by the clinically "benign" action of adding trazodone as a hypnotic, for example, to an SSRI regimen (George and Godleski 1996; Nisijima et al. 1996; Reeves and Bullen 1995) or to nefazodone (Margolese and Chouinard 2000), or by using SSRIs with buspirone (Goldberg 1992). A synopsis of the serotonin syndrome and its distinction from neuroleptic malignant syndrome can be found in Appendix 7 of this volume.

Other Antidepressants

Figure 9–3, "Summary of Psychopharmacology for HIV and AIDS Patients," summarizes recommendations for use of other antidepressants as well as those discussed above.

Venlafaxine (Effexor). Venlafaxine has few interactions with antiretroviral medications and is well tolerated in this population. In order to minimize the gastrointestinal upset that occurs initially with this medication, patients should be started at low doses of the extended-release preparation (i.e., 37.5 mg Effexor XR). The dose can then be increased slowly as the patient accommodates to side effects. Venlafaxine also has sexual side effects.

Bupropion (Wellbutrin, Wellbutrin SR). Bupropion does not produce sexual dysfunction and has activating properties that may be useful when apathy and fatigue occur. In a prospective study, sustained-release bupropion at a mean daily dose of 265 mg was shown to be effective and well tolerated for the treatment of depression in HIV-positive patients, regardless of HIV clinical staging (Currier et al. 2003). It was formerly contraindicated with ritonavir (Norvir) because of the latter's presumed potential to cause bupropion toxicity and induce seizures in an already neurologically vulnerable population. These recommendations have since been modified to advise caution in coadministering the two medications, now that the details of bupropion's metabolism have been refined to show its dependence on the 2B6 isoenzyme rather than the 2D6 (Chuck et al. 1998). Although some studies showed that nonnucleoside reverse transcriptase inhibitors significantly interfere with the metabolism of bupropion in vitro by inhibiting the cytochrome 2B6 isoenzyme (Hesse et al. 2001), in clinical practice bupropion does not appreciably interact with other antiviral medications.

Nefazodone (Serzone). Nefazodone also avoids sexual side effects, and anxious patients may benefit from its sedative properties. Fulminant hepatotoxicity has led to a black box warning. In a recent 12-week open trial in 15 HIV-positive outpatients, nefazodone was demonstrated to have a high rate of efficacy regardless of HIV-related immunosuppression or stage of illness; 73% of the patients were found to be responders, and few adverse effects were noted (Elliot et al. 1999). However, there is potential interaction between nefazodone and several protease inhibitors. For example, because they are both substrates for the cytochromes 3A4 and 2D6, nefazodone is contraindicated with ritonavir because of the risk of a dose-related toxicity (Elliot et al. 1999).

Mirtazapine (Remeron). Mirtazapine has a side effect profile that can be beneficial in HIV patients by promoting weight gain, decreasing nausea, and producing sedation that may help insomnia (Elliot and Roy-Byrne 2000).

Tricyclic antidepressants. Although the SSRIs have largely replaced TCAs as first-line antidepressants, there is a literature on the effectiveness of TCAs for HIV-infected individuals. Their side effect profile limits them, however. TCAs rely principally on cytochrome 2D6 for clearance, so if they are coadministered with protease inhibitors (which inhibit this isoenzyme), one must pay particular attention to monitoring the ECG (to detect potential delayed cardiac conduction) and plasma levels of the TCA. Patients with advanced disease have more severe side effects and make fewer therapeutic gains with TCAs than do healthier HIV-infected individuals. The highly anticholinergic TCAs, such as amitriptyline (Elavil, Endep) and imipramine (Tofranil), should be avoided in cognitively impaired or demented HIV patients because they will worsen confusion. Nortriptyline (Aventyl, Pamelor) and desipramine (Norpramin) minimize anticholinergic side effects; nortriptyline produces fewer problems with orthostatic hypotension. (See also the section on TCAs in Chapter 3, "The Patient With Cardiovascular Disease.")

Psychostimulants. Psychostimulants, which are discussed in the section on HADC, are effective in depressed HIV-positive patients, particularly when symptoms of fatigue, apathy, withdrawal, anorexia, and neurocognitive impairment are prominent. They are especially helpful for producing a rapid antidepressant effect, particularly when psychomotor retardation interferes with the patient's medical care (Pereira and Bruera 2001) (e.g., when the patient cannot cooperate with physical therapy or is too fatigued to get out of bed). Note that the stimulants usually improve appe-

1. **PSYCHOSIS**

DDx:
Assume secondary psychotic disorder (see Appendix. 4, "VINDICTIVE MADS")	**NOTES** (avoid anticholinergic meds like diphenhydramine)

Assume secondary psychotic disorder
(see Appendix. 4, "VINDICTIVE MADS")

Consider: 1st: Delirium
            2nd: Dementia (HADC)
            3rd: Other etiologies
Last: Primary psychiatric etiology

NOTES (avoid anticholinergic meds like diphenhydramine)
➤ For EPS: amantadine (Symmetrel) is less anticholinergic
   than benztropine (Cogentin) or trihexyphenidyl (Artane),
   but it is a dopamine agonist & may precipate delusions; monitor!

Rx:
Avoid conventional (e.g., haloperidol) or depot neuroleptics because of ↑ sensitivity to EPS and NMS
Atypical agents are preferred ("start low, go slow")

2. **HADC Fatigue**

DDx:
Assume medical causes of fatigue
(see Appendix 4, "VINDICTIVE MADS")

Consider: 1st: Delirium (hypoactive)
            2nd: Dementia (HADC)
            3rd: Other etiologies

NOTES
➤ Also consider whether patient has coexisting mood disorder,
   such as depression

Rx:
Psychostimulants e.g., methylphenidate 5 mg bid before 1 P.M., slowly titrate upward
   (increase by 5 mg every 1–2 days until a good response occurs, or dose-limiting side effects occur)
   (may also use the sustained-release formulation for longer therapeutic effect)

3. **DEPRESSION**

DDx:
Assume secondary mood disorder
(see Appendix 4, "VINDICTIVE MADS")

Consider: 1st: Delirium (e.g., hypoactive)
            2nd: Dementia (HADC)
            3rd: Other etiologies
Last: Primary psychiatric etiology

Primary psychiatric etiologies:
Adjustment disorder with depressed mood
Major depressive episode, unipolar
Bipolar disorder, depressed phase
Dysthymic dirsorder
Bereavement; anger; despondency; demoralization

Rx (1st Line):
SSRIs
➤ Side effects: GI, dry mouth, headache, anxiety: usually subside 7–10 days after dose increase
➤ Dose-dependent: decreased libido, problems with erection, orgasm

Venlafaxine: few interactions with HIV meds; nausea may be a problem, so start at 37.5 mg XR preparation
Bupropion: activation useful for apathy & fatigue; no sexual side effects; ritonavir may cause toxicity, so avoid
   combination if possible; OK to use with other antivirals

Rx (2nd Line):
Nefazodone: no sexual side effects; sedation may be helpful; but many drug-drug interactions
   Black box warning about hepatoxicity

Monitor:
WATCH FOR SEROTONIN SYNDROME! (see Appendix 7)
Monitor for additive toxicity (e.g., trazodone for sleep, buspirone for anxiety, triptans for migraine)

Protease inhibitors (esp. ritonavir) will tend to increase psychotropic blood levels.
➤ When adding a psychotropic to a protease inhibitor: *Start low, go slow.*
➤ When adding a protease inhibitor to a psychotropic: *Decrease psychotropic.*

Figure 9–3.   Summary of psychopharmacology for HIV and AIDS patients.
Abbreviations: AZT=zidovudine; CBC=complete blood count; DDx=differential diagnosis; EPS=extrapyramidal symptoms; GI=gastrointestinal; HADC=HIV-associated dementia complex; HIV=human immunodeficiency virus; NMS=neuroleptic malignant syndrome; SSRIs=selective serotonin reuptake inhibitors.

4. **MANIA**

DDx: Assume secondary mood disorder
(see Appendix 4, "VINDICTIVE MADS")
Consider: 1st: Delirium
2nd: Dementia (HADC)
3rd: Other etiologies
Last: Bipolar disorder, manic phase

NOTES
➤ Prevalence increases with HIV disease progression
  ➤ Late-onset mania: patients usually have HADC & 2° mood disorder no personal or family history of mood disorder
  ➤ Early-onset mania: patients more closely resemble patients with 1° mood disorder, usually have personal or family history of mood disorder; no comorbid HADC

Rx: **Divalproex sodium (Depakote):** 250–500 mq PO HS initially, ↑ 250 mq/day q2–4 days until symptomatic control; monitor blood levels, liver function, CBC, especially platelets. Safely used with antiretrovirals, does not alter their metabolism, but ↑ AZT levels.

Lamotrigine, gabapentin, clonazepam: safe in HIV patients; not very helpful in acute mania

With caution: **Lithium:** toxicity, including encephalopathy, occurs at normal therapeutic blood levels; poor oral intake, diarrhea & vomiting ↑ toxicity
Carbamazepine: unknown safety in HIV; risk of bone marrow toxicity; may ↓ protease inhibitor levels, with loss of viral suppression

Figure 9–3. Summary of psychopharmacology for HIV and AIDS patients. *(continued)*

tite in anorexic, fatigued medical patients. In addition, psychostimulants potentiate the effects of narcotic analgesics, reduce narcotic requirements, and oppose the CNS-depressant effect of narcotics. However, psychosis is a possible side effect due to dopamine agonism, especially in patients with primary psychotic disorders such as schizophrenia. Avoid psychostimulants, or use them judiciously, in patients with a history of substance use (particularly amphetamine abuse).

Electroconvulsive therapy. ECT has been administered safely in the setting of HIV and AIDS (American Psychiatric Association 2001).

■ MANIA

Differential Diagnosis

Differential diagnosis of mania in the setting of HIV is as follows: delirium (brain failure); mood disorder due to HADC; effects of medications (especially steroids, antiretroviral medications), illicit drugs, or alcohol withdrawal states; bipolar disorder, manic phase.

Primary Manic Syndromes

Primary manic syndromes are more likely to occur in the context of an established personal or family history of bipolar disorder.

Secondary Manic Syndromes

Secondary manic syndromes, known as HIV-associated mania or "AIDS mania," often result from direct HIV infection of the brain or the multiple infectious, metabolic, neoplastic, and pharmacologic insults to the brain occurring with HIV disease (Mijch et al. 1999; Robinson and Qaqish 2002). Secondary mania is a distinct clinical entity. Although primary mania in an HIV patient would not necessarily correlate with illness variables, AIDS mania usually occurs late in the course of the illness and often correlates with AIDS dementia and structural changes on brain MRI (Angelino and Treisman 2001). Patients with AIDS mania are less likely to have family history of bipolar disorder. They present with more irritability than euphoria, are less overly talkative, and have more psychomotor slowing and cognitive impairment compared with the presentation of primary mania. Secondary mania also takes a more chronic course, with fewer spontaneous episodes of remission and more frequent relapses (Mijch et al. 1999). Antiretroviral medications (particularly zidovudine, didanosine, and efavirenz), neoplasms, and opportunistic infections of the CNS (such as cryptococcal meningitis) also have been implicated in causing secondary mania (DuPont Pharmaceuticals 1998; Ellen et al. 1999).

• *Bottom line:* New-onset mania in an HIV-infected patient should signal a workup for a medical etiology.

Treatment

Primary Mania

The treatment of primary manic syndromes in HIV-infected patients is similar to that in other medically ill patients. Mood stabilizers such as lithium, valproic acid, and carbamazepine are useful, as are neuroleptic medications, especially atypical neuroleptics like risperidone. However, specific side effects must be considered, as discussed below.

Neuroleptics.   Antipsychotics are useful in treating mania in the setting of HIV (Ellen et al. 1999). Neuroleptics seem to reduce symptoms faster than mood stabilizers or sedatives. Monotherapy is preferred to avoid multiple drug interactions (Angelino and Treisman 2001; Ferrando and Wapenyi 2002). (See the preceding section on preferred antipsychotic agents.)

Lithium.   Usually the gold standard for treating bipolar illness, lithium is poorly tolerated by AIDS patients. Dehydration due to severe diarrhea (e.g., such as occurs in cryptosporidial infection, CMV enteritis, or colitis), poor intake, or vomiting can precipitate lithium toxicity. In addition, HIV nephropathy may also reduce lithium clearance. Even at normal therapeutic blood levels, cognitively impaired patients may become delirious on lithium, complicating their medical and psychiatric management (Angelino and Treisman 2001). If possible, alternative mood stabilizers should be used.

Valproic acid (Depakote, Depakene).   Valproic acid is an effective, usually well tolerated mood stabilizer in this population. Starting doses should be around 250–500 mg at night, increased every 2–4 days until achieving symptomatic control. Baseline liver function tests are necessary, as valproic acid has been associated with non-dose-related hepatic failure. Remaining alert for clinical signs of hepatoxicity is considered more relevant than routine laboratory monitoring of liver enzymes, which has little predictive value. The divalproex sodium (Depakote) preparation has fewer gastrointestinal side effects such as dyspepsia or nausea. Significant weight gain, which would be helpful in cachectic patients, occurs commonly, independent of dose. Valproic acid has been associated with changes in platelet counts, but clinically significant thrombocytopenia is rare. Valproic acid is relatively contraindicated in patients with hepatitis or liver disease; if it is used in this population, it must be with the ongoing consultation of a gastroenterologist. Of some concern are reports that valproic acid can stimulate HIV replication in vitro; although this has not yet

proven to be clinically significant, some recommend closer viral load monitoring (Robinson and Qaqish 2002).

Carbamazepine (Tegretol).   Carbamazepine causes induction of 1A2, 2C9, 2C19, and, most significantly, 3A4, potentially lowering serum levels of protease inhibitors and thus producing loss of viral suppression (Cozza et al. 2003). It is associated with the potential for neutropenia, anemia, and thrombocytopenia. Alternatives to this medication are preferable.

Gabapentin (Neurontin).   Of limited value in acute mania, gabapentin is renally excreted and is usually well tolerated. It has anxiolytic and sedative properties, with few drug-drug interactions.

Clonazepam (Klonopin).   Also of limited value in acute mania, clonazepam is a benzodiazepine without active metabolites that is useful for sedation. It undergoes only part of its metabolism via 3A4 and then is acetylated (Cozza et al. 2003). Parenchymal liver disease does not directly affect its metabolism.

Lamotrigine (Lamictal).   Of limited value as monotherapy in acute mania, lamotrigine is gaining use as an add-on agent or for hypomania. It has been tested mainly in the context of HIV-associated neuropathic pain, where it appears to be well tolerated and effective for patients receiving neurotoxic antiretroviral therapy (Simpson et al. 2003). There has been only one case in the literature of prolonged hypersensitivity syndrome related to lamotrigine in a patient with HIV (Beller and Boyce 2002).

Topiramate (Topamax).   No reports of use in HIV were located.

Secondary Mania

There has been little independent research on treatment specifically of secondary mania as distinguished from primary mania in this population. The side effects of the traditional mood stabilizers are magnified by the fragility of the patients, who often have advanced disease. Low-dose, high-potency neuroleptics and atypical neuroleptics (e.g., risperidone and olanzapine) appear to be effective (Robinson and Qaqish 2002). Because secondary mania is connected with the progression of HIV disease, antiretrovirals with good CNS penetration may prove to be protective against secondary mania, resulting in significant improvement. With the widespread use of HAART, the incidence of HIV-associated mania appears to be declining (Ferrando and Wapenyi 2002). Mania is less likely

to recur once viral load is reduced to undetectable levels or if cryptococcal meningitis is successfully treated (Cohen and Jacobson 2000).

ANXIETY AND ADJUSTMENT DISORDERS

Anxiety disorders and anxiety symptoms are fairly common in the HIV spectrum. In a large, nationally representative study of adults receiving care for HIV infection, the prevalence of generalized anxiety disorder was estimated at 15.8%, and the prevalence of panic attacks was 10.8% (Bing et al. 2001; Penzak et al. 2001). Not surprisingly, patients with HIV report more anxiety symptoms than HIV-negative patients (Sewell et al. 2000).

Differential Diagnosis

The differential diagnosis of anxiety states in an HIV-infected person should include the following: delirium, agitation due to HADC, substance-induced reactions (medications, illicit drugs, and alcohol withdrawal states), mood disorders (major depressive disorder, bipolar disorder), anxiety disorders (generalized anxiety disorder, panic disorder, obsessive-compulsive disorder), and adjustment disorders.

Anxiety usually accompanies other psychiatric conditions, such as adjustment disorders or major depression. Secondary anxiety reactions may be precipitated by medications, such as antiviral therapy—particularly zidovudine, efavirenz (Lochet et al. 2003), abacavir (Colebunders et al. 2002), and indinavir (Harry et al. 2000)—and steroids. Patients should also be screened for withdrawal from narcotics, alcohol, and other psychoactive substances. *Drug withdrawal reactions are likely to occur early in a hospitalization and may mimic anxiety reactions.*

Patients with HIV-related neurocognitive impairment often retain insight about their physical deterioration. Adjustment disorders occur quite frequently, prompted by the succession of stressors and losses. Note that the early stages of delirium may resemble adjustment disorders; both may present with irritability, anxiety, tearfulness, agitation, and insomnia.

AIDS Anxiety Versus AIDS Phobia

Realistic worry about AIDS may overlap with phobic anxiety. In the mid-1980s, a subgroup of medically healthy individuals who were anxious about having

AIDS was dubbed the "worried well" (Forstein 1984). These patients had HIV risk factors but remained convinced of infection despite negative medical findings, including serological testing. The "worried well" remained chronically ruminative about HIV infection despite counseling, physical examination, and repeated negative antibody screening. They were unshakably convinced that certain somatic complaints were due to HIV, and complained of nonspecific somatic symptoms (e.g., fatigue, sweating, skin rashes, muscle pains, diarrhea, "swollen glands," sore throat, slight weight loss, dizziness). This conviction has been framed as an anxiety disorder, termed *AIDS phobia* (Harrell and Wright 1998).

The "worried well" often exhibit obsessive-compulsive symptomatology concerning AIDS contagion and death, guilt over high-risk sexual practices, and preoccupation with the dirtiness or infectivity of body fluid. Their distress can be functionally debilitating. Frequent trips to a primary care physician for reassurance and repeated antibody testing are common.

The psychiatric differential diagnosis includes obsessive-compulsive disorder, delusional disorder with somatic symptoms, hypochondriasis, Munchausen's syndrome (factitious disorder), and affective disorders.

Treatment

In addition to the recommendations below, see Chapter 1, "The Delirious Patient," and Chapter 5, "The Patient With Pulmonary Disease," on managing anxiolytic treatment in patients with pulmonary opportunistic infections such as tuberculosis or *Pneumocistis carinii* pneumonia.

Benzodiazepines

Benzodiazepines are useful for the short-term treatment of acute anxiety in this population. Complications include the potential for respiratory depression in patients with respiratory insufficiency, and especially with long-acting benzodiazepines. Lorazepam (Ativan) is usually the "as-needed" benzodiazepine of choice for acute anxiety, given its intermediate half-life, flexibility of administration, and absence of active metabolites. Many patients also do well on buspirone (BuSpar), which must be taken regularly, not prn. In order to limit tolerance and abuse potential, SSRIs remain first-line agents for chronic anxiety disorders.

- Alprazolam (Xanax), diazepam (Valium), midazolam (Versed), and triazolam (Halcion) are significantly inhibited by certain protease inhibitors (ritonavir and amprenavir) (Greenblatt et al. 2000a, 2000b; McNicholl and Peiperl 2003) and nonnucleoside reverse transcriptase inhibitors (efavirenz and delavirdine) (McNicholl and Peiperl 2003; von Moltke et al. 2001) through the cytochrome 3A4 system, potentially leading to respiratory insufficiency, depressive symptoms, fatigue, and cognitive-motor side effects in vulnerable patients (e.g., those with HIV dementia, MCMD, intracranial lesions, or delirium). It is best to avoid these anxiolytics.

- Lorazepam (Ativan), oxazepam (Serax), and temazepam (Restoril) bypass oxidative metabolism, thereby avoiding interactions with antiretrovirals. These agents also have the advantage of short to intermediate half-lives.
- When agitation approaches panic or accompanies delusions, neuroleptic medication may be helpful (Fernandez and Levy 1994). Atypical antipsychotics are also favored over benzodiazepines (which may have a disinhibiting effect) for patients in the early stages of delirium and those with HADC accompanied by anxiety or restlessness (see Chapter 1, "The Delirious Patient").

Buspirone (BuSpar)

Buspirone is well tolerated and has a low risk for drug reactions, with only rare case reports of problems associated with the setting of HIV (Clay and Adams 2003; Trachman 1992). Fernandez and Levy (1994) found that buspirone was best tolerated by patients who either were asymptomatic or had limited disease. When buspirone was coadministered with zidovudine, patients on lower doses of zidovudine (<300 mg/day) fared better. These patients typically required buspirone in the higher therapeutic range (45–60 mg/day).

SSRIs

The starting dosages of SSRIs for anxiety disorders are lower than for depression. Some protease inhibitors, especially ritonavir, are inhibitors of 2D6 and 3A4, which are responsible for metabolism of most SSRIs. Check for potential drug-drug interactions that might result in increased serum levels of antidepressants (Farber and McDaniel 2002; Karasic and Dilley 2003).

Trazodone (Desyrel)

Anxious HIV patients with neuropsychiatric and/or neuromuscular complications have been found to re-

spond well to trazodone in low doses (25–200 mg/day in divided doses) without adverse side effects (Fernandez and Levy 1994). Unlike buspirone, which has no immediate sedative effect, trazodone has a quick-sedating and relaxing effect, mimicking that of the benzodiazepines, but without respiratory depression or the risk of habituation. Notably, ritonavir impairs the metabolism of trazodone and leads to increased sedation, fatigue, and performance impairment (Greenblatt et al. 2003). Orthostatic hypotension and priapism in males are potential adverse side effects.

Antihistamines

Antihistamines such as diphenhydramine (Benadryl) and hydroxyzine (Vistaril, Atarax) are mild anxiolytics, but they should be avoided in the setting of cognitive vulnerability or delirium because they are anticholinergic and may exacerbate cognitive problems.

■ INSOMNIA

Alterations in sleep architecture occur in asymptomatic, seropositive patients and include decreased sleep efficiency, increased stage 1 shifts, and increased amounts of slow-wave sleep in the second half of the night (Norman et al. 1988, 1992; White et al. 1995). It has been suggested that immune dysregulation and/or cytokines, such as tumor necrosis factor-alpha or interleukin-1-beta, disrupt sleep in persons with HIV/AIDS (Darko et al. 1998). However, other factors may also contribute to insomnia, such as viral progression, infection, fatigue, mood disorders, psychological stress, drug side effects, and environmental disruption (e.g., HAART's rigid schedules). Psychological distress may affect the immune system because of its effects on sleep quality (Cruess et al. 2003).

Often, the underlying causes of HIV-related insomnia are not correctable. Treatment should start by correcting potentially reversible, secondary causes and using behavioral interventions, such as improving sleep hygiene, regulating sleep-wake cycles, and relaxation techniques (Reite et al. 2002). Many medications used to treat HIV/AIDS disturb sleep and cannot be discontinued. It is particularly important to eliminate other sleep-disrupting substances, such as alcohol, caffeine, nicotine, or drugs of abuse.

Sedative-hypnotics (benzodiazepine and nonbenzodiazepine) can be prescribed in this population as needed (Halman et al. 2002). There is a small but distinct risk of priapism in males taking trazodone. Although short-term medication management is the usual goal, the benefits of medically supervised, long-term hypnotic treatment sometimes outweigh the risks because persistent insomnia undermines quality of life. See Appendix 13, "Commonly Used Drugs With Sedative-Hypnotic Properties," in this volume.

DECISIONS ABOUT TREATMENT TERMINATION

Consulting psychiatrists regularly encounter HIV patients who are refusing medical treatment, bringing into question the patient's capacity to make rational, informed decisions about his or her medical care. The potential for HADC complicates this assessment. Accurate decisional capacity and suicide assessments are crucial. However, many ethical issues are specific to the patient learning to live with HIV and AIDS and have been detailed by other authors (Anderson and Barret 2001; Bennett and Erin 2001; Bonde 2001; Kopp 2003).

• *Caution:* Thoughts about rational suicide can be expected throughout the course of serious illnesses like AIDS. However, depression affects decision making about rational suicide; a classic study showed that clinically depressed patients who were refusing life-sustaining interventions changed their minds when depression resolved, even though the medical prognosis had not changed (Fogel and Mor 1993). Mood disorders should be carefully considered when evaluating the patient's decision-making capacity. (Chapter 12 in this volume presents some of the basic issues in assessing decisional capacity in medical patients.)

SUICIDE

Estimates of the suicide rate vary across studies of individuals who are HIV-positive and those who have frank AIDS. Before antiretroviral treatments existed in the 1980s, reported rates of completed suicide in HIV-positive patients were as high as 36 times that of the general population (Marzuk et al. 1988). However, more recent data demonstrate only modestly elevated suicide rates, comparable with those of other medically ill populations. For example, in a study of suicide victims among New York City residents in the early 1990s, almost 9% were HIV-positive; after demo-graphic adjustment, these estimates suggested that a positive HIV serostatus confers a twofold-higher risk for suicide (Marzuk et al. 1997). This finding was similar to the twofold-higher risk of suicide among HIV-positive military applicants (Dannenberg et al. 1996).

The following have been linked to suicide risk in HIV-positive patients (Kelly et al. 1998): substance abuse; major depressive disorder; previous suicide attempts; family psychiatric history; family history of attempted suicide; and antisocial personality disorder. Psychosocial factors such as decline in physical functioning, a history of multiple HIV-related losses, lack of social support, and financial losses have also been linked to suicide risk.

OTHER FACTORS AFFECTING HIV

Psychological Factors: The Knowledge–Behavior Gap

Many investigations with different sample populations have supported the same discouraging finding: increased knowledge of high-risk sexual behavior does not necessarily translate into meaningful reduction in risky behaviors (Brathwaite 2001; Butts and Hartman 2002; Levounis et al. 2002). Why?

The following summaries may be useful in your consultations:

• Box 9–2. "Assessing HIV Risk Behavior: A Checklist of Behaviors and Attitudes"
• Table 9–7. "Risk of HIV Transmission Associated With Various Sexual Activities"
• Chapter 13. "Psychological Issues in Medical Patients: Autonomy, Fatalism, and Adaptation to Illness"
• Chapter 14. "When Patients Ask About the Spiritual: A Primer"

Highly Active Antiretroviral Therapy

One unexpected culprit in the persistence of risky behaviors is HAART, which in some ways has limited its own efficacy. Optimism and misunderstanding about HAART account for a decline in safe sex practices. For example, unprotected anal intercourse in men who have sex with men has increased according to some reports, accompanied by a parallel increase in the annual HIV incidence in this population, particularly in young men. Those more likely to report unprotected sex implicate HAART for reducing their concern about becoming infected (Ostrow 2002).

Table 9–7.   Risk of HIV transmission associated with various sexual activities

Risk level	Sexual activity
No risk	Dry kissing Body-to-body rubbing (frottage) Massage Nipple stimulation Using unshared inserted sexual devices Being masturbated by partner without semen or vaginal fluids Erotic bathing and showering Contact with feces or urine on intact skin
Theoretical risk	Wet kissing Cunnilingus with barrier Anilingus ("rimming") Digital-anal and digital-vaginal intercourse, with or without glove Using shared but disinfected inserted sexual devices
Low risk	Sharing undisinfected personal hygiene items (razors, toothbrushes) Cunnilingus without barrier during or outside of menstruation Fellatio and ejaculation, with or without ingestion of semen Fellatio, with or without condom Penile-vaginal intercourse with condom Penile-anal intercourse with condom
High risk	Penile-vaginal intercourse without condom Penile-anal intercourse without condom Coitus interruptus (intercourse with withdrawal before ejaculation)

Source.   Adapted from American Psychiatric Association: "Practice Guideline for the Treatment of Patients With HIV/AIDS." *American Journal of Psychiatry* 157:1–62, 2000. (Available at: http://www.psych.org/aids.)

Another study assessing the impact of HIV treatment advances on HIV-seropositive individuals demonstrated the following erroneous beliefs: that AIDS is less of a health risk than before (33% of subjects); that HAART reduces the risk of HIV transmission (15%); that there is now less need to observe safe sex practices (10%). About one-fourth of the sample practiced safer sex significantly less often since HAART was introduced (Demmer 2002).

Finally, HAART has been associated with adverse side effects, which may reduce the motivation of affected individuals to adhere to its rigid regimen (Duran et al. 2001; Proctor et al. 1999). The lipodystrophy syndrome (LDS) is characterized by the redistribution of body fat and by metabolic abnormalities. Patients develop a characteristic body habitus, consisting of truncal obesity (including a dorsocervical fat pad, or "buffalo hump," and enlargement of the breasts) and peripheral wasting (of arms, legs, buttocks, and particularly noticeable in the face). There is no treatment. Many patients are upset by LDS, particularly when it affects the face. Patients often feel that LDS "advertises" their positive serostatus, impinging on their privacy. Many LDS patients report feeling more stigma-

tized, particularly in communities that correctly "read" the underlying etiology for the changes (Oette et al. 2002; Riley 2002). One study described the shock, depression, isolation, and rejection experienced by LDS patients, accompanied by efforts to conceal or alter their appearance to reduce stigmatization (Riley 2002). Many study subjects felt that their health care providers were not sufficiently empathic with their predicament.

Sociocultural Factors

Culture and Attitude

The attitudes toward a particular illness are often culturally determined and psychologically fixed, and they may be maintained independently of factual knowledge. The concept of autonomy relative to illness first appeared in the research literature as "health locus of control" (HLOC) (Wallston et al. 1978). An "internally directed" system drives the individual who takes responsibility for his or her health and believes that personal actions have an impact. An "externally directed" system occurs in the fatalistic person who believes that health and illness are influenced by sources beyond personal control (e.g., fate, chance, or other people). Assessments of HLOC are strong independent predictors of health-related behaviors, such as acquiring AIDS knowledge, with high "externality" associated with less knowledge (Aruffo et al. 1993). (For further discussion of psychological issues pertaining to health-related behavior, see Chapter 13.)

Culture and Lifestyle

Culture also influences behavior and attitudes toward sex, and therefore potential vulnerability to HIV infection. In addition, denial and disavowal of personal medical risk often attaches itself to "the other guy." Some people imagine that "somebody else" will get lung cancer from smoking or die from driving drunk; they are immune. Vulnerability to HIV may be displaced onto stigmatized groups, such as injection drug users or men who have sex with men, or fantasized to be limited to the distant continents of Africa and Asia. This is a bit like bird-watching on the good ship Titanic: HIV infection continues to spread, and unfortunately it is here to stay for all of us.

Summaries of this important research area sometimes risk generating the very stereotypes we seek to avoid. To do it justice would require a separate textbook. A few examples may suffice.

Intracultural homophobia. Although homophobia is by no means exclusive to these cultures, African American and Latino men who have sex with men face particular taboos against male-to-male sexuality within their culture. Cooperating with or receiving services from the supportive gay, predominantly white community may be perceived as a racial betrayal (Denizet-Lewis 2003). A man facing this type of sociocultural bias might adapt by pursuing a double life: marriage to a woman to save cultural face; covert sexual relationships with men for gratification. Clearly, this type of behavior has an impact on the epidemiology of HIV in the female partners of these men (see Denizet-Lewis 2003).

Racial bias. Culture mediates sexual attitudes as well. Country of birth (U.S.-born or immigrated) predicts differences in the sexual practices among men of the same ethnic background, such as marital status while engaging in covert sex with other men (Diaz et al. 1993). In a classic early study, the perception of risk was partially related to the race of the sexual partner, with nonwhite race conferring the illusion of less risk (Peterson and Marin 1988). It is now recognized that

there are special HIV prevention needs for men of color who have sex with men (MSM) and those who have sex with men and women (MSM/W). It is important to be familiar with at least three key areas in HIV prevention research for this population: 1) social, contextual, and cultural factors and their relationship to increased risk behaviors among MSM and MSM/W; 2) characteristics of MSM and MSM/W of color that place them at risk for HIV; and 3) HIV prevention strategies targeting MSM and MSM/W of color (Brooks et al. 2003). (See also National Minority AIDS Council, http://www.nmac.org. Accesed July 2004.)

Gender. Gender differences affect perception about prevention. For example, the female condom (FC) is potentially a highly effective method for preventing the spread of HIV and other sexually transmitted diseases. Studies have shown that FC-focused interventions significantly increase condom use among women at high risk for HIV infection (Hardwick 2002). However, there are attitudinal problems for some women concerning the use of FCs, related to aesthetics, previous difficulties with the male condom, anticipated reactions by a male partner, and doubts about efficacy (Hirky et al. 2003). Efforts are under way to develop vaginal microbicides to create a chemical barrier to prevent the virus from getting to or infecting its target cells. This would create a female-controlled HIV prevention technology, especially for women who cannot induce their partners to use condoms.

Comment: Studies of public health interventions have found greater effectiveness when programs are culturally appropriate and gender-tailored, particularly with high-risk populations (e.g., female crack cocaine users with paying sex partners [Sterk et al. 2003]). These findings have immediate relevance for the consulting physician: If doctor and patient are from discordant ethnocultural backgrounds, assume that cultural differences may play a role in the patient's perception of risk, sexuality, and illness. Do some research; ask for help from other knowledgeable professionals from the same background as the patient. Better yet, ask the patient to explain to you. ("I'm interested in learning more. Could you help me understand how people from your country/culture think about…? Is it ever acceptable to…," etc.) Generic interventions or interviews based on the majority culture or on ethnic stereotypes are primed to fail.

The Center for AIDS Prevention Studies at the University of California–San Francisco provides fact sheets that help update clinical knowledge and are appropriate for distributing to patients. Fact sheets are available in English and Spanish, and selected ones are available in Kiswahili (http://www.caps.ucsf.edu/FS-index.html; accessed July 2004). A partial list of topics: What are the HIV prevention needs of…Women? Women who have sex with women? Men who have sex with women? Men who have sex with men? Young men who have sex with men? Adolescents? Young women? Adults over 50? African Americans? U.S. Latinos? Asian and Pacific Islanders? American Indian and Alaskan Natives?

■ REFERENCES

American Psychiatric Association: Diagnostic and Statistical Manual of Mental Disorders, 4th Edition, Text Revision. Washington, DC, American Psychiatric Association, 2000a

American Psychiatric Association: Practice Guideline for the Treatment of Patients With HIV/AIDS. Am J Psychiatry 157:1–62 (http://www.psych.org/aids), 2000b

American Psychiatric Association: The Practice of Electroconvulsive Therapy: Recommendations for Treatment, Training, and Privileging. A Task Force Report of the American Psychiatric Association. Washington, DC, American Psychiatric Association, 2001

Anderson J, Barret R (eds): Ethics in HIV-Related Psychotherapy: Clinical Decision Making in Complex Cases. Washington, DC, American Psychological Association, 2001

Angelino A, Treisman G: Management of psychiatric disorders in patients infected with human immunodeficiency virus. Clin Infect Dis 33:847–856, 2001

Aruffo J, Coverdale J, Pavlik V, et al: AIDS knowledge in minorities: significance of locus of control. Am J Prev Med 9:15–20, 1993

Bartholow B, Doll L, Joy D, et al: Emotional, behavioral and HIV risks associated with sexual abuse among adult homosexual and bisexual men. Child Abuse Negl 9:747–761, 1994

Beckett A, Summergrad P, Manschreck T, et al: Symptomatic HIV infection of the CNS in a patient without clinical evidence of immune deficiency. Am J Psychiatry 144:1342–1343, 1987

Beller TC, Boyce JA: Prolonged anticonvulsant hypersensitivity syndrome related to lamotrigine in a patient with human immunodeficiency virus. Allergy Asthma Proc 23:415–419, 2002

Bennett R, Erin C (eds): HIV and AIDS: Testing, Screening, and Confidentiality (Issues in Biomedical Ethics). New York, Oxford University Press, 2001

Berghuis J, Uldall K, Lalonde B: Validity of two scales in identifying HIV-associated dementia. J Acquir Immune Defic Syndr Hum Retrovirol 21:134–140, 1999

Bing E, Burnam M, Longshore D, et al: Psychiatric disorders and drug use among human immunodeficiency virus-infected adults in the United States. Arch Gen Psychiatry 58:721–728, 2001

Boccellari A, Zeifert P: Management of neurobehavioral impairment in HIV-1 infection. Psychiatr Clin North Am 17:183–203, 1994

Bonde L: The effects of grief and loss on decision making in HIV-related psychotherapy, in Ethics in HIV-Related Psychotherapy: Clinical Decision Making in Complex Cases. Edited by Anderson JR, Barret B. Washington, DC, American Psychological Association, 2001, pp 83–98

Brathwaite K: HIV/AIDS Knowledge, Attitudes, and Risk-Behaviors Among African-American and Caribbean College Women. Int J Adv Couns 23:115–129, 2001

Breitbart W, Rosenfeld B, Kaim M, et al: A randomized, double-blind, placebo-controlled trial of psychostimulants for the treatment of fatigue in ambulatory patients with human immunodeficiency virus disease. Arch Intern Med 161:411–420, 2001

Brooks R, Rotheram-Borus MJ, Bing EG, et al: HIV and AIDS among men of color who have sex with men and men of color who have sex with men and women: an epidemiological profile. AIDS Educ Prev 15:1–6, 2003

Buhrich N, Cooper D, Freed E: HIV infection associated with symptoms indistinguishable from functional psychosis. Br J Psychiatry 152:649–653, 1988

Butts JB, Hartman S: Project BART: effectiveness of a behavioral intervention to reduce HIV risk in adolescents. MCN Am J Matern Child Nurs 27:163–169, 2002

Catz SL, Gore-Felton C, McClure JB: Psychological distress among minority and low-income women living with HIV. Behav Med 28:53–59, 2002

Centers for Disease Control and Prevention: HIV AIDS Surveill Rep 9:10, 1998

Centers for Disease Control and Prevention: U.S. HIV and AIDS cases reported through June 2001. HIV AIDS Surveill Rep 13, 2002

Chuck S, Rodvold K, von Moltke LL, et al: Pharmacokinetics of protease inhibitors and drug interactions with psychoactive drugs, in Psychological and Public Health Implications of New HIV Therapies. Edited by Ostrow D, Kalichman S. New York, Plenum, 1998, pp 33–60

Ciesla J, Roberts J: Meta-analysis of the relationship between HIV infection and risk for depressive disorders. Am J Psychiatry 158:725–730, 2001

Clay PG, Adams MM: Pseudo-Parkinson disease secondary to ritonavir-buspirone interaction. Ann Pharmacother 37:202–205, 2003

Cohen M, Jacobson J: Maximizing life's potentials in AIDS: a psychopharmacologic update. Gen Hosp Psychiatry 22:375–388, 2000

Colebunders R, Hilbrands R, De Roo A, et al: Neuropsychiatric reaction induced by abacavir (letter). Am J Med 113:616, 2002

Cournos F, McKinnon K, Rosner J: HIV among individuals with severe mental illness. Psychiatric Annals 31:50–56, 2001

Cozza KL, Armstrong SC, Oesterheld JR: Concise Guide to Drug Interaction Principles for Medical Practice: Cytochrome P450s, UGTs, P-Glycoproteins, 2nd Edition. Washington, DC, American Psychiatric Publishing, 2003

Cruess DG, Antoni MH, Gonzalez J, et al: Sleep disturbance mediates the association between psychological distress and immune status among HIV-positive men and women on combination antiretroviral therapy. J Psychosom Res 54:185–189, 2003

Currier M, Molina G, Kato M: A prospective trial of sustained-release bupropion for depression in HIV-seropositive and AIDS patients. Psychosomatics 44:120–125, 2003

Dannenberg A, McNeil J, Brundage J, et al: Suicide and HIV infection: mortality follow-up of 4,147 HIV-seropositive military service applicants. JAMA 276:1743–1746, 1996

Darko D, Mitler M, Miller J: Growth hormone, fatigue, poor sleep, and disability in HIV infection. Neuroendocrinology 67:317–324, 1998

Demmer C: Impact of improved treatments on perception about HIV+ safer sex among inner-city HIV-infected men and women. J Community Health 27:63–73, 2002

Denizet-Lewis B: Living (and dying) on the down low: double lives, AIDS, and the black homosexual underground. New York Times Magazine, August 3, 2003, pp 28–33, 48–53

Diaz T, Chu S, Frederick M, et al: Sociodemographics and HIV risk behaviors of bisexual men with AIDS: results from a multistate interview project. AIDS 7:1227–1232, 1993

Duggan J, Peterson WS, Schutz M, et al: Use of complementary and alternative therapies in HIV-infected patients. AIDS Patient Care STDS 15:159–167, 2001

DuPont Pharmaceuticals: Sustiva [efavirenz; product information]. Wilmington, DE, DuPont Pharmaceuticals, 1998

Duran S, Saves M, Spire B, et al: Failure to maintain long-term adherence to highly active antiretroviral therapy: the role of lipodystrophy. AIDS 15:2441–2444, 2001

Dybul M: Guidelines for using antiretroviral agents among HIV-infected adults and adolescents. Ann Intern Med 137:381–433, 2002

Ellen S, Judd F, Mijch A, et al: Secondary mania in patients with HIV infection. Aust N Z J Psychiatry 33:353–360, 1999

Elliot A, Roy-Byrne P: Mirtazapine for depression in patients with human immunodeficiency virus. J Clin Psychopharmacol 20:265–267, 2000

Elliot A, Russo J, Bergam K, et al: Antidepressant efficacy in HIV-seropositive outpatients with major depressive disorder: an open trial of nefazodone. J Clin Psychiatry 60:226–231, 1999

Farber E, McDaniel J: Clinical management of psychiatric disorders in patients with HIV disease. Psychiatr Q 73:5–16, 2002

Fauci A, Lane H: Human immunodeficiency virus—HIV disease: AIDS and related disorders, in Harrison's Principles of Internal Medicine, 15th Edition. Edited by Braunwald E, Fauci A, Kasper D. New York, McGraw-Hill Medical, 2001, pp 1852–1913

Fernandez F, Levy J: Psychopharmacology in HIV spectrum disorders. Psychiatr Clin North Am 17:135–148, 1994

Ferrando S, Wapenyi K: Psychopharmacological treatment of patients with HIV and AIDS. Psychiatr Q 73:33–48, 2002

Fogel B, Mor V: Depressed mood and care preferences in patients with AIDS. Gen Hosp Psychiatry 15:203–207, 1993

Forstein M: AIDS anxiety in the "worried well," in Psychiatric Implications of Acquired Immune Deficiency Syndrome. Edited by Nichols S, Ostrow D. Washington, DC, American Psychiatric Press, 1984, pp 50–60

Foster R, Olajide D, Everall I: Antiretroviral therapy-induced psychosis: case report and brief review of the literature. HIV Med 4:139–144, 2003

George T, Godleski L: Possible serotonin syndrome with trazodone addition to fluoxetine. Biol Psychiatry 39:383–386, 1996

Gnam W, Flint A, Goldbloom D: Isoniazid-induced hallucinosis: response to pyridoxine (letter). Psychosomatics 34:537–539, 1993

Goldberg R: Serotonin syndrome from trazodone and buspirone. Psychosomatics 35:235–236, 1992

Goodman LA, Fallot RD: HIV risk-behavior in poor urban women with serious mental disorders: association with childhood physical and sexual abuse. Am J Orthopsychiatry 68:73–83, 1998

Greenblatt D, von Moltke L, Harmatz J, et al: Alprazolam-ritonavir interaction: implications for product labeling. Clin Pharmacol Ther 67:335–341, 2000a

Greenblatt D, von Moltke L, Harmatz J, et al: Differential impairment of triazolam and zolpidem clearance by ritonavir. J Acquir Immune Defic Syndr 24:129–136, 2000b

Greenblatt D, von Moltke L, Harmatz J, et al: Short-term exposure to low-dose ritonavir impairs clearance and enhances adverse effects of trazodone. J Clin Pharmacol 43:414–422, 2003

Halevie-Goldman B, Potkin S, Poyourow P: AIDS-related complex presenting as psychosis (letter). Am J Psychiatry 144:964, 1987

Halman MH, Bialer P, Worth JL, et al: HIV disease/AIDS, in The American Psychiatric Publishing Textbook of Consultation-Liaison Psychiatry: Psychiatry in the Medically Ill, 2nd Edition. Edited by Wise MG, Rundell JR. Washington, DC, American Psychiatric Publishing, 2002, pp 807–851

Halstead S, Riccio M, Harlow P: Psychosis associated with HIV infection. Br J Psychiatry 153:618–623, 1988

Hardwick D: The effectiveness of a female condom intervention on women's use of condoms. Can J Hum Sex 11:63–76, 2002

Harrell J, Wright L: The development and validation of the Multicomponent AIDS Phobia Scale. Journal of Psychopathology and Behavioral Assessment 20:201–216, 1998

Harris M, Jeste D, Gleghorn A, et al: New-onset psychosis in HIV-infected patients. J Clin Psychiatry 52:369–376, 1991

Harry T, Matthews M, Salvari I: Indinavir use: associated reversible hair loss and mood disturbance. Int J STD AIDS 11:474–476, 2000

Hays R, Turner H, Coates T: Social support, AIDS-related symptoms, and depression among gay men. J Consult Clin Psychol 60:463–469, 1992

Heaton R, Grant I, Butters N, et al: The HNRC 500: neuropsychology of HIV infection at different disease stages. J Int Neuropsychol Soc 1:231–251, 1995

Hesse L, von Moltke L, Shader R, et al: Ritonavir, efavirenz, and nelfinavir inhibit CYP2B6 activity in vitro: potential drug interactions with bupropion. Drug Metab Dispos 29:100–102, 2001

Hirky A, Kirshenbaum SB, Melendez RM, et al: The female condom: attitudes and experiences among HIV-positive heterosexual women and men. Women Health 37:71–89, 2003

Holmes T, Sabaawi M, Fragala M: Psychostimulant suppository treatment for depression in the gravely ill (letter). J Clin Psychiatry 55:265–266, 1994

Holmes V: Treatment of monosymptomatic hypochondriacal psychosis with pimozide in an AIDS patient (letter). Am J Psychiatry 146:554–555, 1989

Hutton H, Treisman G, Fishman M, et al: HIV risk behaviors and their relationship to posttraumatic stress disorder among women prisoners. Psychiatr Serv 52:508–513, 2001

Jay C: Neurological manifestations of human immunodeficiency virus infection, in Neurology in Clinical Practice, 3rd Edition. Edited by Bradley W, Daroff R, Fenichel G, et al. Boston, MA, Butterworth-Heinemann, 2000, pp 1407–1422

Jones B, Teng E, Folstein M, et al: A new bedside test of cognition for patients with HIV infection. Ann Intern Med 119:1001–1004, 1993

Jover F, Cuadrado JM, Andreu L, et al: Reversible coma caused by risperidone-ritonavir interaction. Clin Neuropharmacol 25:251–253, 2002

Kalichman SC, Weinhardt L, DiFonzo K, et al: Sensation seeking and alcohol use as markers of sexual transmission risk behavior in HIV-positive men. Ann Behav Med 24:229–235, 2002

Karasic D, Dilley J: HIV-Associated Psychiatric Disorders. USCF HIV InSite Knowledge Base, 2003. Available at: http://hivinsite.ucsf.edu. Accessed May 1, 2003.

Kelly B, Raphael B, Judd F, et al: Psychiatric disorder in HIV infection. Aust N Z J Psychiatry 32:441–453, 1998

Kelly D, Beiqui L, Bowmer M: Extrapyramidal symptoms with ritonavir/indinavir plus risperidone. Ann Pharmacother 36:827–830, 2002

Kopp C: The New Era of AIDS: HIV and Medicine in Times of Transition (International Library of Ethics, Law, and the New Medicine, Vol 15). Dordrecht, The Netherlands, Kluwer Academic, 2003

Lagana L, Chen X, Koopman C, et al: Depressive symptomatology in relation to emotional control and chronic pain in persons who are HIV positive. Rehabil Psychol 47:402–414, 2002

Lee S, Klesmer J, Hirsch B: Neuroleptic malignant syndrome associated with use of risperidone, ritonavir and indinavir: a case report. Psychosomatics 41:453–454, 2000

Lenderking W, Wold C, Mayer K, et al: Childhood sexual abuse among homosexual men. Prevalence and association with unsafe sex. J Gen Intern Med 12:250–253, 1997

Levounis P, Galanter M, Dermatis H, et al: Correlates of HIV transmission risk factors and considerations for interventions in homeless, chemically addicted and mentally ill patients. J Addict Dis 21:61–72, 2002

Lochet P, Peyriere H, Lotthe A, et al: Long-term assessment of neuropsychiatric adverse reactions associated with efavirenz. HIV Med 4:62–66, 2003

Lyketsos CG, Hoover DR, Guccione M, et al: Changes in depressive symptoms as AIDS develops. The Multicenter AIDS Cohort Study. Am J Psychiatry 153:1430–1437, 1996

Maj M: Depressive syndromes and symptoms in subjects with human immunodeficiency virus (HIV) infection. Br J Psychiatry Suppl 30:117–122, 1996

Mandell W, Kim J, Latkin C, et al: Depressive symptoms, drug network, and their synergistic effect on needle-sharing behavior among street injection drug users. Am J Drug Alcohol Abuse 25:117–127, 1999

Marder K, Albert S, McDermott M: Prospective study of neurocognitive impairment in HIV (DANA cohort: dementia and mortality outcomes). DANA Consortium on Therapy for HIV Dementia and Related Disorders. J Neurovirol 4:358, 1998

Margolese HC, Chouinard G: Serotonin syndrome from addition of low-dose trazodone to nefazodone (letter). Am J Psychiatry 157:1022, 2000

Marzuk P, Tierney H, Tardiff K, et al: Increased risk for suicide in persons with AIDS. JAMA 259:1333–1337, 1988

Marzuk P, Tardiff K, Leon A, et al: HIV seroprevalence among suicide victims in New York City, 1991–1993. Am J Psychiatry 154:1720–1725, 1997

McKinnon K, Rosner J: Severe mental illness and HIV-AIDS. New Dir Ment Health Serv Fall (87):69–76, 2000

McKinnon K, Wainberg ML, Cournos F: HIV/AIDS preparedness in mental health care agencies with high and low substance use disorder caseloads. J Subst Abuse 13:127–135, 2001

McKinnon K, Cournos F, Herman R: HIV among people with chronic mental illness. Psychiatr Q 73:17–31, 2002

McNicholl I, Peiperl L: Database of Antiretroviral Drug Interactions. UCSF HIV InSite Knowledge Base. 2003. Available at: http://hivinsite.ucsf.edu. Accessed May 1, 2003.

Mijch A, Judd F, Lyketsos C, et al: Secondary mania in patients with HIV infection: are antiretrovirals protective? J Neuropsychiatry Clin Neurosci 11:475–480, 1999

Miller M: A model to explain the relationship between sexual abuse and HIV risk among women. AIDS Care 1:3–20, 1999

Navia B, Jordan B, Price R: The AIDS dementia complex, I: clinical features. Ann Neurol 19:517–524, 1986

Nisijima K, Shimizu M, Abe T, et al: A case of serotonin syndrome induced by concomitant treatment with low-dose trazodone and amitriptyline and lithium. Int Clin Psychopharmacol 11:289–290, 1996

Norman SE, Chediak AD, Freeman CA: Sleep disturbances in men with asymptomatic human immunodeficiency (HIV) infection. Sleep 15:150–155, 1992

Norman SE, Resnick L, Cohn MA, et al: Sleep disturbances in HIV-seropositive patients (letter). JAMA 260:922, 1988

Oette M, Juretzko P, Kroidl A, et al: Lipodystrophy syndrome and self-assessment of well-being and physical appearance in HIV-positive patients. AIDS Patient Care STDS 16:413–417, 2002

Ostrow D: Attitudes towards highly active antiretroviral therapy are associated with sexual risk taking among HIV-infected and uninfected homosexual men. AIDS 16:775–780, 2002

Penzak S, Lawhorn W, Hon Y, et al: Influence of ritonavir and CYP1A2 genotype on olanzapine disposition in healthy subjects (abstract #A-493). 41st Interscience Conference on Antimicrobial Agents and Chemotherapy, Chicago, IL, December 16–19, 2001

Pereira J, Bruera E: Depression with psychomotor retardation: diagnostic challenges and the use of psychostimulants. J Palliat Med 4:15–21, 2001

Perry S, Jacobsberg L, Card C, et al: Severity of psychiatric symptoms after HIV testing. Am J Psychiatry 150:775–779, 1993

Peterson J, Marin G: Issues in the prevention of AIDS among black and Hispanic men. Am Psychol 43:871–877, 1988

Petrak J, Byrne A, Baker M: The association between abuse in childhood and STD/HIV risk behaviors in female genitourinary (GU) clinic attendees. Sex Transm Infect 6:457–461, 2000

Peyriere H, Mauboussin J, Rouanet I, et al: Management of sudden psychiatric disorders related to efavirenz. AIDS 15:1323–1324, 2001

Power C, Selnes O, Grim J, et al: HIV Dementia Scale: a rapid screening test. J Acquir Immun Defic Syndr Hum Retrovirol 8:273–278, 1995

Power R, Gore-Felton C, Vosvick M, et al: HIV: effectiveness of complementary and alternative medicine. Prim Care 29:361–378, 2002

Proctor VE, Tesfa A, Tompkins DC: Barriers to adherence to highly active antiretroviral therapy as expressed by people living with HIV/AIDS. AIDS Patient Care STDS 13:535–544, 1999

Rabkin JG, Rabkin R, Wagner G: Effects of fluoxetine on mood and immune status in depressed patients with HIV illness. J Clin Psychiatry 55:92–97, 1994

Rabkin JG, Ferrando SJ, Jacobsberg LB, et al: Prevalence of Axis I disorders in an AIDS cohort: a cross-sectional, controlled study. Compr Psychiatry 38:146–154, 1997

Rabkin JG, Wagner JG, Rabkin R: Fluoxetine treatment for depression in patients with HIV and AIDS: a randomized, placebo-controlled trial. Am J Psychiatry 156:101–107, 1999

Reeves R, Bullen J: Serotonin syndrome produced by paroxetine and low-dose trazodone. Psychosomatics 3:159–160, 1995

Reite M, Ruddy J, Nagel K: Evaluation and Management of Sleep Disorders, 3rd Edition. Washington, DC, American Psychiatric Publishing, 2002

Riley SP: Lipodystrophy and the psychosocial effects of stigma in a sample of HIV-positive gay men (immune deficiency). Dissertation Abstracts International: Section B: the Sciences and Engineering 62:4233. Ann Arbor, MI, University Microfilms International, 2002

Robinson M, Qaqish R: Practical psychopharmacology in HIV-1 and acquired immunodeficiency syndrome. Psychiatr Clin North Am 25:149–175, 2002

Ross MW, Rosser BR: Measurement and correlates of internalized homophobia: a factor analytic study. J Clin Psychol 52:15–21, 1996

Ross MW, Wodak A, Gold J, et al: Differences across sexual orientation on HIV risk behaviours in injecting drug users. AIDS Care 4:139–148, 1992

Royall D, Mahurin R, Gray K: Bedside assessment of executive cognitive impairment: the Executive Interview. J Am Geriatr Soc 40:1221–1226, 1992

Sabin T: AIDS: the new "Great Imitator." J Am Geriatr Soc 35:467–471, 1987

Scamvougeras A, Rosebush P: AIDS-related psychosis with catatonia responding to low-dose lorazepam (letter). J Clin Psychiatry 53:414–415, 1992

Schillerstrom J, Deuter MS, Wyatt R, et al: Prevalence of executive impairment in patients seen by a psychiatry consultation service. Psychosomatics 44:290–297, 2003

Schwartz T, Masand P: The role of atypical antipsychotics in the treatment of delirium. Psychosomatics 43:171–174, 2002

Semple S: Motivations associated with methamphetamine use among HIV+ men who have sex with men. J Subst Abuse Treat 22:149–156, 2002

Sewell D, Jeste D, Atkinson J, et al: HIV-associated psychosis: a study of 20 cases. Am J Psychiatry 151:237–242, 1994

Sewell M, Goggin K, Rabkin J, et al: Anxiety syndromes and symptoms among men with AIDS: a longitudinal controlled study. Psychosomatics 41:294–300, 2000

Simpson DM, McArthur JC, Olney R, et al: Lamotrigine for HIV-associated painful sensory neuropathies: a placebo-controlled trial. Neurology 60:1508–1514, 2003

Snyder S, Prenzlauer S, Maruyama N, et al: Catatonia in a patient with AIDS-related dementia (letter). J Clin Psychiatry 53:414, 1992

Sterk CE, Theall KP, Elifson KW: Effectiveness of a risk reduction intervention among African American women who use crack cocaine. AIDS Educ Prev 15:15–32, 2003

Stiffman AR, Dore P, Cunningham RM, et al: Person and environment in HIV risk behavior change between adolescence and young adulthood. Health Educ Q 22:211–226, 1995

Trachman S: Buspirone-induced psychosis in a human immunodeficiency virus-infected man. Psychosomatics 33:332–335, 1992

Treisman G, Kaplin A: Neurologic and psychiatric complications of antiretroviral agents. AIDS 16:1201–1215, 2002

Treisman G, Fishman M, Lyketsos C, et al: Evaluation and treatment of psychiatric disorders associated with HIV infection, in HIV, AIDS and the Brain. Edited by Price R, Perry S. New York, Raven, 1994, pp 239–250

Trobst K: Personality pathways to unsafe sex: personality, condom use, and HIV risk behaviors. J Res Pers 36:117–133, 2002

Upadhyaya M, Chaturvedi S: Psychosis and antituberculosis therapy. Lancet 2:735–736, 1989

Volkow N, Harper A, Munnisteri D, et al: AIDS and catatonia (letter). J Neurol Neurosurg Psychiatry 50:104–118, 1987

von Moltke L, Greenblatt D, Granda B, et al: Inhibition of human cytochrome P450 isoforms by nonnucleoside reverse transcriptase inhibitors. J Clin Pharmacol 41:85–91, 2001

Wallston K, Wallston B, Devellis R: Development of the Multi-dimensional Health Locus of Control (MHLC) scales. Health Educ Monogr 6:161–170, 1978

White J, Darko D, Brown S, et al: Early central nervous system response to HIV infection; sleep distortion and cognitive-motor decrements. AIDS 9:1043–1050, 1995

The Patient With Hepatitis C

Silvia Hafliger, M.D.

Hepatitis C is a silent epidemic that afflicts 4 million people in the United States and 170 million people worldwide. In the next decade, more Americans will die of hepatitis C, cirrhosis, and hepatocellular cancer than of HIV infection. Hepatitis C is a single-stranded RNA virus whose replication and mode of entry have been difficult to study because of the lack of an animal model. There is considerable genomic heterogeneity. The virus is currently classified into six genotypes, with genotype 1 being the most common but the least responsive to treatment. The virus was discovered in 1989, and commercial testing became available in 1991.

■ TRANSMISSION

Hepatitis C is transmitted in blood. Most patients acquire the virus from injection drug use, pre-1992 blood transfusion, body piercing or tattoos (via infected ink or needles), intranasal cocaine use (via infected straw), sharing of toothbrushes or razors, or vertical transmission during vaginal delivery. Sexual transmission is rare and carries a 5% lifetime risk.

Unlike hepatitis B, which resolves in 85% of patients after acute infection, 85% of infected hepatitis C

patients will become chronic carriers. The incubation period is approximately 6 weeks. Viral infection causes few symptoms, and liver function tests (LFTs) are unreliable for diagnosis. The following profile adds to the difficulty of diagnosis:

- 30% of those infected will have normal LFT results and be asymptomatic.
- 50% of those infected will have minimal LFT elevation, yet be asymptomatic.
- Only 20% will have symptoms, such as fatigue or mild upper quadrant pain, with minimal elevations in ALT and AST, usually two to three times normal.
- Most acute infections go unrecognized, and diagnosis is made 20 to 30 years later by antibody detection (Jacobson 2001).

■ COMPLICATIONS

Hepatitis C is a neurotropic virus, and it has been detected in the cerebrospinal fluid and brain tissue of infected patients (Laskus et al. 2002). Its proclivity for the central nervous system, like that of HIV, possibly contributes to the high prevalence of depression, fatigue, and mild cognitive dysfunction in hepatitis C

Wyszynski AA, Wyszynski B (eds.): *Manual of Psychiatric Care for the Medically Ill.* Washington, D.C., American Psychiatric Publishing, Inc., 2005

patients (Kramer et al. 2002). It is the most common reason for liver transplantation in the United States, because 20% of chronic carriers will progress to cirrhosis. Unfortunately, transplantation is not a cure; the lifelong immunosuppression following transplantation increases the likelihood of reinfection of the new liver due to unchecked viral replication.

■ DIAGNOSIS

A liver biopsy is the only way to predict progression to cirrhosis and serves as a guide for treatment. Inflammation and fibrosis are measured and rated from 1 to 4. *Grade* refers to inflammatory changes seen on biopsy, and *stage* to the amount of fibrosis.

Enzyme-linked immunosorbent assay (ELISA) antibody testing detects hepatitis C. False positives occur in patients with autoimmune illnesses. False negatives occur in immunosuppressed and dialyzed patients. A positive antibody test indicates the need for further blood work to obtain viral load and genotype (Jacobson 2001).

■ TREATMENT

Treatment of hepatitis C currently uses interferon alpha and ribavirin.

Interferon alpha is a cytokine with antiviral, antiproliferative properties. It binds to cell surface receptors and initiates second messengers, which signal the production of antiviral proteins. Interferon is administered by injection three times a week. A long-acting product, pegylated interferon, has received approval and is injected weekly. Interferon undergoes renal clearance and does not have major drug interactions except with coadministration of zidovudine, lamivudine, and other nucleoside reverse transcriptase inhibitors.

Ribavirin, a nucleoside analogue, inhibits RNA polymerase and depletes intracellular guanosine triphosphate. It undergoes hepatic and renal clearance. There are no P450 interactions. The half-life of ribavirin is greater than 200 hours.

Side effects of interferon and ribavirin are constitutional (flu-like) symptoms and late-onset neuropsychiatric problems (occurring 6–12 weeks into treatment). Early constitutional symptoms include fatigue, chills, myalgia, nausea, headache, low-grade fever, and anorexia. There is also the risk of bone marrow suppression with anemia, thrombocytopenia, and neutropenia.

Hypo- and hyperthyroidism occur in subsets of patients.

■ NEUROPSYCHIATRIC COMPLICATIONS OF TREATMENT

Approximately 20% of psychiatrically asymptomatic patients will develop neuropsychiatric complications on the interferon and ribavirin regimen, most notably the following:

- Depression
- Mood lability
- Irritability
- Insomnia
- Cognitive dysfunction (e.g., decreased short-term memory, generalized slowing, word-finding difficulties)
- Decreased fine motor control

Patients with a history of substance abuse are at risk of experiencing increased drug cravings and relapse.

The specific mechanisms for the development of neuropsychiatric complications are unknown. However, interferon causes a dysregulation of the neuroendocrine, neurotransmitter, and cytokine pathways. Administration of interferon leads to lowering of serotonin levels, which may explain the observed irritability, crying, rage, and decreased frustration tolerance (Bonaccorso et al. 2002). Dopamine systems are equally dysregulated. Prolonged administration of interferon alpha most likely decreases dopamine levels and may account for cognitive slowing, decreased attention, and lower motivation. Interferon induces secondary cytokines, including interleukin (IL)–1, IL-2, IL-6, and tumor necrosis factor alpha, which in turn influence the hypothalamic-pituitary-adrenal axis (Dieperink et al. 2000; Lerner et al. 1999; Trask et al. 2000).

■ PSYCHIATRIC MANAGEMENT

Psychiatric intervention is often crucial in supporting patients through the year-long treatment for hepatitis C. Treatment with selective serotonin reuptake inhibitors (SSRIs) diminishes depression, irritability, and mood swings (Farrah 2002; Kraus et al. 2002; Loftis and Hauser 2003; Musselman et al. 2001; Ondria 1999).

All SSRIs seem to have efficacy in this setting, but comparative studies are lacking. Patients who currently are depressed should be treated with an SSRI prior to starting treatment with interferon (Dieperink et al. 2003; Hauser et al. 2000, 2002).

A history of traumatic brain injury or structural CNS abnormalities presents a greater risk for developing a delirium and impulsive self-injurious behavior on interferon (Adams et al. 1988).

Modafinil (Provigil) or methylphenidate (Ritalin) is useful for treating fatigue or cognitive slowing (Schwartz et al. 2002).

Interferon and SSRIs in combination may precipitate mania in vulnerable patients. Gabapentin (Neurontin) and olanzapine (Zyprexa) are reportedly helpful (Altingdag 2001; Greenberg et al. 2000).

Supportive psychotherapy often focuses on the shame and stigma of having an infectious disease.

■ REFERENCES

Adams F, Fernandez F, Mavligit G: Interferon-induced mental disorders associated with unsuspected pre-existing neurologic abnormalities. J Neurooncol 6:355–359, 1988

Altingdag A: Interferon alpha induced mood disorder with manic features. Gen Hosp Psychiatry 23:168–170, 2001

Bonaccorso S, Marino V, Puzella A, et al: Increased depressive ratings in patients with hepatitis C receiving interferon-alpha based immunotherapy are related to interferon-alpha induced changes in the serotonergic system. J Clin Psychopharmacol 22:86–90, 2002

Dieperink E, Willenbring M, Ho S: Neuropsychiatric symptoms associated with hepatitis C and interferon alpha: a review. Am J Psychiatry 157:867–876, 2000

Dieperink E, Ho S, Thuras P, et al: A prospective study of neuropsychiatric symptoms associated with interferon alpha-2b and ribavirin therapy for patients with chronic hepatitis C. Psychosomatics 44:104–112, 2003

Farrah A: Interferon-induced depression treated with citalopram. J Clin Psychiatry 63:166–167, 2002

Greenberg D, Jonasch E, Gadd M, et al: Adjuvant therapy of melanoma with interferon alpha-2b is associated with mania and bipolar syndromes. Cancer 89:356–362, 2000

Hauser P, Soler R, Reed S, et al: Prophylactic treatment of depression induced by interferon alpha. Psychosomatics 41:439–441, 2000

Hauser P, Khosla J, Aurora H, et al: A prospective study of the incidence and open-label treatment of interferon-induced major depressive disorder in patients with hepatitis C. Mol Psychiatry 7:942–947, 2002

Jacobson I: Managing chronic hepatitis C infection. Hosp Physician 37:34–41, 2001

Kramer L, Bauer E, Funk G, et al: Subclinical impairment of brain function in chronic hepatitis C infection. J Hepatol 37:349–354, 2002

Kraus M, Schafer A, Faller H, et al: Paroxetine for the treatment of interferon alpha induced depression in chronic hepatitis C. Aliment Pharmacol Ther 16:1091–1099, 2002

Laskus T, Radkowski M, Bednarska A, et al: Detection and analysis of hepatitis C virus sequences in cerebrospinal fluid. J Virol 76:10064–10068, 2002

Lerner D, Stoudemire A, Rosenstein D: Neuropsychiatric toxicity associated with cytokine therapies. Psychosomatics 40:428–435, 1999

Loftis J, Hauser P: Co-management of depression and HCV treatment. Psychiatric Annals 33:385–391, 2003

Musselman D, Lawson D, Gumnick J, et al: Paroxetine for the prevention of depression induced by high dose interferon alpha. N Engl J Med 344:961–965, 2001

Ondria G: Five cases of interferon alpha induced depression treated with antidepressant therapy. Psychosomatics 40:510–512, 1999

Schwartz A, Thompson J, Masood N: Interferon-induced fatigue in patients with melanoma: a pilot study of exercise and methylphenidate. Oncol Nurs Forum 29:E85–E90, 2002

Trask P, Esper P, Riba M, et al: Psychiatric side effects of interferon therapy: prevalence, proposed mechanisms, and future directions. Clin Oncol 18:2316–2326, 2000

Chapter

11

A Primer on Solid Organ Transplant Psychiatry

Silvia Hafliger, M.D.

Few treatments in medicine are as dramatic as solid organ transplantation in restoring quality of life to a person ravaged by the consequences of end organ failure. Organ transplantation began in the early 1950s, but success was limited by ineffective immunosuppressive agents; patients died of organ rejection or overwhelming infections. A succession of immunosuppressant drugs was developed, culminating in the discovery in 1972 of cyclosporine, isolated from a soil fungus. Cyclosporine was first used in humans in 1978. It was approved by the U.S. Food and Drug Administration in 1983, ushering in a new era of successful solid organ transplantation.

Today, more than 80,000 patients in the United States are on the national organ waiting list. Except for kidney recipients, priorities are stratified according to patients' health status, their immediate probability of dying, and their waiting time on the list. Sicker patients receive transplants first. Every 14 minutes a new name is added to the list. Unfortunately, the demand greatly outstrips supply; 11 people die each day while waiting for transplants. At the end of 2002, more than 50,000 patients were awaiting kidney transplantation, more than 17,000 needed a liver, 4,000 were waiting for lungs and another 4,000 for hearts (UNOS 2002). These totals do not include patients who are likely to benefit from transplantation but are not referred to a center for evaluation.

■ ORGAN ALLOCATION

The United Network for Organ Sharing (UNOS), a private, nonprofit organization, is responsible for allocation of organs within the United States. UNOS oversees the national waiting list and coordinates organ donation. Within the United States, there are more than 40 organ procurement organizations (OPOs) responsible for organ recovery. Currently, there is mandatory reporting of imminent brain death. If there is a potential organ donor, the hospital first contacts the organ procurement organization. The OPO's staff evaluates the potential donor, asks for family consent, and reports to UNOS, which identifies possible matching recipients. This information is relayed back to the OPO, which then contacts the transplant center with the next eligible recipient.

Wyszynski AA, Wyszynski B (eds.): *Manual of Psychiatric Care for the Medically Ill.* Washington, D.C., American Psychiatric Publishing, Inc., 2005

Organ availability is regional despite the national waiting list. There are three potential solid organ donor sources:

- *Brain-dead donor:* Two physicians, one of them a neurologist, determine brain death, which is defined as the cessation of all brain function, including that of the brainstem. This meets legal criteria of death, and a certificate is issued. A brain-dead donor can save up to seven lives by the harvesting of heart, kidneys, lungs, pancreas, and intestine. Each year, there are at least 20,000 potential cadaveric donors secondary to brain death, but only 10%–20% become donors. Even if there is a signed donor card, procurement of organs is difficult. Families have the final veto power. Many of these potential donors are young, victims of accidents or cerebral aneurysms, whose bodies "look healthy" to their families—still with a heartbeat, "still breathing." Signing the consent for organ donation is difficult for families, who may feel this is abandonment of care, or mutilation. All major religions allow organ donation, but cultural barriers do exist. For example, the Japanese find cadaveric donation nearly impossible because it is considered disrespectful to the dead.
- *Nonbeating-heart donor:* When brain death does not occur but the patient is in a persistent terminal, vegetative state, the family gives permission to discontinue life support, resulting in cardiac arrest of the patient. After 5 minutes, the kidney and liver can be harvested.
- *Living donation:* A part or whole organ from a healthy person is removed. Living donation is now possible for kidney, lung, and liver transplantation.

Liver Transplantation

Thomas Starzl performed the first liver transplant in 1967. Early 1-year survival rates were around 25%. By 1995, there were 3,882 liver transplants, with 80%–90% 1-year survival. Today, the average waiting time for a liver transplant for a person with blood group O is 2–5 years. The most common indication for liver transplantation in the United States today is for hepatitis C–induced cirrhosis (see Chapter 10, "The Patient With Hepatitis C"), followed by cirrhosis due to alcohol, autoimmune hepatitis, primary biliary cirrhosis, and cryptogenic cirrhosis. Transplantation is not a cure for hepatitis C, and viral reinfection of the liver graft may lead to renewed organ failure over time.

The highest priority in organ allocation is assigned to patients with acute organ failure (e.g., those with acetaminophen overdose, drug reaction, idiopathic failure, or acute severe hepatitis A). For chronic liver disease, values of bilirubin, prothrombin time, and kidney function are used to calculate the Model for Endstage Liver Disease score (MELD score, 6–40) to predict mortality within the next few weeks. Higher scores represent greater probability of dying within the next few weeks if a liver transplant is not performed.

The number of adult patients needing liver transplantation is rapidly growing because of hepatitis C cirrhosis. The first living related transplant occurred in 1989 between a parent and child, and this has since become the standard of care for pediatric liver transplantation (Emond 2001; Singer et al. 1989). For the parent who donates 20% of his or her liver, the surgery is well tolerated with few postoperative complications.

The first published reports of adult-to-adult living donation occurred in Australia in 1996, followed by Colorado in 1999. The donor's entire right lobe (60% of hepatic mass) is removed to ensure adequate graft size for the recipient. Regeneration of the liver to about 80%–90% of its original size requires 6–8 weeks. Estimated donor mortality is 0.4%. Most deaths have been secondary to pulmonary embolism, liver failure, or hemorrhage. Morbidity ranges from 5% to 20% and includes risk of bile leak, biliary stricture, wound infection, and incisional hernia. Postoperative pain can be severe. Donors must plan on a minimum of 2 months' recovery at home (Trotter et al. 2002).

Kidney Transplantation

End-stage renal disease secondary to diabetes mellitus is the most common indication for kidney transplantation (42%), followed by hypertension (26%) and glomerulonephritis (11%).

Although dialysis keeps patients with renal insufficiency alive, even the most efficient dialysis removes only about 20% of solutes when averaged over time. Patients on dialysis still have impaired quality of life, with mild uremic symptoms and high rates of depression and sexual dysfunction. Patients struggle with muscle cramps, postdialysis fatigue, malaise, nausea, and vascular access complications. Transplantation offers improvement of quality of life with greater energy, improved cognitive function, and more independence. Recipients of kidneys from living donors have a 97% 1-year survival rate and a 91% 5-year survival rate; cadaver kidney recipients have 1- and 5-year survival rates of 94% and 81%, respectively. These survival rates exceed those of matched patients who remain on dialysis.

Patients with kidney transplants have the shortest hospital stay and the easiest postoperative course compared with the other solid organ transplants. Kidney transplant patients also tend to have fewer neuropsychiatric complications and to function well on discharge. Cardiovascular disease, including myocardial infarction and stroke, and peripheral vascular disease due to hyperlipidemia, hypertension, and diabetes are the most common causes of death in renal transplant recipients (Bartucci 2002).

Joseph Murray performed the first successful living related kidney transplantation in 1954, between monozygotic twins at the Peter Bent Brigham Hospital in Boston, Massachusetts. Because the kidney is considered a "quality-of-life organ" as opposed to a "life-saving" organ, there is no scoring system to predict mortality. The kidney is more immunogenic than the liver. Organs are allocated based on blood type compatibility, with points assigned for human leukocyte antigen match and waiting time. The average waiting time is about 7 years for a cadaveric donor. Living donation is encouraged in all recipients (Cupples and Ohler 2002). The number of living related kidney donor procedures now exceeds cadaveric transplantation. Mortality for the donor is low—estimated to be 0.03%–0.05%. Morbidity is approximately 4% and includes, in order of decreasing frequency, pneumonia, urinary tract infection, wound complications, deep vein thrombosis, and pulmonary embolism (Bia 1998; Kasiske 1998).

The majority of donors report a positive experience, with enhanced self-esteem and stronger bonding with the recipient, feeling that if they had it to do over again, they would make the same decision about donation. A negative experience of donation correlates with female gender and perioperative complications (Johnson 1999).

Guidelines have been published for conducting a psychiatric evaluation of unrelated kidney donors (Leo et al. 2003).

Lung Transplantation

Lung transplants are the most challenging of the transplants discussed in this chapter, with the highest post-transplant mortality. The 1-year survival is approximately 75%, with a 50% survival rate at 5 years. The most common indications for single lung transplantation, in descending order, are chronic obstructive pulmonary disease (COPD), idiopathic pulmonary fibrosis, primary pulmonary hypertension, and cystic fibrosis. Indications for double lung transplant are cystic fibrosis, COPD, and primary pulmonary hypertension.

Acute rejection is quite common following lung transplantation. The lung is the only transplanted organ with direct communication to the external environment. Rates of infection are high. Recurrent pulmonary infection with cytomegalovirus, pseudomonas, candida, and aspergillus are frequent challenges. Chronic rejection or bronchiolitis obliterans syndrome will affect approximately 50% of patients and will lead to progressive deterioration in lung function and death. Patients with lung transplants need to be vigilant. Long-term monitoring for infection and decreased lung function is essential.

From a psychiatric viewpoint, delirium rates are high, both pre- and post-transplant. Hypoxia plays an important role. Anxiety disorders and depression also occur frequently in this population.

James Hardy performed the first single lung transplant in 1963; the patient survived 18 days. Successful bilateral sequential single lung transplant occurred in 1989. Vaughn Starnes performed the first living lobar donor lung transplant, involving the right lower lobe donated by a mother to a 12-year-old daughter, in 1990. Over the next 10 years, 450 lung transplants were completed, with 1- and 5-year survival rates of 83% and 54%, respectively (Turka and Norman 2001). Today, lung transplantation is indicated for patients who have significant functional limitations and high risk of mortality. There is no point system or priority given for severity of illness. The average waiting time is about 1–2 years.

Living, related donation occurs at only a few centers in the United States, usually for cystic fibrosis. Two living donors are required, one for the right lower lobe and the other for the left lower lobe. There have been no reports of donor mortality, but very few of these procedures have been performed. Morbidity includes persistent air leaks requiring prolonged use of a postoperative chest tube, Dressler's syndrome (postpericardiotomy syndrome), and pulmonary artery thrombosis. In the donor, a 17% decrease in forced vital capacity and a 16% decrease in total lung capacity from preoperative values occurs 2 years postdonation (Schenkel et al. 2001).

Heart Transplantation

Ischemic (45%) and nonischemic (44%) cardiomyopathy account for most heart transplantation, followed by congenital abnormalities, severe valvular disease, and retransplantation. The patient survival rate is 86%

at 1 year and 80% at 3 years. Cardiac allograft vasculopathy is an accelerated form of coronary artery disease and is one of the main causes of graft failure after transplantation.

Patients with advanced congestive heart failure are now considered for implantation of a left ventricular assist device (LVAD). Cannulae are inserted through a median sternotomy into the left ventricle and ascending aorta; the other ends of the tubes connect to a pumping device implanted below the diaphragm. Transcutaneous wires connect to external batteries, which are worn as a belt. Patients leave the hospital and return to a reasonably normal life including some sports and work. These devices were considered initially to be a transition to transplantation. Because of severe organ shortages, however, some patients live with LVADs as their only means of improved functioning (Querques and Stern 2002; Rose et al. 2001). In LVAD patients, rates of cognitive dysfunction due to microembolism are high, as are rates of delirium, depression, and anxiety disorders. Infections secondary to the presence of the device are common and can lead to sepsis and mediastinitis.

Rates of depression are high in patients awaiting heart transplants; one in five patients will have experienced a major depressive disorder (MDD). The prevalence of depression increases after transplant, according to one study (Dew et al. 2001); one in four post-transplant patients will receive a diagnosis of MDD within the first 3 years after transplant. Post-traumatic stress disorder related to the transplant occurs especially in the first year after transplant. Patients experience intrusive thoughts and flashbacks about the waiting and perioperative periods.

Heart transplant patients, probably more than other organ recipients, are preoccupied with the personal characteristics of the donor. The heart has symbolic meaning for many recipients, representing the "seat of the soul," emotions, and life itself. The kidney or liver usually has less metaphoric importance. It is more challenging for some to accept a heart transplanted from someone else as part of the "self."

Christiaan Barnard performed the first human cardiac transplant in Cape Town, South Africa, in 1967; the patient survived 18 days and died of septicemia. Early survival statistics were grim, but cardiac transplantation has since flourished and improved. Ninety heart transplants were performed worldwide in 1980. By 1995, 2,369 heart transplants had been completed in the United States, with a 1-year survival rate of 90%. Today, priorities for receiving a transplant are stratified according to severity of heart failure. Status 2 indicates necessity of a heart transplant; status 1b re-

quires inotropic therapy (i.e., continuous dobutamine or milrinone infusion), and status 1a indicates a critically ill patient in the intensive care unit. Status 2 patients usually wait more than 1 year before receiving a transplant.

■ THE MULTIDISCIPLINARY TRANSPLANT TEAM

Successful organ transplantation requires teamwork and coordination of care. Many specialists care for a patient referred to a transplant center, including a hepatologist, cardiologist, nephrologist, pulmonologist, immunologist, interventional radiologist, and several surgeons. Transplant coordinators, most of whom are nurse practitioners, serve as liaisons between the patient and the team, manage the day-to-day flow of information, screen test results, and monitor immunosuppression and graft function. The financial cost of transplantation can be overwhelming; financial and billing specialists coordinate payment with insurance companies and are part of the team.

Most transplant teams have a working relationship with a psychiatrist to provide pre- and post-transplant psychiatric assessment and treatment of psychiatric disorders. Knowledge of systems theory, family dynamics, and medical illness improves psychiatric effectiveness. A major role of the transplant psychiatrist is to treat the psychiatric complications arising from transplant surgery and its treatment. Often the psychiatrist helps the patient cope with the psychological demands of his or her illness and helps translate medical facts for the patient and family. Once a patient qualifies for transplantation, a long-term relationship between the psychiatrist and patient is often established. Social workers assist in providing additional social and educational interventions.

■ GENERAL SCREENING OF CANDIDATES FOR TRANSPLANT

Transplant evaluation consists of three areas of assessment: medical, economic, and psychosocial.

Medical Testing

Cancer or severe organ disease (of any organ other than the one being replaced) may make transplantation impossible. Presence of human immunodeficiency virus (HIV) infection or chronic progressive neurological illnesses may also be contraindications. Some transplant centers now accept selected HIV-positive patients for liver transplant as part of a National Institutes of Health protocol.

Economic Feasibility

Transplantation surgery costs over $200,000, and posttransplant immunosuppressive therapy costs about $3,000 a month. Transplantation is covered by most insurance, including Medicaid and Medicare.

Psychosocial Evaluation

The psychiatric evaluation usually lasts 60–90 minutes and uses the clinical psychiatric interview as the main screening tool. More formal instruments such as the Psychosocial Assessment of Candidates for Transplant (PACT) and the Transplant Evaluation Rating Scale (TERS) (Levenson and Olbrisch 2000) are used mainly in the research setting to quantify screening results. Most patients have some degree of neuropsychiatric impairment due to end organ failure. Neuropsychiatric impairments are greatest in patients with end-stage liver disease. Cognitive deficits, such as impairments in attention, concentration, and memory, usually improve after transplantation. Active substance abuse or dependence, untreated psychiatric illness, and lack of adherence to medical or psychiatric care may be psychosocial contraindications. Included in the evaluation are practical considerations such as adequacy of family support, safety of the home environment, and availability of transportation, as discussed under Social Support below.

■ PRETRANSPLANT PSYCHIATRIC EVALUATION ISSUES

For many patients, the transplant psychiatrist is the first mental health professional they have ever met. There is often some opposition to meeting the psychiatrist; patients may be anxious that they will be considered "crazy" or that the psychiatrist will "mind-read." The presence of a family member during the interview is often comforting and can also provide important collateral information.

Social Support

Prospective transplant candidates are usually very ill. Years of end organ failure have taken a neuropsychi-

atric toll, especially in patients with hepatic failure. It is imperative that family or care partners be present during patient evaluations. During this evaluation, care partners also benefit, frequently learning about the illness, the prognosis, necessary lifestyle changes, risks and benefits of transplantation, and immunosuppression. Since they will assume a large part of the patient's pre- and postprocedure care, care partners must be taught about medications, dietary restrictions, and warning signs of worsening illness, such as delirium, medication side effects, depression, and recurrent substance abuse.

The post-transplant challenges are far-reaching, and usually patients cannot meet them alone. For example, patients are discharged on multiple medications and must make return visits to the transplant clinic once or twice weekly for blood work, medical visits, or biopsies. They may need extensive wound care or intravenous antiviral or antibiotic medications. Sometimes patients are emergently admitted to a local community hospital and become incapacitated; someone knowledgeable must be able to contact the transplant center as soon as possible. The care partner (usually a family member or friend) assumes responsibility temporarily until the patient is well enough to function independently. A nurse's aide or home attendant is not considered an adequate substitute for the care partner. The transplant team sees patients only for short periods; unfortunately, at most programs, patients who have no family or care partners *are not usually candidates for transplantation*.

Psychiatric Disorders

Depression, anxiety disorders, and denial are quite common in patients awaiting a transplant. Several issues warrant emphasis:

- *Depression* may impede motivation to cooperate with the many tasks required of the patient post-transplant, such as interacting with a complex medical system, keeping medical appointments, and adhering to medication.
- *Denial* about the seriousness of the illness impairs insight and judgment. It can affect decisions about when to pursue medical care for complications or make lifestyle changes. Denial has been linked to pretransplant patient mortality because some patients seek medical care too late in their illness. When they finally do seek out care, complications are too advanced or they have neglected to make adequate financial preparation for the procedure.

- *Severe mental illnesses,* such as bipolar illness or schizophrenia, must be stable and must be actively treated by a community psychiatrist, with family support available. The suitability of mentally ill patients for transplantation is determined on an individual basis. There are few data on transplant outcomes in these patients.

Informed Consent

Patients frequently have minimal understanding of the risks and benefits of transplantation. Often they do not understand the procedure, despite having consulted many health care providers. For example, some patients think that only the "bad part" of an organ is "cut out" and that a new organ is placed next to the old one. Patients with hepatitis C often think that liver transplantation will cure them, not realizing that the virus persists after organ replacement. Conversely, many think the transplanted organ will last only a year or two. Others have unrealistic expectations about their transplanted organ, fantasizing that life will improve in improbable ways. Many individuals do not understand that immunosuppression therapy is permanent and brings its own complications. The patient and family must be prepared for the reality that the eagerly anticipated surgery is only the beginning of recovery, bringing a new set of demands.

Ability to Comply With Medical Care

Prospective transplant candidates must demonstrate that they can work with the medical team and adhere to complicated medical regimens. This capability is difficult to assess in one visit. Collateral history from the referring physician is quite helpful and includes information such as the patient's reliability about keeping appointments, the ability to follow instructions, and his or her typical adherence to medication schedules. The patient must be reliable about taking medications and communicating side effects or changes in health. Patients who formerly took medications only for symptomatic relief must be willing to adhere to lifelong immunosuppressive regimens.

The clinic patient without a relationship to a primary care doctor is at a disadvantage. Such patients tend to operate in a "crisis mode" and to know less about their illness and medications. This approach will not succeed for the transplant patient, who must be knowledgeable about the illness, health status, and medications and must carry a medication list at all times.

Psychological Challenges of the Waiting Period

Severe organ shortages result in a wait of several years for transplantation. Deteriorating health, financial hardships, and development of psychiatric problems such as depression impose significant burdens. Many patients experience sexual dysfunction, which further strains their primary relationship. Care partners are at risk for burnout and for becoming psychiatrically symptomatic themselves.

It is unfortunate that some patients will not receive an organ despite having "met all requirements." Patients and families must learn to live with uncertainty. They must cope with the possibility of the patient's death yet remain hopeful and proactive regarding medical care. Waiting patients and families are encouraged to stay as active as possible, and they often benefit from attending support groups with other transplant candidates and recipients. Some type of work or volunteer activity is recommended whenever it is possible for a chronically ill patient to participate.

Potential Living Donors

Donation by a living donor has many advantages over the long wait for cadaveric donors. However, living adult organ donation also puts enormous pressure on the donor, family, and recipient. It is an asymmetrical transaction, often surrounded by a kind of gift-giving ritual, with health care professionals positioned as its gatekeepers (Russell and Jacob 1993).

All donors undergo psychiatric evaluation to screen for depression, anxiety disorder, psychosis, past or current substance abuse, and personality disorder. Donors must be at least 18 years of age, with rare exceptions, and demonstrate adequate decision-making abilities and appreciation of the potential risks of the surgery (i.e., morbidity, mortality, need for postoperative recovery). The financial impact of the procedure on the donor is evaluated. Often the same family will be burdened with caring for both patients who have had major surgery. Donor discussions include the possibility of graft failure and risk of recurrent illness in the recipient (e.g., secondary to substance abuse and/or hepatitis C) and the possible need for retransplantation.

It is crucial to understand the donor-recipient family dynamics. The donor's decision-making process is carefully screened for potential coercion. For example, is the donor attempting "redemption" for some past transgression by giving the organ to the family member? Is there the fantasy of undoing "black sheep" status, or gaining love and acceptance from the recipient or the family? If the recipient develops complications or dies, how will the donor deal psychologically with the issue of the "flawed gift"? Will the donor feel that his or her transplanted organ hastened the recipient's death?

Donors have the option at any time in the evaluation process to withdraw consent, assured of strict confidentiality. A medical excuse may be offered as the reason for the withdrawal. There must be a minimum of a 2-week waiting period between consent and surgery, in order to allow the donor sufficient time to decide whether or not to proceed. If a prospective donor decides to withdraw, there arise many "no-win" psychological issues, such as guilt, "loss of face," questions from the family, and the enduring consequences of the decision not to donate.

Living organ donors are frequently parents of young children, and their decisions may have complicated repercussions for the family. For example, if the prospective donor is the mother of young children, the risk of surgery may bring up fears of leaving her children motherless. If the donor's spouse objects but the donor proceeds against the spouse's wishes, the entire family is affected. Ongoing psychological support for the donor and nondonors is essential (Fox and Swazey 1992; Simmons 1977).

The organ recipient also faces psychological pressures from living donation. Usually the recipient is older, with complicated feelings about accepting a "gift" from a child, spouse, or sibling. Recipients may feel guilty and ashamed about their primary illness, particularly if they perceive it to be self-induced (e.g., a consequence of substance use). They may struggle with the desire for personal survival as weighed against the need to protect the donor. How difficult will it be for the recipient to live with this "gift" and the burden of indebtedness?

Counseling should be available to recipients, donors, and those who decline donation, to help them through these difficult issues.

■ SPECIAL POPULATIONS

Patients undergoing transplantation must be able to demonstrate abstinence from alcohol, nicotine, and illicit drugs. This requirement is challenging for certain populations, who nonetheless may undergo successful transplantation with psychiatric help.

Patients With Alcohol Dependence

Approximately 20%–40% of all liver transplants are for cirrhosis resulting from alcohol dependence. Pa-

tients in this category generally do as well as other transplant patients, with the same 1-year survival of 80%–90% (Beresford 1994). However, coinfection with hepatitis C accelerates the rate of progression to cirrhosis. Moreover, women are at risk for developing cirrhosis if they drink more than two servings of alcohol a day, even though they do not meet diagnostic criteria for alcohol dependence or abuse.

Patients with diagnosed alcohol dependence have an estimated relapse rate of 20%–30%. Direct questioning by the clinician on each visit to the transplant center seems to be the best method to monitor for relapse (DiMartini et al. 2001).

Most transplant centers require a 6-month abstinence period before accepting an alcohol-dependent patient for transplantation. Ideally, patients have begun specific treatment for their dependency prior to transplantation. Abstinence achieved in the setting of serious medical complications of end organ failure does not appear to predict sustained abstinence after transplantation.

A frequently used evaluation tool for the selection of candidates is the Michigan Alcoholism Prognosis Scale developed by Beresford (Beresford 1994, 2001). This scale examines six areas: Do the patient and the family accept a diagnosis of alcoholism? Has the patient found a substitute activity to drinking? Will there be behavioral consequences to resumed drinking? Does the patient have renewed hope or self-esteem? Is there a stable social relationship? Is there social stability, that is, stable work and residence? (DiMartini and Trzepacz 2000)

A history of polysubstance dependence carries a greater risk of post-transplantation relapse. A patient who has been dependent on cocaine or heroin should demonstrate a minimum of 1 year of abstinence in a documented relapse prevention program. Substance abuse counselors must fax monthly urine toxicology results and attendance records to the psychosocial team. Families are educated about the warning signs of relapse on the first visit. They are encouraged to contact the transplant center immediately at the first signs of possible return to drinking or drug use.

A multicenter prospective study is in progress in order to validate scales that will more closely predict abstinence and assist in the selection of transplant candidates.

Patients With Nicotine Dependence

Patients must stop smoking in order to qualify as candidates for lung, heart, or liver transplantation. Cigarette smoking increases the likelihood of heart disease and malignancies, among the most common causes for mortality after transplantation. It also adds to the risk of developing hypertension, which can occur with immunosuppressive medications such as cyclosporine (Sandimmune, Neoral) or tacrolimus (Prograf).

Patients are encouraged to seek nicotine replacement strategies, such as the patch or gum and/or treatment with bupropion (Zyban). Urine toxicology tests screen for nicotine metabolites (cotinine levels) to monitor abstinence (Hertz 2001).

Patients in Methadone Maintenance

Patients participating in a licensed methadone program are considered increasingly as candidates for transplantation. They do not have to taper off methadone but should receive maintenance doses that keep them comfortable and craving-free (Koch and Banys 2001). Acute postoperative pain management for these patients may include morphine or an increased dose of methadone given every 6 hours for pain control.

Patients With Severe Mental Illness

Patients must be able to form trusting, stable relationships with the transplant team or at least one team member; severe Axis II pathology will interfere with this process. Patients with borderline personality disorder tend to cope poorly both before and after transplant. Impulsivity, noncompliance, substance abuse, and self-destructive behavior impair recovery (Shapiro et al. 1995). Splitting and projection can be difficult to handle in a medical/surgical setting. Narcissistic patients and those with paranoid characters will also be disruptive. Early diagnosis and psychiatric referral of patients with character pathology can minimize the negative impact, but usually these problems require long-term treatment.

Patients with schizophrenia or bipolar disorder must be in a working relationship with a community psychiatrist. If their illness is stable and under control, schizophrenia patients may become transplant candidates. Their workability within a transplant team is assessed on an individual basis.

■ POST-TRANSPLANT ISSUES

Most patients experience joy and intense relief after successfully surviving the transplant surgery. The improvement in their health is frequently dramatic. For example, after liver transplant, the patient's energy level increases, and pruritus, encephalopathy, and ascites dissipate. Most patients consider their recovery

miraculous and are extremely grateful. The event of transplantation is usually celebrated as a "second birthday." Many individuals write a thank-you note to the donor family. Their notes are written anonymously, but there is often great curiosity about the life and characteristics of the donor. The donor families are sometimes equally curious about the recipient, and often the family write back. Rarely, recipient and donor family meet.

Patients are routinely told the sex and age of the cadaveric donor. For some, this can be difficult if the organ donor was not of the same gender. Male patients may joke about becoming "like a woman" or vice versa. Donated livers can be up to 90 years old because the liver is less subject to aging than donated hearts or kidneys. (The liver has a double blood supply and minimal arteriosclerosis.) An organ donated from a 24-year-old may be perceived differently than one from a 92-year-old, perhaps as more vital. For liver recipients who feel guilty about their previous drug or alcohol use, expressing thanks may be very difficult, and some recipients will feel that someone had to die for them to live. This perspective is not limited to those whose primary illness was self-induced. Clarification of these issues is often the focus of psychological intervention.

Patients who receive a heart transplant experience different psychological issues because the heart often carries different psychological weight than other organs. It is often called the "seat of the soul." The transplanted heart is perceptible and feels "alive" in the chest. Heart patients are usually more preoccupied with the personal characteristics of the donor than other organ recipients and wonder how these traits may have been "transplanted" along with the organ. Organ recipients vary in their focus on their transplanted organ; some even name their organ, referring to it as their "baby"; most, however, either adapt silently or do not make their fantasies accessible to the transplant team.

After the "honeymoon period" ends, patients must confront issues that had been put on hold by their illness. Frequently, they have been ill for so many years that dealing with financial, insurance, work, and relationship matters is overwhelming. The fantasy that "everything will be better" dissolves, and recipients begin to face past failures and disappointments. Psychological preparation prior to transplantation assists in developing realistic expectations.

Disappointment and disillusionment are especially troubling when recovery is hampered by organ rejection or exacerbations of other illnesses. There is often the feeling of living on borrowed time. For example, recipients with hepatitis C have to live with the possibility of recurrent hepatic fibrosis secondary to the virus. Those with cancer often worry about the activation of previously dormant malignancies, since occult lesions will grow more rapidly in the setting of immunosuppression.

Patients without major complications are encouraged to return to work or some activity within 6 months after surgery. This transition may be difficult for those who have not worked in years or have been receiving disability payments. Loss of the familiar sick role and the prospect of vocational training may be psychologically stressful. The care partner also has to shift focus, defining new personal goals.

Common Psychiatric Problems

The first year after transplantation is difficult. Patients have to relearn bodily signals, distinguishing normal aches and pains from serious symptoms such as incipient graft rejection or infection. The most common post-transplant psychiatric problem is depression. The selective serotonin reuptake inhibitors (SSRIs) are preferred medications for depression in this setting. Nefazodone (Serzone) should be avoided because of its strong inhibition of cytochrome P450 3A4, which is involved in cyclosporine/tacrolimus metabolism.

Supportive psychotherapy is often helpful. Some patients with difficult hospitalizations have symptoms similar to those of posttraumatic stress disorder, such as vivid dreams and preoccupation with the traumatic events. Supportive counseling and treatment with an SSRI or an antianxiety agent such as clonazepam (Klonopin) or lorazepam (Ativan) are quite useful. (See also the section Transplant Psychopharmacology later in this chapter.)

Patients with a history of alcohol or chemical dependence are at greater risk for relapse as contact with the transplant team diminishes. Recurrent substance abuse can result in nonadherence to the post-transplant medication regimen, leading to mortality from graft rejection. The motivation for substance abuse treatment after transplantation is reduced because the patient now has the transplant, and this complicates the medical management.

Common Medical Problems

Post-transplant immunosuppression is lifelong. It carries several risks, including higher rates of cancer, lymphoproliferative disorders, chronic renal insufficiency, and heart disease. There are also complications secondary to the recurrence of the underlying disease, such as hepatitis C. Patients may require readmission for treatment of chronic organ rejection, infection, or surgical complications. Other medical complications common after transplant include weight gain (a complication of steroids), osteoporosis, insulin-dependent diabetes mellitus (a complication of medications), glaucoma and cataracts, and heightened vulnerability to skin cancer. Return to smoking also increases the risk of heart disease and lung cancer.

Patients can return to normal sexual activity approximately 6–8 weeks after transplantation. Use of birth control is encouraged. Pretransplant infertility in both sexes due to chronic illness may resolve. Improved general health restores sperm count and ovulation. Women can become pregnant after transplantation and receive care from an obstetrician familiar with transplant issues. At present no teratogenic problems, developmental delays, or learning disabilities have been reported in children exposed to cyclosporine in utero. Women on immunosuppression are at higher risk for preterm delivery, low-birthweight infants, and cesarean section (Coscia et al. 2002). Sexual dysfunction is not uncommon, particularly in heart transplant recipients.

Pain Management

Actual pain from the transplant surgery is usually minimal. The transplanted organ is without afferent nerves. Pain usually is from the incision or is musculoskeletal. Back pain is not uncommon. Patients use morphine in the early postoperative period but quickly switch to a less potent narcotic analgesic. Patients on methadone maintenance will need additional medication to cover the acute pain. If methadone is used for pain control, it must be given at 6-hour intervals.

For patients requiring long-term narcotic analgesic medications, administration should be centralized, usually with the transplant psychiatrist. This method avoids overprescribing and iatrogenic dependency. Gabapentin (Neurontin) and SSRIs are often used to enhance analgesia.

Palliative Care

There is a fine line between the need for organ transplantation and palliative care; patients awaiting transplant are terminally ill and will die without an organ. Those patients judged to be inappropriate for transplantation will require palliative care, with adequate pain control and management of symptoms of end organ failure. Recurrent cancer after transplant can be emotionally devastating, requiring the active involvement of the psychosocial team.

Patient death after transplantation is a painful loss for everyone, including the transplant team, whose members require support as well. Moreover, organ shortages increase the risk of dying from end organ failure while "waiting for a miracle." Understandably, families may be shocked, and even enraged, when their loved one dies while waiting. It is unfortunate when anger is displaced onto the transplant team, creating management problems that may be difficult to resolve.

Neuropsychiatric Complications

The neuropsychiatric complications of end organ failure include hepatic encephalopathy (see Chapter 2), uremic encephalopathy (see Chapter 4), congestive heart failure (see Chapter 3), respiratory failure (see Chapter 5), and toxic leukoencephalopathy (see below).

Cyclosporine, tacrolimus, metronidazole (Flagyl), drugs of abuse, alcohol, and cocaine can cause structural alteration in the cerebral white matter, mainly demyelination, detectable on magnetic resonance imaging. Cognition, emotions, movement, vision, and sensation depend on the integrity of white matter. Leukotoxic agents disrupt neuronal transmission, manifested as changes in mental status, confusion, and inattention, and possibly progressing to abulia and stupor. If there is a suspicion of demyelination, the offending drug is discontinued. Atypical neuroleptics are effective for treating agitation, visual hallucinations, and paranoia (Beresford 2001; Filley and Kleinschmidt-DeMasters 2001; Strouse et al. 1998; Wijdicks 2001).

■ TRANSPLANT PHARMACOLOGY

Allograft rejection caused by cell-mediated immunity involves T lymphocytes, macrophages, dendritic cells, antigen-presenting cells, and natural killer cells. All immunosuppressant medications modulate and interfere with T-cell activation, differentiation, and receptor binding or cytokine release.

Most patients will be taking one to three immunosuppressant drugs for the rest of their lives. Higher doses are used in the early postoperative period. Depending on the graft function, medication tapering occurs within 6 months, balancing the risks of rejection and infection. Most patients will initially be on steroids and two other antirejection drugs. Steroids are often tapered early, when possible, because of multiorgan side effects (Vierling 1999).

Cytomegalovirus infection is the most common opportunistic infection in immunocompromised transplant patients. Infections with herpesviruses may result in post-transplant lymphoproliferative disorder (secondary to Epstein-Barr virus) and varicella zoster infection, which are potentially life-threatening in the immunocompromised patient (Hayden 2001). As mentioned, hepatitis C cirrhosis is the cause for most liver transplants performed in the United States, and viral reinfection of the liver graft may lead to renewed organ failure. Interferon alpha and ribavirin are the treatment for hepatitis C both pre- and post-transplant. They are discussed in more detail in Chapter 10, "The Patient with Hepatitis C."

Hepatitis B infection had a poor prognosis until the introduction of prophylactic treatment with hepatitis B immune globulin and lamivudine (Epivir, 3TC). Hepatitis B immune globulin provides passive immunity for patients exposed to hepatitis B. It contains antibodies to hepatitis B surface antigen, which is prepared from plasma donated from people with high anti–hepatitis B titers. It may protect naive hepatocytes by blocking the hepatitis B virus receptors; it also neutralizes circulating virions through immune precipitation and immune complex formation.

Steroids are used extensively in the transplant setting because of their powerful immunosuppressive properties. They are associated with many neuropsychiatric side effects (see Chapter 8, "The Patient Using Steroids").

Several of the antiviral agents have adverse neuropsychiatric side effects. Lamivudine is a nucleoside reverse transcriptase inhibitor, active against the hepatitis B virus (which is a double-stranded DNA virus), as well as against HIV-1 and HIV-2. Other antiviral agents include adefovir, acyclovir/valacyclovir, and ganciclovir/valganciclovir. Discussion of the many other medications used in transplant medicine is beyond the scope of this chapter. Table 11–1 lists selected drugs that are associated with adverse neuropsychiatric reactions or interactions with psychotropic medications. Note that most drug interactions involve cytochrome 3A4.

■ TRANSPLANT PSYCHOPHARMACOLOGY

It is recognized that chronically ill patients have higher rates of depression and anxiety disorders than the general population. Loss of independence, work, and uncertainty about the future weigh heavily on patients and families. It is challenging to differentiate the secondary effects of end organ failure from primary

Table 11–1. Selected transplant medications with adverse neuropsychiatric reactions and drug-drug interactions

Medication	Drug-drug interactions relevant to psychiatry	Adverse neuropsychiatric reactions
Cyclosporine (Sandimmune, Neoral)	P450 3A4 interactions: Inhibitors: paroxetine (weak), nefazodone, fluvoxamine, citalopram Inducers: carbamazepine	Anxiety, restlessness, delirium, visual hallucinations Paresthesias, tremor, seizures, ataxia, cortical blindness
FK-506 (tacrolimus, Prograf)	P450 3A4 interactions: Inhibitors: nefazodone, fluvoxamine	Insomnia, tremor, delirium, paranoia, akinetic mutism, leukoencephalopathy
Sirolimus (Rapamycin, Rapamune)	P450 3A4 interactions	
Prednisone	(See also Chapter 8, "The Patient Using Steroids")	Irritability, restlessness, anxiety, insomnia Affective disorders (manic>depressive); psychosis; delirium; impaired cognition, memory and concentration
Penicillins		Seizures and delirium
Norfloxacin, ciprofloxacin	P450 1A2 interactions (↑ clozapine levels)	Delirium, visual hallucinations
Macrolide antibiotics (e.g., erythromycin)	P450 3A4 interactions	
Lamivudine (Epivir, 3TC)	None reported	Headache, insomnia, fatigue
Ribavirin	None reported	Irritability, depression, suicidality, fatigue, insomnia, anxiety. Increased neurotoxicity with interferon.
Acyclovir/valacyclovir	None reported	Delirium, depression, visual hallucinations
Ganciclovir/valganciclovir	None reported	Headache, convulsions, nightmares, visual hallucinations

psychiatric illness, particularly when there is symptomatic overlap with depression.

Patients with a history of psychiatric illness such as depression or bipolar illness are vulnerable to posttransplant recurrence, potentially exacerbated by medications. These patients require close monitoring for emergence of mood symptoms.

Patients with end organ failure—particularly cirrhosis—and psychiatric illness are frequently undertreated because of concerns about causing further organ damage. However, with cautious titration of medication and careful observation, psychopharmacological treatment is usually safe, and its use should not be limited by fear of exacerbation of the underlying disease. The guiding principle of psychopharmacology in patients with end organ failure is "start low, go slow." Baseline liver and kidney function should be checked prior to starting psychotropic medications.

Liver Transplantation

Depression

Symptoms of chronic hepatic encephalopathy are especially challenging because they are frequently mistaken for depression. Serotonin reuptake inhibitors are the most frequently used medications for depression and anxiety symptoms in this population. The medication dose should be slowly titrated upward until there is improvement of target symptoms. Drug-drug interactions may become clinically relevant because most immunosuppressive medications, including prednisone, are metabolized by 3A4 isoenzymes (Cozza et al. 2003), which also degrade many psychotropic medications.

Citalopram (Celexa), escitalopram (Lexapro), and sertaline (Zoloft) are particularly good choices because they are associated with fewer drug-drug interactions (Liston et al. 2001). Fluoxetine (Prozac) is no longer the antidepressant of choice because of its long half-life and potential for drug-drug interactions, but it has been used safely in organ transplant patients (Strouse et al. 1996). Nefazodone (Serzone) should be avoided because of its risk of hepatotoxicity and strong inhibition of P450 3A4 (Aranda-Michael et al. 1999; Campo et al. 1998). Methylphenidate (Ritalin) has been successful in the amotivated, fatigued post-transplant patient (Plutchik 1998).

Delirium

Delirium is quite common in the early postoperative period, especially in liver transplant patients. Patients and family must be educated about its warning signs. The etiology is multifactorial and includes delayed graft function, acid-base and electrolyte imbalance, infection, and prolonged hypotension during the surgery.

Recommended treatment involves haloperidol (Haldol) or atypical neuroleptics. *Caution:* Liver transplant patients are more vulnerable to developing extrapyramidal side effects (EPS) because of prolonged chronic hepatic encephalopathy and impaired basal ganglia function. Choosing an atypical antipsychotic instead of haloperidol to treat agitated delirium may lower the risk of EPS. As a result, haloperidol use is limited to post-transplant delirium, when a parenteral agent is needed; once the patient can take oral medication, atypical neuroleptics are recommended.

In many transplant centers, olanzapine (Zyprexa) has become the treatment of choice because of its minimal EPS and efficacy in mood stabilization (Breitbart et al. 2002; Schwartz and Masand 2002). However, olanzapine may worsen glucose intolerance and hyperglycemia, further exacerbating steroid effects. Caution is necessary. Risperidone (Risperdal, the most potent dopamine D_2 antagonist of the atypical neuroleptics, has been noted to cause EPS. There are insufficient data on the use of ziprasidone (Geodon) or aripiprazole (Abilify).

Chapter 1, "The Delirious Patient," provides an extensive discussion of the management of the delirious patient.

Anxiety

Benzodiazepines are to be avoided in patients with liver failure because they will worsen or precipitate hepatic encephalopathy. Low-dose tricyclic antidepressants and atypical neuroleptics such as quetiapine (Seroquel) (25–50 mg/day) and gabapentin (Neurontin) (titrated to symptoms) are safe alternatives.

Insomnia secondary to hepatic encephalopathy is common. Treatment with zolpidem (Ambien) or benzodiazepine hypnotics such as temazepam (Restoril) is not advised. Low-dose doxepin 25–50 mg/day, trazodone 25–50 mg/day, or atypical antipsychotics (e.g., quetiapine, olanzapine) are helpful and do not worsen encephalopathy.

Mania

Irritability, mood lability, insomnia, anxiety, racing thoughts, and feeling jittery or "on fire" are common steroid- or immunosuppressant-induced complaints. Early detection and treatment will prevent progression into full-blown mania or psychosis. Patients with a history of bipolar illness are at risk for cycling into mania or depression.

Atypical neuroleptics such as olanzapine and quetiapine are first-line medications to treat hypomania or mania in the first postoperative months. Mood symptoms often abate after lowering doses of steroids and immunosuppressive drugs. Certain immunosuppressant drugs (e.g., cyclosporine, FK-506 [tacrolimus]) produce end-stage renal disease at a rate that approaches 5%–10% 10 years post-transplant.

It is preferable to find alternatives to long-term use of lithium for patients taking these immunosuppressants, because of the possible double burden on the kidney. In the short run, however, lithium alone or in combination with atypical neuroleptics is acceptable in patients with known bipolar illness. However, lithium should not be the first choice in drug-induced mania.

The addition of valproic acid (Depakote, Depakene) in the immediate postoperative period is not advised because serum levels of this agent may mask causes of enzyme elevation other than drug-induced liver toxicity, such as perfusion injury, bile duct obstruction, rejection, or recurrent hepatitis C. Valproic acid can cause hyperammonemia and should be used cautiously in brittle, pretransplant cirrhotic patients. When liver enzyme levels stabilize and the risk of rejection decreases, valproic acid can be added for persistent mood symptoms. Valproic acid does not inevitably worsen liver function in patients with hepatitis C (Felker 2003).

Carbamazepine (Tegretol) and oxcarbazepine (Trileptal) are not recommended for transplant recipients. Carbamazepine may be hepatotoxic; oxcarbazepine may exacerbate the risk of hyponatremia in patients with portal hypertension and fluid overload. Clonazepam (Klonopin) and, anecdotally, gabapentin (Neurontin) are helpful if anxiety is the predominant mood symptom.

Kidney Transplantation

Depression

SSRIs are safe for kidney transplant recipients but require caution when coadministered with medications that cause P450 3A4 inhibition (Murphy 2001). Refer to Chapter 4, "The Patient with Kidney Disease," for information on treating the patient on dialysis.

Delirium

Delirium following kidney transplantation is relatively uncommon. Anecdotal reports seem to point to steroid-induced psychosis as the main culprit. Refer to Chapter 8, "The Patient Using Steroids."

Anxiety

Benzodiazepines safely treat patients with renal disease, although dosing should consider prolonged half-life in this setting. Short-acting benzodiazepines such as lorazepam or oxazepam are preferred (Murphy 2001) (see also Chapter 4, "The Patient With Kidney Disease").

Mania

Mood symptoms induced by steroid or immunosuppressive drugs are best treated with atypical neuroleptics. Valproic acid is the preferred long-term medication for mood stabilization at many centers. As reviewed in Chapter 4, "The Patient With Kidney Disease," long-term use of lithium, particularly in patients who require serum levels at the higher end, has been associated with renal insufficiency. Chronic allograft nephropathy is a feared cause of graft failure. Risk factors include hypertension, hyperlipidemia, smoking, and nephrotoxicity due to immunosuppressant medication. Lithium can cause a progressive combined glomerular and tubulointerstitial nephropathy. Avoid combining cyclosporine or tacrolimus with lithium, because these combinations put the patient at higher risk for graft failure (Markowitz et al. 2000; Tariq et al. 2000).

Heart Transplantation

Depression

The techniques for using antidepressants are the same in heart transplant patients as in cardiac patients who have not had transplant surgery. A review of these methods and medications can be found in Chapter 3, "The Patient With Cardiovascular Disease." SSRIs are preferred over the more cardiotoxic tricyclic antidepressants. Sertraline (Zoloft), venlafaxine (Effexor), and citalopram (Celexa) have been use safely in cardiac patients (Glassman et al. 2002; Querques and Stern 2002; Shapiro et al. 1999). The psychostimulants methylphenidate and dextroamphetamine have been successfully used after heart transplant with minimal effect on heart rate and blood pressure (Kaufman et al. 1984; Masand and Tesar 1996).

Delirium

Delirium is common following heart transplant and has multiple etiologies, such as CNS microembolism due to a heart bypass pump, cross-clamping of the aorta, hypoxemia, steroids, and infection. As discussed in Chapter 1, "The Delirious Patient," haloperidol in combination with lorazepam, and the atypical antipsychotics, are safe treatment interventions. Significant QT prolongation with antipsychotics is unusual and is easily monitored in the postoperative care setting.

Anxiety

Anxiety disorders are very common in cardiac patients awaiting transplant and in those after surgery. Tachycardia, shortness of breath, angina, pulmonary embolism, and chest tightness due to worsening of heart failure may mimic anxiety or panic disorder. The treatment of anxiety in patients with cardiac disease is presented in detail in Chapter 3. Clonazepam (Klonopin) and lorazepam (Ativan) have also been beneficial in treating excessive anxiety both before and after cardiac transplant (Shapiro 1996).

Mania

Mood symptoms secondary to steroid use or immunosuppression are treated with atypical neuroleptics or clonazepam. The techniques for using mood stabilizers are the same in heart transplant patients as in cardiac patients who have not had transplant surgery. These methods and medications are reviewed in detail in Chapter 3.

Lung Transplantation

Depression

There are no published data on antidepressant use in lung transplant patients. Anecdotal reports favor the use of SSRIs.

Delirium

Delirium following lung transplant is secondary to hypoxemia, hypercapnia, and infection. Treatment of choice involves the antipsychotics (Craven 1990), as discussed in detail in Chapter 1. Use caution with the usual technique of combining haloperidol with lorazepam (Ativan); as a member of the benzodiazepine class of medications, lorazepam has the potential for respiratory depression in patients with chronic lung disease (see Chapter 5, "The Patient With Pulmonary Disease"). A sedating atypical neuroleptic may be a better choice in this vulnerable population.

Anxiety

Chronic shortness of breath and fear of suffocation lead to high rates of anxiety disorders both before and after lung transplant. Bronchodilators and steroids contribute to anxiety as well (see also Chapter 5). A low-dose sedating atypical neuroleptic is the preferred medication to treat anxiety when there is concern about CO_2 retention. Experts in the field of lung transplantation also use lorazepam (Ativan) and clonazepam (Klonopin) for anxious patients without CO_2 retention (David Federonko, M.D., personal communication, October 2003).

Mania

Atypical neuroleptics effectively treat steroid-induced mood symptoms (see Chapter 8, "The Patient Using Steroids"). There appears to be no contraindication to using valproic acid. Lithium should be used with caution because of its potential to produce renal dysfunction.

■ REFERENCES

Aranda-Michael J, Koehler A, Bejarano P, et al: Nefazodone-induced liver failure: report of three cases. Ann Intern Med 130:285–288, 1999

Bartucci M: Kidney transplantation, in Solid Organ Transplantation. Edited by Cupples SA, Ohler L. New York, Springer, 2002, pp 189–222

Beresford T: Overt and covert alcoholism, in Liver Transplantation: The Alcoholic Patient. Edited by Lucey M, Merion R, Beresford T. Cambridge, England, Cambridge University Press, 1994, pp 6–28

Beresford T: Neuropsychiatric complications of liver and other solid organ transplantation. Liver Transpl 7:S36–S45, 2001

Bia M: Pretransplant evaluation of the living donor, in Primer on Transplantation. Edited by Norman D, Suki W. Mt. Laurel, NJ, American Society of Transplant Physicians, 1998, pp 191–196

Breitbart W, Tremblay A, Gibson C: An open trial of olanzapine for the treatment of delirium in hospitalized cancer patients. Psychosomatics 43:175–182, 2002

Campo J, Smith C, Perel J: Tacrolimus toxic reaction associated with the use of nefazodone: paroxetine as an alternative agent. Arch Gen Psychiatry 55:1050–1052, 1998

Coscia L, McGrory C, Philips L, et al: Pregnancy and transplantation, in Solid Organ Transplantation. Edited by Cupples SA, Ohler L. New York, Springer, 2002, pp 373–393

Cozza KL, Armstrong SC, Oesterheld JR: Concise Guide to Drug Interaction Principles for Medical Practice: Cytochrome P450s, UGTs, P-Glycoproteins, 2nd Edition. Washington, DC, American Psychiatric Publishing, 2003

Craven JL: Postoperative organic mental syndromes in lung transplant recipients. Toronto Lung Transplant Group. J Heart Transpl 9:129–132, 1990

Cupples SA, Ohler L (eds): Solid Organ Transplantation. New York, Springer, 2002

Dew MA, Kormos RL, DiMartini AF, et al: Prevalence and risk of depression and anxiety -related disorders during the first three years after heart transplantation. Psychosomatics 42:300–313, 2001

DiMartini A, Trzepacz P: Alcoholism and organ transplantation, in The Transplant Patient. Edited by Trzepacz P, DiMartini A. Cambridge, England, Cambridge University Press, 2000, pp 214–238

DiMartini A, Day N, Dew M, et al: Alcohol use following liver transplantation. Psychosomatics 42:55–62, 2001

Emond J: Living-related liver transplantation: selection of recipients and donors, in Primer on Transplantation, 2nd Edition. Edited by Norman D, Turka L. Mt. Laurel, NJ, American Society of Transplantation, 2001, pp 529–535

Felker B: The safety of valproic acid use for patients with hepatitis C infection. Am J Psychiatry 160:174–178, 2003

Filley C, Kleinschmidt-DeMasters B: Toxic leukoencephalopathy. N Engl J Med 345:425–431, 2001

Fox RC, Swazey JP: Organ transplantation as gift exchange, in Spare Parts: Organ Replacement in American Society. New York, Oxford University Press, 1992, pp 31–42

Glassman AH, O'Connor CM, Califf RM, et al: Sertraline treatment of major depression in patients with acute MI or unstable angina. JAMA 288:701–709, 2002

Hayden F: Antiviral agents, in Goodman and Gilman, Pharmacological Basis of Therapeutics, 10th Edition. Edited by Hardman J, Limbird L. New York, McGraw-Hill, 2001, pp 1313–1347

Hertz M: Lung Transplant Medical Care. Minneapolis, MN, Fairview Publications, 2001

Johnson E: Long-term follow-up of living kidney donors: quality of life after donation. Transplantation 67:717–721, 1999

Kasiske B: The evaluation of prospective renal transplant recipient and donor. Surg Clin North Am 11:27–39, 1998

Kaufman M, Cassem N, Murray G, et al: The use of methylphenidate in depressed patients after cardiac surgery. J Clin Psychiatry 45:82–84, 1984

Koch M, Banys P: Liver transplantation in opioid dependence. JAMA 285:1056–1058, 2001

Leo R, Smith B, Mori D: Guidelines for conducting a psychiatric evaluation of the unrelated kidney donor. Psychosomatics 44:452–460, 2003

Levenson J, Olbrisch M: Psychosocial screening and selection of candidates for organ transplantation, in The Transplant Patient. Edited by Trzepacz P, DiMartini A. Cambridge, England, Cambridge University Press, 2000, pp 21–41

Liston H, Markowitz J, Hunt N, et al: Lack of citalopram effect on pharmacokinetics of cyclosporine. Psychosomatics 42:370–372, 2001

Markowitz G, Radhakrishnan J, Kambhan N, et al: Lithium nephrotoxicity: a progressive combined glomerular and tubulointerstitial nephropathy. J Am Soc Nephrol 11:1439–1448, 2000

Masand P, Tesar G: Use of stimulants in the medically ill. Psychiatr Clin North Am 19:515–547, 1996

Murphy K: Psychiatric aspects of kidney transplantation, in Handbook of Kidney Transplantation. Edited by Danovitch G. Philadelphia, PA, Lippincott Williams & Wilkins, 2001, pp 365–379

Plutchik L: Methylphenidate in post liver transplant patients. Psychosomatics 39:118–223, 1998

Querques J, Stern T: Mind and heart, in Cutting Edge Medicine, Vol 21. Edited by Scotland N. Washington, DC, American Psychiatric Publishing, 2002, pp 1–21

Rose SM, Turka L, Kerr L, et al: Advances in immune-based therapies to improve solid organ graft survival. Adv Intern Med 47:293–331, 2001

Russell S, Jacob R: Living related organ donation: the donor's dilemma. Patient Educ Couns 21:89–99, 1993

Schenkel F, Barr M, Starnes V: Living-donor lobar lung transplantation: donor evaluation and selection, in Primer on Transplantation, 2nd Edition. Edited by Norman D, Turka L. Mt. Laurel, NJ, American Society of Transplantation, 2001, pp 645–647

Schwartz T, Masand P: The role of atypical antipsychotics in the treatment of delirium. Psychosomatics 43:171–174, 2002

Shapiro PA: Psychiatric aspects of cardiovascular disease. Psychiatr Clin North Am 19:613–629, 1996

Shapiro PA, Williams DL, Foray AT, et al: Psychosocial evaluation and prediction of compliance problems and morbidity after heart transplantation. Transplantation 60:1462–1466, 1995

Shapiro PA, Lesperance F, Frasure-Smith N, et al: An open-label preliminary trial of sertraline for treatment of major depression after acute myocardial infarction (the SADHAT trial). Sertraline Anti-Depressant Heart Attack Trial. Am Heart J 137:1100–1106, 1999

Simmons R: Living related donors: costs and gains, in Gift of Life. Edited by Simmons RG, Klein SD, Simmons RL. New York, Wiley, 1977, pp 153–197

Singer P, Siegle M, Whitington P, et al: Ethics of liver transplantation with living donors. N Engl J Med 321:620–621, 1989

Strouse T, Fairbanks L, Skotzko C, et al: Fluoxetine and cyclosporine in organ transplantation: failure to detect significant drug interactions or adverse clinical events in depressed organ recipients. Psychosomatics 37:23–30, 1996

Strouse T, El-Saden S, Glaser N, et al: Immunosuppressant neurotoxicity in liver transplant recipients. Psychosomatics 39:124–133, 1998

Tariq M, Morais C, Sobki S, et al: Effect of lithium on cyclosporine induced nephrotoxicity in rats. Ren Fail 22:545–560, 2000

Trotter J, Wachs M, Everson G, et al: Adult to adult transplantation of the right hepatic lobe from a living donor. N Engl J Med 346:1074–1082, 2002

Turka L, Norman D (eds): Primer on Transplantation. Mt. Laurel, NJ, American Society of Transplantation, 2001

UNOS: United Network for Organ Sharing. 2002. Available at: http://www.unos.org. Accessed December 13, 2002.

Vierling J: Immunology of acute and chronic hepatic allograft rejection. Liver Transpl Surg 5:S1–S20, 1999

Wijdicks E: Neurotoxicity of immunosuppressive drugs. Liver Transpl 7:937–942, 2001

Assessing Decisional Capacity and Informed Consent in Medical Patients

A Short, Practical Guide

Antoinette Ambrosino Wyszynski, M.D.
Carol F. Garfein, M.D.

■ DECISIONAL CAPACITY (COMPETENCY) AND INFORMED CONSENT

This discussion is a quick outline of some of the basic concepts in informed consent and decisional capacity. In-depth reviews may be found in volumes by Berg et al. (2001) and Grisso and Appelbaum (1998a).

All adults are presumed to be competent until proven otherwise. Competency is usually specific and defined in relation to a specified act, such as competency to make a will (*testamentary capacity*), to testify in court (*testimonial capacity*), or to consent to or refuse treatment (*decision-making capacity*). Being competent to perform one act does not mean that one is necessar-

ily competent to perform another. Unlike testamentary competency to make a will, for example, decisional capacity to refuse medical treatment is not subject to a uniform legal standard across the United States. Table 12–1 outlines a set of requirements for decisional capacity (Grisso and Appelbaum 1998a).

Doctors may be involved in expressing an opinion regarding the functioning and the abilities of an individual, but *competence* is a legal, not a medical concept, *decided by a judge, not a physician*. In the medical setting, a "competency" determination is more accurately an assessment of a patient's decision-making *capacity* (Grisso and Appelbaum 1998a). Requests to psychiatrists for evaluations are most frequently made for the following:

Wyszynski AA, Wyszynski B (eds.): *Manual of Psychiatric Care for the Medically Ill.* Washington, D.C., American Psychiatric Publishing, Inc., 2005

Table 12–1. Psychiatric requirements for decisional capacity

Required criterion	Operational description	Sample questions	Conditions that might interfere[a]
Factual understanding[b]	To understand the illness and its prognosis To understand the risks and benefits of treatment options, including nontreatment	Assess patient's understanding of: *The diagnosis:* "Please tell me in your own words: what do you believe is wrong with your health?" *Symptoms:* "What are some of the symptoms of your condition?" *Recommended [test/treatment]:* "What is the next step that the doctors have recommended to [treat or diagnose] your condition?" *Potential benefits:* "How do you think that the [treatment/test] the doctors are suggesting might help you? Even if you don't want it, can you explain how it *might* help someone?" *Potential risks:* "What are some of the risks of the [test/treatment]? Why do you believe it will have that effect?" *Consequences without treatment:* "What do you believe will happen if you are not treated? What will happen if you decide not to go along with your doctor's recommendation? How will this affect you at home or at work or with your family?" *Available choices:* "Let's review once more all the treatment options/ choices that you have. Can you list them for me?"	Low IQ Low education level Poor attention span Dementia Receptive aphasia Undiagnosed hearing loss
Insight and appreciation	To recognize that his/her welfare is affected by outcome of the decision To appreciate that he/she will benefit or suffer from the consequences of the decision	Patient's appreciation of the personal relevance of diagnosis: "Do you have doubts about how the doctors' diagnosis actually applies to you? If so, could you explain your doubts to me?"	Denial Delusions Suicidal intent Confabulation
Reasoning	To be realistic in his/her decision making To use the information logically to reach a decision	*Comparative reasoning:* "Let's go over the choice you prefer. Tell me why this choice seems best for you compared with the others we discussed." *Consequential reasoning:* "How do you think the treatment you want might affect your everyday life, like at home, or at work, or with your family?" *Ability to reason with relevant information:* "Tell me how you decided to [accept/reject] the recommended treatment. What factors were important in reaching the decision? How did you balance them?"	Psychosis Impaired memory Poor information processing Other cognitive deficits

Table 12–1. Psychiatric requirements for decisional capacity (*continued*)

Required criterion	Operational description	Sample questions	Conditions that might interfere[a]
Evidencing a choice or preference	To minimally be able to express a consistent preference or decision for or against something. (A person who is unable or unwilling to express a preference presumably lacks the capacity to make a choice.)	*Ability to express choice:* "Which one choice [of treatments] seems best for you?" *Quality of reasoning in arriving at final choice:* "When we started talking today, you favored [insert patient's preferred treatment, or state, 'you had difficulty deciding']. What do you think now, after discussing everything? What do you want to do?"	Muteness Inability to write, gesture, or signal Catatonia Unintelligibility Pathological ambivalence

[a]Although uncommon in most hospital settings, malingering may complicate and render decisional capacity evaluations invalid.
[b]The patient need not possess this level of understanding upon admission; he or she need only be able to receive and retain it in some reasonable form *during* the decision-making process.
Source. Adapted from material in Grisso and Appelbaum 1998a.

- Refusing treatment or disposition
- Signing out against medical advice
- Giving informed consent for a procedure

Decisional capacity for medical situations is considered an "acute" concept, applying to the person's ability at a particular point in time (Reid 2001). For example, capacity may fluctuate depending on the treatment (e.g., anesthesia or pain medication) or the illness (e.g., waxing or waning as in psychosis or delirium, or relatively stable as in dementia) (Reid 2001).

■ EXCEPTIONS TO INFORMED CONSENT

There are four situations in which informed consent is not necessary: waiver, incompetency, therapeutic privilege, and emergencies ("WITE") (Rundell and Wise 2000). They are explained in Table 12–2.

■ INCAPACITY, THE CONSULTANT, AND THE MEDICAL TEAM

When patients are in *agreement* with a proposed treatment or procedure, capacity assessments are not always requested, although this is not ideal ethically or from the risk management standpoint. Often, requests for assessments come at times of contention and tension, such as when a difficult patient is demanding to sign out of the hospital against medical advice or is re-fusing a procedure that is potentially life-preserving but may not be a clear-cut emergency.

As a consultant, one is often tempted to make a determination consistent with what will meet the recommendations of the medical team. Alternatively, one might be distracted by a personal formulation of what is "in the best interests of the patient."

Trainees are often most articulate about their potential for bias. One psychiatric resident who was learning to conduct capacity evaluations asked, "But what if I don't agree with the procedure that the surgeons want to do?"

Matters become more complicated. The discovery of disruptions in mental status that impair capacity is often greeted by immediate demands for "transfer to psychiatry." If the patient is too ill for such a transfer to be feasible, then an atmosphere of contention may invade the relationship with the consultant.

Several points bear emphasis:

- The role of the consultant is to *assess the mental status*. Psychiatrists participate in assessing decisional capacity specifically because of their expertise in the mental status.
- The psychiatrist's opinion must focus on *the patient's fitness to make a specific medical decision*. Opinions about the fitness of the procedure, and about what would be the best overall outcome for the patient, the medical-surgical team, and the hospital, are distractions. They are often subtle and hard to resist; however, they are irrelevant to the patient's decisional capacity and must be isolated out of the evaluation.

Table 12–2.   Exceptions to informed consent ("WITE")

Waiver	A patient competently, knowingly, and voluntarily has waived his or her right to receive information (e.g., a patient does not want information on drug side effects or on a possible negative surgical outcome).
Incompetency	Legal incompetency or lack of decisional capacity renders a person incapable of giving informed consent. [Options: see Table 12–5]
Therapeutic privilege	This is the most difficult of the four exceptions to apply. Informed consent is not required if a psychiatrist determines that a complete disclosure of possible risks and alternatives might have an adverse effect on the patient's health and welfare. If there is no specific case law or statute relevant to such a decision, the physician must be able to substantiate the patient's psychological inability to withstand being informed of the proposed treatment.
Emergencies	The law typically "presumes" that consent is granted when emergency treatment is necessary to save a life or prevent imminent serious harm and it is impossible to obtain either the patient's consent or that of someone authorized to provide consent for the patient. Two qualifications must be fulfilled: 1) the emergency must be serious and imminent; and 2) the patient's condition (and not other circumstances; e.g., adverse environmental circumstances) must determine that an emergency exists.

Source.   Adapted from Rundell and Wise 2000; Simon 2002.

- Remaining focused on the mental status is easier to advise in a handbook than it is to achieve in practice, particularly during an urgently called consultation. Be alert to potential confounders of objectivity, such as being cued by what the consultees want to hear or trying to avoid administrative headaches (e.g., "turf" battles, delays in routine treatment, the need for adjudication by a court). As Shouton et al. (1991) pointed out:

> [In the end,] the consultant must keep in mind that he [or she] is that: a consultant whose job it is to advise and not decide. The consultee may choose to disregard an assessment that a patient is incompetent [i.e., lacks capacity] to make treatment decisions and proceed with treatment. It is the treating physician who assumes both the legal and moral liability of his [or her] own actions. The consultant can only serve as a guidepost. (p. 635)

■ PRACTICAL ADVICE FOR EVALUATING CAPACITY

- Review the patient's medical history and current medical condition. Look especially for a history of changes in orientation and cognition.
- Perform a thorough clinical interview and mental status exam, looking for evidence of impaired cognition or a specific psychiatric disorder.
- Try to carry out the evaluation as a *dialogue,* rather than a mechanical question-and-answer session (Deaton et al. 1993). The ability to form an alliance with the examiner often predicts the patient's ability to engage in a course of treatment, a kind of "interpersonal competency" (Bursztajn and Hamm 1982). Encourage the patient to ask questions and volunteer thoughts or feelings about the particular procedures; this allows a more natural way of assessing thought process and content.

A 1991 paper by Campbell discussed pitfalls to avoid when discussing treatment options. Although originally written for nephrologists discussing dialysis treatment options, several of her warnings—which are really about maintaining neutrality—are also helpful to psychotherapeutic work, particularly while assisting patients in exploring medical treatment decisions:

- The *"I'll compare both treatments" trap:* Although physicians may be tempted to use this approach because it seems so logical and time-efficient, "pa-

tients may end up confused or glassy-eyed while nodding and agreeing that of course, they understand" (Campbell 1991, p. 176). To medically ill, anxious people, there is nothing more confusing than an approach that details comparisons. Explain treatment options individually first, and then compare them sparingly to allow the patient to review.
- *The trap of complex explanations:* It is easier for health care professionals to speak the technical shorthand that they use with colleagues. It takes more work to distill complicated medical concepts into simple explanations for the patient, whose concentration is already burdened by illness and fear.
- *The trap of prejudging who would or would not do well:* It is hard not to prejudge who would or would not do well with particular treatments on the basis of previous experiences with other patients. Every patient is unique and should not be judged on first impressions. Try to give patients the chance to make an educated decision for themselves.
- *The trap of deciding what you think would be best:* Patients often ask their physicians, including their psychiatrists, "Yes, but what do *you* think I should do? What treatment is best?" Beware of offering a quick opinion; there are pitfalls if you do so, such as the patient's continued dependency on "experts" and abdication of making responsible decisions.
- *Other pitfalls:* Finally, be careful of making sweeping generalizations, creating bias with length of discussion time (e.g., directing a patient to a particular decision by providing more details and discussion about it than about the alternatives), or using biased wording that propels the patient down one decision path and not another. Table 12–3 provides a checklist of pitfalls in assessing patients' decision-making capacity.

Grisso and Appelbaum (1998a) suggested several specific interview techniques for assessing competency. They recommended that the consultant, after becoming familiar with the medical chart, interviewing the care staff, and reviewing the medical disclosure, explain the disclosure to the patient again. Their recommendations are listed in Table 12–4.

The ultimate determination of decision-making capacity is based on the clinical judgment of the examiner. Figure 12–1 provides a worksheet for organizing the historical, mental status, and capacity-specific interview data. There are also sample questions for assessing capacity (i.e., factual understanding, reasoning, insight and appreciation, and the ability to evidence a choice or preference).

Table 12–3. Practitioner's checklist: pitfalls in assessing patients' decision-making capacity

Practitioner assumes that if the patient lacks capacity for one type of medical decision, the patient lacks capacity for all medical decisions.

Practitioner does not understand that capacity (or incapacity) is not "all or nothing" but specific to a decision.

Practitioner confuses legal competence, as decided by a formal judicial proceeding, with clinical determination of decision-making capacity.

Practitioner fails to ensure that the patient has been given relevant and consistent information about the proposed treatment before making a decision.

As long as a patient agrees with the practitioner's health care recommendations, the practitioner fails to consider that the patient may lack capacity for decisions.

When evaluating a patient's ability to return to independent living, the practitioner assesses only what the patient says, and fails to have the patient's functional abilities and living situation evaluated.

In assessing capacity to make medical decisions, the practitioner gives greater weight to the patient's final decision than to the process the patient uses in coming to that decision.

Practitioner assumes that if a patient has the diagnosis of dementia, even if mild, the patient lacks capacity for making all medical decisions.

Practitioner does not understand that criteria for determining capacity to make decisions vary with the risks and benefits inherent in the decision.

Practitioner believes that if a patient has a mental illness such as schizophrenia, the patient lacks capacity to make any medical decisions.

Practitioner lacks knowledge of emergency procedures for treating medically ill patients who lack decision-making capacity.

Practitioner assumes that if a past evaluation indicates lack of capacity to make medical decisions, the patient is decisionally incapacitated for similar decisions in the future.

Practitioner does not understand his or her obligation to maximize a patient's capacity to make decisions (even if this requires extra effort).

Practitioner believes that evaluation of cognition—for example, by using the Mini-Mental State Examination—is the appropriate method for determining capacity to make medical decisions.

Source.   Adapted from Ganzini L, Volicer L, Nelson W, et al: "Pitfalls in Assessment of Decision-Making Capacity." *Psychosomatics* 44:237–243, 2003.

Table 12–4. Interview techniques for assessing decisional capacity

(a) Explain the medical disclosure	❏ "Start from scratch" by explaining the medical/surgical disclosure to the patient again, discussing the patient's diagnosis and the proposed procedure and/or treatment. Review the potential risks and benefits as they have been explained to you by the primary care physician. Ask if there are any questions.
(b) Inquire	❏ Tell the patient that you want to make sure that he/she has understood what you have described. Ask the patient to describe to you his/her understanding of the information—what the disorder is called, what is wrong with him/her, what will happen if it is not treated, etc.
(c) Probe	❏ When the patient omits information, assist recall by using prompts from the disclosure segment of the interview. If the patient seems misinformed, challenge the patient's assumptions to see how rigidly they are kept, and on what basis.
(d) Re-explain	❏ Re-explain anything that has been misunderstood or is unclear. Re-inquire as in (b) above.

Source.   Adapted from Grisso and Appelbaum 1998a.

- Do not hesitate to seek legal consultation or contact the hospital's or organization's risk management department for counsel if there is particular difficulty, uncertainty, or ambiguity in the case.

Structured instruments such as the MacArthur Competence Assessment Tool for Treatment (Mac-CAT-T; Grisso and Appelbaum 1998a) seek to improve interrater reliability and focus on specific skills within domains of competency. The MacCAT-T is a semistructured interview that addresses the patient's understanding, appreciation, reasoning, and expression of a choice regarding treatment options. A manual and standard record form are available to guide the numerical rating of patient responses (Grisso and Appelbaum 1998b). A videotape is also available demonstrating an actual administration of the MacCAT-T by the authors (Grisso and Appelbaum 1999).

Strict Versus Lenient Standards of Competency: Factors Affecting Choice

Risk/Benefit

A sliding scale for strictness of standards is often used, based on the favorability of the risk/benefit outcome for the patient (Roth et al. 1977).

- *Favorable risk/benefit outcome:* A *strict* standard of capacity is used if the patient is *refusing* a treatment that has high likelihood of a favorable outcome with relatively low risk (e.g., intravenous antibiotics for an infected toe in a diabetic patient). A *lenient* standard is used if the patient is *consenting* to such a treatment.
- *Unfavorable risk/benefit outcome:* A *strict* standard is used if the patient is *consenting* to a treatment that carries a high risk with minimal or no benefit likely (e.g., experimental chemotherapy with high toxicity, for someone with disseminated cancer); a *lenient* standard is used if the patient is *refusing* such a treatment.

Comment: This approach has been criticized as allowing the patient to be manipulated by a well-meaning but paternalistic physician. On the other hand, its proponents feel it permits the better-informed physician to triage risk for patients, increasing the likelihood that those patients will be able to make their own truly informed decisions about their medical care. Reid (2001) has explained the situation most succinctly:

Interventions that are not likely to harm the patient or that involve a great preponderance of benefit and very little risk are not generally seen as matters that justify much testing of competence. The level of competence required for consenting to them is often very low....[For example,] almost any adult, even with substantial psychiatric symptoms or mental retardation, may often be allowed to consent to low-risk procedures and treatments [e.g., simple venipuncture, physical exam] by simply expressing agreement, and sometimes by merely expressing a choice or participating voluntarily....Some procedures have very significant consequences but the decision process involving them is pretty simple. (p. 277)

Complexity of Decision

The most illuminating example of this dilemma is given by Reid (2001). There are two 35-year-olds with mild mental retardation. One develops severe traumatic gangrene of her foot and requires amputation in order to survive. The second develops breast cancer and has to choose lumpectomy, mastectomy, chemotherapy, and/or radiation. The first is a yes-or-no decision to amputate; it is a major life event and a procedure with a clear life-or-death outcome of the decision. The second situation is more ambiguous; the woman must be able to process the pros and cons of different types of treatment and their statistical uncertainty, as well as their impact on appearance, future fertility, and statistical survival. The level of competence required to evaluate any of the possible treatment options and compare them with the others is substantial. Reid (2001) noted:

In the first example (trauma-related gangrene and amputation), the law may allow considerable mental incapacity before questioning the patient's competence. In the second (complex breast cancer), some substitution of judgment (e.g., by a guardian) is likely to be required. (p. 278)

Competence to Consent Versus Competence to Refuse

As any consultant knows, things really get murky when patients refuse a lifesaving procedure (like amputating a gangrenous limb). Sometimes, *informed refusal* may require a much higher level of competence than informed consent. The sliding scale of risk is often inescapable for setting strictness or lenience of standards in determining decisional capacity for medical decisions.

Patient: _____   Date: _____

STAFF INTERVIEW & CHART REVIEW

(1)	**HIGH-PRIORITY QUESTIONS** ⇨	Is this an emergency? ❑ yes ❑ no If yes, why?	Will the patient die without treatment? ❑ yes ❑ no
(2)	Medical diagnosis		Proposed treatment

(3)	Risks of treatment (How likely is each?) 1. _____ 2. _____ 3. _____	Consequences of refusing treatment 1. _____ 2. _____ 3. _____	Treatment options 1. _____ 2. _____ 3. _____

(4) Reasons for psychiatric consultation?

RED FLAGS ⇨	Psychosis? ❑ yes ❑ no	Suicidal ideation? ❑ yes ❑ no	Delirium? ❑ yes ❑ no	Dementia? ❑ yes ❑ no

(5) What do the primary care staff think might be causing the difficulties with capacity?

GENERAL MENTAL STATUS EXAM

SENSORIUM: alert   drowsy   fluctuating   other

APPEARANCE	SPEECH
MOOD/AFFECT	**Suicidal ideation?** ❑ yes ❑ no **Homicidal ideation?** ❑ yes ❑ no
THOUGHT PROCESS/CONTENT	**ORIENTATION** Person? ❑ yes ❑ no Time? year___ season___ date___ day___ month___ Place? state___ country___ town____ hospital___ floor___

CONCENTRATION Serial 7s 100 __93 __86 __79 __72 __65 Or *WORLD* backwards D_ L_ R_ O_ W_	**REGISTRATION** Give patient 3 objects to repeat. ___ **RECALL:** __ objects in __ minutes	**FOLLOW A 3-STAGE COMMAND** "Take a paper in your right hand, fold it in half, and put it on the floor."
NAME a pencil, and a watch. **REPEAT:** "No ifs, ands, or buts."	**READ** and obey the following: "Close your eyes."	**WRITE** a sentence. Subject __ Verb__ Makes sense?__
OTHER:		

CAPACITY-SPECIFIC INTERVIEW (sample questions)

(1) "Please tell me in your own words: what do you believe is wrong with your health?"

Patient's understanding of the diagnosis is   Satisfactory   Impaired   Unsatisfactory   Bizarre

(2) "Do you have doubts about how the doctors' diagnosis actually applies to you? If so, could you explain your doubts to me?"

Patient's appreciation of the personal relevance of diagnosis is   Satisfactory   Impaired   Unsatisfactory   Bizarre

(3) "What are some of the symptoms of your condition?"

Patient's understanding of symptoms is   Satisfactory   Impaired   Unsatisfactory   Bizarre

(4) "What is the next step that the doctors have recommended to [treat or diagnose] your condition?"

Patient's understanding of recommended [test/treatment] is   Satisfactory   Impaired   Unsatisfactory   Bizarre

(5) | "How do you think that the [treatment/test] the doctors are suggesting might help you? Even if you don't want it, can you explain how it *might* help someone?"

Patient's understanding of potential benefits is   Satisfactory   Impaired   Unsatisfactory   Bizarre

(6) | "What are some of the risks of the [treatment/test]? Why do you believe it will have that effect?"

Patient's understanding of potential risks is   Satisfactory   Impaired   Unsatisfactory   Bizarre

(7) | "Your doctor (or I) told you of a (percentage/likely/unlikely] chance that [named risk] might occur with this [treatment/test]. In your own words, how probable is it?"

Patient's understanding of the likelihood of risks is   Satisfactory   Impaired   Unsatisfactory   Bizarre

(8) | "What do you believe will happen if you are not treated? What will happen if you decide not to go along with your doctor's recommendation? How will this affect you at home or at work or with your family?"

Patient's understanding of consequences without treatment is   Satisfactory   Impaired   Unsatisfactory   Bizarre

(9) | "Let's review once more all the treatment options/choices that you have. Can you list them for me?"

Patient's understanding of available choices is   Satisfactory   Impaired   Unsatisfactory   Bizarre

(10) | "Which one choice [from #(9) above] seems best for you?"

Can the patient express a choice?   **Yes   No**

Patient's ability to express choice is   Satisfactory   Impaired   Unsatisfactory   Bizarre

(11) | "Let's go over the choice you prefer. Tell me why this choice seems best for you compared to the others we discussed."

Can the patient compare at least 2 treatment options, specifying at least some difference between them?   **Yes   No**

Patient's comparative reasoning is   Satisfactory   Impaired   Unsatisfactory   Bizarre

(12) | "How do you think the treatment you want [i.e., preferred treatment chosen in #10] might affect your everyday life, like at home, or at work, or with your family?"

Patient thinks of at least 1 practical outcome of preferred treatment; does not merely repeat back the original disclosure.   **Yes   No**

Patient's consequential reasoning is   Satisfactory   Impaired   Unsatisfactory   Bizarre

(13) | "Tell me how you decided to [accept/reject] the recommended treatment... What factors were important in reaching the decision? How did you balance those factors?"

Patient's ability to reason with relevant information is   Satisfactory   Impaired   Unsatisfactory   Bizarre

(14) | "When we started talking today, you favored [insert patient's preferred treatment, or state, 'you had difficulty deciding.'] What do you think now, after discussing everything? What do you want to do?"

Does the patient's final choice follow logically from previous reasoning, with no distortion of reality?   **Yes   No**

FINAL DETERMINATION about patient's decision-making capacity for the specific treatment or procedure	Satisfactory Impaired Unsatisfactory Bizarre
	Date: Time:

Figure 12–1.   Worksheet for decision-making capacity: organizing the data.

Source.   Devised by A.A. Wyszynski from the work of Grisso and Appelbaum (1998a), pp. 77-99, with permission of the authors.

Documentation

Use phrases such as the following when documenting your findings in the patient's chart (Deaton 2000):

- "The patient appears to have X diagnosis because…"
- "Treatment will be instituted so that…"
- "This treatment has the following risks…; nonetheless, the risks are outweighed by the following benefits:…"
- "The patient has been informed of the above treatment plan, as well as of the following treatment option:…"
- "As evidenced by the following, the patient has the capacity to give informed consent:…"

Modify the scheme accordingly when the patient is giving "informed refusal," or when the patient is found to lack the capacity ("is not competent") to give consent.

The Patient Who Lacks Mental Capacity for Health Care Decisions

There are several options for patients who lack decisional capacity for health care decisions, as listed in Table 12–5.

Table 12–5. Health care consent options for patients who lack decisional capacity

- Advance directives (living wills, durable power of attorney, health care proxy)
- Statutory surrogates (spouse or court-appointed guardians)[a]
- Substituted judgment of a family member (proxy consent)
- Substituted judgment by the court
- Adjudication of incompetence with appointment of a guardian
- Institutional administrators or committees
- Treatment review panels

---

[a]Some states (but not all) permit proxy decision making through their medical statutory surrogate laws that specific relatives (usually next of kin, e.g., spouse; may also be court-appointed guardian) may authorize consent on behalf of the incompetent patient. In many states, proxy consent is limited to medical conditions and is not available for patients with psychiatric conditions.
Source. Adapted from Simon 2002. Used with permission.

Substituted Judgment

Sometimes the process of obtaining an adjudication of incompetence (and the appointment of a guardian) is burdensome and costly and takes so long that it interferes with the timely provision of care. A common solution is to seek *proxy consent* of a family member serving as a guardian. The standard generally applied by the law for surrogate decision making is that of "*substituted judgment.*" The standard requires the appointed agent to make medical decisions as the patient would choose to make them, not as the agent would make them. The agent must be able to synthesize the diverse values, beliefs, practices, and prior statements of the patient for a specific circumstance (Emanuel and Emanuel 1992).

- *Caution:* Not all states permit proxy consent without going to court (i.e., "by statute"); when there is doubt about the legality of proxy consent, it is unwise to rely on the good-faith consent of the next of kin without obtaining legal counsel (Macbeth et al. 1994).

Nonurgent Treatment

Physicians are authorized to institute treatment in emergencies when the patient lacks decisional capacity (e.g., when delirium is present). However, if there is no emergency or advance directive but there is a need to treat (e.g., for dementia), it is best to obtain legal counsel as quickly as possible. *Exceptions:* some states automatically empower next of kin or other individuals to give consent for an incapacitated individual (Deaton 2000).

Advance Directives

By law, the competent patient always retains the right to make his or her own medical decisions and to contravene or even revoke the advance directive. Laws regarding advance directives are made at the state level. Several types of advance directives are discussed below.

- The *living will* is a legal document that pertains exclusively to the issue of withholding or withdrawing life-support systems. Its twofold purpose is 1) to express a person's desire whether or not to be kept alive by artificial means and 2) to protect the physician who makes the decision to withhold treatment (Deaton 2000).
- The *durable power of attorney for health care* goes beyond the living will, granting the right to control all aspects of personal care and medical treatment,

including treatment refusal and withdrawal. Unlike the traditional power of attorney, the "durable" version remains valid even when the individual lacks the capacity to make decisions.

- The *health care proxy* is a legal instrument similar to the durable power of attorney but is specifically created for health care decision-making.

When evaluating someone who plans to execute an advance directive, the consultant should perform the usual evaluation for capacity, exploring the individual's understanding and reasoning that underlie treatment requests or refusals. Clinical impressions should be documented in case there is a dispute about the validity of the directive or a disagreement with the patient's appointed proxy about decision-making capacity (Schneiderman and Teetzel 1995).

The application of advance directives to patients with psychiatric syndromes becomes complicated. For example, a patient with a mental disorder due to a general medical condition may be asymptomatic when he or she executes a durable power of attorney agreement or healthy care proxy directing, "If I become mentally unstable again, administer medications even if I strenuously object or resist" (Simon 2002). However, advance directives are easily revoked, and if this occurs, it may be necessary to honor the patient's refusal even if there is evidence that the patient lacks decisional capacity. These complexities are beyond the scope of this limited summary; legal consultation should be sought in these situations.

Do-Not-Resuscitate (DNR) Orders

Any competent patient has the right to reject or to insist on resuscitative treatment. Terminally ill patients with intact decisional capacity can generally decline further medical intervention with informed consent. If a patient is incapacitated, the state must sustain life support unless specific instructions from the patient, when competent, are available stating his or her wishes (Simon 2002). As set forth in the landmark *Cruzan* decision by the U.S. Supreme Court (1990), the state may refuse to remove food and water without clear and convincing evidence of the patient's wishes to withhold treatment, even to the exclusion of the family's wishes. This ruling compelled physicians to seek clear and competent instructions for the patient regarding foreseeable treatment decisions (Simon 2002).

Once made by a person with intact capacity, the DNR decision can rarely be overruled. If the patient ei-

ther requests or declines resuscitation and later becomes incapacitated, the court (not the family) may be the only party able to reverse the patient's original decision. (However, some states permit the family, a significant other, a physician, and/or the hospital ethics committee to intervene to resuscitate the patient who has become incapacitated, if a chance of recovery exists.)

- *Note:* If a person with a severe psychiatric disorder, such as major depression, refuses resuscitation because death is an "appropriate, deserved" outcome, he or she is considered to be incapacitated.

■ PHYSICIAN-ASSISTED SUICIDE

Physician-assisted suicide (PAS) is a highly controversial topic currently receiving tremendous attention from both the public and the medical community. The legal and ethical aspects of PAS range beyond the scope of this review. Very briefly, as PAS gains increasing legal recognition, psychiatrists are likely to be called in for consultation to determine the terminally ill patient's capacity to commit suicide. The presence of a psychiatric illness associated with suicide, such as a treatable major depressive episode, must be ruled out as the driving factor behind PAS (Deaton 2000; Simon 2002).

■ REFERENCES

Berg J, Appelbaum P, Lidz C, et al (eds): Informed Consent: Legal Theory and Clinical Practice. New York, Oxford University Press, 2001

Bursztajn H, Hamm R: The clinical utility of utility assessment. Med Decis Making 2:161–165, 1982

Campbell A: Strategies for improving dialysis decision making. Perit Dial Int 11:173–178, 1991

Deaton R: Medical-legal issues and psychiatric consultation, in Psychiatric Care of the Medical Patient. Edited by Stoudemire A, Fogel B, Greenberg D. New York, Oxford University Press, 2000, pp 1135–1144

Deaton R, Colenda C, Bursztajn H: Medical-legal issues, in Psychiatric Care of the Medical Patient. Edited by Stoudemire A, Fogel B. New York, Oxford University Press, 1993, pp 929–938

Emanuel E, Emanuel L: Proxy decision making for incompetent patients—an ethical and empirical analysis. JAMA 267:2067–2071, 1992

Grisso T, Appelbaum P: Assessing Competence to Consent to Treatment. New York, Oxford University Press, 1998a

Grisso T, Appelbaum P: MacArthur Competence Assessment Tool for Treatment (MacCAT-T) (manual and record form). Sarasota, FL, Professional Resource Press, 1998b. Available at: http://www.prpress.com.

Grisso T, Appelbaum P: MacArthur Competence Assessment Tool for Treatment (MacCAT-T) (videotape). Sarasota, FL, Professional Resource Press, 1999. Available at: http://www.prpress.com.

Macbeth J, Wheeler A, Sither J, et al: Legal and Risk Management Issues in the Practice of Psychiatry. Washington, DC, Psychiatrists Purchasing Group, 1994

Reid W: Competence to consent. J Psychiatr Pract 7:276–278, 2001

Roth L, Meisel A, Lidz C: Tests of competency to consent to treatment. Am J Psychiatry 134:279–284, 1977

Rundell JR, Wise MG: Concise Guide to Consultation Psychiatry, 3rd Edition. Washington, DC, American Psychiatric Press, 2000

Schneiderman LJ, Teetzel H: Who decides who decides? When disagreement occurs between the physician and the patient's appointed proxy about the patient's decision-making capacity. Arch Intern Med 155:793–796, 1995

Shouton R, Groves J, Vaccarino J: Legal aspects of consultation, in Massachusetts General Hospital Handbook of General Hospital Psychiatry, 3rd Edition. Edited by Cassem N. St. Louis, MO, Mosby-Year Book, 1991, pp 619–638

Simon R: Legal and ethical issues, in The American Psychiatric Publishing Textbook of Consultation-Liaison Psychiatry: Psychiatry in the Medically Ill, 2nd Edition. Edited by Wise MG, Rundell JR. Washington, DC, American Psychiatric Publishing, 2002, pp 167–186

Chapter 13

Psychological Issues in Medical Patients

Autonomy, Fatalism, and Adaptation to Illness

Antoinette Ambrosino Wyszynski, M.D.

The attitudes of autonomy and fatalism relative to illness are often culturally determined and psychologically fixed. Moreover, these attitudes may be maintained independently of factual knowledge. The concept of health-related autonomy first appeared in the research literature as "health locus of control" (HLOC; Wallston et al. 1978). An "internally directed" system characterizes the individual who takes responsibility for his or her health and believes that personal actions have an impact. An "externally directed" system occurs in the fatalistic person who believes that health and illness are influenced by sources beyond one's control (e.g., fate, chance, "other people"). Assessments of HLOC are strong independent predictors of health-related behaviors, with high "externality" associated with less knowledge of illness prevention (Aruffo et al. 1993).

Often there are mixtures of these two attitudes that shift, depending on stage of illness, phase of life, and personality variables. If the patient's beliefs about his or her illness are ignored by the physician because they seem "irrational," then rapport will be difficult to establish and medical advice may fall on polite but deaf ears. Misunderstandings are particularly likely if the doctor and patient come from different cultures.

■ THE "I TAKE CHARGE" PATIENT

Patient's self-defense strategy: "If I can maintain the belief that I control my illness, then I will be less terrified about sickness and dying" (autonomous; internal health locus of control).

Wyszynski AA, Wyszynski B (eds.): *Manual of Psychiatric Care for the Medically Ill.* Washington, D.C., American Psychiatric Publishing, Inc., 2005

Sample statements (Aruffo et al. 1993):

- "If I take care of myself, I can avoid illness."
- "Whenever I get sick, it's because of something I've done or not done."
- "People's ill health results from their own carelessness."
- "I am directly responsible for my health."
- "When I feel ill, I know it is because I have not been getting the proper exercise or eating right."

Individuals with this approach are proactive about maintaining their health. The belief in their own autonomy makes them participate in staying healthy and take advantage of information that promotes good health. Unfortunately, when illness occurs, these patients are vulnerable to feeling guilty that they have not tried hard enough, were not vigilant enough, or "didn't have the right attitude." If their particular beliefs are at odds with the medical system (e.g., the belief in "healing crystals" as a substitute for chemotherapy), then medical interventions may be rejected as attempts to make them "submit to the system." Management entails exploring patients' convictions about why they became sick and what *they* believe will be therapeutic (e.g., "I got diabetes because I ate too much sugar. I don't want insulin because everyone I know who took it wound up with an amputation and died. I'd rather avoid sugary foods than take insulin."). Without empathic understanding regarding patients' beliefs, attempts to "talk them out of" their convictions or provide alternative explanations may alienate patients and could jeopardize treatment.

■ THE "WISH UPON A STAR" PATIENT

Patient's self-defense strategy: "If I can maintain the belief that I have little impact on my illness, then I will be less terrified about sickness and dying" (fatalistic; external health locus of control).

Sample statements (Aruffo et al. 1993):

- "Good health is largely a matter of good fortune."
- "No matter what I do, if I am going to get sick I will get sick."
- "Most people do not realize the extent to which their illnesses are controlled by accidental happenings."
- "I can only do what my doctor tells me to do."

- "There are so many strange diseases around that you can never know how or when you might pick one up."
- "People who never get sick are just plain lucky."

Fatalistic patients believe that health and illness are influenced by sources beyond their control, such as chance. Fatalists have the advantage of being less likely to blame themselves for medical outcomes, compared with their more autonomous counterparts. They will be most likely to follow medical advice if they identify the physician as the "externalized" authority who controls their health. However, the physician may be obliged to assume an authoritarian role, with the patient as passive participant. If the physician attempts to "force" a fatalistic patient into autonomous decision making (e.g., into participation in informed discussions), antagonism often results (e.g., "the doctor is making me listen to things I would just rather not know"). Fatalistic people also may resist changing their behavior to promote health, particularly if the changes are inconvenient or unpleasurable (e.g., using condoms, going for mammograms, exercising). Management entails exploring the underlying belief in "fate" with the patient first (e.g., "What are the advantages of avoiding yearly mammograms? How do you know that it is your fate to avoid the test, rather than to discover what it reveals? How does the unknown make you worry less, compared with knowing something and taking action to fix it?"). Paradoxically, the helpless surrender to "fate" often helps the person feel *less* helpless because the denial diminishes anxiety. Interventions that ignore the psychological need for passivity and denial will be disregarded, or will make the patient become angry and possibly abandon treatment.

■ STAGES IN PSYCHOLOGICIAL ADAPTATION TO SERIOUS ILLNESS

Four stages have been defined in the psychological adaptation to serious illness (Nichols 1985). Although these stages may occur simultaneously or in any order, they are helpful in orienting clinicians as they work with seriously ill patients. The following material is a summary of an outline by Nichols (1985).

Initial Crisis Stage

The effects of the diagnosis register on the patient, family, and friends. Denial predominates, sometimes alternating with intense emotions (shock, anxiety, guilt, fear, anger, sadness). Denial may be so intense that the patient may adopt an attitude of indifference. As long as the patient is following medical advice and is adapting reasonably, there is no need to attempt to dislodge denial. Patients at this stage typically have difficulty retaining information and may distort what they are told regarding their illness. For transmittable illnesses such as AIDS or hepatitis, the reactions may be more intense because of the fear of contagion and the need to manage risky behaviors.

Transitional Stage

This stage begins when denial gives way to alternating feelings of guilt, anger, self-pity, and anxiety, often with ruminations about past behavior. This is a period of distress, confusion, and disruption. Depression, suicidal ideation, and lashing out at family and caregivers often ensue. In cases of an HIV-positive diagnosis, for example, there is sometimes drug use and/or sexual acting out. In situations where comprehension is impaired, the clinician should advise accompanied medical visits to be sure that the patient understands and adheres to instructions.

Acceptance Stage

The patient begins to form a new identity, integrating the acceptance of the illness and its implications. Patients may describe appreciating the quality of life rather than quantity of years. Some individuals develop a fighting spirit toward the illness, reassess former values, and sometimes feel a new sense of spirituality and concern for others. They feel less victimized by life, become less egocentric, and find satisfaction in altruistic and community activities. However, it has been noted that acceptance is "a deficiency state, … as is evidenced by losses of health, energy, income, and independence. Under these circumstances, the human spirit's ability to marshal such inner resources is remarkable" (Fernandez and Nichols 1990, p. 31).

Preparatory Stage

At this stage, patients often fear becoming too dependent on others. They take care of unfinished practical business (e.g., making wills, attending to finances) and confront lingering emotional issues with loved ones. It is crucial for patients to have opportunities to discuss their feelings about dying and death if they wish. Although suicidal ideation occurs fleetingly

throughout all stages, and some may consider suicide preferable to intolerable dependency, most patients continue to fight for life. It has been shown that people who suffer life-threatening complications may believe that good times lie ahead and that life continues to be worthwhile (Rabkin et al. 1993).

The clinician should watch for acting out of some of the unresolved conflicts from earlier stages of coping. For example, the patient who has seemingly accepted the inevitability of dying from a serious illness may embark upon a long-term project that he or she cannot possibly live to finish (e.g., buying a house, adopting a child, planning to coach next summer's Little League). Such actions can be very distressing to family members because they seem "crazy." Family members often respond by saying nothing because they do not want to "take away hope," but privately grieve again. One therapeutic strategy would be to explore the patient's feelings and hopes about the new project, without attempting to influence the patient's actions. There will usually be opportunities to demonstrate the contrast between the patient's hopeful fantasies (i.e., that he or she will live much longer than is expected) and the difficult reality (i.e., that the remaining time is very limited). Clinicians must be prepared for the patient's reexperience of the initial crisis stage (shock, anxiety, guilt, fear, anger, sadness). It is often another opportunity to help the patient (and family) through the stages of transition, acceptance, and preparation.

◼ TREATMENT GOALS FOR PEOPLE LEARNING TO LIVE WITH SERIOUS ILLNESS

Psychotherapy with patients who are learning to live with a serious medical illness requires flexibility and knowledge of the illness's medical, psychiatric, and psychological impact. Issues seemingly resolved at one phase of treatment may emerge again with intensity as changes in physical and cognitive status occur.

Zegans et al. (1994) summarized treatment goals as follows:

1. Help patients maintain control of their lives.
2. Assist them in finding healthy coping skills, especially when confronting the many stresses of their illness.
3. Work to lessen feelings of anger, denial, panic, and despair when they are disruptive to patients' treatment or quality of life.

4. Enable patients to establish and maintain feelings of self-respect by working through issues connected with guilt, shame, and self-blame.
5. Facilitate communication with family, partners, and friends about the disease.
6. Address fears of rejection and abandonment in the context of terminal illness.
7. Assist the patient in maintaining good interpersonal and sexual relationships whenever possible.
8. Collaborate in developing strategies to deal with real and anticipated crises in the health and socioeconomic spheres.
9. Help identify and address the "unfinished business" in patients' lives.
10. Work together with the patient to explore the meaning of death.

■ REFERENCES

Aruffo J, Coverdale J, Pavlik V, et al: AIDS knowledge in minorities: significance of locus of control. Am J Prev Med 9:15–20, 1993

Fernandez F, Nichols S: Psychiatric complications of HIV disease, in AIDS Primer. Edited by American Psychiatric Association AIDS Education Project. Washington, DC, American Psychiatric Association, 1990, pp 29–33

Nichols S: Psychosocial reactions of persons with the acquired immunodeficiency syndrome. Ann Intern Med 103:765–767, 1985

Rabkin JG, Remien R, Katoff L, et al: Resilience in adversity among long-term survivors of AIDS. Hosp Community Psychiatry 44:162–167, 1993

Wallston K, Wallston B, Devellis R: Development of the Multi-dimensional Health Locus of Control (MHLC) scales. Health Educ Monogr 6:161–170, 1978

Zegans L, Gerhard A, Coates T: Psychotherapies for the person with HIV disease. Psychiatr Clin North Am 17:149–162, 1994

Chapter 14

When Patients Ask About the Spiritual

A Primer

Stanley Grossman, M.D.

Antoinette Ambrosino Wyszynski, M.D.

Leonard Barkin, M.D.

Victor Schwartz, M.D.

Few psychiatrists learn how to deal with or even think about the spiritual issues that arise as people cope with the tragic things that happen to them. However, psychological trauma is often all about the personally tragic. For those facing the immediate tragedy of serious illness, spirituality and religious faith can be powerful allies. Spiritual beliefs often buffer and facilitate the transition from the initial shock of diagnosis to the eventual acceptance of the illness and its implications. Even if dormant for most of adulthood, spiritual thoughts and feelings are catalyzed by illness—whether it be in renewal of previously discarded beliefs, affirmation of currently held ones, or sometimes angry disavowal of it all. As patients grapple with anger and doubt, difficult psychotherapy-specific questions arise, of a kind that most psychiatrists feel ill trained to answer. For example:

- Doctor, why would God do this to me?
- Why do bad things happen to good people?
- Should I pray? Aren't there studies that show that prayer helps?
- Do you believe in the power of prayer, doctor?
- Do you think that something better waits for me in another life, when my suffering will be over?
- Shouldn't we leave it to God to decide further treatment?

Sometimes these questions do not allow much time for premeditated response. What do you say? How do you say it? Do you dodge the question? Refuse to answer? Answer everything by asking "What comes to mind?" Try to reassure the patient? Refer everything to a pastoral counselor? Where do you draw the line between what is helpful to answer at the bedside and what is not?

Wyszynski AA, Wyszynski B (eds.): *Manual of Psychiatric Care for the Medically Ill.* Washington, D.C., American Psychiatric Publishing, Inc., 2005

■ IS IT EVER APPROPRIATE FOR DOCTORS TO SPEAK ABOUT RELIGION WITH A PATIENT?

It has been said that there are no atheists in foxholes, or on the deathbed. However, opinions vary about the appropriateness of discussing religious questions with patients. Some feel that it is better left to a rabbi, imam, minister, or priest and that a trained spiritual counselor is a necessary part of the therapeutic team. Others disagree, proposing that it can be helpful to explore patients' religious faith in the context of a specific medical issue if it comforts them, particularly as they struggle with the distress of a new diagnosis or proposed procedure (Ehman et al. 1999; Hebert et al. 2001).

The doctor's role as the patient's protector in the fight against illness dovetails with the universal desire for a powerful guardian during times of mortal crisis. Patients understandably turn to physicians with questions about divine guardianship when they are made anxious by their medical illness. Usually religion is mentioned briefly, with the patient seeking physician-assisted support, not theological advice. In psychotherapy, questions about God, prayer, and religion are more complex, containing levels of meaning and personal history for the patient.

Although prayer, religion, and spirituality deal with the indefinable, for these discussions with medical patients it is important to maintain concrete goals (Lo et al. 2002):

- Clarify the patient's concerns, beliefs, and needs about spiritual or religious issues to determine the appropriateness of a pastoral referral.
- Help the patient identify goals for medical care.
- Assist the patient in making medical decisions.

There are a number of helpful interview questions for asking about religion and spirituality in a psychological interview, as listed in Table 14–1.

One major pitfall in physician-patient discussions about spiritual and religious issues involves *trying to resolve unanswerable questions for the patient rather than elicit the patient's feelings about them.* There are others:

- Being sidetracked from the psychological to the theological; for example, focusing on the patient's spiritual dilemmas at an intellectual level rather than exploring feelings and meanings
- Providing inappropriate reassurance
- Subtly imposing one's beliefs—or skepticism—on the patient

"Doctor, aren't there studies that show that prayer helps?"

What is the best way to field questions about the value of prayer for medical outcome? Most practitioners follow the guideline of supporting what reassures the patient, as long as it does no harm and does not interfere with medical interventions. Some highly controversial studies, such as those on intercessory prayer, in which others pray for the patient, have suggested that prayer does help (Harris et al. 1999; Sloan and Bagiella 2002). There is less contention about the beneficial general effects of personal rhythmic prayer (Bernardi et al. 2001), transcendental meditation (Zamarra et al. 1996), and positive outlook (Ironson et al. 2002). Prayer and spirituality often assist in reducing anxiety. They also help the patient to regain a sense of control over the illness.

Table 14–1. Directive questions for doctor-patient discussions about religion and spirituality

- Some people find that religion or spirituality is helpful for coping and others do not. What has been your experience?
- Has religion or spirituality helped you, and if so, how?
- Has religion or spirituality hurt you in any way, and if so, how?
- How have your beliefs influenced your behavior during this illness?
- Are you part of a spiritual or religious community? Is this a support to you?
- Which religion did your family practice when you were growing up?
- How have those beliefs affected your life? Have they changed over time?
- What religion do you practice/follow now? How important is it to you?
- Do you believe in God or a higher power?
- What does your belief in God (or a higher power) mean to you?
- How would you like me, your health care provider, to address these issues in your care?

Source. Adapted from Larson et al. 1997 and Breitbart 2001.

"What religion are you, doctor?"

If possible, try to follow the model "I will be glad to answer, but please tell me, what does my religious background [mean to you, make you feel]? Why is that important to you?" The goal here is to provide an opportunity for the patient to talk about anxieties and concerns before being "reassured" by your immediate answer, and no further discussion seems necessary. It is important to foster rapport and a bond with the patient by not being defensive. If the patient comments on your religious differences, with statements like "I was raised as an 'x', and you are a 'y'. I don't think you can understand me," you might respond, "If I don't understand something, I will be sure to ask you. If I can't answer some questions to your satisfaction, we'll call in someone who can be more specific [like a member of the clergy]. It will be helpful for me too, so that I can further help you."

■ ILLNESS AND REGRESSION

Medical patients are said to "regress." Regress to where? Why does that happen? Where does religion fit in?

Serious illness strips people of adult identity, particularly as the illness advances. The patient experiences multiple losses: of physical functions, emotional stability, bodily integrity, and contact with familiar people. Seriously ill patients often mourn the loss of the "ordinary": the repetitive, mundane, day-to-day details that lend emotional security to psychological life. Religion plays an important role in countering this aspect of regression; it reaffirms belonging and orderliness through ritual and custom. Each person will experience illness uniquely and will construct personal, if unspoken narratives about it. Childhood fears emerge as a consequence of this assault on adult identity, producing several of the commonly observed regressive attitudes in adult medical patients, such as

- Passivity, often in excess of physical debility
- The wish to be nurtured (often in a childlike manner)
- The yearning for a powerful protector
- A childlike preoccupation with guilt and forgiveness for past mistakes

"Is there an afterlife, doctor?"
"Do you think that something better waits for me in another life, when my suffering will be over?"

Start by considering what the patient is really asking you for; it is usually for some type of reassurance. For dying patients, questions about an afterlife are often attempts to bridge a sense of profound isolation, linking them to a future and to hope. Preparation of concrete symbols, such as diaries, legacies, and memorials, do something very similar. For example, in ancient Egypt, tombs were equipped with funerary objects to care for the "spirit" as a way to link the dead with the past as well as the future. (When we hold on to items of our deceased loved ones, we too are linking with them.) Many religions readily lend themselves to symbols such as God as omnipotent protector or forgiver of sins and the person as a child of God, potentially granted immortal life. The promise of a better life that follows the misery of this one holds special appeal for someone who is suffering from illness.

With this in mind, the therapist or clinician might respond, "I'm not sure about it myself, but can you tell me what would be comforting to you about an afterlife? How do you feel life after this one would be different? How do your religious or spiritual beliefs guide you?"

Theology-focused questions should be referred to a pastoral counselor. Table 14–2 lists information on how to locate faith-specific pastoral counselors and palliative care resources.

■ ILLNESS AND GUILT

Why do medical patients so frequently feel that they are being punished? Punished for what?

Coping with illness is often described as a battle. The "fight" metaphor sometimes implies that on one side stands Good (patient, doctor, medicines), while on the opposing side rises Bad, the enemy (illness and death). If illness is an evil to be battled, then a negative moral value may accrue to being sick, "staying" sick, or being "defeated" by the illness and death. Many patients experience their poor health as punishment for having transgressed in the past ("What did I do to deserve this?"). If the patient does not get better, his or her guilt often intensifies, creating the feeling of disappointing caregivers and letting everyone down. Guilt from previous life events becomes displaced onto the illness, which is experienced as punishment for mistakes and transgressions of the past. For some people, guilt and punishment help them cope with the sense of the random, arbitrary, and meaningless in regard to the illness: "I became ill because I sinned" replaces "I became ill because anyone can become ill; it is random, and it has no meaning." Excessive guilt may also be a symptom of a major depressive episode and indicate the need for antidepressant therapy.

Table 14–2. How to locate faith-specific pastoral counselors and palliative care resources

American Association of Pastoral Counselors (AAPC)	Referral service: http://www.aapc.org Telephone 703-385-6967 (specify patient's religious affiliation and geographic area) Contains a membership directory of more than 500 members from more than 100 faith communities, with credentials (e.g., licensure as a psychologist, psychiatrist, family therapist) Pastoral counseling centers can also be found in the Yellow Pages or on the Internet. Many centers are accredited by the AAPC. To be certified, a pastoral counselor must have a theology-based master's or doctoral degree or a comparable degree in pastoral counseling. AAPC members receive clinical pastoral education that is closely supervised, usually through a hospital chaplain, with classroom instruction.
International Psycho-Oncology Society	http://www.ipos-society.org Contains educational materials and links targeting the psychosocial aspects of patient care.
Pallium	http://www.pallium.ca (temporarily relocated to http://www.virtualhospice.ca) A Web-based professional community of clinicians, educators, and academicians collaborating in Canada's palliative care system
Project on Death in America	http://www.soros.org/death Provides a broad range of resources related to palliative care, including funding initiatives, educational materials, and summaries of international efforts related to end-of-life care

Note.   All sites accessed July 2004.

■ STARTING PSYCHOTHERAPY WITH SERIOUSLY ILL MEDICAL PATIENTS

How do you begin psychotherapy with seriously ill medical patients? Do you get them to talk about the illness first? Or try to distract them?

Although potentially curable or at least manageable, most medical illnesses elicit feelings about mortality and life's meaning. The following lead questions may be used to explore the "life narrative," which provides the context for the meanings of the illness for a particular person (Viederman 2003a, 2003b). Although the questions are derived from palliative care medicine, whose mission is to help people "die with dignity," the goal of psychotherapy for patients who will survive is to help them "live with dignity," medical illness and all. The questions are adapted from the work of Chochinov (2002):

1. Can you tell me a little about your life, particularly those parts that you either remember most or think are the most important?
2. When in your life have you felt most "alive" or happy?
3. Are there specific things that you would want your family to know about you? Are there particular things you would want them to remember?
4. What are the most important roles (e.g., family, vocational, community service) you have played so far in your life? Why are they so important to you, and what do you think you accomplished in those roles? Are there particular things that you feel still need to be done?
5. What are your most important accomplishments, and what do you feel most proud of? Are there particular things that you feel still need to be achieved in your life?
6. Are there particular things that you feel still need to be said to your loved ones, or things that you would want to take the time to say once again?
7. What are your hopes and dreams for your loved ones?
8. What have you learned about life so far that you would want to pass along to others? What advice or words of guidance would you wish to pass along to your [son, daughter, husband, wife, parents, others]?
9. [For terminally ill patients] Are there words or perhaps even instructions you would like to offer your family, in order to provide them with comfort or solace? In creating this permanent record, are there other things that you would like to include?

"Why do bad things happen to good people?"

Sometimes when the patient gets really bad news, difficult questions arise about God, and it's hard to know what to say. *Try shifting from looking for things to say to asking thought-provoking questions.* Keep the time frame day by day. Consider what the patient is really seeking in the questions about God or "good people." Frequently, there is the feeling of having lost the protection of a divine friend, a presence who was perhaps taken for granted but was subliminally "always there" until illness destroyed it, along with normal life and good health. Medical patients often feel horribly alone in a hostile universe that has engulfed them. Although technical medical advances have extended lives, they also sometimes diminish the quality of life for sick people. Patients consistently describe feeling dwarfed, isolated, and dehumanized by medical procedures and diagnostic equipment. As one patient with recurrent cancer said so poignantly, "It's not that I fear dying. It's the machines, it's the procedures, and it's the faces without any expression. If I knew how to pray, I would."

People are looking for comfort from their physicians and for insight, not theology, from their psychotherapists. When the condition worsens or gets more complex, focus on what is psychologically attainable for that patient, on that day, in that session. Sometimes one can only keep watch, sitting vigil with the patient during the grief or rage about what has befallen him or her. Sometimes clinicians must endure listening to material about religion, spirituality, or God that they find personally offensive or blasphemous. However, maintaining the "watch" with the patient who rages in anguish often produces therapeutic rewards. For example, one patient who survived a serious medical illness returned several years later, in good health. She said that what had been most helpful about psychotherapy was that she had not felt alone, and that she did not have to protect the therapist from her feelings (as she did her family, pastor, and friends). She said that the therapist "had kept her company" during one of the most angry, frightened, and disoriented periods of her life. The consistency of psychotherapy had helped maintain hope.

Try to refrain from being drawn into discussions of the mystical, good and evil, or the infinite—anxiety usually worsens when such matters are discussed, and psychiatric training rarely prepares us to tread these profound spaces in 50-minute sessions. Focus instead on understanding the here and now. The mundane is usually reassuring when people have been given bad news: "O.K. That was tough going today. But let's put together our game plan for this week."

There will certainly be common elements among patients with the same illness (for example, fears of dying, burial, and suffocation are ubiquitous among lung cancer patients). However, a seemingly obvious psychological or medical symptom can be overdetermined; that is, it can have a number of meanings, including those that are unexpected, unpredicted, and highly individual to a particular patient. Often there is unconscious overlap between preexisting psychological conflicts and current reactions to the medical situation; the past merges with the present reality to intensify the traumatic experience. For example, a patient was one of three sisters who had recently been given diagnoses of breast cancer. She felt despairing because she had the *least* aggressive form of cancer. The oncologist requested psychiatric consultation because the patient often "forgot" her oncology appointments and was jeopardizing her chance of a cure. Psychological exploration revealed that her "survivor guilt" extended to her early history, in which she was the only sister to escape her father's abusive behavior as his "favorite" (Wyszynski 1990).

Questions about spirituality and religion in psychotherapy may be attempts to make sense of it all and to find solace. Two goals for psychotherapy are relatively universal:

- To help transform the metaphor of illness as punishment to illness as a punishment-neutral misfortune, having nothing to do with "badness" or "sin"
- To help the patient reclaim his or her identity as a person, not a depersonalized cog in the medical system machinery, by exploring personal narrative with the doctor

◼ PROMOTING RESILIENCE

The construct of resilience can be used to explore questions about spirituality. *Resilience* has been defined as the capacity to emerge from adversity stronger and more capable than before. James Griffith has developed a series of questions designed to foster resilience by encouraging self-reflection (Griffith 2001; Griffith and Griffith 2002). He has suggested the following sets of questions to help start the dialogue:

To foster a sense of belonging, and counter a sense of *isolation*:

- Who really understands your situation?
- When you have difficult days, with whom do you talk?
- In whose presence do you feel a sense of peace? [Would you consider contacting that person directly again?]
- [If religious] What does God know about your experience that other people don't understand?

To foster hope, and counter *despair:*

- From what sources do you draw hope?
- On difficult days, what keeps you from giving up?
- What has been your experience of living in relationship to this illness?
- What has it cost in your personal relationships? Professional life? Your sense of self as a person? Your dreams or vision of the future?
- Who have you known in your life who would not be surprised to see you hopeful amidst adversity? What did this person know that other people might not have known about you?

To foster assertiveness, and counter *helplessness:*

- What should I know about you as a person that goes beyond your illness?
- What most helps you to stand strong against the challenges of this illness?
- How have you kept this illness from taking charge of your whole lifestyle and identity?

To foster a sense of purpose, and counter a sense of *meaninglessness:*

- What keeps you going on difficult days?
- For whom, or for what, does it matter that you continue to live?
- What do you hope to contribute with your life in the time you have remaining?
- [If religious] What does God hope you will do with your life in days to come?

To foster joy, and counter feelings of *sorrow:*

- For what are you most deeply grateful?
- What sustains your capacity to experience joy in the midst of pain?
- If you could look back on this experience of illness from some future time, what would you say that you took from the experience that added to your life?

Also see the work of Breitbart (2002) on meaning-centered group psychotherapy for advanced cancer patients.

■ COUNTERTRANSFERENCE ISSUES

Countertransference issues that may arise during doctor-patient discussions of religion and spirituality include *skepticism, tactlessness, proselytizing,* and *avoidance.*

Patients' need for religious or spiritual discussions at times of medical crisis may dredge up deep reactions within the clinician. Formal religion may have been hurtful or offensive to the doctor. In such cases, it will be hard to suppress *skepticism* that religion could be comforting to anyone, or to tolerate spiritual discussions for the sake of patient coping. *Tact* may be consequently hard to muster and sustain:

> For the [clinician] who at one time had a religious affiliation, and now no longer has one, the problems posed by religion encountered [in the patient] are even more challenging....Guilt over desertion, apostasy or heresy is often experienced. There may be anger toward former beliefs and practices, and toward those who hold these beliefs and practices. (Lovinger 1984, pp. 16–17)

Conversely, *proselytizing,* or an overly positive attitude about spirituality, may put the patient on guard, prompting avoidance or defensiveness. The patient may "tune out the pep talk" if it is overly enthusiastic, or may experience it in unexpected ways. For example, inquiring about God or religion without any cue from the patient may be off-putting and may also alarm the patient about his or her prognosis (Ehman et al. 1999).

Finally, the clinician may *avoid* spiritual or religious discussions because these topics raise the clinician's anxiety about his or her own mortality. A physician's repeated exposure to profound questions about why bad things happen may make it difficult to maintain neutrality without feeling personally vulnerable. Incurable illness may challenge our identity as healers and our unconscious denial of mortality for ourselves and the people we love. If the patient can lose God's protection, then we can, too; if illness truly is not punishment, but random, then it can strike us, too. Medical science itself is not immune to the pull of spiritual metaphor; most doctors have succumbed at times to the wish to "rescue" patients, by staging an "assault" on the sickness, equipped with "weapons" from the "armamentarium." This is no easy job; the physician is trying to battle illness, and to avoid the pitfall of "playing God," while staring at his or her own mortality mirrored back in the sick patient. The reflex response may be to beat a retreat, triaging the remotely theological by "calling in the clergy."

A psychological paradox may ensue: the doctor may feel compelled to "do something" but simultaneously feel therapeutically paralyzed. *All-or-nothing themes* may begin to appear as the physician struggles with contradictory feelings of being "powerful but helpless" in response to the disease, the patient, and the family. These responses are not limited to psychiatrists but are also observed in other medical professionals. Examples of all-or-nothing themes:

- The patient has failed all chemotherapy, is aware that he or she is dying, and yet wants to "keep trying." The doctor has discussed the grave prognosis with the patient, yet still feels there is dishonesty in continuing a treatment that will not save the patient. (Possible subtext: I am a doctor. I'm only supposed to do what is proven beneficial in clinical trials.)
- The doctor goes blank and is unable to find anything to say to a patient who is dying. (Possible subtext: How can I possibly find the right words to help? Worse, if I say the wrong thing will it devastate the patient?)
- The doctor finds it difficult to answer the family's questions at the bedside of a dying patient. He or she often "runs out of time" on rounds, particularly during visiting hours. (Possible subtext: If I let them lean on me, will I lessen their grief and pain? Or will I become trapped in these difficult feelings myself, and never break free?)

Realistically, no person can wield the power described in the last two subtexts above. They are examples of magical thinking, which defends against feeling helpless. If the physician does not recognize and adjust for these psychological strategies, personal discomfort actually intensifies. Therapeutic powerlessness and confusion may result. For example, the physician may overidentify with the patient's predicament and become excessively involved, making it difficult to maintain therapeutic objectivity. Alternatively, the physician may avoid the patient in order to feel less helpless, inadvertently making the patient feel emotionally abandoned.

Other types of countertransference reactions that interfere with the doctor-patient relationship in the medical setting are discussed in Chapter 15, "The Seriously Ill Patient: Physician Factors in the Doctor-Patient Relationship."

■ REFERENCES

Bernardi L, Sleight P, Bandinelli G, et al: Effect of rosary prayer and yoga mantras on autonomic cardiovascular rhythms: comparative study. BMJ 323:1446–1449, 2001

Breitbart W: Spirituality and meaning in supportive care: spirituality- and meaning-centered group psychotherapy interventions in advanced cancer. Support Care Cancer 10:272–280, 2002

Chochinov H: Dignity-conserving care—a new model for palliative care: helping the patient feel valued. JAMA 287:2253–2260, 2002

Ehman J, Ott B, Short T, et al: Do patients want physicians to inquire about their spiritual or religious beliefs if they become gravely ill? Arch Intern Med 159:1803–1806, 1999

Griffith J[L]: Brief therapy at the bedside: psychotherapy today in consultation-liaison psychiatry. Presented at the 154th annual meeting of the American Psychiatric Association, New Orleans, LA, May 2001

Griffith JL, Griffith ME: Encountering the Sacred in Psychotherapy: How to Talk With People About Their Spiritual Lives. New York, Guilford, 2002

Harris W, Gowda M, Kolb J, et al: A randomized, controlled trial of the effects of remote, intercessory prayer on outcomes in patients admitted to the coronary care unit. Arch Intern Med 159:2273–2278 [erratum: 160:1878], 1999

Hebert R, Jenckes M, Ford D, et al: Patient perspectives on spirituality and the patient-physician relationship. J Gen Intern Med 16:685–692, 2001

Ironson G, Solomon GF, Balbin EG, et al: The Ironson-Woods Spirituality/Religiousness Index is associated with long survival, health behaviors, less distress, and low cortisol in people with HIV/AIDS. Ann Behav Med 24:34–48, 2002

Larson D, Lu F, Swyers J, et al (eds): Appendix A: questions for assessing patients' religious beliefs and their influences on patients, in Model Curriculum for Psychiatric Residency Training Programs: Religion and Spirituality in Clinical Practice. Rockville, MD, National Institute for Healthcare Research, 1997

Lo B, Ruston D, Kates L, et al: Discussing religious and spiritual issues at the end of life: a practical guide for physicians. JAMA 287:749–754, 2002

Lovinger R: Working With Religious Issues in Therapy. New York, Jason Aronson, 1984

Sloan R, Bagiella E: Claims about religious involvement and health outcomes. Ann Behav Med 24:14–21, 2002

Viederman M: Life Passage in the Face of Death, Vol I: A Brief Psychotherapy (videotape). Washington, DC, American Psychiatric Publishing, 2003a

Viederman M: Life Passage in the Face of Death, Vol II: Psychological Engagement of the Physically Ill Patient (videotape). Washington, DC, American Psychiatric Publishing, 2003b

Wyszynski A: Managing noncompliance in the "difficult" medical patient: the contributions of insight. Psychother Psychosom 54:181–186, 1990

Zamarra J, Schneider R, Besseghini I, et al: Usefulness of the transcendental meditation program in the treatment of patients with coronary artery disease. Am J Cardiol 77:867–870, 1996

Chapter

15

The Seriously Ill Patient: Physician Factors in the Doctor-Patient Relationship

A Short, Practical Guide

Antoinette Ambrosino Wyszynski, M.D.
Bernard Wyszynski, M.D.

■ PSYCHOLOGICAL REACTIONS IN CLINICIANS WORKING WITH SERIOUSLY ILL PATIENTS

Caring for people with any serious medical illness confronts the doctor with challenges that are sometimes personally disturbing. Three commonly occurring reactions in clinicians working with seriously ill patients are physician burnout, avoiding the bad news, and disapproval of the patient.

Physician Burnout

Burnout is a significant occupational hazard. It is likely that you are experiencing burnout if you find yourself stuck in or wavering between emotional extremes: feeling easily overwhelmed, even by minor events, or feeling psychologically numbed and unable to respond to the emotional needs of family, friends, or patients. "Burnout" is not a DSM-IV-TR diagnostic category, but it has been experienced by just about everyone who has practiced medicine or psychiatry. The diminished psychological reserve characteristic of burnout is unmistakable:

- Emotional exhaustion (experienced as cynicism, a lack of capacity to offer psychological support to others)
- Quick anger or frustration
- Emotional numbness, apathy, or boredom

Wyszynski AA, Wyszynski B (eds.): *Manual of Psychiatric Care for the Medically Ill*. Washington, D.C., American Psychiatric Publishing, Inc., 2005

- Feeling a lack of personal accomplishment
- Feeling hopeless
- Somatic symptoms (fatigue, insomnia, headache, appetite changes)

No particular personality pattern or work style appears to predispose to burnout. In physicians, attitudes such as the need to be constantly available to patients, the need to cure, and the denial of personal feelings seem to set the stage for burnout later on (Demmer 2002; Shirom 2003; Spickard et al. 2002).

Simple burnout can be "treated" with remedies that are simple but hard to come by: time off and diminished workload. Regular discussions with a colleague help. Mood or anxiety disorders, if they occur, should be treated with medication and, if desired, psychotherapy. Treatment of patients with relapsing or progressing illnesses (such as AIDS, certain neurological illnesses, and cancer) can exact a psychic toll on medical caregivers. Clinicians who frequently deal with these patients are prone to developing the coping mechanisms of intellectualization and repression. Unhappily, these defensive strategies by the physician are a setup for doctor-patient misunderstandings; the "well-defended" doctor may come across to patients as "cold," callous, and lacking in compassion.

A physician's experience of patients' neediness as overwhelming or intolerable may be another sign of burnout. If the physician feels it necessary to respond by limiting the patient's access to him or her, conflict may result, producing antagonism that may damage the treatment. If medical complications occur later on, patients and their families may express their anger as litigiousness.

Avoiding the Bad News

Bad news is difficult to manage, even if the patient has already been told it by another physician. Psychiatric clinicians often grapple with the problem of "what to do" when the patient has heard bad medical news delivered by an internist or surgeon: Bring it up? Avoid it? Wait until the patient says something? There is no rule of technique, only the following caution: sometimes the dilemma arises because it is too personally upsetting *for the doctor* to experience the patient's reactions. The illness itself may have personal meaning that prompts avoidance, or the clinician may fear being at a loss for "what to say" to help the patient through the crisis.

Sometimes countertransference avoidance may be concealed under cover of "tact" (e.g., not wishing to make the patient feel worse) or "technique" (e.g., wait-ing for the patient to bring up the difficult material). It may take several other forms in the clinical setting: for example, the doctor may have trouble making time for the patient, or forget appointments, or book two patients for the same appointment. Occasionally, avoidance may also be experienced as its opposite, namely, preoccupation—for example, repeatedly dreaming or "obsessing" about the patient's situation outside the office or hospital. The opposites of forgetting and ruminating are linked psychologically; both are attempts by the physician to cope with what is psychologically painful about the patient.

A clinician's failure to bring up obvious issues, such as noticeable hair loss from chemotherapy or the poor prognosis implied by a new test result, can make the patient feel isolated and alone. Medical patients have an uncanny way of knowing what is happening to them, and sensing what you know, even when it is left unsaid. Patients who receive bad news often try to protect their families, their friends, their business associates, and even their religious beliefs from the implications of terrifying information. The doctor's silence may be misinterpreted to mean that what has happened is too terrifying for *anyone* to talk about; the patient concludes that the doctor must be protected, too. This predicament may intensify the patient's loneliness and isolation.

There is no formula for sharing information with patients, particularly when medical events are evolving rapidly. A good policy is to use tactful honesty and allow the patient's psychology to do the rest. Psychological defenses usually filter what the patient is ready to discuss. In cases where repression and denial of information create problems in following medical advice, a thorough psychiatric evaluation may reveal an Axis I condition.

Be cautious about making statements that the patient "is a better/stronger/saner person" for having been ill (unless, of course, such descriptions come from the patient). Many patients report that such statements are infuriating. The "emphasize-the-positive" comments are sometimes reassuring to the doctor, who has found something optimistic to say, but can feel dismissive of the patient's despair and struggle. Such comments may also be experienced as the physician's avoidance of emotional engagement with the patient's predicament.

Disapproval of the Patient

Emotions of anger, dislike, and the wish to quit a case are familiar to most experienced physicians. Such reactions, however, do not feel compatible with the

Hippocratic oath. Every doctor has experienced aversion to certain patients or their lifestyles. The temptation is for physicians to disapprove of their own disapproval because it seems unprofessional.

Two patient triggers that often prompt this response in physicians are nonadherence to medical advice and the threat of self-harm. For example, the doctor may personally condemn the HIV patient's ongoing drug use or become furious at a lung cancer patient's smoking. In addition, threats of suicide by seriously ill patients can also be quite unsettling and may induce an uncomfortable reaction in the physician, such as the wish to abandon the case.

Personal reactions of the physician are inevitable and unavoidable. When they go unrecognized by the doctor, they are more likely to color the interaction and thus to impede clinical effectiveness. Recognizing and working with one's own feelings of disapproval or condemnation toward the patient is challenging, but preferable to having these feelings sneak into patient interactions.

Generally, sharing specific personal reactions with the patient is not a useful strategy. It burdens the patient, does nothing to promote medical adherence, and potentially increases the tension between doctor and patient. It is possible, for example, to give a recommendation to stop smoking, or to explore why an individual continues to have unsafe sex, without offering how it makes you feel. In fact, these direct discussions with patients may be more effectively conducted *after* figuring out privately why the particular patient or behavior is so personally disturbing. Often a trusted colleague is a more appropriate sounding board, particularly if he or she knows you and has experienced similar reactions.

■ THE QUESTIONS PATIENTS ASK: A PRETEST OF COUNTERTRANSFERENCE FOR CLINICIANS

Medical patients often ask questions that verge on the existential. Few people—especially if blessed with good health—reflect on these uncomfortable issues before being personally confronted with them. Countertransference creates problems when acted out by the unaware clinician. Consider the following questions in order to explore your own "gut responses." The questions are adapted from an exercise that was originally developed by Winiarski (1991) for psychotherapists working with HIV-infected patients. This

exercise is useful preparation as well for other clinicians who work with any seriously ill patient.

Why Me?

What is your gut response? Be alert to statements that carry value judgments, especially in illnesses like AIDS, substance abuse, or lung cancer, in which behavior has played a role in the patient's becoming ill. Responses to "Why me?" that imply blame (e.g., "Because you smoked"; "Because you were promiscuous and had anal intercourse"; "Because you shot up drugs") will affect how safe the patient feels with you. These statements are variations of "Because you did not follow the rules." The converse is, "Those who followed the rules did not become ill." Where do you stand on rules and social norms? Are you a rule follower, and uncomfortable with those who are not? Do you become angry with those who flout convention? Do you protect yourself with the fantasy that illness "happens" only to those who invite or "deserve" it?

Explore your own attitudes regarding drug use, especially if you work with HIV-infected patients. Is drug use a symptom of a personality disorder? Is a person responsible for having a personality disorder? Is it a result of the person's environment?

Will I Die in Pain?

This is the one of several questions concerning fears of dying. If you do not know the answer, how willing are you to learn the medical facts? To learn about pain control? Have you thought of what you personally fear about dying? About death? What are your attitudes regarding pain control for medical patients? For medically ill substance abusers? Are you the kind of person who will not take an aspirin and who frowns at others for "overmedicating"?

People experience pain differently, but can you remain nonjudgmental with the patient who has a low pain threshold? Injection drug users, in particular, report low pain thresholds. Yet they are least likely to be treated for pain, because their physicians fear being manipulated. As the psychiatric consultant, how would you negotiate this dilemma?

Will I Die Alone?
Will You Stay With Me Until the End?

The request to the clinician is easy to miss in the first of these questions, which is a subtle version of the more obvious plea in the second question (Winiarski

1991). At one level, the patient may be asking, "Will you abandon me as others have, or as I fear others will?" Alternatively, "Will you be by my bedside and see me through this ordeal?" Think through your responses—practical and emotional—beforehand. Are you willing to visit a deteriorating patient in the hospital? Where do you draw the line relative to the dictates of your schedule? If your vacation were planned, would you change it if your patient were dying? How would you respond to direct queries such as "Yes, your schedule is busy, but can't you get to the hospital?" What stops you? What fears of loss and impotence may underlie your inability to "stay until the end" of a terminal illness? These questions tap how close you can be to your patient and how much loss you can tolerate. If you find it hard to tolerate loss, do you disparage yourself and, possibly, the patient?

On the other hand, is the "caregiver" in you being manipulated? What lies behind your eagerness to stand by and hold the patient's hand? Is there grandiosity or a rescue fantasy? Beware! Both may render a clinician ineffectual. Are you overinvolved? Is your overinvolvement a reaction to negative feelings about the patient? What might these be? Would your answer differ depending on the patient's gender or illness? For psychiatrists: do you believe it is the function of a psychotherapist to be at the bedside until the patient dies?

Can You Stand to Look at Me?

Privately, what is your honest response? For example, Kaposi's sarcoma lesions may cause severe swelling of arms, legs, and face. Cancer patients often lose their hair and become cachectic. Neurosurgical patients and those with head and neck malignancies are often disfigured. These are not easy sights for anyone. How necessary is it for you to have a patient who appears attractive or normal? What feelings and fears are elicited in you when you imagine being with someone disfigured?

Wouldn't You Kill Yourself If You Were Me?

This is one of the most difficult and provocative of questions. You should be clear regarding your response *before* you start treatment with a patient. Your beliefs in the quality and quantity of life—your despair and optimism—are tapped by this question. Do you believe in the individual's right to commit "rational" suicide? Or do you feel that no suicidal ideation

is rational, that it reflects a severe psychiatric disturbance, no matter how thoughtful the patient appears? Would you be willing to collude in the suicide of a terminally ill patient if you were certain you would not suffer professional or legal repercussions? Or are you convinced that you would intervene to prevent a suicide under any circumstances? If you would intervene to block a suicide under any circumstances, should you state this at the beginning of treatment? How do you manage the patient's potential reply of "Sure, I'll talk to you about my life, except for my considerations of suicide." How does cutting off the possibility of that discussion limit the effectiveness and relevance of the treatment for the patient?

A religious perspective may or may not be helpful:

> While we may have some religious or ethical considerations regarding suicide, we may be confused about whether to apply these [clinically]. One [clinician], working with a Catholic patient considering suicide, may attempt to dissuade him or her by raising the issue of mortal sin. Another practitioner may feel more comfortable steering clear of religious issues. (Winiarski 1991, p. 123)

Finally, do you think you might consider killing yourself in the patient's situation? How does your answer to this question influence your ability to facilitate the discussion with the patient?

Since I Can't Be Cured, Wouldn't It Be Better to Give Up?

Do you believe a person's life—even a disfigured or terminally ill person's life—is worth fighting for? Is each life equal to the next? If you believe in rational suicide, would you elect not to intervene in a passive suicide (e.g., noncompliance with medical regimens, signing out of a hospital against medical advice, or refusing emergency treatment)? Deferring intervention may involve avoiding certain questions because you would rather not hear the answers.

Is There a God?
Why Would God Put Me Through This?

Do you restrict yourself to exploring the psychodynamics of this question? Attempt to address it on a religious level? Collaborate with a member of the clergy? How self-revealing is it appropriate to be?

> In [clinician] and [patient] alike, the asking and responding to this question raises profound questions

of life's meaning and possibilities of connections with larger realities. This is the same question that arises during any tragedy. In the face of tragedy, can we believe in a benevolent deity? What role does the concept of God have in our lives? Is he or she a rescuer, or a fellow sufferer whose divine presence gives us courage? If God is a rescuer and we are not rescued, are we undeserving? (Winiarski 1991, p. 123)

Am I Forgiven?

If there is the need for forgiveness, what is the transgression? Who is it that eventually forgives? Are you in a position to offer forgiveness? Are you angry at the patient for being sick? Does the patient sense this? Do you need to be forgiven for some of your feelings regarding the patient?

What Will Happen to My Family?

Countertransference reactions to this question can be particularly difficult if the patient's behavior contributed to contracting or maintaining the illness (e.g., AIDS, cigarette-induced lung cancer or emphysema, alcohol-induced cirrhosis):

> This question can raise feelings of punitiveness in the [clinician], due to a sense that the [patient] may be responsible for his or her own plight and, especially, the plight of family members, including children. [Clinicians] who have lost parents or friends due to perceived "carelessness" may have difficulty empathizing with a person who has been careless about his or her health and therefore has "caused" others' suffering. (Winiarski 1991, p. 124)

Why Should I Tell Anyone?

Think through your stance on whether the patient should tell others about the illness—especially for patients with communicable illnesses or patients whose cancer has metastasized. Do you believe that no secrets should be kept? Can there be exceptions? Why should the patient confide in a family member who has always been rejecting or untrustworthy? Be alert to potential incongruity between the patient's goals for comfort and your goals for communication and reunion. With HIV-infected individuals, what is your reaction to the person who insists on maintaining the secret, even though others may be injured? What of the man who continues to have unsafe sex or share needles, thus spreading HIV? What about the HIV-positive woman who chooses to bring the fetus to term, with the possibility that the child may be HIV-positive? What do you do about warning the partner?

■ REFERENCES

Demmer C: Stressors and rewards for workers in AIDS service organizations. AIDS Patient Care STDS 16:179–187, 2002

Shirom A: Job-related burnout: a review, in Handbook of Occupational Health Psychology. Edited by Quick J, Tetrick L. Washington, DC, American Psychological Association, 2003, pp 245–264

Spickard A, Gabbe S, Christensen J: Mid-career burnout in generalist and specialist physicians. JAMA 288:1447–1450, 2002

Winiarski M: AIDS-Related Psychotherapy. Elmsford, NY, Pergamon, 1991, pp 121–124

Chapter

16

Epilogue: The Physician as Comforter

Salvatore V. Ambrosino, M.D.

The quality of mercy is not strained…: it is twice blessed;
It blesseth him that gives and him that takes.

Medical illness imposes loss—of health, of life, and often the painful loss of loved ones. Surreptitious in onset, or striking suddenly, illness makes both the afflicted and those close to them begin to recognize that life is finite, and to acknowledge our human days are numbered. For some, illness may be experienced as death waiting quietly behind the curtain. Then the questions flow:

- "Why me?"
- "Are the doctors right?"
- "Can I be cured?"
- "Will it affect my job?"
- "What will happen to my wife? My husband? My children?"
- "What was life all about?"

As a nation saw on September 11, 2001, personal tragedy happens in the social context of a culture and its civilization. At the moment of tragedy, people turn to their belief systems to fix their existence in a continuity of life. The atheist sees the implications of illness as a biological end, while the theist sees death as a bi-

ological passageway to another world, another consciousness. Often, human beings cling to the idea of being invulnerable and immortal.

Illness can shatter these human props. A person may be confronted with pangs of remorse, regret, or, for the fortunate, feelings of fulfillment upon looking back. At that time, the physician's role may shift from diagnostician to comforter. We may find ourselves called upon to bring closure to the therapeutic efforts concerning the illness. The goal becomes one of helping the patient, and the family who suffers with the patient, to respond to the "traumatic command" of the illness—to weather the early storms of discovery and to integrate the illness with its consequences into the fabric of their mutual history. The challenge is to help the patient accept the losses of illness and death not as a loss of *love*, but a loss of *time*.

Patients who will fare better psychologically are those who possess a good balance between denial and reality, as well as a clear sense of self, and can balance the good with the bad in what they feel toward people who are important to them. For these individuals, there often arises the conviction that although death

Wyszynski AA, Wyszynski B (eds.): *Manual of Psychiatric Care for the Medically Ill.* Washington, D.C., American Psychiatric Publishing, Inc., 2005

may put an end to time, love endures. Those patients who have fulfilled their personal goals and who have had lives of personal choice are best prepared to deal with the inevitable regrets as life ends. They are the individuals who rise to the "traumatic command" of the illness as it ushers in another phase of life.

The family is often the forgotten casualty of serious illness. When a loved one is hospitalized, the most difficult problem confronting a family is the baffling nature of the disease. They seek hope and reassurances. A family with misapprehensions of the disease and a remote, hurried treating physician create a terrible mix. Physicians must sit down with the family and give them their undivided attention—inviting questions, staying alert to anxieties, and discussing the "realities" in a way that is appropriate for the family hearing them. Although a family's resilience cannot be created in crisis, the family may have to be the first to be confronted with the details of treatment and prognosis. If the family has strong religious or spiritual beliefs, these may be called upon to help the patient struggle with the "now" and the "what may be" in the future. The family and patient lacking formal religious beliefs may nonetheless find reassurance in sharing kindness and good memories with each other.

There is no substitute for the availability of the physician in this difficult process. Such an involvement is costly—in time, often in self-reflected anguish. As the patient faces death, we physicians are also confronted with our own mortality, as well as our helplessness. Accustomed to seeking "cure," we must now shift gears, bringing peace and solace to patients and to those who love them.

There arises another problem: How does all of this fit into the corporate restraint imposed by managed care? How do solace and commitment fit into a procedure code? In the days before doctors were hounded by administrators who were never at a bedside and team reviewers without medical degrees, physicians were honored if they spent more, not less, time with very ill patients. To be at the bedside of a mortally ill human being was, and still is, a privilege. *The physician is not an employee.* I pose the following question: When these cost-containment people find themselves in similar circumstances—as we all inevitably must—how will they wish themselves and their own families to be treated?

When I was a young intern on morning rounds in 1953 with my fellow housestaff, an eighty-year-old woman lay in bed riddled with carcinomatosis. She smiled when she saw us and said in a weak voice, "You are my white angels." I never forgot her courage and kindness. We did not cure her, but we somehow brought her comfort. From that day forth, I tried not to be obstructed by the reality that I would not cure many of my patients, and that many would die despite my efforts. I have tried to remember that doctors sustain patients both in their suffering and in their hope. I believe that a physician must remain the one who would dare to walk "where the angels tread," preserving the patient's dignity and easing the patient's sorrow.

Indeed, after fifty years of practicing medicine and psychiatry, I would never try to drag any patient into my personal view of heaven. I have espoused, however, that "the inevitable hour" does not have to lead to the grave alone; and I have tried to keep this promise to my patients: that I will do my best to be at their bedside at the end, sometimes against all odds, remaining always their physician, ever involved and, even now, listening.

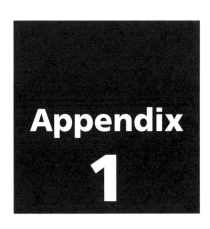

Appendix 1

American Psychiatric Association Guidelines for Assessing the Delirious Patient

Checklist

Wyszynski AA, Wyszynski B (eds.): *Manual of Psychiatric Care for the Medically Ill*. Washington, D.C., American Psychiatric Publishing, Inc., 2005

American Psychiatric Association Guidelines for Assessing the Delirious Patient: Checklist

---

History
- ✓ Changes in behavior and mentation
- ✓ Blood transfusions
- ✓ High-risk sexual behavior
- ✓ Drug and alcohol use
- ✓ General medical records (anesthesia record, if postoperative)
- ✓ Medications (types, doses; do changes correlate with behavioral shifts?)

Physical Status
- ✓ Physical examination
- ✓ Neurological examination
- ✓ Review of vital signs

Mental Status
- ✓ Interview
- ✓ Cognitive testing

Basic Lab Tests for All Patients With Delirium
- ✓ Complete blood count (CBC)
- ✓ Electrolytes (including calcium, magnesium, phosphorus)
- ✓ Glucose
- ✓ Blood urea nitrogen (BUN), creatinine
- ✓ Liver function tests (AST, ALT, alkaline phosphatase, bilirubin)
- ✓ Thyroid function tests (TFTs) [not included in the original APA guideline]
- ✓ B_{12} and folate levels
- ✓ Electrocardiogram
- ✓ Chest X ray
- ✓ Measurement of arterial blood gases or oxygen saturation
- ✓ Urinalysis

Additional Laboratory Tests, Ordered as Indicated by Clinical Condition
- ✓ Urine culture and sensitivity
- ✓ Urine drug screen
- ✓ Blood cultures
- ✓ Measurement of serum levels of medications, e.g., cyclosporine, digoxin, phenobarbital, theophylline
- ✓ Blood tests, e.g., Venereal Disease Research Laboratory (VDRL), heavy metal screen, lupus erythematosus (LE) prep, antinuclear antibodies (ANA), serum ammonia, human immunodeficiency virus (HIV)
- ✓ Urinary porphyrins
- ✓ Lumbar puncture (LP)
- ✓ Brain computed tomography (CT) or magnetic resonance imaging (MRI)
- ✓ Electroencephalogram (EEG)

Note. AST (formerly "SGOT")=aspartate aminotransferase; ALT (formerly "SGPT")=alanine aminotransferase.

Source. Adapted from American Psychiatric Association, "Practice Guideline for the Treatment of Patients With Delirium." *American Journal of Psychiatry* 156:1–20, 1999. Used with permission.

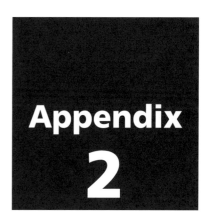

Worksheet for Organizing Medical Chart Information

The Initial Psychiatric Consultation

Wyszynski AA, Wyszynski B (eds.): *Manual of Psychiatric Care for the Medically Ill*. Washington, D.C., American Psychiatric Publishing, Inc., 2005

Worksheet for Organizing Medical Chart Information: The Initial Psychiatric Consultation

Patient's Name: _____   **Date:** _____

CHART REVIEW	MEDICAL	NEUROPSYCHIATRIC
Chief complaint		
Past history	Cancer (esp. Lung, Breast, Melanoma)? Blood transfusions (surgery before 1985)? High-risk sexual behavior?	Neurological Illness? Dementia? HIV? Head Trauma? Pregnancy: Prior postpartum episodes? EtOH? Drugs? Last drink/drug:____ Psychiatric hospitalizations? Suicidality? Screening for bipolar spectrum disorder (see p. 321)
Current course		Date psychiatric symptoms started:____ Change in behavior? Personality? Mood? Thought content? Anxiety? Cognition?
Staff comments		Especially: Fluctuating MSE? Sundowning?
Patient's medications (circle those affecting MSE)	Steroids Cyclosporine Antiarrhythmics Anticholinergics NSAIDs Antihypertensives Interferon Analgesics Propranolol Theophylline Anticonvulsants Antiretrovirals Antibiotics, high-dose (postpartum: metronidazole) H2 antagonists (peptic ulcers/reflux)	Especially: Serotonergics Benzodiazepines Antiparkinsonians
Recent medication changes (dates)		
Notable test results (check normal; circle abnormal; underline not done)	Vital signs CBC Na/K/Ca/Mg B$_{12}$/Folate Toxicology screen Glucose LFTs Serum albumin BUN/creatinine UA TFTs ABGs HIV VDRL ANA ESR Serum ammonia Other: CXR ECG Blood cultures NOTES:	Neurological exam LP EEG Head CT/MRI Other:
Risk factors for delirium (circle all that apply)	Elderly Severe illness, esp. cancer or cardiac arrest Dementia Terminal illness Fever	Azotemia Hypoalbuminemia Hyponatremia Multiple medications Hypothermia Poor hearing and/or vision
Questions & notes		

Note. ABG=arterial blood gas; ANA=antinuclear antibodies; BUN=blood urea nitrogen; CBC=complete blood count; CT/MRI=computed tomography/magnetic resonance imaging; CXR=chest X ray; ECG=electrocardiogram; EEG=electroencephalogram; ESR=erythrocyte sedimentation rate; ETOH=beverage alcohol; HIV=human immunodeficiency virus; LFTs=liver function tests; LP=lumbar puncture; MSE=mental status examination; NSAIDs=nonsteroidal anti-inflammatory drugs; TFTs=thyroid function tests; UA=urinalysis; VDRL=Venereal Disease Research Laboratory test.

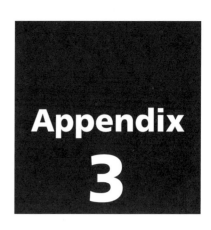

Decision Tree for Psychiatric Differential Diagnosis of Medically Ill Patients

Decision Tree for Psychiatric Differential Diagnosis of Medically Ill Patients

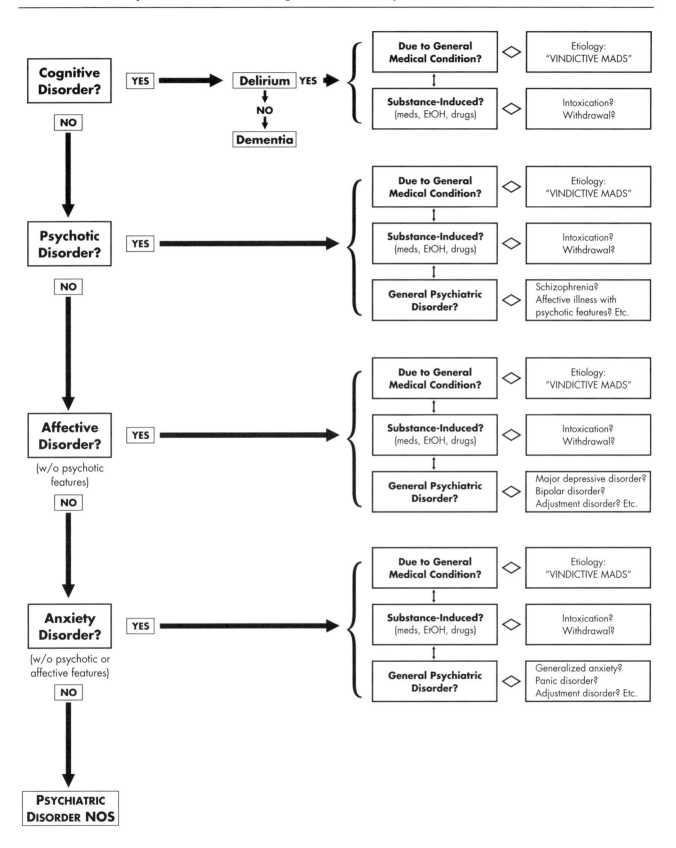

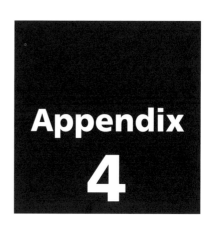

"VINDICTIVE MADS"

Differential Diagnosis of Mental Status Changes

Wyszynski AA, Wyszynski B (eds.): *Manual of Psychiatric Care for the Medically Ill.* Washington, D.C., American Psychiatric Publishing, Inc., 2005

"VINDICTIVE MADS": Differential Diagnosis of Mental Status Changes

Etiology	Diagnosis
VASCULAR	Hypertensive encephalopathy; cerebral arteriosclerosis Intracranial hemorrhage or thromboses Emboli from atrial fibrillation, patent foramen ovale, or endocarditic valve Circulatory collapse (shock) Lupus cerebritis (including postpartum psychosis); polyarteritis nodosa; thrombotic thrombocytopenic purpura; hyperviscosity syndrome; sarcoid
INFECTIOUS	Sepsis/encephalitis/meningitis (bacterial/viral/fungal/parasitic) Abscess (brain/epidural/subdural) General paresis; malaria; Lyme disease; typhoid fever; Behçet's; mumps HIV/AIDS: *Systemic infections:* disseminated herpes zoster; *Mycobacterium avium-intracellulare;* candidiasis; pneumonia. *CNS infections:* neurosyphilis; cytomegalovirus encephalitis; herpes simplex encephalitis; cryptococcal meningitis; progressive multifocal leukoencephalopathy (papovavirus); toxoplasmosis; tubercular meningitis; Creutzfeldt-Jakob disease
NEOPLASTIC	1°: gliomas, meningiomas, etc.; 2°: metastases; carcinomatous meningitis; paraneoplastic syndromes HIV/AIDS: CNS lymphoma; Kaposi's sarcoma (rarely metastasizes, but forms multiple 1° tumors)
DEGENERATIVE	Dementias 2° to Alzheimer's, Pick's, Parkinson's, Huntington's, Creutzfeldt-Jakob, Wilson's diseases, etc. HIV/AIDS: HIV-associated dementia complex (HADC); HIV-associated minor cognitive-motor disorder (MCMD)
INTOXICATION (AND WITHDRAWAL)	*Medications:* steroids; HIV antiretrovirals; antibiotics; antifungals; antituberculars; anticholinergics; serotonergics ("serotonin syndrome"); analgesics; neuroleptic malignant syndrome HIV/AIDS: any and all of the above Illicit drugs or alcohol (intoxication and withdrawal, esp. DTs)
CONGENITAL DEFECTS/STATES	Inborn errors of metabolism; structural defects: e.g., aneurysm, heart defects
TRAUMATIC	Head trauma: e.g., subdural and epidural hematomas; contusion; laceration Postoperative trauma; fat emboli syndrome; heatstroke
INTRAVENTRICULAR	Normal-pressure hydrocephalus
VITAMIN DEFICIENCY	Thiamine (Wernicke-Korsakoff); niacin (pellagra); B_{12} (esp. atrophic gastritis in the elderly); folate. Monitor especially in patients who are cachectic or have had gastric surgery, malabsorption syndromes, etc.
ENDOCRINE/METABOLIC	Hypoglycemia (HIV/AIDS: 2° to pentamidine and protease inhibitors) Organ failure: brain/kidney/hepatic failure (esp. hepatic encephalopathy) Electrolyte or acid-base disturbances (see Appendix 17) Other: diabetes (coma/shock); hypo/hyperthyroid; hypo/hyperparathyroid, hypo/hyperadrenal; carcinoid; Whipple's disease
METALS	Lead, manganese, mercury, other toxins
ANOXIA	Anoxia and hypoxia 2° to cardiac failure or pulmonary infection/failure; anesthesia; anemia
DEPRESSION/PSYCHIATRIC CONDITIONS	1° psychiatric conditions causing mental status changes: e.g., poor concentration ("pseudodementia") 2° to depression; mania; catatonia, etc.
SEIZURES	Acquired seizures 2° to any etiology; postictal states; complex partial status

Note. 1°=primary; 2°=secondary; CNS=central nervous system; DTs=delirium tremens; esp.=especially; HIV/AIDS=human immunodeficiency virus/acquired immunodeficiency syndrome.

Source. Adapted from Ludwig AM: *Principles of Clinical Psychiatry.* New York, Free Press, 1980.

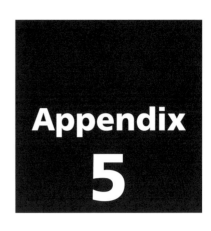

Appendix 5

A Short, Practical Guide to Treating Dementia-Related Behavioral Problems in the Medical Setting

Ceri Hadda, M.D.

Diagnosis is challenging when delirium and dementia occur simultaneously, especially when delirium is of the hypoactive type. Both disorders target elderly persons. Both attack cognition. Both produce behavioral disinhibition, particularly at night ("sundowning"). The state of consciousness distinguishes one from the other. The patient with dementia is usually *consistently alert,* albeit cognitively impaired. The alertness of the delirious patient *shifts throughout the day.* Longitudinal information-gathering from the observations of friends, family, and staff helps establish the pattern.

The following quick reference guide to managing dementia-related behavioral problems in the medical setting was derived from practice guidelines of the American Psychiatric Association and the American Academy of Neurology.

■ MEDICAL WORKUP OF DEMENTIA

For All Patients:

- Laboratory tests: complete blood count (CBC); electrolyte and metabolic panels; B_{12} and folate levels; rapid plasma reagin titer; urinalysis; urine toxicology, if indicated
- More specific tests depending on history and pattern of cognitive deficits, such as erythrocyte sedimentation rate, antinuclear antibodies test, Lyme titer, antiphospholipid syndrome test, anti-Hu antibody test
- Electrocardiogram
- Chest X ray, if indicated
- Test for human immunodeficiency virus
- Computed tomography (CT) of head—to rule out

Wyszynski AA, Wyszynski B (eds.): *Manual of Psychiatric Care for the Medically Ill.* Washington, D.C., American Psychiatric Publishing, Inc., 2005

recent bleed or mass lesion, normal-pressure hydrocephalus
- Magnetic resonance imaging of head—same benefits as CT but increased sensitivity for ischemia or infarct involving subcortical and brainstem areas or demyelinating lesions
- Electroencephalography
- Lumbar puncture
- Positron emission tomography scan

PRINCIPLES OF SYMPTOM MANAGEMENT

For symptom management in dementia, a multimodal approach using behavioral and pharmacological treatments ensures optimal results.

- Many symptoms of dementia, including wandering, perseverative behavior, and impaired social skills, do not respond to medications and may even be exacerbated by them.
- When at all possible, use nonpharmacological interventions to deal with symptoms, to avoid unnecessary side effects from medication as well as polypharmacy.

A WORD ABOUT "AGITATION"

Agitation is not a diagnostic term, but rather is often used to describe a cluster of behaviors including repetitive verbal, vocal, or motor activity that is disruptive to others. Some behaviors are best managed with nonpharmacological treatment. Others—especially those that are distressing or threatening harm to the patient and others—may warrant pharmacological intervention.

Behavior is typically clustered into subtypes, including 1) physically aggressive behavior such as biting and kicking; 2) physically nonaggressive behavior such as pacing; 3) verbally aggressive behavior such as cursing and screaming; and 4) verbally nonaggressive behavior such as perseverative speech and questioning.

Etiology of the above behaviors is often multifocal and may include cognitive impairment, preexisting psychiatric illness, medical disorders and their treatment, pain, and functional disability.

- When called regarding an "agitated" patient, first determine the disturbance in behavior and then begin to investigate potential causes.

- Potentially reversible common causes of agitation—such as urinary tract infections, constipation, chronic pain, initiation of new medication, a recent change in environment or withdrawal from alcohol, and illicit drugs or medications—must be appropriately evaluated and treated first.

NONPHARMACOLOGICAL METHODS OF SYMPTOM MANAGEMENT

In addition to memory impairment and symptoms warranting medication management, dementias usually involve multiple behavioral disturbances that are best handled in nonpharmacological ways. Disturbances of this type include 1) wandering and pacing, 2) hoarding and hiding things, 3) perseverative thoughts and actions, 4) regressive behavior such as neediness, and 5) inappropriate social interactions. If no reversible cause of behavioral disturbance is found, nonpharmacological methods are best for these types of behaviors. Interventions may focus on sensory, environmental, or behavior modalities.

- *Sensory interventions* include music therapy; aromatherapy; bright-light therapy (in the evening for sundowning; in the morning for agitation with sleep dysregulation); examination of glasses, dentures, and hearing aids; pain assessment; and light exercise to promote regularity and a sense of well-being.
- *Environmental strategies* include promoting personal space for patients; reducing disruptive stimuli such as noise from other patients, loudspeakers, and equipment/machinery; providing safe venues for wandering; and pet therapy.
- *Behavioral approaches* include providing praise and encouragement for positive behavior; redirecting negative behavior; reality orientation; and approaching the patient in a calm, soft-spoken manner rather than a confrontational, seemingly punitive one.
- Remember that caregivers—both family and staff—need support, too.

GENERAL PHARMACOLOGICAL PRINCIPLES

- When at all possible, use nonpharmacological interventions to deal with symptoms in order to avoid excessive medication and polypharmacy.

- Treat coexisting symptoms, such as depression or psychosis, with appropriate medication.
- Medication may be necessary when 1) nonpharmacological treatments do not work, 2) reversible causes for the behavioral disturbances have not been found, and/or 3) the symptoms are dangerous or distressing to the patient or others.
- Statistically, dementia patients are elderly, with decreased renal clearance and slowed hepatic metabolism consistent with normal aging. Multiple medical problems common in older patients often lead to polypharmacy, setting the stage for drug-drug interactions. In addition, cognitive impairment creates an even greater sensitivity to medications and susceptibility to increased confusion.
- Medicating the psychiatric symptoms of dementia requires a delicate hand. Starting doses should be reduced to ¼ to ½ those given to younger adults; each increase in dose should be small; and longer periods should elapse between increases.
- Avoid anticholinergic medications that can promote confusion and worsen preexisting symptoms such as urinary retention or blurry vision.
- All elderly patients, but particularly those with dementia, are particularly prone to extrapyramidal side effects. Medications with extrapyramidal side effect profiles must be prescribed with extra caution and observation (e.g., when pacing dose increases, carefully evaluate for akathisia).
- Be wary of medications associated with CNS suppression. They may increase the risk of falls, exacerbate respiratory depression, and increase confusion.

■ PHARMACOLOGICAL TREATMENTS FOR SPECIFIC SYMPTOMS

Psychosis

Delusions, hallucinations, and other types of psychosis may be treated with atypical antipsychotics such as olanzapine (Zyprexa), quetiapine (Seroquel), and ziprasidone (Geodon). Watch for excessive sedation, parkinsonism, and the tendency to fall. Regarding other antipsychotics, note the following:

- *Risperidone (Risperdal):* There is a large literature on the use of risperidone for patients with dementia. However, in 2003 the manufacturer revised recommendations to physicians about using risperidone for elderly patients with dementia-related psycho-

sis. These recommendations were based on data from a study of 1,230 patients with dementia in four placebo-controlled trials conducted in elderly patients with dementia. Cerebrovascular adverse events (i.e., stroke, transient ischemic attacks), including fatalities, were reported in trials of risperidone in elderly patients with dementia-related psychosis. The manufacturer specifically states that risperidone is not safe or effective in the treatment of dementia-related psychosis.
- *Aripiprazole (Abilify):* Information was just beginning to accumulate on the use of this novel antipsychotic at the time of this writing.

Mood Disturbances

In assessing possible depression, take note that patients with dementia may be *apathetic* rather than truly depressed. If you have determined that the patient is probably depressed, choose a medication to target particular symptoms, as you would with cognitively intact patients:

- Use antidepressants such as selective serotonin reuptake inhibitors (SSRIs), bupropion (Wellbutrin), mirtazapine (Remeron), or venlafaxine (Effexor) for depression, with or without irritability and anxiety.
- Common side effects of antidepressants include gastrointestinal upset; headache; falls, sedation (with mirtazapine and paroxetine [Paxil]); sedation or activation and possible increased blood pressure (with venlafaxine); hyponatremia (with SSRIs); and tremor (with bupropion).
- Use certain side effects and features to advantage: trazodone (Desyrel) promotes sleep; bupropion is beneficial for the patient with amotivation and decreased daytime activity; mirtazapine promotes both sleep and appetite. Use once-a-week formulation fluoxetine (Prozac Once A Week) for those patients who have difficulty with daily medication administration. Sertraline (Zoloft) and citalopram (Celexa) have relatively few drug-drug interactions; paroxetine is the most anticholinergic of the SSRIs. With trazodone, which was originally developed as an antidepressant, there are potential problems with orthostatic hypotension and priapism. However, trazodone remains an effective hypnotic in low doses.
- Improvement in mood with antidepressant medication may not be apparent for 4 to 6 weeks.
- Consider electroconvulsive therapy (ECT) for medication-refractory cases of depression, as well as cases in which medication is contraindicated. ECT

promotes both decreased motor symptoms and improved mood in patients with Parkinson's disease.

Mood Lability and Impulsivity

- Use mood stabilizers such as valproic acid (Depakote, Depakene) or carbamazepine (Tegretol). Side effects include sedation, ataxia, tremor; thrombocytopenia/anemia and liver function test abnormalities (with valproic acid); and leukopenia (with carbamazepine). Monitor CBC, liver function, and drug levels.
- Use atypical antipsychotics such as olanzapine, quetiapine, or ziprasidone in patients with mood lability and concurrent psychosis. (See the earlier description of problems associated with risperidone.)
- Lithium is potentially problematic because of the vulnerability of elderly patients to dehydration-induced toxicity and drug-drug interactions.
- There are anecdotal reports, but no controlled studies, suggesting that off-label use of gabapentin (Neurontin) is helpful in some patients.

Anxiety

- The same medications used for depression may be used for anxiety.
- Buspirone (BuSpar) is also helpful for anxiety in this setting.
- If possible, avoid benzodiazepines, which can worsen confusion, cause paradoxical agitation, and increase risk of falls and respiratory suppression.

Physical Aggression and Disinhibition

- Use mood stabilizers such as valproic acid or carbamazepine. Side effects include sedation, ataxia, tremor; thrombocytopenia/anemia and liver function test abnormalities (with valproic acid); and leukopenia (with carbamazepine). Monitoring of CBC, liver function, and drug levels are necessary. Lithium is potentially problematic because of the vulnerability to dehydration-induced toxicity and drug-drug interactions.
- Atypical antipsychotics may also be necessary if aggression is severe or is not responding quickly enough to mood stabilizers.
- There are anecdotal reports, but no controlled studies, that off-label use of gabapentin is helpful in some patients.

Sleep Difficulties

Insomnia, nocturnal confusion, and interrupted sleep commonly occur in dementia. Simple sleep hygiene may suffice if sleep dysregulation is mild or does not cause disruption to family/caregivers, especially if the risk of medication side effects outweighs the sleep problem. Sleep hygiene includes regular sleep and waking times, restricted caffeine intake, limited napping, regular exercise and social stimulation during the day, avoidance of fluids in the evening, and soothing bedtime rituals. Occasionally, medical causes of sleep dysregulation—such as sleep apnea—require attention.

- Use of hypnotic medications should be tailored to clinical needs of patients. Trazodone and zolpidem (Ambien) are often used as hypnotics, but zolpidem may cause confusion. Mirtazapine is indicated for depressed patients with sleep and concurrent appetite difficulties. Psychotic patients with sleep disturbances may benefit from olanzapine. Patients with mood lability and difficulty sleeping should receive a larger bedtime dose of their mood stabilizer to promote improved sleep.
- Benzodiazepines are second-line agents for sleep in patients with dementia because they can exacerbate sleep apnea and confusion and can cause paradoxical activation/disinhibition, rebound insomnia, daytime sleepiness, and increased risk of falls. Use these agents only when absolutely necessary. Avoid long-acting benzodiazepines and stay with those that bypass first-pass liver metabolism—lorazepam (Ativan), oxazepam (Serax), and temazepam (Restoril)—to avoid accumulation of active metabolites. Avoid triazolam (Halcion) because its ultrashort half-life is associated with amnesia.
- Avoid diphenhydramine (Benadryl) because it is anticholinergic and can worsen confusion.

■ RECOMMENDED READINGS

American Psychiatric Association: Practice guideline for the treatment of patients with Alzheimer's disease and other dementias of late life. Am J Psychiatry 154:1–39, 1997

Coffey CE, Cummings JL, Lovell MR, et al (eds): The American Psychiatric Press Textbook of Geriatric Neuropsychiatry, 2nd Edition. Washington, DC, American Psychiatric Press, 2000

Cummings J, Mega M (eds): Neuropsychiatry and Behavioral Neuroscience. New York, Oxford University Press, 2003

Doody RS, Stevens JC, Beck RN, et al: Practice Parameter: Management of Dementia (An Evidence-Based Review). Report of the Quality Standards Subcommittee of the American Academy of Neurology. Saint Paul, MN, AAN Enterprises, 2002

Jacobson S, Pies R, Greenblatt D: Handbook of Geriatric Psychopharmacology. Washington, DC, American Psychiatric Publishing, 2002

Lantz M: Options for the treatment of behavioral disturbances in dementia. Clinical Geriatrics 11:34–36, 2003

Nasr S, Osterwell D: The nonpharmacological management of agitation in the nursing home: a consensus approach. Annals of Long-Term Care 7:171–180, 1999

Weiner M, Lipton A (eds): The Dementias: Diagnosis, Treatment and Research, 3rd Edition. Washington, DC, American Psychiatric Publishing, 2003

Yudofsky SC, Hales RE (eds): The American Psychiatric Publishing Textbook of Neuropsychiatry and Clinical Neurosciences, 4th Edition. Washington, DC, American Psychiatric Publishing, 2002

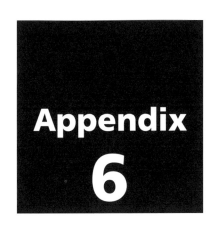

Appendix 6

A Guide to Herbal Supplements in the Medical Setting

Nancy Forman, M.D.

The World Health Organization estimates that 75%–80% of the world's population, or about 4 billion people, rely on traditional medicines, most commonly involving the use of plant extracts, for their medicinal needs (Li et al. 2000; Weiss and Fintelmann 2000). In the United States, it is estimated that 15%–30% of the general population, and a higher percentage in some ethnic groups, use herbal medications (Callaway and Grob 1998). About 42% of Americans take some form of complementary or alternative medicine (CAM); roughly two-thirds have used CAM at least once in their lifetime (Cupp 1999).

The following account for more than half of all the single-herb medications used in the United States: echinacea, ephedra, garlic, ginkgo, ginseng, kava, saw palmetto, St. John's wort, and valerian (Blumenthal et al. 2000; Ernst 2002; Stedman 2002).

Some individuals use herbal medicines because they believe these medications are safer, since they are "natural." However, herbs contain active chemical compounds that are not inherently less toxic than those found in synthesized pharmaceuticals. Herbal medications may be adulterated with pharmaceuticals, contaminated with heavy metals, or toxic themselves (Galluzzi et al. 2000). Studies have suggested that the majority (up to 70%) of patients do not reveal their use of herbal medications to their allopathic practitioners (Callaway and Grob 1998). Given these findings and the potential for complications, it is important to inquire, routinely and specifically, about patients' use of herbal medications (Blumenthal et al. 2000). (*Note:* Ephedra sales have been prohibited in the United States as of 2004.)

The following chart is intended to alert practitioners to the adverse effects of herbs and to flag known or suspected drug–herbal medicine interactions that have been described in the English-language medical literature. Because herbal products are not subject to the same standards as medications licensed by the U.S. Food and Drug Administration, it is impossible to make this list complete; adulteration and contamination have the potential to further complicate an already complex situation.

Additional resources that may be helpful include the following:

- *http://nccam.nih.gov* (National Center for Complementary and Alternative Medicine of the National Institutes of Health). A Web site containing fact sheets, databases, and consensus reports about alternative therapies.
- *http://consumerlab.com* (ConsumerLab). The Web site of a laboratory that performs independent testing on herbal medications and other supplements and health products.
- *http://www.herbmed.org* (HerbMed). An interactive Web site that contains information about specific herbal medications, including research summaries and MEDLINE links.

■ REFERENCES

Adusumilli PS, Lee B, Parekh K, et al: Acalculous eosinophilic cholecystitis from herbal medicine: a review of adverse effects of herbal medicine in surgical patients. Surgery 131:352–356, 2002

Ang-Lee M, Moss J, Yuan C-S: Herbal medicines and perioperative care. JAMA 286:208–216, 2001

Blumenthal M, Goldberg A, Brinckmann J (eds): Herbal Medicine: Expanded Commission E Monographs. Newton, MA, Integrative Medicine Communications, 2000

But PP, Tomlinson B, Cheung KO, et al: Adulterants of herbal products can cause poisoning (letter). BMJ 313:11, 1996

Callaway JC, Grob CS: Ayahuasca preparations and serotonin reuptake inhibitors: a potential combination for severe adverse interactions. J Psychoactive Drugs 30:367–369, 1998

Crone C, Gabriel G: Herbal and nonherbal supplements in medical-psychiatric patient populations. Psychiatr Clin North Am 25:211–230, 2002

Cupp M: Herbal remedies: adverse effects and drug interactions. Am Fam Physician 59:1239–1244, 1999

Doyle H, Kargin M: Herbal stimulant containing ephedrine has also caused psychosis (letter). BMJ 313:756, 1996

Ernst E: The risk-benefit profile of commonly used herbal therapies: ginkgo, St. John's wort, ginseng, echinacea, saw palmetto and kava. Ann Intern Med 136:42–52, 2002

Galluzzi S, Zanetti O, Binetti G, et al: Coma in a patient with Alzheimer's disease taking low dose trazodone and ginkgo biloba. J Neurol Neurosurg Psychiatry 68:679–680, 2000

Garges HP, Varis I, Doraiswamy PM: Cardiac complications and delirium associated with valerian root withdrawal. JAMA 280:1566–1567, 1998

Gold JL, Laxer DA, Dergal JM, et al: Herbal-drug therapy interactions: a focus on dementia. Curr Opin Clin Nutr Metab Care 4:29–34, 2001

Haller C, Benowitz N: Adverse cardiovascular and central nervous system events associated with dietary supplements containing ephedra alkaloids. N Engl J Med 343:1833–1838, 2000

Horowitz RS, Feldhaus K, Dart R, et al: The clinical spectrum of Jin Bu Huan toxicity. Arch Intern Med 156:899–903, 1996

Ioannides C: Pharmacokinetic interactions between herbal remedies and medicinal drugs. Xenobiotica 32:451–478, 2002

Jacobs KM, Hirsch KA: Psychiatric complications of Ma-huang. Psychosomatics 41:58–62, 2000

Josefson D: Herbal stimulant causes US deaths. BMJ 312:1441, 1996

Larkin M: Surgery patients at risk for herb-anaesthesia interactions. Lancet 354:1362, 1999

Li AM, Chan MH, Leung TF, et al: Mercury intoxication presenting with tics. Arch Dis Child 83:174–175, 2000

McRae S: Elevated serum digoxin levels in patients taking digoxin and Siberian ginseng. CMAJ 155:293–295, 1996

Miller LG: Herbal medicinals: selected clinical considerations focusing on known or potential drug-herb interactions. Arch Intern Med 158:2200–2211, 1998

Miller LG, Murray WJ (eds): Herbal Medicinals: A Clinician's Guide. New York, Pharmaceutical Products Press, 1998

Morelli V, Zoorob R: Alternative therapies, part 1: depression, diabetes and obesity. Am Fam Physician 62:1051–1060, 2000

Nierenberg A, Burt T, Matthews J, et al: Mania associated with St. John's wort. Biol Psychiatry 46:1707–1708, 1999

PDR for Herbal Medicines, 2nd Edition. Montvale, NJ, Medical Economics, 2000

Pribitkin E, Boger G: Herbal therapy: what every facial plastic surgeon must know. Arch Facial Plast Surg 3:127–132, 2001

Spoelhof G, Foerst L: Herbs to magnets: managing alternative therapies in the nursing home. Annals of Long-Term Care 10:51–57, 2002

Stedman C: Herbal hepatotoxicity. Semin Liver Dis 22:195–206, 2002

Stewart MJ, Steenkamp V, Zuckerman M: The toxicology of African herbal remedies. Ther Drug Monit 20:510–516, 1998

Warber SL, Bankroft J, Pedroza J: Herbal Appendix. Clinics in Family Practice 4:1045–1068, 2002

Weiss RF, Fintelmann V: Herbal Medicine, 2nd Edition. New York, Thieme, 2000

Herbal Supplements in the Medical Setting

NAME	ALSO KNOWN AS	COMMON USES AND PROPERTIES	ADVERSE EFFECTS	DRUG INTERACTION	REFERENCES
Aga	*Amanita muscaria*	Neuralgia, fever, anxiety, alcohol poisoning, joint pain	Dizziness, vomiting, abdominal pain, movement disorders, muscle cramps, psychic stimulation followed by deep sleep, confusion, mania, unconsciousness, coma, death		Herbal PDR (2000)
American hellebore	*Veratrum viride*	Historically, used internally to treat pneumonia, peritonitis, epilepsy, pain, asthma, colds, cholera, croup, etc.	Sneezing, lacrimation, salivation, vomiting and diarrhea, inability to swallow, paresthesias, vertigo, blindness, convulsions, bradycardia, hypotension, cardiac death		Herbal PDR (2000)
Anemarrhena	Zhi-mu, *Anemarrhena asphodeloides*	Agitation	In overdose, gastroenteritis, intestinal colic, diarrhea		Herbal PDR (2000)
Angelica	*Angelica archangelica, Angelica officinalis*	Fevers, colds, urinary tract infections, dyspepsia, loss of appetite	Dermatophotosensitivity		Herbal PDR (2000)
Angel's trumpet	*Datura brugmansia*		Hallucinogenic, anticholinergic (see also Malpitte, *Datura stramonium*)		Larkin (1999); Stewart et al. (1998)
Areca nut	*Areca catechu*, betel nut, pinang	Intoxicating qualities; stimulant, euphoriant			Herbal PDR (2000); Weiss and Fintelmann (2000)
Ayahuasca		Hallucinogen		Has potent MAOI activity and should be avoided in combination with any medication that interacts adversely with MAOIs, such as SSRIs	Callaway and Grob (1998)
Betel (see areca nut)					
Borage	*Borago officinalis*	Depression	Hepatotoxicity, lowers seizure threshold		Weiss and Fintelmann (2000)

Herbal Supplements in the Medical Setting *(continued)*

NAME	ALSO KNOWN AS	COMMON USES AND PROPERTIES	ADVERSE EFFECTS	DRUG INTERACTION	REFERENCES
Chamomile		Sedative, antispasmodic	Contact irritant, esp. eyes; allergy common, with symptoms including abdominal cramps, sensation of tongue thickness, tight sensation in throat, angioedema of lips and eyes, diffuse pruritis, generalized urticaria, upper airway obstruction, pharyngeal edema	*Note:* Chamomile contains coumarin. If used with anticoagulants, monitor coagulation profile carefully.	Miller (1998); Spoelhof and Foerst (2002)
Cola	*Cola acuminata*	Lack of stamina; CNS stimulant	Insomnia, hyperexcitability, restlessness (contains caffeine)		Herbal PDR (2000)
Ephedra (see ma-huang)					
Evening primrose oil	*Oenothera biennis*	Diabetic neuropathy, multiple sclerosis, Sjögren's syndrome, ADHD	Hepatotoxicity; lowers seizure threshold; gastrointestinal disturbances, headache	Phenothiazines, anticonvulsants, NSAIDs, steroids, β-blockers, anticoagulants	Adusumilli et al. (2002); Miller (1998); Warber et al. (2002)
Feverfew	*Tanacetum parthenium*	Migraines	Upon abrupt discontinuation, post-feverfew syndrome (nervousness, headache, insomnia, stiffness, joint pains, tiredness). Inhibits platelet activity.	Concurrent use of NSAIDs may decrease effectiveness. Contains tannin, so may decrease iron absorption. May increase anticoagulant effect of warfarin.	Stedman (2002)
Ginger	*Zingiber officinale*	Antinauseant (including nausea related to kinetosis), antispasmodic	Prolongs bleeding time through inhibition of thromboxane synthetase	Antiplatelet agents, anticoagulants	Warber et al. (2002)
Ginkgo biloba		Dementia, memory impairment, cognitive decline	Gastrointestinal upset, platelet inhibition, headache	Anticoagulants: increases anticoagulant effect of warfarin. May decrease effectiveness of anticonvulsants (due to presence of ginkgotoxin, a known neurotoxin). Use care also with medications known to decrease seizure threshold. Trazodone: increased sedation and coma. Interactions expected with MAOIs.	Gold et al. (2001); Miller (1998); Stedman (2002)

Herbal Supplements in the Medical Setting *(continued)*

NAME	ALSO KNOWN AS	COMMON USES AND PROPERTIES	ADVERSE EFFECTS	DRUG INTERACTION	REFERENCES
Ginseng	*Panax*, various species	Endurance, stress resistance enhancer; improved concentration, adaptogen, aphrodisiac	Hypertension, vomiting, epistaxis, headache, moderate estrogen effect, question of neonatal androgenization, CNS stimulant with nervousness, sleeplessness	Increased digoxin level (probably just in assay, without causing clinical toxicity [see McRae 1996]), headache, tremulousness, mania in patients on phenelzine, decreased INR in patients with stable coagulation profiles on warfarin. *Note:* Platelet effects appear to be species specific and occur with Asian but not Siberian ginseng (see Pribitkin et al. 2000). May interfere with antihypertensives and with glycemic control in diabetic patients.	Cupp (1999); Gold et al. (2001); McRae (1996); Miller (1998); Pribitkin and Boger (2001); Stedman (2002); Weiss and Fintelmann (2000)
Goldenseal	*Hydrastis canadensis*	Antidiarrheal, topical antiseptic	Seizures in high doses	Opposes anticoagulation	Spoelhof and Foerst (2002)
Hops	*Humulus lupulus*	Mild sedation may help to decrease male libido through its anaphrodisiac effect.		Potentiates sedatives	Adusumilli et al. (2002); Weiss and Fintelmann (2000)
Horseradish		Antiseptic with circulatory and digestive stimulation effects, diuretic	May depress thyroid function		Miller (1998)
Jin bu huan	Active agent: *l*-tetrahydro-palmatine	Sedative, analgesic	Depressed mental status, fatigue, hypertension, acute or chronic hepatitis		Horowitz et al. (1996); Stedman (2002)
Kava	*Piper methysticum*, kava-kava	Antianxiety, muscle relaxant, sedative	EPS, dermopathy, diffuse hepatocellular necrosis	Benzodiazepines (alprazolam mentioned specifically): excess sedation, lethargy, disorientation. Alcohol: increased toxicity. Anesthetics: prolongs effects of some. Effectiveness of L-dopa decreased. Possible additive effects with antiplatelet agents.	Cupp (1999); Gold et al. (2001); Larkin (1999); Miller (1998); Stedman (2002)
Kelp		Weight loss	Can cause hypo- or hyperthyroidism	Use with known stimulant could be dangerous	Miller (1998)
Khat	*Catha edulis*, Bushman's tea	Hallucinogen, CNS stimulant (used in Africa)	Hallucinogenic		Stewart et al. (1998); Weiss and Fintelmann (2000)
Licorice	*Glycyrrhiza*, various species	Antispasmodic, anti-inflammatory; gastritis, peptic ulcer disease		Glycyrrhizin in licorice has MAOI activity	Miller (1998); Warber et al. (2002)

Herbal Supplements in the Medical Setting *(continued)*

NAME	ALSO KNOWN AS	COMMON USES AND PROPERTIES	ADVERSE EFFECTS	DRUG INTERACTION	REFERENCES
Ma-huang	Ephedra, herbal fen-phen, Herbal Ecstasy, Cloud 9, Ultimate Xphoria	Weight reduction, appetite suppressant, decongestant, bronchodilator, stimulant	Anxiety, tremulousness, insomnia, palpitations, personality changes, mania, psychosis, hypertension, CVA, myocardial infarction, cardiac arrhythmias, sudden death	May interact with antidepressants or antihypertensives to cause increase in blood pressure and/or heart rate. Additive effects with other stimulants. Life-threatening interactions.	Adusumilli et al. (2002) ; Ang-Lee et al. (2001); Cupp (1999); Doyle and Kargin (1996); Haller and Benowitz (2000); Jacobs and Hirsch (2000); Josefson (1996); Larkin (1999); Morelli and Zoorob (2000)
Malpitte	*Datura stramonium,* jimson weed, thornapple, deadly nightshade	Hallucinogen; active components: scopolamine, hyoscyamine	Marked aggression, dilated pupils, tachycardia		Larkin (1999); Stewart et al. (1998)
Podophyllum hexandrum	*P. emodi,* gwai-kou, Himalayan mayapple	Found as adulterant of lung-dam-cho (*Gentiana,* various species) and of wai-ling-sing	Neuropathy, encephalopathy		But et al. (1996)
Saw palmetto	*Serenoa repens*	Prostatic hypertrophy, antiandrogenic effects, diuretic, urinary antiseptic, anabolic properties	Gastrointestinal upset, headaches, diarrhea	May interact with other androgen therapies; may be additive with other hormone therapies (estrogen replacement, oral contraceptives)	Miller (1998); Miller and Murray (1998)
Sceletium, various species		Hallucinogenic			Stewart et al. (1998)

Herbal Supplements in the Medical Setting *(continued)*

NAME	ALSO KNOWN AS	COMMON USES AND PROPERTIES	ADVERSE EFFECTS	DRUG INTERACTION	REFERENCES
St. John's wort	*Hypericum perforatum*	Depression, anxiety, sleep disturbances, viral infections	Mania	Diabetes medications; decreases cyclosporine levels (thereby decreasing immunosuppression). Contains tannin, so may decrease iron absorption. Enhances metabolism of oral contraceptives, tricyclic antidepressants. Decreases theophylline levels. Decreases levels of protease inhibitors, including amprenavir, ritonavir, saquinavir, nelfinavir, and indinavir; may have similar effect on nonnucleoside transcriptase inhibitors, including delavirdine, efavirenz, nevirapine. Decreases digoxin levels. Enhanced effects of SSRIs/SNRIs, resulting in serotonin syndrome. Interactions also described with anticoagulants (may decrease INR), antiplatelet agents, MAOIs, steroids, calcium channel blockers, benzodiazepines. Mechanism of action unknown, thought to have MAOI properties from quercitrin content, and possibly SSRI activity as well. Prudent to avoid with MAOIs, β-sympathomimetics (including ma-huang and pseudoephedrine), and SSRIs until status/mechanism further clarified.	Adusumilli et al. (2002); Gold et al. (2001); Ioannides (2002); Miller (1998); Nierenberg et al. (1999); Spoelhof and Foerst (2002)
Valerian	*Valeriana officinalis*	Hypnotic, muscle relaxant	Headache, paradoxical stimulant effect, abnormal liver function tests. Benzodiazepine-like acute withdrawal.	Potentiates action of sedatives, benzodiazepines, alcohol, barbiturates. Prolongs thiopental/ pentobarbital-induced sleep.	Ang-Lee et al. (2001); Crone and Gabriel (2002); Garges et al. (1998); Gold et al. (2001); Miller (1998); Spoelhof and Foerst (2002)
Watermelon frost		Pain/healing of mucosal lesions. A Chinese herbal medicine containing mercury.	Motor/vocal tics in high doses in children		Li et al. (2000)
Wormwood		Appetite stimulant	Lowers seizure threshold		Miller (1998); Miller and Murray (1998)

Note. ADHD=attention-deficit/hyperactivity disorder; CNS=central nervous system; CVA=cerebrovascular accident; EPS=extrapyramidal side effects; INR=international normalized ratio (a standardized measurement of warfarin therapy effectiveness); MAOI=monoamine oxidase inhibitor; NSAIDs=nonsteroidal anti-inflammatory drugs; SNRI=selective norepinephrine reuptake inhibitor; SSRI=selective serotonin reuptake inhibitor.

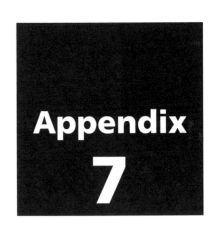

Appendix 7

Worksheet for Diagnosing and Comparing Serotonin Syndrome and Neuroleptic Malignant Syndrome

Wyszynski AA, Wyszynski B (eds.): *Manual of Psychiatric Care for the Medically Ill.* Washington, D.C., American Psychiatric Publishing, Inc., 2005

Worksheet for Diagnosing and Comparing Serotonin Syndrome and Neuroleptic Malignant Syndrome

	Serotonin syndrome[1]	**Neuroleptic malignant syndrome[2,3]**
Necessary criteria	*Prior to onset of signs and symptoms:* ❑ Addition/increase of serotonergic agent ❑ Absence of change in a neuroleptic ❑ Other etiologies have been ruled out ❑ ***At least 3 of the 11 shaded features with boxes, below***	*All 5 criteria required concurrently:* ❑ Neuroleptic treatment within 7 days of onset (within 2–4 weeks for depot neuroleptics) ❑ Hyperthermia ≥38°C (100.4°F) ❑ Muscle rigidity ❑ Other etiologies have been ruled out ❑ ***At least 5 of the 10 shaded features with boxes below***
	↓↓↓↓	↓↓↓↓
Mental status	❑ Mental status changes	❑ Mental status changes
Behavioral	❑ Restlessness, agitation	Restlessness, agitation
Autonomic	❑ Hyperthermia ❑ Diaphoresis ❑ Shivering	☑ ***Hyperthermia*** (necessary criterion) ❑ Diaphoresis or sialorrhea ‡
	❑ Some form of autonomic nervous system dysfunction[a] Labile blood pressure changes Tachycardia Dilated pupils (mydriasis)	Specific autonomic nervous system dysfunction ❑ Labile blood pressure changes ❑ Tachycardia Dilated pupils (mydriasis)
	‡ ‡	❑ Tachypnea or hypoxia ❑ Incontinence
Physical exam	❑ Myoclonus ❑ Hyperreflexia ❑ Tremor ❑ Incoordination ❑ Muscle rigidity[a] ‡	‡ ‡ ❑ Tremor ‡ ☑ ***Muscle rigidity*** (necessary criterion) Extrapyramidal symptoms
Laboratory values	Elevations uncommon; usually normal CPK, WBC, LFTs	❑ ↑ CPK or myoglobulinuria ❑ Leukocytosis ❑ Metabolic acidosis
Miscellaneous	Diarrhea[b]	‡

Note. CPK=creatine phosphokinase; LFTs=liver function tests; WBC=white blood count.

‡Variable or not present.

[a]Substituted for diarrhea in the proposed revisions to the 1991 Sternbach criteria for serotonin syndrome. Proposed by Mann SC, Caroff SN, Keck PE, Lazarus A: *Neuroleptic Malignant Syndrome and Related Conditions,* 2nd Edition. Washington, DC, American Psychiatric Publishing, 2003.

[b]Dropped at the suggestion of Mann et al. (see above) from the 1991 Sternbach criteria because of low prevalence rate (8%) in a series of 168 cases of serotonin syndrome reviewed since 1991.

Source. Adapted from Mann SC, Caroff SN, Keck PE, Lazarus A: *Neuroleptic Malignant Syndrome and Related Conditions,* 2nd Edition. Washington, DC, American Psychiatric Publishing, 2003, pp. 18, 84, 86, 88. Used with permission.

[1]Sternbach H: "The Serotonin Syndrome." *American Journal of Psychiatry* 148:705–713, 1991.

[2]Caroff SN, Mann SC, Lazarus A: "Neuroleptic Malignant Syndrome: Diagnostic Issues." *Psychiatric Annals* 21:130–147, 1991.

[3]Neuroleptic Malignant Syndrome Information Service Hotline: 1-888-NMS-TEMP (1-888-667-8367) [Outside the United States: 1-315-428-9010].

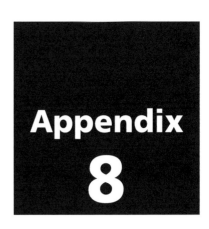

Delirium Rating Scale-Revised-98

Wyszynski AA, Wyszynski B (eds.): *Manual of Psychiatric Care for the Medically Ill.* Washington, D.C., American Psychiatric Publishing, Inc., 2005

Delirium Rating Scale-Revised-98 ©Trzepacz 1998

Patient's Name: _____ Date/Time: _____

1. **Sleep-wake cycle (SWC)**	0 Not present 1 Mild sleep continuity disturbance at night or occasional daytime drowsiness 2 Moderate disorganization (e.g., falling asleep during conversations, daytime napping, several brief nighttime awakenings with confusion/behavioral changes or very little nighttime sleep) 3 Severe disruption (e.g., day-night reversal of SWC, severe circadian fragmentation with multiple periods of sleep & wakefulness, or severe sleeplessness)	○ Naps ○ Day-night reversal ○ Nocturnal disturbance only

2.
Perceptual disturbances & hallucinations
	0 Not present
	1 Mild perceptual disturbances (e.g., a sound, noise, color, spot, flashes, etc.)
	2 Illusions present
	3 Hallucinations present (e.g., voices, music, people, animals, scenes, etc.)
		Type:
		  ○ auditory
		  ○ visual
		  ○ olfactory
		  ○ tactile
		○ Simple: uncomplicated
		○ Complex: multidimensional

3.
Delusions
	0 Not present
	1 Mildly suspicious, hypervigilant, or preoccupied
	2 Unusual/overvalued ideation not of delusional proportions; could be plausible
	3 Delusional
		Type:
		  ○ persecutory
		  ○ grandiose
		  ○ somatic
		  ○ poorly formed
		  ○ systematized
		Reported by:
		  ○ patient
		  ○ family
		  ○ staff
		  ○ caregiver

4.
Lability of affect
	0 Not present
	1 Affect somewhat altered or incongruent to situation; changes over course of hours; emotions are mostly under self-control
	2 Affect often inappropriate to situation & intermittently changes over course of minutes; emotions not consistently under self-control, though respond to redirection by others
	3 Severe & consistent disinhibition of emotions; affect changes rapidly, inappropriate to context, does not respond to redirection by others
		Rate patient's outward emotional presentation, rather than a description of what patient feels.
		Type:
		  ○ angry
		  ○ anxious
		  ○ elated
		  ○ irritable
		  ○ dysphoric

5.
Language
Assess fluency, grammar, comprehension, semantic content, & naming (e.g., pen, parts of watch)
	0 Normal language
	1 Mild impairment, including word-finding difficulty or problems with naming or fluency
	2 Moderate impairment, including comprehension difficulties or deficits in meaningful communication (semantic content)
	3 Severe impairment including nonsensical semantic content, word salad, muteness, or severely reduced comprehension
		Rate spoken/written/sign language abnormalities not attributable to dialect or stuttering.
		If necessary, test comprehension & naming nonverbally: have patient follow commands or point.
		Check if:
		  ○ intubated
		  ○ mute

Delirium Rating Scale-Revised-98 ©Trzepacz 1998 *(continued)*

6. Thought process abnormalities	0 Normal thought processes 1 Tangential or circumstantial 2 Associations loosely connected occasionally, but largely comprehensible 3 Associations loosely connected most of the time	Base on verbal or written output. If patient does not speak or write, don't rate this item. Check if: ◯ intubated ◯ mute
7. Motor agitation	0 No restlessness or agitation 1 Mild restlessness of gross motor movements or mild fidgetiness 2 Moderate motor agitation including dramatic movements of extremities, pacing, fidgeting, removing intravenous lines, etc. 3 Severe motor agitation, e.g., combativeness or need for restraints/seclusion	◯ Check here if restrained. Type:_____ OMIT: dyskinesia, tics, chorea Rate by direct observation or from other sources (family, staff, etc.)
8. Motor retardation	0 No slowness of voluntary movements 1 Mildly reduced frequency, spontaneity, or speed of motor movements, sufficient to interfere somewhat with the assessment 2 Moderately reduced frequency, spontaneity, or speed of motor movements, sufficient to interfere with participation in activities or self-care 3 Severe motor retardation with few spontaneous movements	◯ Check here if restrained. Type:_____ OMIT: drowsiness, sleep, retardation 2° to parkinsonian symptoms. Rate by direct observation or from other sources (family, staff, etc.).
9. Orientation	0 Oriented to person, place, time 1 Disoriented to place or time (>2 days; or wrong month; or wrong year), but not both 2 Disoriented to time & place 3 Disoriented to person (not recognizing familiar persons; may be intact even if the patient has naming difficulty but recognizes the person)	Date:_____ Place:_____ Person:_____ If can't speak, give visual or auditory multiple choice options. If hospitalized>3 weeks, allow wrong date up to 7 days instead of 2 days.
10. Attention *(e.g., months of year backwards; digit span)*	0 Alert & attentive 1 Mildly distractible or mild difficulty sustaining attention, but able to refocus with cueing. On formal testing, makes only minor errors & is not significantly slow in responses. 2 Moderate inattention with difficulty focusing & sustaining attention. On formal testing, makes numerous errors & requires prodding to focus or finish the task. 3 Severe difficulty focusing &/or sustaining attention, with many incorrect or incomplete responses, or inability to follow instructions. Distracted by noises/events.	Do not use writing as testing modality for patients with sensory deficits, who are intubated, or whose hand movements are constrained.
11. Short-term memory *Recall of 3 items presented either verbally or visually after a delay of 2–3 minutes*	0 Short-term memory intact 1 Recalls 2/3 items; may be able to recall third item after category cueing 2 Recalls 1/3 items; may be able to recall other items after category cueing 3 Recalls 0/3 items	# trials for registration of items:_____ Category cueing helped? ◯ yes ◯ no When formally tested, info must be registered adequately first before recall is tested. Distract patient during delay period & do not allow rehearsal.

Delirium Rating Scale-Revised-98 ©Trzepacz 1998 *(continued)*

12.
Long-term
memory
Recall of 3 items after 5 minutes (visual or verbal) or culturally or personally relevant info that can be corroborated
	0 No significant long-term memory deficits
	1 Recalls 2/3 items; &/or has minor difficulty recalling details of other long-term info
	2 Recalls 1/3 items; &/or has moderate difficulty recalling other long-term info
	3 Recalls 0/3 items; &/or has severe difficulty recalling other long-term info
		Category cueing helped?
		   ○ yes
		   ○ no
		When formally tested, registration of info must be adequate before testing recall. Distract patient during 5-minute delay & do not allow rehearsal.
		For general info questions, make allowances for mental retardation or limited education.

13. **Visuospatial** **ability** *(e.g., draw: intersecting pentagons, clock face)*	0 No impairment 1 Mild impairment such that overall design & most details or pieces are correct; &/or little difficulty navigating in his/her surroundings 2 Moderate impairment with distorted appreciation of overall design &/or several errors of details or pieces; &/or needing repeated redirection to keep from getting lost in a newer environment; trouble locating familiar objects in immediate environment 3 Severe impairment on formal testing; &/or repeated wandering or getting lost	○ Unable to use hands Assess informally: patient's difficulty navigating living areas or environment (e.g., getting lost). Assess formally: drawing or copying a design, arranging puzzle pieces, drawing a map & identifying major cities, etc. 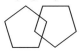

Severity Score *(items 1–13)*	(cutoff for delirium=15)

Use these optional diagnostic items for delirium diagnosis. Add to severity score to produce a total score.

14. **Temporal** **onset of** **symptoms**	0 No significant change from usual or long-standing baseline behavior 1 Gradual onset of symptoms, occurring over period of several weeks to a month 2 Acute change in behavior/personality occurring over days to a week 3 Abrupt change in behavior occurring over several hours to a day	○ Check if symptoms appeared on a background of other psychopathology. Rate acuteness of onset, not duration, of current episode's initial symptoms. Distinguish onset of delirium-related symptoms from other, preexisting psychiatric disorder(s).
15. **Fluctuation of** **symptom** **severity** *Usually cognition, affect, intensity of hallucinations, thought disorder, or language disturbance*	0 No symptom fluctuation 1 Symptom intensity fluctuates in severity over hours 2 Symptom intensity fluctuates in severity over minutes	○ Check here if symptoms only appear at night Rate waxing & waning of symptom(s) for a specific time interval. NOTE: Perceptual disturbances usually occur intermittently, but might become more intense when other symptoms fluctuate in severity.
16. **Physical** **disorder**	0 None present or active 1 Presence of any physical disorder that might affect mental state 2 Drug, infection, metabolic disorder, CNS lesion or other medical problem that specifically can be implicated in causing the altered behavior or mental state	Rate: Can a physiological or pharmacological problem be implicated in causing the symptoms? Implicated medical disorder(s): _____

Total Score *(items 1–16)*	(cutoff for delirium=18)

Source.   Adapted from Trzepacz PT, Mittal D, Torres R, et al.: "Validation of the Delirium Rating Scale-Revised-98: Comparison With the Delirium Rating Scale and the Cognitive Test for Delirium." *Journal of Neuropsychiatry and Clinical Neurosciences* 13:229–242, 2001. Used with permission.

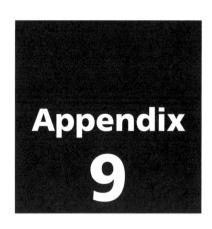

Appendix
9

The Confusion Assessment Method (CAM) Instrument

Wyszynski AA, Wyszynski B (eds.): *Manual of Psychiatric Care for the Medically Ill*. Washington, D.C., American Psychiatric Publishing, Inc., 2005

The Confusion Assessment Method (CAM) Instrument

Patient's name: _____ Date and time of assessment: _____

	Clinical Assessment	Yes	No	Uncertain
Need 1 & 2 for Dx — **Feature 1: Acute onset & fluctuating course** (assess for at least one →)	Is there evidence of an acute change in mental status from the patient's baseline? (Sources: family members, nurses)	Yes	No	Uncertain
	Does the abnormal behavior fluctuate during the day (come & go)?	Yes	No	Uncertain
	Does the abnormal behavior fluctuate in intensity (improve then worsen)?	Yes	No	Uncertain
Feature 2: Inattention	Does the patient have difficulty focusing attention (being easily distractible, have difficulty keeping track of what is being said?)	Yes: mild / marked	No	Uncertain
Need 3 or 4 for Dx — **Feature 3: Disorganized thinking**	Was the patient's thinking disorganized or incoherent, e.g., rambling or irrelevant conversation, unclear or illogical flow of ideas, switching from subject to subject?	Yes: mild / marked	No	Uncertain
Feature 4: Altered level of consciousness	Overall, how would you rate the patient's level of consciousness? [Vigilant: hyperalert, oversensitive to environmental stimuli, easily startled] [Lethargic: Drowsy, easily aroused. Stupor, coma: unarousable]	Vigilant / Lethargic / Stupor, coma	Alert	Uncertain
Other features of interest (no norms) — **Feature 5: Disorientation**	Was the patient disoriented at any time during the interview, e.g., thinking that they were in the wrong bed, or misjudging the time of day?	Yes: mild / marked	No	Uncertain
Feature 6: Memory impairment	Did the patient demonstrate any memory problems during the interview, e.g., inability to remember events in the hospital or difficulty remembering instructions?	Yes: mild / marked	No	Uncertain
Feature 7: Perceptual disturbances	Did the patient have any evidence of perceptual disturbances, i.e., illusions, hallucinations, or misinterpretations (e.g., thinking something was moving when it was not)?	Yes: mild / marked	No	Uncertain
Feature 8: Psychomotor activity	**Agitation:** At any time during the interview, did the patient have an unusually increased level of motor activity, such as restlessness, picking at bedclothes, tapping fingers, or making frequent sudden changes of position?	Yes: mild / marked	No	Uncertain
	Retardation: At any time during the interview, did the patient have an unusually decreased level of motor activity, such as sluggishness, staring into space, staying in one position for a long time, or moving very slowly?	Yes: mild / marked	No	Uncertain
Feature 9: Altered sleep-wake cycle	Did the patient have evidence of disturbance of the sleep-wake cycle, such as excessive daytime sleepiness with insomnia at night?	Yes: mild / marked	No	Uncertain

Source. Inouye SK, van Dyck CH, Alessi CA, et al.: "Clarifying Confusion: The Confusion Assessment Method: A New Method for Detection of Delirium." *Annals of Internal Medicine* 113:941–948, 1990. Adapted with permission of the *Annals of Internal Medicine*, American College of Physicians, Independence Mall West, Sixth Street at Race, Philadelphia, PA 19106–1572.

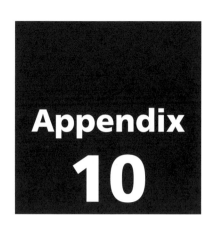

Appendix 10

Memorial Delirium Assessment Scale (MDAS)

Wyszynski AA, Wyszynski B (eds.): *Manual of Psychiatric Care for the Medically Ill.* Washington, D.C., American Psychiatric Publishing, Inc., 2005

Memorial Delirium Assessment Scale (MDAS) ©1996

Instructions: Rate the severity of the following symptoms of delirium based on current interaction with subject or assessment of his/her behavior or experience over past several hours (as indicated in each item).

Item 1 – Reduced level of consciousness (awareness): Rate the patient's current awareness of and interaction with the environment (interviewer, other people/objects in the room; for example, ask patients to describe their surroundings).

0: none	(patient is spontaneously fully aware of environment and interacts appropriately)
1: mild	(patient is unaware of some elements in the environment, or not spontaneously interacting appropriately with the interviewer; becomes fully aware and appropriately interactive when prodded strongly; interview is prolonged but not seriously disrupted)
2: moderate	(patient is unaware of some or all elements in the environment, or not spontaneously interacting with the interviewer; becomes incompletely aware and is appropriately interactive when prodded strongly; interview is prolonged but not seriously disrupted)
3: severe	(patient is unaware of all elements in the environment, with no spontaneous interaction or awareness of the interviewer, so that the interview is difficult-to-impossible, even with maximal prodding)

Item 2 – Disorientation: Rate current state by asking the following 10 orientation items: date, month, day, year, season, floor, name of hospital, city, state, and country.

0: none	(patient knows 9–10 items)
1: mild	(patient knows 7–8 items)
2: moderate	(patient knows 5–6 items)
3: severe	(patient knows no more than 4 items)

Item 3 – Short-term memory impairment: Rate current state by using repetition and delayed recall of 3 words [patient must immediately repeat and recall words 5 minutes later after an intervening task. Use alternate sets of 3 words for successive evaluations (for example, apple, table, tomorrow; sky, cigar, justice).]

0: none	(all 3 words repeated and recalled)
1: mild	(all 3 repeated, patient fails to recall 1)
2: moderate	(all 3 repeated, patient fails to recall 2–3)
3: severe	(patient fails to repeat 1 or more words)

Item 4 – Impaired digit span: Rate current performance by asking subject to repeat first 3, 4, then 5 digits forward and then 3, then 4 backward; continue to the next step only if patient succeeds at the previous one.

0: none	(patient can do at least 5 numbers forward and 4 backward)
1: mild	(patient can do at least 5 numbers forward and 3 backward)
2: moderate	(patient can do 4–5 numbers forward, cannot do 3 backward)
3: severe	(patient can do no more than 3 numbers forward)

Item 5 – Reduced ability to maintain and shift attention: As indicated during the interview by questions needing to be rephrased and/or repeated because patient's attention wanders, patient loses track, patient is distracted by outside stimuli or over-absorbed in a task.

0: none	(none of the above; patient maintains and shifts attention normally)
1: mild	(above attentional problems occur once or twice without prolonging the interview)
2: moderate	(above attentional problems occur often, prolonging the interview without seriously disrupting it)
3: severe	(above attentional problems occur constantly, disrupting and making the interview difficult-to-impossible)

Memorial Delirium Assessment Scale (MDAS) [©]1996 *(continued)*

Item 6 – Disorganized thinking: As indicated during the interview by rambling, irrelevant, or incoherent speech, or by tangential, circumstantial, or faulty reasoning. Ask patient a somewhat complex question (for example, "Describe your current medical condition").

0: none	(patient's speech is coherent and goal-directed)
1: mild	(patient's speech is slightly difficult to follow; responses to questions are slightly off target but not so much as to prolong the interview)
2: moderate	(disorganized thoughts or speech are clearly present, such that interview is prolonged but not disrupted)
3: severe	(examination is very difficult or impossible due to disorganized thinking or speech)

Item 7 – Perceptual disturbance: Misperceptions, illusions, hallucinations inferred from inappropriate behavior during the interview or admitted by subject, as well as those elicited from nurse/family/chart accounts of the past several hours or of the time since last examination.

0: none	(no misperceptions, illusions, or hallucinations)
1: mild	(misperceptions or illusions related to sleep, fleeting hallucinations on 1–2 occasions with inappropriate behavior)
2: moderate	(hallucinations or frequent illusions on several occasions with minimal inappropriate behavior that does not disrupt the interview)
3: severe	(frequent or intense illusions or hallucinations with persistent inappropriate behavior that disrupts the interview or interferes with medical care)

Item 8 – Delusions: Rate delusions inferred from inappropriate behavior during the interview or admitted by the patient, as well as delusions elicited from nurse/family/chart accounts of the past several hours or of the time since last examination.

0: none	(no evidence of misperceptions or delusions)
1: mild	(misperceptions or suspiciousness without clear delusional ideals or inappropriate behavior)
2: moderate	(delusions admitted by the patient or evidenced by his/her behavior that do not or only marginally disrupt the interview or interfere with medical care)
3: severe	(persistent and/or intense delusions resulting in inappropriate behavior that disrupts the interview or interferes with medical care)

Item 9 – Decreased or increased psychomotor activity: Rate activity over past several hours, as well as activity during interview, by circling (a) hypoactive, (b) hyperactive, or (c) elements of both present.

0: none	(normal psychomotor activity)
a b c 1: mild	(Hypoactivity is barely noticeable, expressed as slightly slowing of movement. Hyperactivity is barely noticeable or appears as simple restlessness.)
a b c 2: moderate	(Hypoactivity is undeniable, with marked reduction in number of movements or marked slowness of movement; subject rarely spontaneously moves or speaks. Hyperactivity is undeniable, subject moves almost constantly; in both cases, exam is prolonged as a consequence.)
a b c 3: severe	(Hypoactivity is severe; patient does not move or speak without prodding or is catatonic. Hyperactivity is severe; patient is constantly moving, overreacts to stimuli, requires surveillance and/or restraint; getting through the exam is difficult or impossible.)

Memorial Delirium Assessment Scale (MDAS) ©1996 *(continued)*

Item 10 – Sleep-wake cycle disturbance (disorder arousal): Rate patient's ability to either sleep or stay awake at the appropriate times. Utilize direct observation during the interview, as well as reports from nurse, family, patient, or charts describing sleep-wake cycle disturbance over the past several hours or of the time since last examination. Use observations of the previous night for morning evaluation only.

0: none	(at night, sleeps well; during the day, has no trouble staying awake)
1: mild	(mild deviation from appropriate sleepfulness and wakefulness states: at night, difficulty falling asleep or transient night awakenings, needs medication to sleep well; during the day, reports of drowsiness or, during the interview, is drowsy but can easily fully awaken him/herself)
2: moderate	(moderate deviation from appropriate sleepfulness and wakefulness states: at night, repeated and prolonged night awakening; during the day, reports of frequent and prolonged napping or, during the interview, can only be roused to complete wakefulness by strong stimuli)
3: severe	(severe deviations from appropriate sleepfulness and wakefulness states: at night, sleeplessness; during the day, patient spends most of the time sleeping or, during the interview, cannot be roused to full wakefulness by any stimuli)

Source.   Reprinted by permission of Elsevier Science from Breitbart W, Rosenfeld B, Roth A, et al.: "The Memorial Delirium Assessment Scale." *Journal of Pain and Symptom Management* 13:128–137, 1997. Copyright 1997 by the U.S. Cancer Pain Relief Committee.

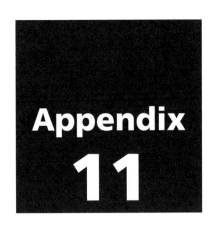

Risk Factors for
Torsades de Pointes

Wyszynski AA, Wyszynski B (eds.): *Manual of Psychiatric Care for the Medically Ill.* Washington, D.C., American Psychiatric Publishing, Inc., 2005

Risk Factors for Torsades de Pointes

CARDIAC CONDITIONS	Bradyarrhythmia Congenital long QT syndrome Congestive heart failure Coronary artery bypass grafting Heart block (sinoatrial or atrioventricular) Hypertension Ischemic heart disease Mitral valve prolapse Myocardial infarction Myocarditis Pacemaker malfunction
MEDICATIONS THAT PROLONG QT$_C$	
ANTIARRHYTHMICS	Group Ia (e.g., disopyramide, procainamide, quinidine) Group III (e.g., N-acetylprocainamide, amiodarone, sotalol)
PSYCHOTROPICS	Butyrophenones (especially droperidol>haloperidol) Phenothiazines (especially chlorpromazine, thioridazine) Tricyclic antidepressants (amitriptyline, desipramine, imipramine, nortriptyline) Ziprasidone
ANTIBIOTICS/ANTIVIRALS	e.g., amantadine, ampicillin, erythromycin, pentamidine, trimethoprim-sulfamethoxazole
VASODILATORS	e.g., bepridil, prenylamine
HYPOLIPIDEMICS	e.g, probucol
TOXIC/METABOLIC DISTURBANCE AND SYSTEMIC DISEASE	Electrolyte disturbances: hypocalcemia, hypokalemia, hypomagnesemia Hepatic dysfunction (e.g., alcohol abuse) Hypothyroidism Renal disease
CENTRAL NERVOUS SYSTEM INSULTS	e.g., subarachnoid hemorrhage, stroke

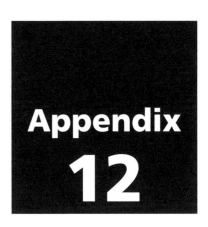

Guidelines for Adult Psychotropic Dosing in Renal Failure

Wyszynski AA, Wyszynski B (eds.): *Manual of Psychiatric Care for the Medically Ill.* Washington, D.C., American Psychiatric Publishing, Inc., 2005

Guidelines for Adult Psychotropic Dosing in Renal Failure

	Half-life (hours)		Adjustment of pre-ESRD dose: GFR (mL/min)		
	Normal	ESRD	>50	10–50	<10
ANTIDEPRESSANTS					
Bupropion (Wellbutrin)[a]	10–21	No data	NAN	NAN	NAN
Citalopram (Celexa)	5–10	32–70	NAN[b]		No data[b]
Escitalopram (Lexapro)	27–32	No data	NAN[b]		No data[b]
Fluoxetine (Prozac)	24–72[c]	Unchanged	NAN	NAN	NAN
Fluvoxamine (Luvox; antiobsessional SSRI)	12–15	Unchanged	NAN	NAN	NAN
Nefazodone (Serzone)	2–4	Unchanged	NAN	NAN	NAN
Paroxetine (Paxil)	10–16	30	NAN	**Decrease to 50%–75%**	**Decrease to 50%**
Sertraline (Zoloft)	24	No data	NAN	NAN	NAN
Venlafaxine (Effexor)	4	6–8	**Decrease to 75%**	**Decrease to 50%**	**Decrease to 50%**
TRICYCLIC ANTIDEPRESSANTS					
Amitriptyline (Elavil)	20–40	Unchanged	NAN	NAN	NAN
Clomipramine (Anafranil)	19–37	No data	No data	No data	No data
Desipramine (Norpramin)	18–26	No data	NAN	NAN	NAN
Doxepin (Sinequan)	8–25	10–30	NAN	NAN	NAN
Imipramine (Tofranil)	12–24	No data	NAN	NAN	NAN
Nortriptyline (Pamelor)	25–38	15–66	NAN	NAN	NAN
Protriptyline (Vivactil)	54–98	No data	NAN	NAN	NAN
ANXIOLYTICS AND BENZODIAZEPINES					
Alprazolam (Xanax)	9.5–19.0	Unchanged	NAN	NAN	NAN
Buspirone (BuSpar)	2–3	5.8	Use with caution (Bristol-Myers Squibb Co., November 2003).		
Chlordiazepoxide (Librium)	5–30	Unchanged	NAN	NAN	NAN
Clonazepam (Klonopin)	18–50	No data	NAN	NAN	NAN
Diazepam (Valium)	20–90	Unchanged	NAN	NAN	NAN
Lorazepam (Ativan)	5–10	32–70	NAN	NAN	NAN
Midazolam (Versed)	1.2–12.3	Unchanged	NAN	NAN	NAN
Oxazepam (Serax)	5–10	25–90	NAN	NAN	NAN
ANTICONVULSANTS AND MOOD STABILIZERS					
Carbamazepine (Tegretol)	25–65	Unchanged	NAN	NAN	NAN
Gabapentin[d] (Neurontin)	5–7	132	**400 mg tid**	**300 mg q12–24h**	**300 mg qod**
Lamotrigine (Lamictal)	25–30	Unchanged	NAN	NAN	NAN
Lithium[d]	14–28	40	NAN	**Decrease maintenance to 50%–75% of usual**	**Decrease maintenance to 25%–50% of usual**
Topiramate[e] (Topamax)	19–23	48–60	NAN	**Decrease to 50%**	**Decrease to 50%**
Valproic acid (Depakote)	6–15	Unchanged	NAN	NAN	NAN

Guidelines for Adult Psychotropic Dosing in Renal Failure *(continued)*

	Half-life (hours)		Adjustment of pre-ESRD dose: GFR (mL/min)		
	Normal	ESRD	>50	10–50	<10
ANTIPSYCHOTICS					
Aripiprazole (Abilify)	75–94	No data	NAN[b]		
Chlorpromazine (Thorazine)	11–42	Unchanged	NAN	NAN	NAN
Clozapine (Clozaril)	4–12	No data	No data	No data	No data
Haloperidol (Haldol)	10–19	No data	NAN	NAN	NAN
Olanzapine (Zyprexa)	21–54	No data	NAN[b]		
Quetiapine (Seroquel)	6	No data	NAN[b]		
Risperidone (Risperdal)	21–30	No data	**Initial dose: 0.5 mg bid; dosage increases ≤0.5 mg bid. Allow at least 1 week for increases above 1.5 mg bid.[b]**		
Ziprasidone (Geodon)	7 MTH	No data	**NAN, but avoid intramuscular form.[b]**		
ANTIPARKINSONIANS					
Amantadine (Symmetrel)	No data	Increases[b]	NAN	Decrease dose[b]	
Benztropine (Cogentin)	No data	No data	No data	No data	No data
Diphenhydramine (Benadryl)	3.4–9.3	No data	NAN	NAN	NAN
Propranolol (for akathisia)	2–6	1–6	NAN	NAN	NAN
Trihexyphenidyl (Artane)	No data	No data	No data	No data	No data
HYPNOTICS					
Estazolam (ProSom)	8–24	No data	NAN	NAN	NAN
Quazepam (Doral)	20–40	No data	No data	No data	No data
Temazepam (Restoril)	4–10	No data	NAN	NAN	NAN
Trazodone (Desyrel)	6–11	No data	NAN	No data	No data
Triazolam (Halcion)	2–4	Unchanged	NAN	NAN	NAN
Zaleplon (Sonata)	1–1.5	No data	NAN[b]		No data[b]
Zolpidem (Ambien)	1.5–4	No data	NAN[b]		

Note. **Boldface type** indicates adjustment for renal failure necessary. ESRD=end-stage renal disease; GFR=glomerular filtration rate; MTH=by mouth; NAN=no adjustment necessary; monitor patient for sensitivity to side effects; SSRI=selective serotonin reuptake inhibitor.
[a]Monitor electrolytes. The electrolyte imbalances of ESRD may predispose to seizures, which could potentiate lowering of the seizure threshold by bupropion.
[b]Manufacturer's information or recommendation.
[c]Half-life of active metabolite is 7–9 days.
[d]Renal route of excretion.
[e] When not used concomitantly with enzyme-inducing drugs, almost 90% eliminated directly through the kidneys. In the presence of enzyme inducers, about 30% of the drug is eliminated by hepatic biotransformation (see Asconape 2002, Chapter 4).
Source (except where indicated).   Adapted from Aronoff GR, Berns JS, Brier ME, et al.: *Drug Prescribing in Renal Failure: Dosing Guidelines for Adults,* 4th Edition. Philadelphia, PA, American College of Physicians, 1999.

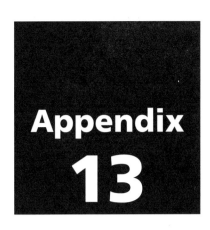

Appendix 13

Commonly Used Drugs With Sedative-Hypnotic Properties

Wyszynski AA, Wyszynski B (eds.): *Manual of Psychiatric Care for the Medically Ill.* Washington, D.C., American Psychiatric Publishing, Inc., 2005

Commonly Used Drugs With Sedative-Hypnotic Properties

Agent	Half-life in healthy people[a] (hours)	Suggested starting dose for medically ill[b] (mg)	Notes
Zaleplon (Sonata)	1–1.5	5	Pyrazolopyrimidine. No active metabolite.
Zolpidem (Ambien)	1.5–4	2.5	Imidazopyridine. No active metabolite.
Triazolam (Halcion)	2–5	AVOID	Ultra-short-acting benzodiazepine hypnotic. Although no active metabolite is an advantage, not a first choice in medically ill because of higher rates of reported amnesia, dissociative episodes.
Temazepam (Restoril)	8–12	7.5	Benzodiazepine. No active metabolite. Undergoes glucuronidation, not oxidation, so unaffected by parenchymal liver disease.
Estazolam (ProSom)	12–20	AVOID	Benzodiazepine. Minimal active metabolite. Poor choice for medically ill because of long half-life.
Oxazepam (Serax)	5–15	10	Benzodiazepine. No active metabolite. Undergoes glucuronidation, not oxidation, so unaffected by parenchymal liver disease.
Alprazolam (Xanax)	12–20	0.125	Benzodiazepine. Has active metabolite. Some reports of difficulty with withdrawal syndromes with alprazolam.
Lorazepam (Ativan)	10–20	0.25	Benzodiazepine. No active metabolite. Undergoes glucuronidation, not oxidation, so unaffected by parenchymal liver disease; often used synergistically with haloperidol to treat "sundowning" in elderly and delirious patients. Advantage of oral, intramuscular, and intravenous administration.
Clonazepam (Klonopin)	22–38	0.125	Benzodiazepine. Undergoes part of its metabolism via 3A4, then is acetylated. No active metabolite. Relatively unaffected by parenchymal liver disease. Available as orally disintegrating tablet.
Diazepam (Valium)	20–50	AVOID	Benzodiazepine; accumulation of active metabolite causes CNS depression, predisposes to falls.
Clorazepate (Tranxene)	60–100	AVOID	Benzodiazepine; accumulation of active metabolite causes CNS depression, predisposes to falls.
Quazepam (Doral)	50–200	AVOID	Benzodiazepine; accumulation of active metabolite causes CNS depression, predisposes to falls.
Flurazepam (Dalmane)	50–200	AVOID	Benzodiazepine; accumulation of active metabolite causes CNS depression, predisposes to falls.

Commonly Used Drugs With Sedative-Hypnotic Properties *(continued)*

Agent	Half-life in healthy people[a] (hours)	Suggested starting dose for medically ill[b] (mg)	Notes
Medications with sedative-hypnotic properties used to treat insomnia[a]			
Gabapentin (Neurontin)	5–7	100	Anticonvulsant. Off-label use is helpful for insomnia in some patients.[a] Renally metabolized and excreted. Unaffected by liver disease.
Haloperidol (Haldol)	10–19	0.25–0.5	Antipsychotic; particularly helpful in delirious or demented patients; disadvantage of EPS.
Quetiapine (Seroquel)	6[d]	25	Atypical antipsychotic; particularly helpful in delirious or demented patients; fewer EPS than haloperidol.
Olanzapine (Zyprexa)	21–54[d]	2.5	Atypical antipsychotic; particularly helpful in delirious or demented patients; fewer EPS than haloperidol.
Risperidone (Risperdal)	21–30[d]	0.25	Atypical antipsychotic; particularly helpful in delirious or demented patients; fewer EPS than haloperidol.
Diphenhydramine (Benadryl)	3.4–9.3	AVOID	Antihistamine; may cause or worsen confusional states due to anticholinergic properties.
Buspirone (BuSpar)	2–3	5	Nonbenzodiazepine anxiolytic. Occasionally effective for nocturnal agitation in elderly patients.
Trazodone (Desyrel)	6–11	AVOID	Cyclic antidepressant; risk of postural hypotension.

Note. CNS=central nervous system; EPS=extrapyramidal side effects.
[a]Data from Reite M, Ruddy J, Nagel K: *Evaluation and Management of Sleep Disorders,* 3rd Edition. Washington, DC, American Psychiatric Publishing, 2002. Used with permission.
[b]Based on the principle that the initial adult dose should be reduced by one-half to two-thirds for a medically fragile patient. Medications that are likely to induce adverse side effects are marked "AVOID."
[c]Data from Aronoff GR, Berns JS, Brier ME, et al.: *Drug Prescribing in Renal Failure: Dosing Guidelines for Adults,* 4th Edition. Philadelphia, PA, American College of Physicians, 1999.
[d]Data from manufacturer.

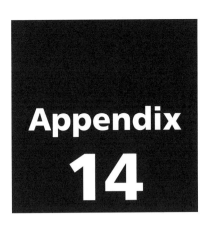

Electroconvulsive Therapy in Medical Illness: Practice Guidelines of the American Psychiatric Association

Wyszynski AA, Wyszynski B (eds.): *Manual of Psychiatric Care for the Medically Ill.* Washington, D.C., American Psychiatric Publishing, Inc., 2005

Electroconvulsive Therapy in Medical Illness: Practice Guidelines of the American Psychiatric Association (see also p. 127)

GENERAL RECOMMENDATIONS

1. There are no "absolute" medical contraindications to ECT.

2. In situations in which ECT is associated with an increased likelihood of serious morbidity or mortality, the decision to administer ECT should be based on the premise that the patient's psychiatric condition is grave and that ECT is the safest treatment available.

3. Careful medical evaluation of risk factors should be carried out prior to ECT, with specific attention to modifications in patient management or ECT technique that may diminish the level of risk.

4. Specific conditions that may be associated with substantially increased risk include the following:
   - Unstable or severe cardiovascular conditions such as recent myocardial infarction, unstable angina, poorly compensated congestive heart failure, and severe valvular cardiac disease
   - Aneurysm or vascular malformation that might be susceptive to rupture with increased blood pressure
   - Increased intracranial pressure, as may occur with some brain tumors or other space-occupying cerebral lesions
   - Recent cerebral infarction
   - Pulmonary conditions such as severe chronic obstructive pulmonary disease, asthma, or pneumonia
   - Patient status rated as a level 4 or 5 on the ASA [American Society of Anesthesiologists] physical status classification [indicating severe cardiopulmonary or other organ system disease]

RECOMMENDATIONS: CONCURRENT MEDICAL ILLNESS

Cardiovascular Disorders

1. Consultation with a physician who has expertise in the assessment and treatment of cardiovascular diseases should be considered if the pre-ECT evaluation suggests significantly increased cardiovascular risk. Conditions associated with increased risk include (but are not limited to) coronary artery disease, active angina, congestive heart failure, valvular heart disease, vascular aneurysms, uncontrolled hypertension, high-grade atrioventricular block, symptomatic ventricular arrhythmias, and supraventricular arrhythmias with uncontrolled ventricular rate. For such patients, the treatment team should request both an evaluation of the risk of the specific conditions and suggestions, if any, for clinical management as well as risk reduction. The team should not request "clearance" for ECT. Consultation should also be considered for patients with demand pacemakers or implanted defibrillators during ECT.

2. All patients referred for ECT who have clinically significant cardiovascular disease should have an ECG, a chest radiograph, and measurement of serum electrolytes as part of the pre-ECT evaluation. A functional cardiac imaging study should be considered if specifically indicated by history or physical examination.

3. Unstable cardiovascular disease should be stabilized as much as possible prior to ECT.

4. When standing and prn cardiovascular medications are likely to decrease the risks of ECT, they should be continued prior to and during the ECT course, including administration of scheduled doses between ECT on treatment days.

5. Additional short-acting cardiovascular medications, including anticholinergics, sympatholytics, nitrates, and other antihypertensive agents, should be considered at the time of ECT if there are specific reasons to believe they will decrease risks. Care should be taken to avoid iatrogenic hypotensive effects. Whenever possible, systemic lidocaine should be avoided until after the induced seizure.

Source.   Reprinted from *A Task Force Report of the American Psychiatric Association: The Practice of Electroconvulsive Therapy. Recommendations for Treatment, Training, and Privileging.* Washington, DC, American Psychiatric Association, 2001, pp. 30, 54. Used with permission.

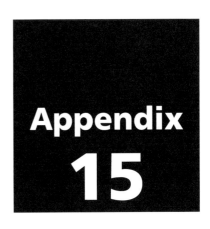

Appendix 15

Diagnosing Depression in the Medically Ill

Several problems complicate the accurate diagnosis of depression in medical patients:

- The effects of impaired cognitive functioning secondary to the medical illness itself
- Realistic threats to survival, making it difficult to distinguish psychological reactions to life-threatening illness from the onset of a depressive syndrome during recovery.
- The ambiguous significance of vegetative symptoms (e.g., weight loss, fatigue, weakness, anorexia) as discriminators of major depression versus the physical illness and its treatments
- Misassumptions that depressive states are "normal" in response to illness

Endicott (1984) advised substituting the following for the "classic" vegetative symptoms (e.g., change in appetite or weight, sleep disturbances, fatigue or loss of energy, diminished ability to think or concentrate, or indecisiveness):

- Tearfulness/depressed appearance
- Social withdrawal/decreased talkativeness
- Brooding/self-pity/pessimism
- Lack of reactivity to environmental events

Subsequently, Cavanaugh (1995) suggested modification of the diagnostic criteria for depression in the medically ill so that they included the following:

- Hopelessness, helplessness, not caring anymore
- Loss of interest, particularly in people
- Feeling bad about oneself, not the situation; feeling that illness is a punishment for wrongdoing
- Diminished ability to think or concentrate not easily explained by delirium, dementia, physical illness, or treatments
- Recurrent thoughts of death—not related to wishing to be dead to end physical suffering, but temporally related to affective and cognitive symptoms of depression
- Vegetative changes (significant weight, sleep, and/or appetite changes; anergia) not easily explained by physical illness, treatments, or hospital environment
- Psychomotor agitation or retardation not easily explained by delirium, dementia, physical illness, or treatments
- Assessment of the patient's sphere of functioning extended to include participation in medical care. The patient is not participating in medical care in spite of his or her ability to do so, is not progressing

Wyszynski AA, Wyszynski B (eds.): *Manual of Psychiatric Care for the Medically Ill*. Washington, D.C., American Psychiatric Publishing, Inc., 2005

despite an improved medical condition, and/or is functioning at a lower level than the medical condition warrants.

This same author and colleagues (Cavanaugh et al. 2001) later sought to determine whether major depressive disorder diagnosed according to DSM-IV criteria (American Psychiatric Association 1994) modified for the medically ill (as above) predicted in-hospital mortality better than major depressive disorder diagnosed according to inclusive DSM-IV criteria, and whether depression predicted mortality independent of severity of physical illness. Of 392 consecutive medical inpatients, 241 (mean age 49.9 years) were interviewed within the first 3 days of admission, and 151 were excluded from the study. A diagnosis of major depressive disorder based on criteria modified for patients with medical illness better predicted mortality than a diagnosis based on inclusive criteria. Severity of medical illness, a diagnosis of major depressive disorder based on modified criteria, and previous depression independently predicted in-hospital mortality in medical inpatients.

■ REFERENCES

American Psychiatric Association: Diagnostic and Statistical Manual of Mental Disorders, 4th Edition. Washington, DC, American Psychiatric Association, 1994

Cavanaugh S: Depression in the medically ill: critical issues in diagnostic assessment. Psychosomatics 36:48–59, 1995

Cavanaugh S, Furlanetto L, Creech S, et al: Medical illness, past depression, and present depression: a predictive triad for in hospital mortality. Am J Psychiatry 158:43–48, 2001

Endicott J: Measurement of depression in patients with cancer. Cancer 53:2243–2247, 1984

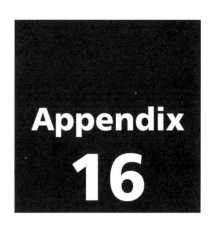

Screening Worksheet for Bipolar Spectrum Disorders

Wyszynski AA, Wyszynski B (eds.): *Manual of Psychiatric Care for the Medically Ill.* Washington, D.C., American Psychiatric Publishing, Inc., 2005

Screening Worksheet for Bipolar Spectrum Disorders

Patient's name: _____   **Date:** _____

	NOTES:
1. Has the patient ever been treated for depression? If so, ask about reactions, as in Question 6, while he/she was taking antidepressants.	
2. Was he/she ever given medication to control his/her mood? For "anxiety"? For "attention deficit disorder" (ADD)? If so, what type of medication?	
3. Has he/she ever seen a mental health professional?	
4. Is there a family history of: Bipolar disorder? Depression? Suicide? Substance abuse? ADD? Psychiatric hospitalizations?	
5. Have family members with such histories ever seen a mental health professional?	

6. Has there ever been a period of time when the patient was not his/her usual self and...	
a. felt so good or so hyper that other people thought he/she was not "normal," or so hyper that he/she got into trouble?	g. was so easily distracted by things that he/she had trouble concentrating or saying on track?
b. was so irritable that he/she shouted at people or started fights or arguments?	h. had much more energy than usual?
c. felt much more self-confident than usual?	i. was much more social or outgoing than usual?
d. got much less sleep than usual and found he/she didn't really miss it?	j. was much more interested in sex than usual?
e. was much more talkative or spoke faster than usual?	k. did things that were unusual for him/her or that other people might have thought were excessive, foolish, or risky?
f. thoughts raced through his/her mind and couldn't be slowed down?	l. spending money got the patient or his/her family into trouble?

NOTES:

7. If patient has experienced more than one symptom in #6, have the symptoms ever occurred during the same time period? Over what interval?	8. How much of a problem did the symptoms in #6 cause the patient? None Mild Moderate Severe

Source.   Questions in item #6 adapted from the Mood Disorder Questionnaire, with permission of the first author. From Hirschfeld RM, Williams JB, Spitzer RL, et al.: "Development and Validation of a Screening Instrument for Bipolar Spectrum Disorder: The Mood Disorder Questionnaire." *American Journal of Psychiatry* 157:1873–1875, 2000.

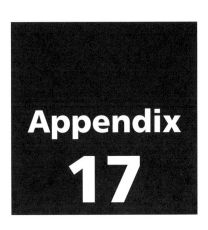

Appendix 17

Neuropsychiatric Effects of Electrolyte and Acid-Base Imbalance

Wyszynski AA, Wyszynski B (eds.): *Manual of Psychiatric Care for the Medically Ill.* Washington, D.C., American Psychiatric Publishing, Inc., 2005

Neuropsychiatric Effects of Electrolyte and Acid-Base Imbalance

Type	Causes	Symptoms	Comments
Hyponatremia	Diuretics, antidepressants, lithium, neuroleptics, excessive parenteral fluids, renal disease, syndrome of inappropriate secretion of antidiuretic hormone (SIADH), polydipsia, carbamazepine	Early: impaired taste, anorexia, fatigue, headache, muscle cramps, thirst, mild confusion Late: confusion (Na<115), delirium, convulsions	Mental symptoms are related to the serum sodium level and the rapidity of its fall. Insidious hyponatremia may be tolerated until Na<100. EEG: loss of alpha activity and irregular discharges of high-amplitude theta waves.
Hypernatremia	Febrile illness with dehydration, diarrhea, CNS lesions, hyperosmolar nonketotic coma, hyperalimentation, severe burns, sodium bicarbonate	Thirst, depression of consciousness (Na>160) Delirium, lethargy, stupor, coma	Mental symptoms are related to the serum sodium level and the rapidity of its rise. Insidious hypernatremia may be tolerated until Na>170. EEG: varying degrees of slow-wave activity, but may be normal.
Hypokalemia	Vomiting, diarrhea, diabetic ketoacidosis, laxative addiction, renal tubular acidosis, diuretics	Muscular weakness and cramps, lethargy, apathy, paresthesias, drowsiness, irritability, hyporeflexia	Symptoms appear with K<3 but vary with the acuteness of onset and the presence/absence of acidosis. ECG changes: T-wave depression, prominent U waves, arrhythmias; predisposes to torsades de pointes (TDP).
Hyperkalemia	Excessive intake of K supplementation or K-containing drugs, nonsteroidal anti-inflammatory agents, K-sparing diuretics, renal failure, trauma	Weakness, hyporeflexia, paresthesias, sensory perception deficits, delirium, cardiac arrhythmias	ECG changes: tall T waves, increased PR interval and QRS widening, fatal arrhythmias.
Hypocalcemia	Hypoparathyroidism, sepsis, renal failure, malabsorption syndrome, drugs (e.g., phenytoin)	Delirium, irritability, fatigue, weakness, depression, muscle cramps, tetany, seizures	Rate of onset may determine appearance of symptoms. Delirium is most likely when onset is acute. EEG: progressive slowing of background activity, as well as low-voltage, fast activity, sharp waves, and spikes. ECG changes: QT elongation; predisposes to TDP.
Hypercalcemia	Malignancy, hyperparathyroidism	Early: anorexia, nausea, vomiting, headache, difficulty walking Delirium (may be the presenting feature), lassitude, drowsiness, anxiety, depression, stupor, coma	Confusion tends to correlate with serum Ca levels. Hypercalcemia presents a life-threatening medical emergency. EEG: diffuse slowing of background activity interrupted by high-voltage bursts of delta waves.

Neuropsychiatric Effects of Electrolyte and Acid-Base Imbalance *(continued)*

Type	Causes	Symptoms	Comments
Hypomagnesemia	Starvation, malabsorption syndrome, chronic alcoholism, diuretics, severe diarrhea, aldosteronism, severe body fluid loss, diabetic acidosis, hyperthyroidism, acute intermittent porphyria	Depression, apathy, anxiety, weakness, tremor, fasciculations, irritability, tetany, seizures, delirium, hallucinations	Magnesium is essential for normal calcium and potassium metabolism. Deficits usually occur in association with other electrolyte abnormalities (e.g., hypocalcemia) and hypokalemia. May be asymptomatic in the absence of other electrolyte abnormalities. Predisposes to TDP.
Hypermagnesemia	Renal failure; magnesium-containing oral purgatives, antacids, or rectal enemas; adrenal insufficiency	Drowsiness, lethargy, weakness; eventual narcosis and coma	—
Hypophosphatemia	Diabetic ketoacidosis, acute and chronic alcoholism, severe burns, respiratory alkalosis, hyperalimentation, phosphate-binding antacids	Mild: weakness, malaise, anorexia, bone pain, joint stiffness, intention tremor. Severe: irritability, apprehension, muscular weakness, numbness, paresthesias, dysarthria, confusion, obtundation, seizures, coma	Hypophosphatemia is common, usually mild, and without consequence.
Hyperphosphatemia	—	Definite clinical manifestations have not been attributed to hyperphosphatemia.	—
Metabolic acidosis	Renal failure, diabetic ketoacidosis, lactic acidosis, intoxications (ammonium chloride, salicylate, methanol), starvation ketosis, alcoholic ketoacidosis, alkali loss (diarrhea, ureteroenterostomy)	Chronic: asymptomatic, or with fatigue and anorexia. Severe: hyperventilation, labored breathing (Kussmaul's respiration), progressive depression of consciousness, stupor, coma, convulsions	Defined as arterial blood pH<7.40. Primary respiratory acidosis: occurs with increased PCO_2. Primary metabolic acidosis: involves compensatory hyperventilation and decreased PCO_2. Symptoms usually difficult to separate from those of the underlying disorder. Depressed levels of consciousness tend to correlate with acidotic cerebrospinal fluid.
Metabolic alkalosis	Vomiting, chloride depletion (gastric drainage, diuretic therapy, post–hypercapnic alkalosis), hyperadrenocorticism, potassium depletion	Lethargy, confusion at pH>7.55. Other: irritability, neuromuscular hyperexcitability, muscle weakness, apathy, stupor. Coexisting hypocalcemia or cerebrovascular disease predisposes to disturbances of consciousness during alkalosis. Hypoventilation secondary to metabolic alkalosis reflects the compensatory need to retain CO_2 and can augment hypoxia and contribute to mental status symptoms.	Defined as arterial blood pH>7.40. Metabolic alkalosis is the acid-base disturbance most often encountered in the hospital setting. Primary respiratory alkalosis: occurs when CO_2 removal by the lungs exceeds its production in the body, with resulting hypocapnia; may be caused by hyperventilation, mechanical overventilation, pneumonia, or hepatic failure.

Note.   CNS=central nervous system; ECG=electrocardiogram; EEG=electroencephalogram; TDP=torsades de pointes.

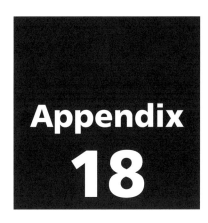

Worksheet for Monitoring Patients Receiving Atypical Antipsychotics

Source. All tables adapted from the recommendations in: American Diabetes Association, American Psychiatric Association, American Association of Clinical Endocrinologists, et al: "Consensus Development Conference on Antipsychotic Drugs and Obesity and Diabetes." *Journal of Clinical Psychiatry* 65:267–272, 2004.

Worksheet for Monitoring Patients Receiving Atypical Antipsychotics

Patient's name: _____   **Height:** _____

	Personal history		Family history	
Overweight (BMI 25.0–29.9)	❏ yes	❏ no	❏ yes	❏ no
Obesity (BMI≥30)	❏ yes	❏ no	❏ yes	❏ no
Diabetes mellitus FPG≥126	❏ yes	❏ no	❏ yes	❏ no
Pre–diabetes mellitus FPG 100–125	❏ yes	❏ no	❏ yes	❏ no
Dyslipidemia	❏ yes	❏ no	❏ yes	❏ no
Hypertension (BP>140/90)	❏ yes	❏ no	❏ yes	❏ no
Cardiovascular disease	❏ yes	❏ no	❏ yes	❏ no

BMI=Body Mass Index; FPG=fasting plasma glucose, in mg/dL; BP=blood pressure, in mm/Hg

Minimum monitoring interval[a]	Weight ❏ lbs ❏ Kg	Body Mass Index	Waist circumference (❏ in/❏ cm)	Blood pressure (mm/Hg)	Fasting plasma glucose (mg/dL)	Fasting lipid profile
Date: _____ Baseline						Chol:_____ HDL:_____ LDL:_____ TG:_____
	Maximum allowed weight gain (baseline + 5%) _____					
Date: _____ 4 weeks						
Date: _____ 8 weeks						
Date: _____ 12 weeks						Chol:_____ HDL:_____ LDL:_____ TG:_____
Date: _____ Month 6						
Date: _____ Month 9						
Date: _____ Year 1						[b] Chol:_____ HDL:_____ LDL:_____ TG:_____
After Year 1 ➡	q3 mo	q3 mo	q12 mo	q12 mo	q12 mo	q5 yr

[a]More frequent assessments may be indicated based on clinical status.

[b]Optional; original recommendations specify once every 5 years after week 12.

Table 1.   Atypical antidepressants and metabolic abnormalities

Risk for weight gain	Clozapine Olanzapine	>	Risperidone Quetiapine	>	Aripiprazole Ziprasidone
Risk for diabetes	Clozapine Olanzapine	>	Risperidone Quetiapine	>	Aripiprazole Ziprasidone
Risk for adverse lipid profile	Clozapine Olanzapine	>	Risperidone Quetiapine	>	Aripiprazole Ziprasidone

Note.   Aripiprazole and ziprasidone are newer drugs (approved 2001–2002) with limited long-term data.

Table 2.   Recommended management for the patient receiving atypical antipsychotics

Clinical problem	Recommended action
Weight gain>5% baseline	Switch to an agent that is weight-neutral
Worsening glycemia	Switch to an agent not associated with diabetes
Dyslipidemia	Switch to an agent that is weight-neutral
Preexisting diabetes	Collaboration with a diabetologist
Hyperglycemia (FSG≥300) Hypoglycemia (FSG≤60)	Immediate medical consultation, whether symptomatic or not
Diabetic ketoacidosis	Emergency medical care

Note.   FSG=fasting serum glucose.

Table 3.   Warning signs of diabetic ketoacidosis

Rapid onset of:	❏ Polyuria, polydipsia	❏ Dehydration
	❏ Weight loss	❏ Rapid respiration
	❏ Nausea, vomiting	❏ Clouding of sensorium

Table 4. Determining Body Mass Index (BMI)

BMI ➡	19	20	21	22	23	24	25	26	27	28	29	30	31	32	33	34	35
Interpretation ➡	Underweight: BMI<18.5 Normal: BMI=18.5–24.9						Overweight: BMI=25–29.9					Obesity: BMI≥30					
Height	Weight (in lbs)																
4'10" (58")	91	96	100	105	110	115	119	124	129	134	138	143	148	153	158	162	167
4'11" (59")	94	99	104	109	114	119	124	128	133	138	143	148	153	158	163	168	173
5' (60")	97	102	107	112	118	123	128	133	138	143	148	153	158	163	168	174	179
5'1" (61")	100	106	111	116	122	127	132	137	143	148	153	158	164	169	174	180	185
5'2" (62")	104	109	115	120	126	131	136	142	147	153	158	164	169	175	180	186	191
5'3" (63")	107	113	118	124	130	135	141	146	152	158	163	169	175	180	186	191	197
5'4" (64")	110	116	122	128	134	140	145	151	157	163	169	174	180	186	192	197	204
5'5" (65")	114	120	126	132	138	144	150	156	162	168	174	180	186	192	198	204	210
5'6" (66")	118	124	130	136	142	148	155	161	167	173	179	186	192	198	204	210	216
5'7" (67")	121	127	134	140	146	153	159	166	172	178	185	191	198	204	211	217	223
5'8" (68")	125	131	138	144	151	158	164	171	177	184	190	197	203	210	216	223	230
5'9" (69")	128	135	142	149	155	162	169	176	182	189	196	203	209	216	223	230	236
5'10" (70")	132	139	146	153	160	167	174	181	188	195	202	209	216	222	229	236	243
5'11" (71")	136	143	150	157	165	172	179	186	193	200	208	215	222	229	236	243	250
6' (72")	140	147	154	162	169	177	184	191	199	206	213	221	228	235	242	250	258
6'1" (73")	144	151	159	166	174	182	189	197	204	212	219	227	235	242	250	257	265
6'2" (74")	148	155	163	171	179	186	194	202	210	218	225	233	241	249	256	264	272
6'3" (75")	152	160	168	176	184	192	200	208	216	224	232	240	248	256	264	272	279
6'4" (76")	156	164	172	180	189	197	205	213	221	230	238	246	254	263	271	279	287

BMI=[(weight in pounds)/(height in inches)^2] × 703   ~OR~   (weight in kilograms)/(height in meters)^2

Source. http://www.cdc.gov/nccdphp/dnpa/bmi/bmi-adult-formula.htm. Accessed July 2004.

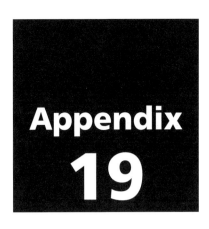

Case Vignettes and Study Guide

■ INTRODUCTION

Our aim in providing study questions for Chapters 2–7 is to place into clinical context certain medical issues of psychosomatic medicine. Rather than making the case write-ups comprehensive, we have intentionally simplified them for this purpose. We have purposely *avoided* modeling question-and-answer strategies based on the board examinations. Instead, the questions raise issues from the literature, and the reader is encouraged to evaluate them on the basis of his or her knowledge. The questions are not intended to resemble an examination; a question may have more than one correct answer. The questions may be used before, after, or as a companion to reading the text.

■ CHAPTER 2

Case Vignette: The Psychotic, Cirrhotic, Alcohol-Dependent Patient

Mr. Psychosis-and-Cirrhosis (P&C) is a 33-year-old man with chronic alcohol abuse and dependence who is well known to the hospital staff. He has frequently been brought to the emergency room acutely intoxicated after menacing passersby. He has had several admissions for hypothermia during the winter months and is marginally compliant with follow-up in the medical clinic for cirrhosis and hypertension. He has demonstrated the stigmata of liver disease for several years, including palmar erythema, spider nevi, and gynecomastia. Physical examination reveals that the liver is not enlarged. There is no psychiatric history other than several admissions for alcohol detoxification. He has never abused drugs.

You are asked to see him approximately 48 hours after admission to the emergency service for workup of hematemesis. Blood and urine tests on admission were negative for drugs or alcohol. He is awaiting transfer to the medical service, but there are no beds. He has been on npo status and has been receiving intravenous hydration. When the resident arrives, the patient is in Posey restraints because of agitation. He has already pulled out his lines twice.

On mental status examination, Mr. P&C appears frightened and his speech is slurred. He intermittently hallucinates, claiming he sees rats and spiders. He is convinced that the staff is trying to poison him. At times, he breaks into inappropriate laughter. He is often alert and then drowsy, and he is oriented for person but not for date or place. Concentration is severely impaired, and he is distractible. Short-term recall is impaired. Remote memory seems grossly intact. He will not cooperate with other aspects of cognitive testing.

Study Questions

(More than one choice may be correct for each question. Choose all that apply.)

Wyszynski AA, Wyszynski B (eds.): *Manual of Psychiatric Care for the Medically Ill.* Washington, D.C., American Psychiatric Publishing, Inc., 2005

1. As you listen to Mr. P&C's psychotic productions, you consider the differential diagnosis of his presentation. Which are true?

   a. The occurrence of vivid visual hallucinations in this setting is pathognomonic of delirium tremens (DTs).
   b. DTs, alcoholic hallucinosis, and hepatic encephalopathy are all considered alcohol withdrawal syndromes.
   c. Paranoid delusions usually precede hallucinations in alcoholic hallucinosis and are related to them thematically.
   d. Had Mr. P&C presented with amusing or playful hallucinations, it would have argued against DTs.
   e. None of the above.

2. You present Mr. P&C with a blank piece of paper and ask him to read what it says; he confabulates that there are instructions to "leave this house of hell." He tries to jump out of bed. What finding(s) would be unique to Wernicke's encephalopathy, as opposed to hepatic encephalopathy, DTs, alcoholic hallucinosis, or the neurological effects of chronic alcohol abuse?

   a. Peripheral neuropathy
   b. Tremor
   c. Sixth-nerve palsy
   d. Confabulation

3. You carefully review the chart. Physical exam: as above. Vital signs: P: 100, R: 22, BP: 160/100, Temp: 99.0. Labs: hematocrit 32, hemoglobin 11. WBC: 6,500 with normal differential. PT/PTT: mildly elevated. Arterial blood gas: pH 7.4, PCO_2 40, PO_2 90. Chemistries: BUN 35, creatinine 1.3, sodium 145, potassium 3.8; calcium, phosphorus, magnesium: normal. Blood alcohol level is zero. Blood and urine for toxicology are negative. AST, ALT, GGTP are mildly elevated. Total bilirubin is minimally elevated. Serum ammonia is pending. Which are true?

   a. The minimally abnormal liver chemistries argue against Wernicke's encephalopathy.
   b. The minimally abnormal liver chemistries argue against hepatic encephalopathy.
   c. Normal brain imaging studies, such as magnetic resonance imaging (MRI), would rule out a secondary psychiatric syndrome.
   d. A normal serum ammonia level would definitively rule out hepatic encephalopathy.
   e. The minimal changes in liver function tests are probably a sign of severe liver failure.

4. Unfortunately, you do not know when Mr. P&C had his last drink. All of the following are true regarding the association between the cessation of drinking and alcohol-associated syndromes *except...*

   a. The risk of DTs is *highest* within the first 24 hours of the last drink.
   b. The risk of alcohol withdrawal seizures is *highest* within the first 24 hours of cessation of drinking.
   c. Alcoholic hallucinosis often follows a prolonged drinking bout.
   d. The onset of hepatic encephalopathy occurs independently of the last drink.
   e. The onset of Wernicke's encephalopathy occurs independently of the last drink.

5. Mr. P&C is disoriented for time and place and has visual hallucinations, sleep-wake cycle disturbance, and psychomotor agitation. Which of the following is the *least* likely diagnosis?

   a. DTs
   b. Hepatic encephalopathy
   c. Alcoholic hallucinosis
   d. Wernicke's encephalopathy

6. Which of the alcohol-related disorders resembles schizophrenia, especially when its association with drinking is not apparent?

   a. DTs
   b. Hepatic encephalopathy
   c. Alcoholic hallucinosis
   d. Wernicke's encephalopathy
   e. Korsakoff's syndrome

7. You consider starting Mr. P&C on a detoxification regimen. Which is an appropriate statement?

   a. Chlordiazepoxide (Librium) would be the detoxification agent of choice for Mr. P&C.
   b. Even without a detoxification regimen, Mr. P&C is probably past the peak time for alcohol withdrawal seizures but still at risk for the occurrence of DTs.
   c. Both DTs and mild withdrawal symptoms resolve within 3–4 days, with or without treatment.
   d. It is contraindicated to begin an alcohol detoxification regimen with chlordiazepoxide at this point.

8. The medical student assigned to Mr. P&C asks you about whether "rum fits" are a form of epilepsy. You respond...

   a. They indicate an underlying seizure disorder that requires continued anticonvulsant prophylaxis.
   b. Patients with preexisting seizure disorders are at greatest risk for alcohol withdrawal seizures.
   c. They present most typically as complex partial seizures.
   d. They are usually self-limited.

9. You learn that the patient is too agitated to cooperate with MRI scan of the head. The nursing staff is pressing you to medicate this patient, pronto! The medical intern awaits your instructions. You respond...

   a. Avoid all medication and use restraints instead.
   b. Because the patient may be in withdrawal and can take nothing by mouth, administer intravenous diazepam (Valium), carefully titrating according to symptoms.
   c. Because the patient may be in withdrawal and can take nothing by mouth, administer intravenous lorazepam (Ativan), carefully titrating according to symptoms.
   d. Sedate the patient with low-dose chlorpromazine (Thorazine)

10. Which of the following are true regarding the pharmacokinetics in liver disease?

    a. Lithium metabolism and dosing remain unchanged in the setting of ascites.
    b. Medications that primarily undergo glucuronidation, rather than oxidation, are more likely to have prolonged half-lives in hepatic failure.
    c. All benzodiazepines undergo Phase I metabolism.
    d. Intramuscular and intravenous administration of drugs bypasses the first-pass metabolism.

11. The benzodiazepines that are safest to use in hepatic failure include the following (choose all that apply):

    a. Lorazepam (Ativan)
    b. Halazepam (Paxipam)
    c. Triazolam (Halcion)
    d. Temazepam (Restoril)

e. Oxazepam (Serax)
f. Alprazolam (Xanax)
g. Prazepam (Centrax)
h. Clorazepate (Tranxene)
i. Clonazepam (Klonopin)

12. Mr. P&C is given three intravenous doses of lorazepam 0.5 mg, which results in a mild reduction of his agitation. The MRI is still pending. Neurological examination shows diffuse hyperreflexia but no focal signs. He continues to hallucinate actively, talking to himself, fearful of taking anything by mouth because he believes it is "living poison of this satanic rite." Which of the following would be typical of a Wernicke's encephalopathic presentation?

    a. Apathetic, detached affect
    b. Psychomotor agitation
    c. History of a drinking binge
    d. Prominent paranoid delusions and auditory or visual hallucinations

13. The most important etiological factor in the development of Wernicke's encephalopathy is...

    a. Vitamin B_{12} deficiency.
    b. Thiamine deficiency.
    c. Folate deficiency.
    d. Alcohol intoxication.
    e. Ammonia load.

14. The medical student is confused about whether Mr. P&C's presentation is an example of "Korsakoff's psychosis." You respond that the term refers to the tendency of these patients to...

    a. Become delusional, with paranoid themes.
    b. Become delusional, with grandiose themes.
    c. Give false accounts of recent experiences.
    d. Resemble the very early visual hallucinatory stage of DTs.

15. All of the following would be true during the examination of a patient with Korsakoff's syndrome *except*...

    a. Concentration deficits evident on digit span testing are fewer than problems with procedural memory.
    b. Alertness is preserved.
    c. Four items are not recalled after 2 minutes.
    d. A catastrophic reaction (e.g., crying) often occurs in response to the memory deficits.
    e. Social behavior is preserved.

16. What additional findings characterize patients with Korsakoff's syndrome?

    a. An inability to learn simple ward routines (procedural memory)
    b. A distortion of the temporal sequence of events
    c. Memory for emotionally charged information consistently better than for neutral material
    d. Blandness of affect and placidity
    e. Deficits similar to those of senile dementia of the Alzheimer type

17. Mr. P&C's cerebrospinal fluid (CSF) examination is normal. Serum ammonia level is still pending because the lab lost the tube. The electroencephalogram (EEG) is read as containing "5- to 7-cps (Hz) theta waves interspersed with alpha rhythm." Mr. P&C appears sedated but is rousable and able to talk. Which of the following is true about this patient's EEG?

    a. It is a normal variant.
    b. It indicates subdural hematoma.
    c. It is an artifact of the lorazepam.
    d. It could indicate impending coma.
    e. It is specific as to etiology.

18. You are paged by a caseworker at the men's shelter, who knows Mr. P&C well and reports that he has been too sick to drink for more than 2 weeks. Mr. P&C has also been acting "peculiarly," with new onset of paranoid ideation. Given this information, the clinical picture, and the test results, which diagnosis is most likely?

    a. Hepatic encephalopathy
    b. DTs
    c. Subdural hematoma
    d. Alcoholic hallucinosis
    e. Wernicke's encephalopathy
    f. Korsakoff's psychosis

19. Precipitants of hepatic encephalopathy include…

    a. Benzodiazepines
    b. Gastrointestinal bleeding
    c. Chlorpromazine (Thorazine)
    d. Constipation
    e. All of the above

20. What is true concerning the neurological examination of patients with hepatic encephalopathy? (choose all that apply):

    a. Rigidity and hyperreflexia that fluctuate in parallel with the psychiatric symptoms are found.
    b. Sensory abnormalities predominate over motor abnormalities.
    c. Extrapyramidal features on motor exam are usually present.
    d. Once neurological signs become evident, there tends to be unremitting progression to coma.
    e. Psychiatric symptoms vary according to the etiology of the underlying liver pathology.

21. Which neurotransmitter has been implicated in the pathogenesis of hepatic encephalopathy?

    a. Serotonin
    b. Gamma-aminobutyric acid (GABA)
    c. Dopamine
    d. Acetylcholine

22. It is quite common to be asked to consult on cirrhotic, alcoholic patients like Mr. P&C when they either are ready for discharge from the medical service or are already ambulatory outpatients. Although these patients have no overt evidence of encephalopathy, they are likely to have neuropsychological deficits that will impair their psychosocial adjustment. This condition has been termed "minimal" encephalopathy. What are true statements about minimal encephalopathy?

    a. Verbal and performance skills (such as short-term visual memory and reaction times) suffer approximately equal decrements.
    b. Performance skills are more often impaired than verbal skills, which may be normal.
    c. There is close correlation between measurements of cerebral morphology on computed tomography (CT) or MRI scans and neuropsychological test performance of these patients.
    d. EEG abnormalities often identify patients with minimal encephalopathy.

Answers

1. e (pp. 29–32)
2. c (p. 36)
3. e (p. 33)
4. b (pp. 30–31)
5. c (pp. 38, 40)
6. c (pp. 38, 40)
7. b, d (pp. 29–32)
8. b, d (p. 30)
9. c (p. 32)
10. d (pp. 46–47)
11. a, d, e, i (p. 46)

12. a (pp. 35–36)
13. b (pp. 35–36)
14. c (pp. 35–36)
15. a, d (pp. 36–37)
16. b, d (pp. 36–37)
17. d (p. 34)
18. a (pp. 32–33)
19. e (p. 33)
20. a, c (pp. 34–35)
21. b (p. 33)
22. b (pp. 37–38)

■ CHAPTER 3

Case Vignette 1: The Patient With Coronary Artery Disease (CAD) and Depression

Mr. Depressed-CAD is a 68-year-old patient with one previous episode of major depression while in his 20s. He has a history of ischemic heart disease and coronary artery disease, and was admitted 1 week ago in congestive heart failure. Furosemide (Lasix) and nitroglycerin are his only medications. He is medically stable. Psychiatric consultation is requested to evaluate the patient for depression. Over the past 3 weeks, his family has noted progressive loss of interest in his usual activities, pervasive sadness, hopelessness, anergy, and tearfulness.

Study Questions

(More than one choice may be correct for each question. Choose all that apply.)

1. The staff taking care of Mr. Depressed-CAD is concerned because he has lost his appetite and does not want to eat. Which of the following are *least* helpful in diagnosing depression in *medically ill* patients?

   a. Vegetative symptoms
   b. Low self-esteem
   c. Guilt
   d. Autonomy of mood

2. Which of the following are true regarding major depression and cardiac morbidity?

   a. Depressed mood appears to predict long-term cardiac mortality following myocardial infarction (MI), *independently* of cardiac disease severity.
   b. Subsyndromal depressive symptoms also correlate with an increased risk of cardiovascular mortality.
   c. Untreated major depression is a risk factor for the development of coronary artery disease.
   d. Depressive illness tends to be overdiagnosed in patients with cardiac disease.

3. According to the recommendations of the International Consensus Group on Depression and Anxiety in General Medicine (2001), what is the preferred treatment for depression and comorbid cardiovascular disease?

   a. The selective serotonin reuptake inhibitors (SSRIs)
   b. The serotonin-norepinephrine reuptake inhibitor venlafaxine (Effexor)
   c. Bupropion (Wellbutrin)
   d. Mirtazapine (Remeron)
   e. Psychostimulants
   f. Electroconvulsive therapy (ECT)

4. SSRIs rarely produce adverse cardiovascular effects. When they do, it is most likely through their impact on…

   a. Cytochrome P450 2D6
   b. Cytochrome P450 3A4
   c. The His bundle
   d. Sodium currents
   e. Calcium channels

5. The patient's wife has heard that fluoxetine (Prozac), and similar medications, "makes people commit suicide." The patient hears this and wishes to take an SSRI, since it will "help me die sooner." The patient's suicidal ideation and lack of concentration have impaired his capacity for making decisions about his medical condition. His wife is his health care proxy and demands to know if treating his depression will improve his medical prognosis. How might you respond?

   a. There is substantial evidence for a relationship between depression and adverse clinical outcomes in cardiac patients.
   b. Treatment of depression in cardiovascular patients improves quality of life and has been shown to *reverse* disease progression.
   c. Treatment of depression in cardiovascular patients improves quality of life and has been shown to *arrest* disease progression.
   d. Treatment of depression in cardiovascular patients improves quality of life but does not appear to *affect* disease progression.

6. The patient has no appetite and stops eating. He states he doesn't have the energy to participate in cardiac rehabilitation. He asks you to leave him alone in peace to die. ECT is "out of the question," according to his wife, who is now willing to try a "quick" treatment to help his depression. Which of the following would be true about using psychostimulants at this point?

   a. They are not effective for depression accompanying medical conditions.
   b. They worsen anergia.
   c. Tolerance tends to develop early.
   d. Worsening anorexia secondary to stimulants like methylphenidate (Ritalin) is a frequent complication.
   e. They improve cognition in medically ill patients.

7. How would you advise the internist regarding psychostimulants for this patient?

   a. The abuse potential of psychostimulants appears to be low in medical patients.
   b. They are relatively contraindicated in elderly depressed patients.
   c. They must be used with caution in patients with congestive heart failure.
   d. Dextroamphetamine (Dexedrine) would be preferred to methylphenidate in a patient like this one.

8. Which of the following are correct statements about psychostimulants in the medical setting?

   a. Dosing should be on a three-times-a-day schedule, with meals.
   b. Failure to respond to the first few psychostimulant doses tends to predict nonresponse to higher doses.
   c. Provided that vital signs are not adversely affected, the medication should be increased until the patient has experienced some medication-related response.

9. The patient cannot tolerate methylphenidate because of jitteriness. He is still quite depressed. He and his family steadfastly refuse ECT. The medical resident has a good alliance with the patient's wife, who has begun to relent a bit in her stance on antidepressants. She has heard of Effexor (venlafaxine) and wants to know more about its appropriateness for her husband. What are treatment considerations for using this medication in patients with comorbid cardiovascular disease?

   a. In medically healthy patients, the incidence of treatment-emergent conduction abnormalities (including QTc prolongation) with venlafaxine does not differ from that with placebo.
   b. Venlafaxine does not appear to have adverse effects on the control of blood pressure for patients with preexisting hypertension.
   c. Venlafaxine's effect on blood pressure appears to be idiosyncratic, rather than dose related.
   d. No specific data on using venlafaxine in patients with recent history of MI or unstable heart disease exist at this time.

10. The patient's wife consents to a trial with an SSRI. Fluoxetine (Prozac) and sertraline (Zoloft) cause the patient headache and gastrointestinal upset and have to be discontinued. Paroxetine (Paxil) makes him too somnolent, even in reduced doses. Mr. Depressed-CAD continues to refuse ECT, stating that he would rather find a less painful way to commit suicide. What are some of the characteristics of bupropion (Wellbutrin) that you could discuss with the cardiologist?

   a. It does not significantly affect pulse rate in cardiovascular patients.
   b. It has been associated with a decline in supine blood pressure in a majority of cardiovascular patients.
   c. It inhibits ejection fraction in patients with left ventricular dysfunction.
   d. It does not significantly prolong cardiac conduction in patients with preexisting bundle branch block.

11. The resident is intrigued by this side effect profile and asks, "Where's the catch?" You respond...

   a. Bupropion has been found to exacerbate preexisting arrhythmias.
   b. It has been associated with inducing higher degrees of atrioventricular block in patients with preexisting bundle branch block.
   c. Patients with preexisting hypertension may experience hypertensive exacerbations secondary to bupropion.
   d. The main noncardiovascular adverse effect is central nervous system (CNS) depression.

12. The patient tolerates bupropion well, but his depression does not respond. Meanwhile, he receives a permanent ventricular demand pacemaker without incident. Subsequently, his wife

convinces him to try ECT. Three days before his first scheduled treatment, however, he experiences several episodes of shortness of breath, chest pain, and light-headedness. He is extremely apprehensive that he is having a heart attack and will die momentarily. Repeated 24-hour ambulatory Holter monitoring during the episodes reveals normal sinus rhythm with minimal rate changes, ranging between 70 and 80 beats per minute. Brief periods of paced rhythm show normal capture and sensing. Premature beats and tachyarrhythmias are absent. The patient becomes even more agitated and fearful, convinced that his pacemaker is "broken" and that the "electric shock" of ECT will further damage it; he withdraws consent for ECT "so I can die in peace." What are some of the management considerations at this point?

a. His symptoms are probably due to erratic functioning of the pacemaker.

b. He probably is having panic attacks.

c. He probably is having further arrhythmic events.

d. ECT is temporarily contraindicated in this setting.

13. ECT is deferred for the time being. The patient is given clonazepam (Klonopin) 0.5 mg orally, two times a day, with rapid resolution of his anxiety symptoms. His wife reports that he has "always been a 'hyper' guy" and that she has "learned to ignore it." What facts would be important regarding the relationship between emotional stress and potential episodes of myocardial ischemia?

a. Emotionally induced cardiac ischemia is often unaccompanied by pain.

b. Mental stress can cause transient episodes of left ventricular dysfunction.

c. As long as psychological stress does not increase heart rate to exertional levels, myocardial ischemia occurs infrequently.

d. None of the above.

14. The patient and his wife finally consent to treatment with ECT with the support of his family. Which of the following are *not* associated with ECT?

a. Hypertension

b. Hypotension

c. Transient tachycardia

d. Transient bradycardia

e. Heart block

Answers

1. a (p. 50)
2. a, b, c (pp. 49–50)
3. a (p. 51)
4. a (p. 55)
5. a, d (pp. 49–50)
6. e (pp. 57–58)
7. a, c (pp. 57–58)
8. c (pp. 57–58)
9. a, b, d (p. 56)
10. a, d (pp. 55–56)
11. c (pp. 55–56)
12. b (p. 51)
13. a, b (p. 50)
14. e (pp. 58–60)

Case Vignette 2: The Depressed, Post–Myocardial Infarction Patient

A cardiologist admits to the coronary care unit Mr. SadHeart, a 57-year-old diabetic man with pneumococcal pneumonia who sustained an inferior-wall myocardial infarction (MI) 3 weeks ago. Mr. SadHeart had been maintained on sertraline (Zoloft) 150 mg/day prior to admission for depression and insomnia before his MI, with good therapeutic effect. Two weeks after admission, the medical resident requests a psychiatric consultation to determine if sertraline should be started again, since it was not given on admission to the coronary care unit.

The patient is stable clinically with no evidence at present of arrhythmias, congestive heart failure, or angina. Medications include the β-blocker atenolol, aspirin, penicillin, and digoxin. The electrocardiogram (ECG) shows changes consistent with inferior-wall MI, and a rate-corrected QT interval (QTc) of 400 milliseconds (440 ms is the upper limit of normal). Resting pulse is 80 and regular. Supine blood pressure is 140/90. Standing blood pressure is 120/88.

Past psychiatric history is notable for depression with no response to fluoxetine (Prozac), paroxetine (Paxil), and bupropion (Wellbutrin).

Study Questions

(More than one choice may be correct for each question. Choose all that apply.)

1. Mr. SadHeart has lost the will to live. He states that God is punishing him for all the wrongs he has committed in his life. He admits to pervasively low mood that is unresponsive to events, such as seeing pictures of his new grandson. He is always criticizing himself. Although he expresses no active suicidal intent, he hopes that

"nature will take its course" and states that it would "serve him right" to die from his illness. So far, Mr. SadHeart has been compliant with his medical regimen. There are no psychotic symptoms. He is cognitively intact except for diminished concentration. Although he has no appetite, his wife successfully encourages him to eat low-salt food that she brings from home. Assuming that he refuses ECT, what advice would you give the house staff about reinstituting sertraline?

a. Tell the resident that sertraline has been shown to be safely prescribed in post-MI patients.

b. Discuss how in post-MI patients sertraline has a high incidence of sinus tachycardia, even in the absence of orthostatic hypotension, and could potentially increase myocardial oxygen demand.

c. Explain that sertraline may have negative inotropic effects on the heart.

d. Caution that sertraline has been associated with aggravating preexisting ventricular irritability and heart block.

2. The decision is made to restart sertraline because of Mr. SadHeart's previous therapeutic response and the exacerbation of his depression when it was stopped. The cardiologist agrees to monitor the patient closely. All of the following are true about the research on sertraline administered post-MI *except...*

a. Treatment with sertraline was initiated an average of 14 days following acute MI and found to be safe.

b. Post-MI sertraline was shown to be safe even in alcohol-dependent patients.

c. Compared with placebo, sertraline had no statistically significant effects on mean left ventricular ejection fraction.

d. The safety of sertraline in the early post-MI period (before 2 weeks) remains unclear.

e. It is uncertain whether the findings on sertraline are generalizable to other SSRIs.

3. What are *false* statements about the following alternatives to sertraline for patients with cardiovascular disease?

a. Mirtazapine (Remeron) has a favorable cardiac profile.

b. Nefazodone (Serzone) does not appear to affect the ECG but is a second-line agent in medically ill patients for other reasons.

c. Trazodone's cardiac profile at higher doses makes it useful for depressed post-MI patients who need a combined antidepressant-hypnotic effect.

d. Tricyclic antidepressants are problematic because of their effect on blood pressure, but they spare conduction, making them useful for patients with heart block.

e. The most common effect of MAOIs on blood pressure is orthostatic hypotension.

4. Mr. SadHeart develops persecutory ideation and psychomotor agitation. He endlessly complains about the overhead lighting in his room, stating that people are "outlined" in "the red light of Satan." He is otherwise medically stable and has had no changes in his vital signs or medication regimen. Serum digoxin level, electrolytes, and thyroid function tests are normal. His neurological exam and brain MRI are normal. The house staff inquires about transfer to psychiatry for recurrent depression, since he is medically cleared. Which of the following considerations are true?

a. The mental status changes are consistent with serotonin syndrome.

b. The mental status changes could be attributable to digoxin.

c. Partial complex status epilepticus should be evaluated with extended video-EEG monitoring.

d. Major depression with psychotic features is the most reasonable diagnosis at this point.

5. Which of the following psychiatric symptoms occur at *therapeutic* digoxin levels?

a. Delirium
b. Hallucinations
c. Depression
d. All of the above
e. None of the above

6. Which of the following is/are *most* characteristic of digoxin toxicity?

a. Mania
b. Auditory disturbances
c. Visual distortions
d. Paranoid delusions

7. Mr. SadHeart's sertraline is stopped and antipsychotic treatment initiated. All of the following are true about Mr. SadHeart's management with antipsychotics *except...*

a. Early in treatment, he is at risk for orthostatic hypotension with risperidone (Risperdal).
b. Haloperidol would be unlikely to worsen his baseline orthostatic changes.
c. He would be at heightened risk of antipsychotic-induced arrhythmias if he had a history of alcohol dependence.
d. The probability of producing significant antipsychotic-induced ECG changes is dose related, rather than medication specific.

8. Which of the following atypical antipsychotics are most likely to induce the "acquired" prolonged QT syndrome?

a. Risperidone (Risperdal)
b. Ziprasidone (Geodon)
c. Quetiapine (Seroquel)
d. Olanzapine (Zyprexa)
e. None of the above

9. Which of the following are potential problems with *both* conventional and atypical antipsychotics in cardiovascular patients?

a. Alpha-1-adrenergic blockade
b. Prolongation of baseline QTc interval
c. Prolongation of PR interval
d. Drug-induced hyperglycemia

10. Alpha-1-adrenergic blockade results in all of the following clinical problems *except*...

a. Orthostatic hypotension
b. Susceptibility to anginal episodes in vulnerable patients due to increased cardiac workload stemming from drops in blood pressure
c. Palpitations due to prolonged cardiac conduction time
d. Increased rate of injury from falls secondary to dizziness

11. The atypical antipsychotic that has been found to run the greatest overall risk of cardiotoxicity is...

a. Clozapine (Clozaril)
b. Risperidone (Risperdal)
c. Ziprasidone (Geodon)
d. Quetiapine (Seroquel)
e. Olanzapine (Zyprexa)

12. The conventional antipsychotic that has been found to run the greatest overall risk of cardiotoxicity is...

a. Thiothixene (Navane)

b. Chlorpromazine (Thorazine)
c. Thioridazine (Mellaril)
d. None of the above

13. What is "acquired" in acquired long QT syndrome?

a. Prolonged depolarization of the heart
b. Prolonged repolarization of the heart
c. Structural damage to the His bundle
d. Vulnerability to arrhythmias

14. Factors that have *not* been associated with an increased risk of torsades de pointes include...

a. Mitral valve prolapse
b. CNS insult, such as subarachnoid hemorrhage
c. Male gender
d. Hypertension
e. Hepatic dysfunction

15. In general, a QTc of 440 ms is considered the average upper limit of normal. The *maximum* QTc interval that should prompt a change in treatment is...

a. 400 ms
b. 440 ms
c. 500 ms
d. 540 ms

Answers

1. a (pp. 53–54)
2. a, b (pp. 53–55)
3. c, d (pp. 56–58)
4. b (p. 52)
5. d (p. 52)
6. c (p. 52)
7. d (pp. 60–61)
8. b (p. 61)
9. a, b, d (pp. 60–62)
10. c (p. 60)
11. a (p. 62)
12. c (p. 61)
13. b, d (p. 61)
14. c (p. 305)
15. c (p. 61)

Case Vignette 3: The Bipolar, Diabetic Patient With Hypertension

Ms. Bipolar-Diabetic (BD) is a 45-year-old insulin-dependent woman with a history of juvenile-onset diabetes, panic disorder, and mitral valve prolapse.

She has been maintained for the past 6 months on paroxetine (Paxil) 30 mg/day for panic disorder with complete resolution of panic symptoms. (Clonazepam [Klonopin] was not effective.) She runs a successful retail business, but over the past month she has begun to behave inappropriately with customers. She puns repeatedly in verbal interactions with them, making conversation impossible. At times Ms. BD has given merchandise away, much to the chagrin of her partner. Her bookkeeper notes large expenditures of cash. The patient feels little need for sleep, is distractible, and demonstrates euphoric mood. She has become convinced that she is Mary Magdalene and hears the voices of Jesus and Moses. She acknowledges feeling extremely anxious and has been taking lorazepam (Ativan) 2 mg bid prn for anxiety (approximately double the dose prescribed by her internist). Family history is notable for bipolar affective illness in her father and paternal uncle.

She is admitted to the psychiatry service. The mental status examination reveals an attractive but unkempt woman, heavily made up, with lipstick smeared haphazardly. Speech is pressured, with flight of ideas. Affect is silly. Mood is euphoric. She denies suicidal ideation. Thought content is notable for grandiose delusions of being the Mother of God. She responds to voices telling her to sing hymns and praise the Lord. She denies hallucinations in other modalities. She is alert and fully oriented, and higher cognitive functions are intact except for difficulty concentrating.

Ms. BD's pulse is 80. Standing and supine blood pressures are 160/100. The physical exam is remarkable for mitral valve click. Holter monitoring shows frequent atrial premature beats. ECG reveals a QTc interval of 400 milliseconds (upper limit of normal is 440 ms). Echocardiography confirms the diagnosis of mitral valve prolapse. However, there was no mitral regurgitation. Levels of fasting blood sugar and glycated hemoglobin (HbA1c) reveal diabetes under good control. Lipid profile is unremarkable. Thyroid function, serum B_{12} levels, sedimentation rate, antinuclear antibodies, and MRI scan of the brain are all normal.

Study Questions

(More than one choice may be correct for each question. Choose all that apply.)

1. Which of the following factors most likely account for the patient's mental status abnormalities?

   a. Lorazepam (Ativan)
   b. Paroxetine (Paxil)
   c. Frequent atrial premature beats
   d. Hypertension
   e. Diabetes mellitus

2. Which two (2) of the following atypical antipsychotics are associated with the highest risk for exacerbating or precipitating hyperglycemia?

   a. Clozapine (Clozaril)
   b. Risperidone (Risperdal)
   c. Ziprasidone (Geodon)
   d. Quetiapine (Seroquel)
   e. Olanzapine (Zyprexa)
   f. Aripiprazole (Abilify)

3. Which two (2) of the following atypical antipsychotics are associated with the most weight gain?

   a. Clozapine (Clozaril)
   b. Risperidone (Risperdal)
   c. Ziprasidone (Geodon)
   d. Quetiapine (Seroquel)
   e. Olanzapine (Zyprexa)
   f. Aripiprazole (Abilify)

4. Which two (2) of the following atypical antipsychotics are associated with the greatest likelihood of worsening lipid profiles?

   a. Clozapine (Clozaril)
   b. Risperidone (Risperdal)
   c. Ziprasidone (Geodon)
   d. Quetiapine (Seroquel)
   e. Olanzapine (Zyprexa)
   f. Aripiprazole (Abilify)

5. Which two (2) of the following atypical antipsychotics are associated with the least weight gain, pose the least risk for hyperglycemia, and are least likely to worsen lipid profiles?

   a. Clozapine (Clozaril)
   b. Risperidone (Risperdal)
   c. Ziprasidone (Geodon)
   d. Quetiapine (Seroquel)
   e. Olanzapine (Zyprexa)
   f. Aripiprazole (Abilify)

6. A consensus statement that has been issued by the American Diabetes Association and American Psychiatric Association has recommended which of the following strategies for monitoring patients receiving antipsychotic pharmacotherapy? Obtain...

   a. Weight and height for body mass index calculation at baseline, and then every 6 months for the duration of treatment.
   b. Waist circumference at baseline, then annually for the duration of treatment.

c. Blood pressure at baseline, after the first 12 weeks, and then annually for the duration of treatment.

d. Fasting plasma glucose at baseline and then monthly for the first year of treatment.

e. Fasting lipid profile at baseline, after the first 12 weeks, and then every 5 years for the duration of treatment.

7. A decision is made to start risperidone (Risperdal). All of the following symptoms would indicate the possible development of diabetic ketoacidosis, *except...*

a. Polydipsia
b. Weight gain due to water retention
c. Hyperphagia
d. Slow rate of respiration
e. Clouding of sensorium
f. Polyuria
g. Dehydration

8. Paroxetine and lorazepam are discontinued. Ms. BD's ECG shows persistent runs of atrial premature contractions. Workup of her elevated blood pressure is consistent with essential hypertension. Her manic symptoms continue. The most common effect(s) of therapeutic lithium levels on the ECG of a healthy patient is/are...

a. Tachycardia
b. ST-segment changes
c. Increased QT intervals
d. T-wave flattening or inversion

9. Which of the following are true about lithium and the heart?

a. Lithium most frequently inhibits conduction within the ventricles.
b. Lithium predisposes sinus node dysfunction and first-degree atrioventricular block.
c. Alternatives to lithium should be used in congestive heart failure.
d. Any history of myocardial infarction is a contraindication to lithium.

10. Which mood stabilizer alternative to lithium is the most potentially cardiotoxic?

a. Carbamazepine (Tegretol)
b. Divalproex sodium (Depakote)
c. Lamotrigine (Lamictal)
d. Topiramate (Topamax)

Answers

1. b (p. 63)
2. a, e (p. 62)
3. a, e (p. 62)
4. a, e (p. 62)
5. c, f (p. 62)
6. b, c, e (p. 62)
7. b, c, d (p. 62)
8. d (p. 63)
9. a (pp. 63–65)
10. a (p. 65)

■ CHAPTER 4

Case Vignette: The Bipolar, Lithium-Dependent Patient in Renal Failure

A colleague refers to you Ms. Manic-Uremic (MU), a 65-year-old woman with a 20-year history of bipolar affective illness treated with lithium. On three occasions in the past, the patient had been noncompliant with lithium, become psychotic, and required hospitalization. On several occasions, the patient refused lithium and attempts were made to substitute carbamazepine (Tegretol), divalproex sodium (Depakote), or lamotrigine (Lamictal). These medications had been unsuccessful and resulted in psychiatric hospitalization. Most recently, she responded to a brief course of risperidone (Risperdal) 3 mg twice daily for psychotic ideation.

Ms. MU had been stable for 2 years on lithium carbonate 1,200–1,500 mg/day, with blood levels ranging from 0.9 to 1.2 mEq/L. Several months ago, her internist noted progressively increasing creatinine. Lithium and oxazepam (Serax; given for anxiety) were discontinued, her fluid was restricted, and the patient was placed on a 40-g low-protein diet. It was hoped that dialysis could be avoided. The patient presents you with a printout of the most recent chemistries, remarkable for serum creatinine of 5.5 and a blood urea nitrogen (BUN) of 62. She has no other medical problems and is taking no other medications.

Up to this time, the patient had been maintained on her usual doses of lithium. She has never been lithium toxic, clinically or by blood level, although polyuria has persisted for years. The family reports that recently she has begun wandering around the neighborhood, talking inappropriately to strangers and unable to find her way back home. They say she is "giddy," unable to sleep, and has been making peculiar dietary indiscretions in respect to her strictly kosher diet (such as bringing home a ham sandwich from one of her walks).

On mental status examination, the patient reports feeling "great emotionally" but "tired all the time" and shows pressured speech. Her affect is silly and her mood euphoric. She occasionally breaks into song, singing "Oh, What a Beautiful Morning," ostensibly because she "feels happy." There is no suicidal ideation. Thought process is circumstantial. Thought content is notable for lack of bizarre or idiosyncratic ideation, but the patient insists, in an engaging, likable way, on trying to interview you about your personal life. There are no delusions or hallucinations. She is alert and oriented to person and place but misreports the date by about 3 days. Recent memory, concentration, and recall are mildly impaired. Remote memory is intact. Proverbs and similarities are interpreted humorously but concretely. There is little insight, but she suspects "this visit has something to do with the lithium, which I haven't needed for years and will never take again."

Study Questions

(More than one choice may be correct for each question. Choose all that apply.)

1. You decide to request additional medical workup to evaluate possible etiologies for her mental status change. Assuming that MRI of the head, thyroid function tests, and serum B$_{12}$ and folate levels are normal, what do you consider next?

   a. Ms. MU's mental status is fairly typical of the early changes of chronic renal failure.
   b. Characteristic EEG changes for Ms. MU would include generalized synchronous paroxysmal spike and wave complexes.
   c. Ms. MU's blood urea nitrogen (BUN) at the time of evaluation would more closely predict neuropsychiatric disturbance than would the rate of its change.
   d. Ms. MU's rate of change of BUN would more closely predict neuropsychiatric disturbance than would the BUN value itself.
   e. The EEG changes that would occur in uremic encephalopathy are nonspecific with regard to etiology.

2. Uremia is most likely to produce mental status changes resembling...

   a. Mania
   b. Depression
   c. Anxiety
   d. Schizophreniform psychosis

3. Ms. MU will probably require psychotropic medications. What are true statements regarding medications in the setting of renal failure?

   a. The absorption of some medications by the small bowel increases in renal failure.

   b. Hepatic metabolism of most psychotropic drugs is unchanged by renal failure.
   c. The complications of ascites and edema require the use of lower doses of water-soluble or protein-bound medications.
   d. Dialysis almost completely removes hydrophilic medications (i.e., lithium and gabapentin), but not lipophilic medications.

4. It is important to understand plasma protein binding in order to prescribe medications in renal failure safely. All of the following are true *except*...

   a. Most psychotropics have high protein-binding affinity.
   b. Lithium is not bound to protein.
   c. Hepatic metabolism of medications remains unchanged in renal failure.
   d. The protein binding of drugs by albumin decreases during renal failure.

5. Which of the following are true?

   a. As a rule, the higher the protein-binding activity of a drug, the more dialyzable it is.
   b. The majority of psychotropics are protein-bound and therefore dialyzable.
   c. Albumin is the protein that is exclusively responsible for binding psychotropics.
   d. None of the above.

6. Many clinicians recommend that doses of psychotropics be reduced in renal failure by a factor of approximately...

   a. One-fourth
   b. One-third
   c. One-half
   d. Two-thirds

7. Doses of lipophilic psychotropic medications should be reduced in renal failure because of...

   a. Diminished renal clearance
   b. Heightened sensitivity to side effects
   c. Impairments of cytochrome P450 metabolism
   d. Increased likelihood of toxicity

8. The family corroborate that Ms. MU has never been lithium toxic, but state that she did complain for many years of urinating a lot. Her husband wants to know if the lithium had anything to do with his wife developing kidney disease. To date, she has refused kidney biopsy. You formulate your response, taking into consideration that...

a. Reports of histopathological damage secondary to lithium have been infrequent, considering the widespread use of lithium.
b. A very small group of patients may develop irreversible lithium-induced renal insufficiency.
c. When renal damage occurs, it usually is in the form of glomerulonephritis.
d. When renal damage occurs, it usually is accompanied by proteinuria.

9. Which of the following risk factors appear to be associated with lithium-induced renal impairment?

a. Lithium intoxication (more frequent episodes associated with greater risk)
b. Lithium plasma levels at or above 1.0 mEq/L associated with greater risk
c. Increasing age
d. Number of manic episodes

10. The patient's son wants to know if her "frequent urinating" (polyuria) had anything to do with his mother developing renal failure. Before answering him, you consider that lithium-induced polyuria…

a. Usually requires that lithium be discontinued
b. Is a consequence of diminished sensitivity of the collecting tubule to antidiuretic hormone (ADH)
c. Is usually considered reversible and without histopathological changes
d. Is often accompanied by proteinuria

11. What statements are true regarding lithium-induced nephrogenic diabetes insipidus (NDI)?

a. Lithium accumulates in collecting tubule cells, blocking ADH.
b. Lithium histologically alters collecting tubule cells, impairing their concentrating ability.
c. Lithium-induced NDI is usually temporary, but it is irreversible in a minority of patients.
d. If the patient is rechallenged with lithium, NDI is likely to recur but is no longer treatable.

12. It is agreed that restarting lithium is the treatment of choice for Ms. MU, given the manic recurrence and history of nonresponse to other mood stabilizers. Ms. MU's casual singing blossoms into the delusion that she is Ethel Merman. To the family's chagrin, she serenades the neighborhood nightly after the 11:00 news. The exhausted family and her nephrologist agree that an antipsychotic medication would be helpful. The clearance of which of the following antipsychotics is most reduced (by 60%) in patients with renal disease?

a. Risperidone (Risperdal)
b. Olanzapine (Zyprexa)
c. Quetiapine (Seroquel)
d. Ziprasidone (Geodon)
e. Haloperidol (Haldol)

13. The vulnerability of end-stage renal disease (ESRD) patients to electrolyte shifts may heighten the risk of developing fatal arrhythmias on which one of the following medications in particular?

a. Risperidone (Risperdal)
b. Olanzapine (Zyprexa)
c. Quetiapine (Seroquel)
d. Ziprasidone (Geodon)
e. Haloperidol (Haldol)

14. Which one of the following medications is most likely to aggravate diabetes mellitus, a common comorbidity for many ESRD patients?

a. Risperidone (Risperdal)
b. Olanzapine (Zyprexa)
c. Quetiapine (Seroquel)
d. Ziprasidone (Geodon)
e. Haloperidol (Haldol)

15. The family are unanimously in favor of the decision to start lithium, because they fear another psychiatric hospitalization for the patient without it. She agrees to comply. The nephrologist gives medical clearance to begin lithium and the family sign informed consent. If her usual lithium requirement has been 1,200 mg/day, how should her dosage be adjusted in the setting of renal failure?

a. If glomerular filtration rate (GFR) is greater than 50 mL/minute, her daily dosage should remain 1,200 mg.
b. If GFR is 30 mL/minute, her daily dosage should be 600–900 mg.
c. If GFR is approximately 10 mL/minute, she cannot receive any lithium and it should be discontinued.
d. Patients should not receive lithium at all if they are in chronic renal failure.

16. Over the next 8 months, Ms. MU's psychosis resolves and she becomes euthymic. However, her

creatinine clearance continues to decline and she becomes essentially anuric. The decision is made to begin hemodialysis, which the patient accepts with surprising aplomb. She will be dialyzed three times a week. How should her psychiatric management proceed?

    a. Since lithium is completely dialyzed, it should be administered daily in the mornings at reduced doses.

    b. She should receive a single oral dose only after each dialysis treatment.

    c. Because she is virtually anuric, she is at risk for fluctuating lithium levels between dialysis sessions.

    d. Lithium could be administered in the dialysate if she were undergoing peritoneal dialysis.

17. In her second week of dialysis, the patient is compliant with lithium maintenance, and she arrives to see you soon after her Monday dialysis. She appears disoriented and drowsy and complains of headache. According to her husband, this also occurred last week. Her husband reports that her last dose of lithium was on Friday afternoon after dialysis. She has received no lithium today. The patient is too sleepy to cooperate with your interview. Her lithium medication management has remained unchanged. What are the *most likely* diagnostic considerations at this point?

    a. Lithium toxicity
    b. Subdural hematoma
    c. Dialysis dementia
    d. Dialysis disequilibrium syndrome

18. As you consider dialysis dementia, the trace element that appears to be most consistently implicated is…

    a. Aluminum
    b. Cobalt
    c. Manganese
    d. Magnesium
    e. Iron

19. Ms. MU is medically and psychiatrically stabilized, but she becomes depressed and feels exhausted every morning on awakening. She speaks of the stressors of dialysis during her psychotherapy sessions. Which of the following are true?

    a. Hemodialysis requires a commitment of several hours per treatment, three times a week.

    b. ESRD patients must learn to substitute a vegetarian type of diet that emphasizes fruits and vegetables, with fluid restrictions.

    c. Uremia produces depression-like symptoms.

    d. Body image problems are more common with hemodialysis (because of the necessity of a shunt) than with peritoneal dialysis.

    e. Different treatment modalities (hemodialysis, continuous ambulatory peritoneal dialysis, transplantation) tend to show fairly consistent outcomes on measures of quality of life.

20. All of the following are complications of ESRD *except*…

    a. Insomnia
    b. Sleep apnea
    c. Restless legs syndrome
    d. Narcolepsy

21. Ms. MU feels hopeless, with guilty ruminations that she has "done this to myself." Pharmacological intervention becomes necessary. According to the manufacturer, which of the following antidepressants require dose reduction in the setting of renal disease?

    a. Bupropion (Wellbutrin, Zyban)
    b. Fluoxetine (Prozac)
    c. Sertraline (Zoloft)
    d. Paroxetine (Paxil)
    e. Venlafaxine (Effexor)

22. You learn that the nephrologist has decided to add recombinant erythropoietin. Which of the following would you expect to see as a consequence?

    a. Anergia
    b. Decline in sexual functioning
    c. Worsened depression
    d. Enhanced psychological well-being

23. What potential side effect(s) of bupropion (Wellbutrin) is/are most likely to be exacerbated by ESRD?

    a. Seizures
    b. Hypotension
    c. Delirium
    d. Hypertension
    e. Restlessness

24. The decision is made to use citalopram (Celexa) for Ms. MU. What would be the main concern about using this medication in a patient on dialysis?

a. Interaction with lithium
b. Interaction with analgesics
c. Interaction with warfarin (Coumadin)
d. Increased sensitivity to electrolyte imbalances

25. Ms. MU's anxiety increases during the dialysis runs. Which of the following is true of lorazepam (Ativan) in the setting of renal failure?

a. Doses should be halved for every 10-point reduction of GFR.
b. It is preferred because of its short half-life.
c. It is preferred because of its lack of active metabolites.
d. It is dialyzable.

26. What is true about the half-life of lorazepam in ESRD?

a. It is unchanged as long as hepatic metabolism remains intact.
b. It is shortened.
c. It exceeds the half-life of clonazepam (Klonopin) in healthy patients.
d. In ESRD, it is the only benzodiazepine that maintains its inactive metabolites.

27. What is true about the use of buspirone (BuSpar) in ESRD?

a. It is the anxiolytic of choice because of its side effect profile.
b. It is the anxiolytic of choice because of its pharmacokinetic profile.
c. Hepatic or renal function produces increased plasma levels and a lengthened half-life of buspirone.
d. It should be used with caution in patients with ESRD.

28. All of the following are likely to be true of sexual functioning of ESRD patients *except...*

a. Libido is relatively spared.
b. Orgasmic capacity is relatively spared.
c. There is a high prevalence of physiologically based impotence in male dialysands.
d. There is decreased testosterone and spermatogenesis in males.
e. There is decreased orgasmic capacity for dialysands of both genders.

29. Ms. MU wants to terminate dialysis so that "I can die in peace." Which of the following study findings about decisions to terminate long-term dialysis are *false?*

a. Suicide rate estimates in dialysis patients are higher than those in the general population or in patients with other chronic illnesses.
b. Patients who choose treatment withdrawal are a fairly homogeneous group of depressed individuals who actively want to die.
c. Rational treatment withdrawal is motivated specifically by the wish to die.
d. Patients who are maintained on dialysis because they are not candidates for renal transplantation are considered to be terminally ill.
e. Most completed suicides among terminally ill patients occur in the setting of clinical depression or impaired judgment.

Answers

1. d, e (pp. 69–70)
2. b (p. 69)
3. b, d (p. 71)
4. c (p. 71)
5. d (p. 71)
6. b (p. 71)
7. b (p. 71)
8. a, b, c (pp. 74–75)
9. a, b, c (p. 75)
10. b, c (p. 75)
11. a, c (p. 75)
12. a (p. 73)
13. d (pp. 73–74)
14. b (pp. 61–62, 73)
15. a, b (pp. 76–77)
16. b, d (pp. 76–77)
17. d (p. 77)
18. a (p. 70)
19. a, c (pp. 78–79)
20. d (p. 79)
21. d, e (p. 72)
22. d (p. 79)
23. a (p. 72)
24. c (p. 72)
25. c (pp. 72–73)
26. c (p. 72)
27. c, d (pp. 72–73)
28. a, b (pp. 79)
29. b, c (pp. 82)

■ CHAPTER 5

Case Vignette: The Anxious, Depressed Asthmatic Patient

Ms. Anxious Asthmatic (AA) is a 50-year-old woman with a 5-year history of asthma who is referred by her pulmonologist for evaluation. She feels that she is no longer coping as well as she used to. She lacks energy, is easily tearful, feels demoralized about her asthma, and "can't seem to snap out of it." She wakes up at 3:00 every morning, has diminished appetite (but no weight loss), and finds mornings "intolerable." She acknowledges transient suicidal ideation. Her boss suggested that she take some time off because she has become forgetful and has difficulty concentrating.

Ms. AA has been experiencing repeated exacerbations of asthma requiring intermittent adjustments in her medications (primarily salmeterol and fluticasone [Advair]). She has intermittently been on steroids in the past. She states that her medication dose is adjusted "according to how I feel." Most recently, her blood gases have been normal.

Ms. AA has been hospitalized three times for exacerbations of asthma. Her pulmonologist confirms that there were no medical or neurological sequelae. There are no other medical problems. She did not have asthma as a child.

The patient has been experiencing a very stressful time in the past 6 months. Her son has been having problems with cocaine addiction but recently signed himself into a drug treatment center. Her husband, while quite supportive, is in danger of being laid off due to budget cuts. She works as the manager of a popular restaurant. Although she enjoys her work, she finds it unpredictable and often stressful. Although not a smoker herself, she is exposed to secondhand smoke at work.

There is no past personal or family psychiatric history. There is no alcohol or substance abuse.

Mental status examination reveals an attractive middle-aged woman, well-groomed and fashionably dressed. Her speech is low in volume, slow in rate. Thought process is goal directed, coherent, and logical. Her affect is sad, and mood is depressed. She reports passive suicidal ideation. Thought content reveals no delusions or bizarre ideation. There are no hallucinations. She is alert and oriented to person, time, place, and situation. She scores 27 on the Mini-Mental State Examination, with difficulty in concentration and recall.

Study Questions

(More than one choice may be correct for each question. Choose all that apply.)

1. During your initial interview with her, Ms. AA briefly acknowledges that she nearly died from the acute exacerbation several years ago. Which of the following are true about the potential impact of anxiety on Ms. AA's illness?

   a. Emotional factors are as potent as allergic factors in precipitating asthmatic attacks.
   b. The mortality rate for asthma is relatively high.
   c. Anxiety, but not depression, influences dyspnea.
   d. Both anxiety and depression influence dyspnea.

2. Ms. AA and her pulmonologist have struggled for years to distinguish symptoms of anxiety from exacerbations of her respiratory disorder. For example, "asthma attacks" have been elicited in the doctor's office merely by suggesting that she will experience one. Her physician feels that sometimes her asthma medications may have been inappropriately increased to medicate anxiety-related dyspnea rather than asthma, making the patient even more agitated and uncomfortable. Your help is requested in this dilemma. What are important factors?

   a. The rate of anxiety disorders in asthmatic patients approximates that in the general population.
   b. The induction of an "asthmatic attack" by suggestion points strongly to a component of conversion disorder, which has a higher incidence in asthmatic patients than in the general population.
   c. After medication side effects are corrected for, the evidence argues against asthmatic patients having any greater biological diathesis for anxiety disorders than the general population.
   d. None of the above.

3. You try to determine during your interview with the patient what elicits the feelings of "breathlessness." Which of the following are true about subjective and objectively measured dyspnea?

   a. There is a predictable relationship between the perception of breathlessness and a given forced expiratory volume in 1 second.
   b. The occurrence of depression may complicate the perception of dyspnea.
   c. The consensus across studies shows that patients with greater dyspnea have more impaired pulmonary function tests than those with fewer dyspneic complaints.
   d. None of the above.

4. The patient reports that there are days when she can "barely function" in her domestic and professional duties because everything makes her feel dyspneic. Which of the following are valid considerations?

   a. Ms. AA's level of functional disability would be expected to correlate more closely with her *subjective perception* of dyspnea than with her objective pulmonary function test results.
   b. Ms. AA's level of functional disability would be expected to correlate more closely with her *objective* pulmonary function test results than with her subjective perception of dyspnea.
   c. When complaints of dyspnea disproportionately exceed objective measures of respiratory disease, they most likely indicate malingering.
   d. None of the above.

5. It becomes clear from your interview that the patient suffers from generalized anxiety. In considering anxiolytics, what statements are true about respiratory depression and benzodiazepines?

   a. Benzodiazepines reduce the ventilatory response to hypoxia.
   b. Benzodiazepines depress respiration primarily by causing muscle relaxation.
   c. Benzodiazepines cause respiratory depression mainly by reducing the ability to clear secretions.
   d. The respiratory depressant effects of benzodiazepines can be partially bypassed by administering low-flow oxygen.
   e. Benzodiazepines reduce the ventilatory response to hypercapnia.

6. The benzodiazpine of choice for the treatment of acute anxiety in the setting of asthma or chronic obstructive pulmonary disease (COPD) is low-dose…

   a. Diazepam (Valium)
   b. Alprazolam (Xanax)
   c. Lorazepam (Ativan)
   d. Temazepam (Restoril)
   e. Clonazepam (Klonopin)

7. The medication(s) appropriate for the treatment of chronic anxiety in the setting of asthma or COPD include…

   a. Propranolol (Inderal)
   b. Diphenhydramine (Benadryl) or hydroxyzine (Vistaril, Atarax)
   c. Low-dose lorazepam (Ativan)
   d. Buspirone (BuSpar)
   e. SSRIs
   f. Atypical antipsychotics

8. The patient is quite distraught because of her cognitive problems, and fears she is developing "Alzheimer's disease." She reports difficulties with concentration and recall. Which of the following statements is/are true?

   a. Hypoxia will be reliably accompanied by acute changes in mental status.
   b. The rate of change in level of oxygen saturation (PO_2) is the measure that most closely correlates with the occurrence of acute psychiatric symptoms.
   c. The level of oxygen saturation (PO_2) is the measure that most closely correlates with the occurrence of acute psychiatric symptoms.
   d. The degree of hypoxemia is not reliably congruent with the extent of lung disease.

9. What statements may be true concerning cognitive difficulties in someone like Ms. AA?

   a. Assessing her level of alertness would give an accurate estimate of the degree of hypoxemia.
   b. Perceptual learning and problem solving tend to be preserved even in the setting of moderate hypoxemia (PaO_2 50–59 mm Hg).
   c. Mild hypoxemia produces cognitive changes, such as problems in abstraction.
   d. None of the above.

10. Carbon dioxide retention most closely resembles…

    a. Amphetamine psychosis
    b. Panic disorder
    c. Barbiturate intoxication
    d. Mania

11. The patient's blood gases worsen. Workup reveals the beginnings of COPD, which includes two distinct processes, namely…(choose two)

    a. Asthma
    b. Emphysema
    c. Chronic bronchitis
    d. Bronchiectasis

12. How does COPD compare to asthma?

    a. The clinical course typically deteriorates in COPD, but not asthma.

    b. Both develop from an inflammatory process in the airways and distal airspaces.

    c. Oxidative stress is thought to produce the inflammation of COPD, but not asthma.

    d. Asthma is more associated with the effects of smoking than COPD.

    e. Cough productive of secretions typifies both conditions.

13. In COPD, the onset of morning headaches often signals…

    a. Major depressive disorder

    b. Neurological complications, such as subdural hematoma

    c. Carbon dioxide retention

    d. Hypoxia

14. The patient decides to take a leave of absence from her job because of her worsening pulmonary condition. She becomes more depressed, experiencing transient suicidal ideation, and awakens breathless in the middle of the night. She feels chronically fatigued and has lost interest in her usual activities. She is very afraid of becoming disabled and a burden to her family. The family are frightened by her deterioration. All of the following are true concerning the treatment of depression in asthmatic and COPD patients *except*…

    a. Monoamine oxidase inhibitors should be avoided.

    b. Theophylline is contraindicated during a course of ECT.

    c. SSRIs remain the primary treatment for depression in pulmonary disease.

    d. Any medication with anticholinergic effects may promote drying of bronchial secretions, making them easier to clear.

15. Which of the following are true statements about sleep and respiratory changes?

    a. There is a decrease in respiratory function during sleep, even in individuals without respiratory disease.

    b. Sleep typically improves respiratory function in COPD and asthmatic patients.

    c. Circadian changes in airway caliber, with mild nocturnal bronchoconstriction, occur in asthmatic patients but not in healthy, nonasthmatic subjects.

    d. Rapid eye movement (REM) sleep is associated with the greatest ventilatory changes.

16. Which of the following are the most common causes of the chronic fatigue and lethargy that occur in COPD patients?

    a. Reduced REM

    b. Decreased arousals

    c. Sleep-related hypoxemia

    d. Sleep-related hypercapnia

    e. Sleep apnea

17. Which of the following are true statements about asthma?

    a. Asthma tends to destabilize and worsen at night.

    b. Asthma tends to destabilize and worsen upon awakening.

    c. Nocturnal asthmatic attacks are usually triggered by underlying anxiety disorders.

    d. Nocturnal asthmatic attacks are usually triggered by an increase in airway inflammation and bronchial reactivity.

18. What factors increase the likelihood of an adverse outcome with benzodiazepines?

    a. More advanced pulmonary disease

    b. The presence of hypercapnia

    c. The use of zolpidem (Ambien)

    d. The use of zaleplon (Sonata)

    e. All of the above

19. Which of the following are true about the management of insomnia in COPD patients?

    a. The majority of COPD patients should have baseline sleep studies.

    b. The occurrence of cardiopulmonary failure in a COPD patient should prompt sleep studies.

    c. The occurrence of systemic hypertension in a COPD patient should prompt sleep studies.

    d. None of the above.

20. All of the following are treatment strategies for sleep apnea syndrome *except*…

    a. Weight reduction

    b. Modest amounts of bedtime alcohol in patients without substance use histories

    c. Assumption of the supine (face-up) position when sleeping

    d. Nasal continuous positive airway pressure (CPAP) during sleep

21. Monitor COPD patients who are being treated with hypnotics for all *except*...

    a. Confusion
    b. Morning somnolence
    c. Morning headache
    d. Increased dyspnea
    e. Decreased mucus secretion

Answers

1. a, d (p. 86)
2. d (pp. 86, 89)
3. b (p. 88)
4. a (p. 88)
5. a (p. 89)
6. c (p. 89)
7. d, e, f (pp. 89–90)
8. b, d (p. 88)
9. c (p. 88)
10. c (p. 88)
11. b, c (p. 87)
12. a, c (p. 87)
13. c (p. 87)
14. d (pp. 91–92)
15. a, d (p. 93)
16. a, c, d (p. 93)
17. a, d (p. 93)
18. a, b (p. 93)
19. b, c (p. 96)
20. b, c (p. 96)
21. e (p. 95)

■ CHAPTER 6

Case Vignette: The Patient With Gastrointestinal (GI) and Psychiatric Symptoms

Ms. Distraught-Abdominal-Pain (DAP) is a 39-year-old businesswoman with a long history of GI symptoms, which have recently worsened as her job has become more stressful. Her work is a source of almost constant irritation, and a change in company owners has led to unpredictable challenges to her authority. She feels that her boss undermines her well-organized, smoothly running department and that things have become "chaotic." Ms. DAP is able to function well at her job, but she experiences bouts of abdominal pain accompanied by frequent, mucusy loose stools. The pain is relieved by defecation. It does not awaken her from sleep, but she often notices transient pins and needles in her fingers and toes when it happens. Ms. DAP also complains of urinary frequency, although she has never had a urinary tract infection. The patient has not lost weight nor had a change in appetite. She is afraid that she might have pancreatic cancer like her mother, who died about 20 years ago at the age of 40. Her internist refers the patient to you for evaluation.

Past medical history is otherwise unremarkable. She is taking no medications. The patient denies recent changes in weight or appetite, hopelessness, anhedonia, or persistent depressed mood. She has never been suicidal.

Past psychiatric history is notable for chronic anxiety, tension, intermittent abdominal uneasiness with stress, jumpiness, and irritability for as long as the patient can remember. As a small child, she was afraid of leaving home to go to school, but she has never had any formal psychiatric treatment. Her former internist prescribed alprazolam (Xanax) intermittently in the past for anxiety. There is no history of drug or alcohol dependence. Family psychiatric history is reportedly negative.

Mental status exam reveals an attractive, meticulously groomed woman, obviously tense. Speech is goal directed, coherent, and logical. Affect shows full range; mood is anxious, but appropriate to expressed thought. Thought content shows no delusions or hallucinations. She denies suicidal ideation. The patient is preoccupied with concerns about her health and job, but there are no obsessions or compulsions. She is alert and fully oriented. Cognitive functions are entirely intact.

Study Questions

(More than one choice may be correct for each question. Choose all that apply.)

1. Ms. DAP reiterates that she is terrified that her symptoms are those of pancreatic cancer and that she will die like her mother. She remembers that her mother had been quite depressed and anxious before the cancer was finally diagnosed, "and then it was too late." Which of the following are true of pancreatic cancer?

    a. It has a bleak 5-year survival rate of <1%.
    b. It is decreasing in incidence.
    c. Psychiatric problems occur *without* systemic symptoms.
    d. Psychiatric symptoms are usually in the context of delirium.

2. When psychiatric syndromes occur with pancreatic cancer...

    a. Schizophreniform psychosis is the most frequent.
    b. The symptoms are usually affective.
    c. They are no more common than those occur-

ring with other GI neoplasms.

  d. None of the above.

3. Risk factors for pancreatic cancer include all of the followings *except*…

  a. Advanced age
  b. Female gender
  c. Excessive coffee consumption
  d. Diabetes mellitus
  e. Heavy tobacco use

4. When jaundice does not occur as an obvious warning signal, the initial complaints and findings of pancreatic cancer include…

  a. Fatigue
  b. Weight loss
  c. Anorexia
  d. Vague, intermittent epigastric pain
  e. Anemia

5. Although not relevant to Ms. DAP, acute intermittent porphyria is in the differential diagnosis of abdominal pain and psychiatric symptoms. The most common presentation of acute intermittent porphyria is…

  a. Depression in the setting of painful diarrhea
  b. Delirium in the setting of intense abdominal pain
  c. Psychosis in the setting of bowel obstruction
  d. Anxiety in the setting of jaundice

6. Acute intermittent porphyria may be confused with psychiatric syndromes because…

  a. Attacks may be precipitated by premenstrual hormonal changes.
  b. Attacks may be precipitated by alcohol.
  c. Attacks may first occur during or shortly after pregnancy.
  d. Attacks may be precipitated by low-calorie diets.
  e. None of the above.

7. When delusions or hallucinations accompany acute intermittent porphyria…

  a. They are atypical, because depression is the most frequent psychiatric presentation.
  b. It is late in the course of the illness.
  c. They are almost exclusively in the setting of delirium.
  d. All of the above.

8. What is true of the course of acute intermittent porphyria?

  a. It progresses unremittingly after the initial episode.
  b. It improves with pregnancy.
  c. It is characterized by remissions and exacerbations.
  d. None of the above.

9. Ms. DAP is tearful in the sessions with you as she speaks about her mother's terrible GI symptoms and rapid death. She is otherwise without evidence of endogenous depression. Ms. DAP reveals that she has always been concerned about health and nutrition. She follows a vegetarian diet, supplemented by a vitamin regimen prescribed by a "holistic nutritionist." Her internist feels that the vitamins are unnecessary but benign. You receive a copy of Ms. DAP's laboratory work. Electrocardiogram (ECG) and all lab values are normal, including thyroid function tests and human immunodeficiency virus (HIV) serological testing. Result of routine urinalysis is negative. Colonoscopy result is pending. The internist consults with you and asks if you want any other tests. GI symptoms are not typical, but when psychiatric symptoms accompany B_{12} (cobalamin) deficiency…

  a. Anorexia with moderate weight loss typically occurs.
  b. They are reliably accompanied by macrocytic anemia.
  c. They are reliably predated by neurological symptoms.
  d. A normal serum B_{12} level reliably rules out vitamin deficiency.
  e. None of the above.

10. The *prototypical* psychiatric symptom of B_{12} deficiency is…

  a. Depression
  b. Mania
  c. Schizophreniform psychosis
  d. Paranoid psychosis
  e. Not predictable

11. Which of the following is/are true regarding *clinically significant* B_{12} deficiency?

  a. A low normal serum B_{12} level serves to rule out B_{12} deficiency.
  b. Presence of anemia is necessary, by definition.

c. Macrocytosis may be absent.

d. Tests of serum methylmalonic acid (MMA) and homocysteine levels are reliably diagnostic.

12. The neurological symptoms of B_{12} deficiency classically consist of…

a. Delirium

b. Paresthesias in feet and fingers

c. Disturbed vibratory sense

d. Extrapyramidal features resembling neuroleptic side effects

e. Inability to maintain balance when standing with eyes closed

13. Ms. DAP's workup is completed and she is diagnosed with irritable bowel syndrome (IBS). She knows little about the condition, except that it is considered "psychosomatic." Which of the following are true regarding IBS?

a. It is a type of inflammatory bowel disease.

b. It is a type of structural bowel disease.

c. It is a type of malabsorption syndrome.

d. It is associated with urological symptoms.

e. It is associated with mucus in the stools.

14. All of the following are characteristic of IBS (in the absence of a mood disorder) *except*…

a. Pain relieved by defecation

b. Pain interfering with sleep

c. Weight loss

d. Constipation

e. Diarrhea

f. Variable pain location

15. The diagnosis of IBS is made by characteristic changes seen on…

a. Barium enema

b. Histopathology

c. Sigmoidoscopy

d. Autoimmune studies

e. None of the above

16. Ms. DAP assumes that *psychosomatic* means "imaginary," a common misconception. What are *physiological* characteristics of IBS?

a. Abnormal small intestine motility

b. Abnormal colonic motility

c. Normal esophageal motility

d. Few identifiable physiological changes

17. Ms. DAP notes that her GI symptoms worsen with anxiety and seem to peak every morning right before she leaves for work. Ms. DAP's husband has observed that her symptoms improve on weekends and vacations. He has urged her to "calm down" at work because she is "giving herself" the symptoms. The patient says that she has always been a "nervous person," even as a college student. "I'd worry about my grades. I'd worry about my finances. I liked things to be routine, no changes. I don't do well with change. It makes me very nervous." She also mentions that her father was phobic of bridges and tunnels and was quite hypochondriacal. There is no present or past personal history of depression. What is known about the epidemiology of IBS?

a. Increased prevalence in higher socioeconomic groups.

b. Female predominance across cultures.

c. Incidence declines with advancing age.

d. It is almost exclusively a disease of Western hemisphere nations.

18. The first case-control study (2002) examined the association between functional bowel disorders and previous experiences of sexual abuse. Patients with idiopathic constipation ($n=53$) were compared with matched control groups of 50 IBS patients, 51 Crohn's disease patients, and 53 nonpatient control subjects. Measures of previous sexual abuse experiences in functional bowel disorder patients, measured by questionnaire and a semistructured interview, showed the following:

a. No significant differences were found among groups of IBS, Crohn's, idiopathic constipation, and control subjects for measures of sexual abuse.

b. No significant differences were found among IBS, Crohn's, idiopathic constipation, and control subjects for measures of psychological stress.

c. Findings support the practice among gastroenterologists of questioning IBS patients about sexual abuse experiences.

d. None of the above.

19. Ms. DAP is lost to follow-up for several months. She returns after having failed several trials of antispasmodic and bulking agents. Her anxiety about her health has skyrocketed. All of the following are true *except*…

a. The American Gastroenterological Association does *not* recommend anxiolytics as independent agents for IBS.

b. For patients with predominant diarrhea and depression, the constipating side effects of the tricyclic antidepressants may be helpful.

c. Use of antidepressants should be limited to those IBS patients with concomitant depression or anxiety.

d. For depressed patients with predominant constipation, a selective serotonin reuptake inhibitor would be the preferable treatment.

20. What will characterize the course, treatment, and prognosis of this patient?

   a. Most patients with IBS have poor insight, complicated by a deteriorating medical course.

   b. The goal of psychological management is to frame the irritable bowel as different, not diseased.

   c. The effectiveness of psychotherapy has been limited to those treatments using psychodynamic techniques.

   d. The effectiveness of psychotherapy has been limited to those treatments using behavioral techniques.

   e. The psychiatric consultant should try to effect a "division of labor" with the gastroenterologist, requesting that the patient direct the GI complaints to the medical specialist.

Answers

1. a, c (pp. 106–107)
2. b (p. 107)
3. b, c (p. 107)
4. a, b, c, d (p. 108)
5. b (p. 108)
6. a, b, c, d (p. 108)
7. c (p. 108)
8. c (p. 108)
9. e (pp. 110–111)
10. e (p. 110)
11. c, d (p. 111)
12. b, c, e (p. 110)
13. d, e (p. 101)
14. b, c (pp. 99–101)
15. c (p. 101)
16. a, b (p. 101)
17. c (pp. 101–102)
18. a, b (p. 103)
19. c (pp. 105–106)
20. b (pp. 104–105)

■ CHAPTER 7

Case Vignette 1: The Pregnant, Anxious Patient Who Becomes Depressed

Ms. Sad-Panicked-and-Pregnant (SPP) is a 31-year-old woman who has a 4-year-old son and has worked as a music teacher for many years. She was referred by her internist 2 years ago with symptoms of insomnia and extreme anxiety, marked by panic attacks, palpitations, dry mouth, fear of going crazy, sweating, and a choking sensation. Panic attacks occurred two to three times per week. Symptoms began when she returned to work after an extended maternity leave. Ms. SPP became extremely depressed and felt she could "no longer cope," but she was at no point suicidal. She acknowledged feelings of guilt and complained of difficulty concentrating and of feeling worse in the morning. Cognitive functions were intact except for diminished concentration. Past psychiatric history was remarkable for mild performance anxiety treated with occasional lorazepam (Ativan) 0.5 mg before recitals. Family history was positive for postpartum depression (PPD) in her mother. There was no drug or alcohol history.

Complete medical and neurological workups (including EEG and MRI of the brain) were normal. The diagnoses of panic disorder (without agoraphobia) and major depression were made, and the patient was begun on venlafaxine extended-release (Effexor XR) and as-needed clonazepam. Panic and depressive symptoms disappeared entirely on 225 mg/day of extended-release venlafaxine, and she no longer needed clonazepam. After 1 year in remission, she slowly tapered venlafaxine over 3 months and remained asymptomatic. She and her husband decided that they wanted a second child.

Study Questions

(More than one choice may be correct for each question. Choose all that apply.)

1. The patient and her husband have used a diaphragm and condom as their main form of birth control. She has taken oral contraceptives, which have had the added benefit of lessening her severe menstrual cramping. What statements are true regarding the psychiatric side effects associated with oral contraceptives?

   a. When oral contraceptives produce adverse psychiatric effects, high levels of estrogen are usually the culprit.

b. Newer preparations containing higher estrogen-to-progestin ratios have fewer of these side effects.

c. The psychiatric symptoms most commonly associated with oral contraceptives are anxiety states.

d. The psychiatric side effects of oral contraceptives occur mainly when the woman takes them irregularly, rather than as directed.

2. Ms. SPP is quite concerned about the risk of recurrence of panic disorder and depression. She fears being "trapped" by the horrible symptoms again, this time while pregnant, without help available to her. What factors do you consider as you begin to counsel Ms. SPP and her husband?

a. Pregnancy has been shown to confer a protective effect for the majority of women with panic disorder.

b. It is not possible to predict the course of untreated panic disorder during pregnancy.

c. If Ms. SPP's panic attacks recur during pregnancy, she should be aware that the largest safety record is with the tricyclic antidepressants, such as nortriptyline, and the serotonin reuptake inhibitors, such as fluoxetine.

d. Clonazepam is contraindicated in pregnancy.

3. The husband wants to know the likelihood of his wife's becoming depressed again during pregnancy. Which of the following is/are true?

a. The risk is greater during the first trimester compared with the second trimester.

b. The risk is greater during the second trimester compared with the first and third trimesters.

c. She is at no greater risk than someone without an affective history.

d. The risk of developing depression during pregnancy would be increased by family history of depression (before, during, after, or unassociated with pregnancy).

4. If Ms. SPP had not been unable to discontinue venlafaxine without experiencing a relapse of panic disorder and depression, the preferred management strategy would be to...

a. Wait until she was pregnant and then discontinue the venlafaxine to minimize exposure to an "unknown-risk antidepressant."

b. Stop the medication slowly before conception because any degree of exposure to an antidepressant is unacceptable.

c. Switch to a better-studied antidepressant such as an SSRI as soon as pregnancy was documented.

d. Inform the patient that any medication changes are best accomplished *prior* to conception.

e. Discuss the risks and benefits of using particular antidepressants in both pregnancy and breastfeeding.

5. "Postpartum blues" is a term found throughout the literature on mood disorders in pregnancy. How does DSM-IV-TR classify this condition?

a. It has created a new category, *brief postpartum dysphoric disorder.*

b. It advises classifying it under *adjustment disorder with depressed mood.*

c. It groups it under *mental disorder due to a general medical condition.*

d. It does not specify.

6. All of the following have been associated with the diagnosis of postpartum blues *except* ...

a. Anxiety

b. Insomnia

c. Poor appetite

d. Psychosis

e. Suicidal ideation

7. Ms. SPP wants to know if you will be able to see her while she is in the hospital after the delivery. You tell her you will see her, but in formulating your potential treatment plan, you consider that she would be most at risk for the blues...

a. Within 24 hours of delivery

b. Between postpartum days 3 and 7

c. Between postpartum weeks 2 and 3

d. Between postpartum months 1 and 2

8. If Ms. SPP were to develop postpartum blues, all of the following are treatment considerations, *except*...

a. The condition is a risk factor for postpartum depression.

b. It does not remit without treatment.

c. Low-dose benzodiazepines may be used for insomnia and anxiety.

d. Postpartum blues should be monitored closely in a patient with a prior history of depression.

9. Ms. SPP becomes pregnant almost immediately, but by the seventh week of pregnancy, she notes recurrent anxiety and dysphoria with insomnia, feelings of guilt, diminished self-esteem, and impaired concentration. There is no psychosis, but she experiences transient suicidal ideation. She does not want to take medications. Which of the following statements are true about suicide and pregnancy?

    a. Women *during* pregnancy have a higher risk of suicide in comparison to the general female population.
    b. Despite their high rate of psychiatric morbidity, women in the first year *after* childbirth have a low risk of suicide in comparison to the general female population.
    c. The risk of suicide is slightly lower in pregnant teenagers compared to other pregnant women.
    d. A history of psychiatric admission increases the risk of suicide.

10. Which of the following are risk factors for postpartum depression?

    a. Depression during the index pregnancy
    b. History of depression unassociated with pregnancy
    c. Pregnancy loss within the past 12 months, by miscarriage
    d. Pregnancy loss within the past 12 months, by elective termination
    e. Abrupt or preliminary discontinuation of antidepressants

11. If psychosis complicates depression during pregnancy, it is usually in the form of...

    a. Paranoid delusions about the fetus
    b. Auditory hallucinations concerning the fetus
    c. Paranoid delusions of persecution
    d. Visual hallucinations

12. Which of the following is true regarding the diagnosis of postpartum depression according to DSM-IV-TR?

    a. DSM-IV-TR adds a "postpartum onset" specifier to the *major depressive disorder* diagnosis.
    b. DSM-IV-TR terms it *major depressive disorder due to a general medical condition* (i.e., pregnancy).
    c. DSM-IV-TR has created a separate category of *postpartum depressive disorder*.

    d. DSM-IV-TR classifies it under *mood disorder not otherwise specified.*
    e. DSM-IV-TR does not consider PPD to be a separate class of affective disorder.

13. DSM-IV-TR considers "postpartum" to be within what time interval following delivery?

    a. Within 2 weeks
    b. Within 1 month
    c. Within months
    d. Within 1 year

14. When assessing any depressed patient, it is useful to check thyroid function. What are true statements regarding thyroid function during and after pregnancy?

    a. Although there are numerous changes in levels of T_3, T_4, and thyroid-stimulating hormone during pregnancy, the pregnant woman remains euthyroid by laboratory evaluation.
    b. Thyroiditis occurs relatively commonly postpartum.
    c. Psychosis may complicate hypothyroidism.
    d. None of the above.

15. At week 11 of pregnancy, the patient experiences deepening depression with panic attacks, increasing suicidal ideation, and decreasing ability to care for her son. You have a risk-benefit discussion with her and her husband. They decide to give informed consent to medication treatment. Which of the following should be discussed with them as they consider treatment choices?

    a. The teratogenic potential of SSRIs has been more controversial than that of the tricyclic antidepressants.
    b. SSRI ingestion during the first trimester of pregnancy has been associated with significant fetal morbidity.
    c. Although the tricyclic antidepressants have been used for over 50 years, the newer SSRIs are better studied.
    d. ECT would not be an option until the second trimester.

16. You decide to recommend paroxetine (Paxil). Findings reported in the literature as possible indications of neonatal toxicity occurring with *in utero* paroxetine exposure include which of the following?

    a. Jaundice

b. Respiratory distress
c. Hypoglycemia
d. Small bowel obstruction
e. None of the above

17. Evidence of the negative effects of untreated maternal depression in pregnancy and postpartum on the infant and growing child include...

    a. Infanticide or child abuse
    b. Fewer vocalizations by the infant
    c. Problems in early childhood intellectual development
    d. More behavioral difficulties in the young child

18. After 1 week on paroxetine, the patient is still having panic attacks and difficulty sleeping. You decide to add an anxiolytic. What factor(s) would influence initiating a benzodiazepine?

    a. Diazepam's many years of use in pregnancy make it the preferred benzodiazepine for this population.
    b. The combination of anxiolytics with paroxetine is contraindicated.
    c. The data suggest that benzodiazepines pose little teratogenic risk but are insufficient to conclude that there is no risk.
    d. A useful strategy in anxious pregnant women with insomnia is to add low-dose diphenhydramine (Benadryl) to temazepam (Restoril) at bedtime, helping to reduce daytime medication requirements.

19. Which of the following medications are preferred by experts for the treatment of anxiety and insomnia in pregnant women?

    a. Alprazolam (Xanax)
    b. Temazepam (Restoril)
    c. Clonazepam (Klonopin)
    d. Lorazepam (Ativan)
    e. Diazepam (Valium)

20. What are some of the considerations for women who require benzodiazepines in pregnancy and also plan to breastfeed?

    a. Benzodiazepines are contraindicated in breastfeeding.
    b. Benzodiazepines increase the risk of urinary retention in the neonate.
    c. The main concern is sedation in the newborn.
    d. They produce gastrointestinal complications in the newborn, leading to feeding problems.

21. Environmental manipulation, such as avoiding caffeine and alcohol, and promoting good sleep hygiene are the first line of treatment for insomnia in pregnant patients. For those women requiring medications, which of the following are safe options?

    a. Diphenhydramine (Benadryl)
    b. Triazolam (Halcion)
    c. Temazepam (Restoril)
    d. Clonazepam (Klonopin)
    e. Amitriptyline (Elavil)
    f. Zolpidem (Ambien)
    g. Zaleplon (Sonata)

22. Ms. SPP is due to deliver in about 10 days. Which of the following are true?

    a. Ideally, the medication should be gradually discontinued at this point.
    b. She is past the high-risk period for recurrent depression.
    c. She is at heightened risk for recurrent depression in the postpartum period.
    d. The main adverse side effect of continuing medication up until delivery is neonatal cardiotoxicity.

23. Symptoms that are most useful for distinguishing normal mood changes from postpartum depression in women who have just given birth include which of the following:

    a. A sense of being overwhelmed or unable to care for the baby
    b. Feeling like a failure as a mother
    c. Appetite disturbance
    d. Sleep disturbance
    e. Obsessional thoughts about harming herself or the baby
    f. Loss of libido
    g. Anergia

24. Ms. SPP delivers a healthy baby girl. She agrees to remain on paroxetine but wants to breastfeed. How do you advise her?

    a. The American Academy of Pediatrics classifies antidepressants as "drugs whose effect on the nursing infant is unknown but may be of concern."
    b. The American Academy of Pediatrics classifies antidepressants as "compatible with breastfeeding."

c. Mothers with a history of unipolar depression who refuse antidepressant therapy while breastfeeding are at high risk for relapse.

d. Long-term data are still pending on the developmental effects of SSRI exposure through breast milk, but the little that we have is reassuring.

e. Long-term data are still pending on the developmental effects of SSRI exposure through breast milk, but the little that we have is alarming.

25. Which of the following are in the DSM-IV-TR differential diagnosis of a depressive mood disorder occurring 2 months following delivery?

a. Postpartum blues
b. Mood disorder due to hypothyroidism
c. Mood disorder due to infection with HIV
d. Mood disorder due to systemic lupus erythematosus
e. Substance-induced depressive disorder
f. Mood disorder with postpartum onset
g. All of the above

Answers

1. b (p. 124)
2. b, c (p. 122)
3. d (p. 118, table)
4. d, e (p. 117)
5. d (p. 130)
6. d, e (p. 130)
7. b (p. 130)
8. b (pp. 130–131)
9. b, d (p. 136)
10. a, b, c, d, e (p. 131)
11. a, c (p. 119)
12. a, e (p. 135)
13. b (p. 135)
14. a, b, c (pp. 136–137)
15. c (pp. 125–126)
16. a, b, c (p. 149)
17. a, b, c, d (p. 133)
18. c (pp. 129, 155–156)
19. c, d (pp. 155–156)
20. c (pp. 156–157)
21. a, d, e (pp. 129–130)
22. c (p. 131)
23. a, b, e (p. 133)
24. a, c, d (p. 138)
25. b, c, d, e (p. 133)

Case Vignette 2: The Pregnant, Bipolar Patient Who Becomes Psychotic

Ms. Psychotic-Bipolar-and-Pregnant (PBP) is an attractive 25-year-old aspiring singer who has been marginally followed in the local clinic for 3 years. She had her first manic episode at age 22, when she was hospitalized with flight of ideas, euphoria, and hyperactivity. At that time, she had the delusion that she was the double of the singer Madonna because Marilyn Monroe's voice followed her everywhere telling her to dye her hair blond. The police had brought her in after she created a disturbance at a local record store by attempting to stage her own concert. There was no history of substance abuse. Family history was notable for one grandmother who was institutionalized after she had her second child. Past medical history was negative.

The patient had responded well to a combination of risperidone (Risperdal) 6 mg po qd and lithium 600 mg bid, attaining levels of approximately 1.0 mEq/mL. She was discharged home, where she lived with a succession of boyfriends. She managed to support herself with waitressing jobs, which changed about every 6 months. She was able to book occasional singing gigs at local bars.

Compliance with medications was an ongoing struggle between Ms. PBP and her therapists at the clinic. She was lost to follow-up until 10 months later, when the obstetrics resident called the clinic to report that Ms. PBP was again psychotic after having delivered a healthy baby girl 1 week earlier. She did not know who was the father of the baby. Police had brought her in from a local record store, where she was singing the Madonna song "Like a Virgin" in a loud voice, draped only in a white bedsheet. In the emergency room, she was euphoric and hyperactive and had flight of ideas. She reported that she was "talking to the voice of the Virgin Mary" because she had a baby, "like Madonna's madonna." Although it was early evening when she was brought in, the patient thought that she was leading a morning prayer service at a church.

Study Questions

(More than one choice may be correct for each question. Choose all that apply.)

1. The major risk factors for the occurrence of postpartum psychosis include all of the following *except…*

a. Bipolar disorder
b. Schizophrenia
c. Postpartum psychosis, by personal history
d. Postpartum psychosis, by family history
e. Panic disorder

2. The relative risk of hospital admission for postpartum psychosis varies according to time from delivery in biologically vulnerable individuals. The period of *greatest* vulnerability is…

   a. 12 months postpartum
   b. 6 months postpartum
   c. 3 months postpartum
   d. 1 month postpartum

3. Following uncomplicated childbirth, the increased risk of psychiatric hospitalization persists for up to…

   a. 2 weeks
   b. 2 months
   c. 12 months
   d. 2 years
   e. The risk is no greater than that for nonpregnant women after the first 12 months.

4. How does Ms. PBP's presentation compare with that of other postpartum psychotic syndromes?

   a. It is unusual, in that the majority of patients with postpartum psychosis requiring hospitalization have schizophreniform rather than affective symptoms.
   b. It is fairly typical, in that the majority of postpartum psychoses are affective in nature rather than schizophreniform.
   c. It is not possible to determine, because there is no distinctive pattern to the symptomatology of postpartum psychosis.
   d. Most postpartum psychotic states present within 2 weeks of delivery.

5. Characteristic features of postpartum psychotic syndromes include…

   a. Delirium-like presentation
   b. Psychomotor retardation
   c. Rapidly evolving suicidal and infanticidal ideation
   d. Indolent course

6. Women who suffer pregnancy-related psychotic episodes often want to know their risk for recurrence if they do (or do not) become pregnant again. All of the following trends have been distilled from the literature *except*…

   a. Postpartum psychotic illness predisposes to additional affective episodes unrelated to pregnancy.

   b. After postpartum psychosis accompanied by affective symptoms, the risk of future affective episodes stays higher than for the general population, whether the woman becomes pregnant again or not.
   c. Mothers without psychiatric history prior to their index postpartum psychotic episode seem to have the most benign course.
   d. Pregnancy-related psychotic episodes confer no greater risk of subsequent affective episodes as long as the woman does not become pregnant.

7. The most common characteristics of completed suicide in postpartum women are…

   a. Death by overdose
   b. Death by violent means
   c. Indications that the woman may have been psychotic
   d. Careful planning

8. All of the following are risk factors associated with infanticide, including neonaticide, *except*…

   a. Maternal age 25–35
   b. Little or no prenatal care
   c. Denial of pregnancy
   d. Ego-dystonic ruminations about harming the baby

9. All of the following are diagnostic considerations in evaluating Ms. PBP *except*…

   a. Substance-induced psychotic disorder
   b. Psychotic disorder due to thyroid disease
   c. Postpartum blues
   d. Psychotic disorder due to systemic lupus erythematosus (SLE)
   e. Psychotic disorder due to HIV

10. On the psychiatry service, Ms. PBP preaches "the word of the Lord" to the other patients, while actively hallucinating. She retains some reality testing about her infant and is concerned that her parents take good care of the child. Her parents are extremely upset about her condition and ask how this could have happened. Which of the following are true?

   a. Women with bipolar disorder are at greater risk for postpartum psychosis than those with unipolar depression.
   b. Women with unipolar depression are at greater risk for postpartum psychosis than those with bipolar disorder.

c. Postpartum psychosis may be the first episode of a bipolar disorder, even though it is complicated by delirium-like features.

d. Women who remained well during pregnancy are at a decreased risk of relapse, even though they discontinued lithium prior to pregnancy.

11. If Ms. PBP could be carefully followed upon discharge, which of the following would be true?

   a. Experts would agree that Ms. PBP's lithium should be discontinued prior to planned conception.

   b. Experts would agree that Ms. PBP should remain on maintenance lithium prior to planned conception.

   c. There would be consensus that lithium is less neurotoxic than valproic acid (Depakote, Depakene) or carbamazepine (Tegretol).

   d. If first-trimester antimanic agents were required, most experts would advise valproic acid or carbamazepine instead of lithium.

12. Ms. PBP is discharged home and does well until she is once again lost to follow-up. She reappears in the emergency room about 1 year later, this time 10 weeks pregnant and again hallucinating, delusional, and with irritable mood. Her lithium level is zero. She is alert and oriented to person and date, but not place, shows diminished concentration, and refuses cognitive testing, claiming that the examiner is a "priest of the devil." She does not know who is the father of her baby. Physical exam and lab results are pending. What characterizes the differential diagnosis at this point?

   a. This clinical picture could be consistent with one of the end-organ side effects of *chronic* lithium exposure, even though her present level is zero and acute toxicity is ruled out.

   b. This clinical picture is consistent with consequences of lithium discontinuation in this patient.

   c. Her presentation is congruent with SLE.

   d. Within the spectrum of thyroid disease, *hyper*thyroidism, but not *hypo*thyroidism, could present in this way.

   e. Although she is at risk for HIV infection, manic syndromes are not a presenting feature of HIV infection without other systemic signs.

13. The medical workup, including labs, is completely normal. All of the following treatment guidelines apply to a psychotic pregnant patient like Ms. PBP *except...*

   a. The atypical antipsychotics are the medications of choice in treating psychosis in pregnant women.

   b. The conventional antipsychotics are the medications of choice in treating psychosis in pregnant women.

   c. Electroconvulsive therapy is an effective treatment for mania in pregnancy.

   d. High-potency, conventional antipsychotics (e.g., haloperidol, perphenazine, trifluoperazine, and thiothixene) are less teratogenic than low-potency conventional antipsychotics (e.g., chlorpromazine).

   e. No effects on behavioral, emotional, or cognitive development have been found in human studies of high-potency, conventional antipsychotics, although *prospective* studies are lacking.

14. Which agents are considered to be the treatment of choice for extrapyramidal side effects caused by the conventional antipsychotics in pregnant women?

   a. Amantadine (Symmetrel)
   b. Atenolol (Tenormin)
   c. Benztropine (Cogentin)
   d. Bromocriptine (Parlodel)
   e. Diphenhydramine (Benadryl)
   f. Propranolol (Inderal)
   g. Trihexyphenidyl (Artane)

15. What are treatment recommendations for women who require antipsychotic therapy and also plan to breastfeed?

   a. Breastfeeding while taking antipsychotics is not recommended because of lack of information.

   b. Breastfeeding while taking antipsychotics is not recommended because of consistent evidence of harm to the infant.

   c. Breastfeeding on antipsychotics is recommended because of their benefits to the mother.

   d. Breastfeeding on antipsychotics is recommended because the benefits of breastmilk to the infant outweigh the calculated risk of side effects.

16. Ms. PBP responds partially to clonazepam (Klonopin) 0.5 mg bid and haloperidol (Haldol)

2 mg tid. She becomes assaultive toward another patient, whom she is convinced is part of the satanic plot to undo her "virgin divinity." The euphoric mood persists. If Ms. PBP becomes violent and requires physical restraint, what instructions should be given to the nurses?

a. She should be placed supine.
b. She should be positioned on her right side.
c. She should be positioned on her left side.
d. Her position should be changed frequently.

17. If you could have managed Ms. PBP before her second pregnancy, which of the following strategies would have won consensus approval from the experts?

a. Counsel the patient that lithium at *any* time during pregnancy confers an *equally* high risk of congenital deformities.
b. Advise her that, based on current knowledge, there is no evidence of an increased risk of developmental abnormalities in developing children who were exposed to lithium in utero but were normal at birth.
c. Advise her that, based on current knowledge, there is no evidence of an increased risk of physical abnormalities in developing children who were exposed to lithium in utero but were normal at birth.
d. Explain that her risk of psychiatric relapse exceeds the risk of teratogenicity on lithium.

18. Which of the following are recommendations for the treatment of bipolar disorder in pregnancy?

a. Consider a trial of lithium prior to conception.
b. Consider a trial of anticonvulsant mood stabilizers prior to conception.
c. Discontinue lithium at least 2 months before attempted conception.
d. The anticonvulsant drugs should be used in pregnancy only if better-studied drugs, such as lithium, are ineffective.
e. Lithium should be used in pregnancy only if anticonvulsant drugs are ineffective.

19. The incidence of neural tube defects for patients on anticonvulsants may be reduced by the following strategies:

a. Treatment with thiamine (B_1) from periconception through the end of the first trimester
b. Treatment with pyridoxine (B_6) from periconception through the end of the first trimester

c. Treatment with folic acid (B_9) from periconception through the end of the first trimester
d. Treatment with cobalamin (vitamin B_{12}) from periconception through the end of the first trimester
e. Using the lowest possible dose of drug
f. Using only one anticonvulsant

20. Fetuses of mothers placed on lithium should undergo screening specifically for...

a. Neural tube defects
b. Ceruloplasmin
c. Congenital heart disease
d. Fragile X syndrome
e. Epstein-Barr virus

21. Some patients want to know the alternatives to lithium use in pregnancy. Fetuses of mothers placed on carbamazepine should undergo screening specifically for...

a. Neural tube defects
b. Ceruloplasmin
c. Congenital heart disease
d. Fragile X syndrome
e. Epstein-Barr virus

22. Fetuses of mothers placed on valproic acid (Depakote, Depakene) should undergo screening specifically for...

a. Abnormal karyotype
b. Skeletal deformities
c. Cardiac malformations
d. Alpha-fetoprotein levels
e. Tay-Sachs disease

23. Ms. PBP has been counseled that in utero exposure to lithium may increase the incidence of Ebstein's anomaly. What features are associated with Ebstein's anomaly?

a. Tricuspid insufficiency
b. Mitral stenosis
c. Transposition of the great vessels
d. Cleft palate
e. Mental retardation
f. Viral infection

24. Ultrasonography is recommended for pregnant women on antimanic prophylaxis...

a. Between 10 and 12 weeks
b. Between 16 and 20 weeks
c. between 20 and 22 weeks
d. Only if they are taking lithium

e. Only if they are taking anticonvulsants

f. If they are taking either lithium or anticonvulsants

25. Ms. PBP refuses lithium but responds quickly to ECT and low-dose neuroleptics. She requires antimanic prophylaxis. She is at week 11. What are the current data on the association between in utero lithium and Ebstein's anomaly?

   a. The incidence of lithium-associated Ebstein's anomaly has been revised *down* from the original estimates made in the 1970s.

   b. The incidence of lithium-associated Ebstein's anomaly has been confirmed as greater than the original estimates made in the 1970s.

   c. The risk of Ebstein's anomaly in pregnancy is about equal for each trimester.

   d. Based on currently available data, the risk of bearing a baby with Ebstein's anomaly is about 20 times greater for a woman on lithium than for women in the general population.

26. Which pharmacokinetic changes occur during pregnancy?

   a. If the patient becomes preeclamptic, the lithium dose should be increased to compensate for the expanded volume of distribution.

   b. Early in the third trimester, glomerular filtration rate (GFR) *rises,* predisposing to subtherapeutic lithium levels and heightened risk of manic relapse.

   c. Late in the third trimester, at the time of delivery, changes in GFR predispose to subtherapeutic lithium levels and heightened risk of manic relapse.

   d. If the patient becomes preeclamptic and is placed on a sodium-restricted diet, she is at heightened risk for lithium toxicity if her dose is not reduced.

27. Early into her second trimester, Ms. PBP is discharged home in the care of her parents on lithium 300 mg bid (level: 1.0 mEq/mL) and haloperidol 1 mg po qd. She is compliant with outpatient psychiatric and obstetric follow-up. She asks if she will remain on this lithium dose throughout. She hopes it will not make her baby "sick" when it is born. She asks if she will be able to breast-feed. You respond:

   a. Neonatal lithium toxicity can be avoided as long as maternal blood levels remain in the therapeutic range.

   b. The syndrome of lithium toxicity in neonates resembles that in the adult.

   c. Most of the toxic effects of lithium in the newborn are self-limiting.

   d. The American Academy of Pediatrics considers lithium to be contraindicated during breastfeeding.

   e. The half-life of lithium in newborns is about double that in the adult.

Answers

1. e (p. 135)
2. d (p. 135)
3. d (p. 135)
4. b, d (p. 135)
5. a, c (p. 135)
6. d (pp. 135–136)
7. b, c (p. 136)
8. a, d (p. 136)
9. c (pp. 136–137)
10. a, c (pp. 135–137)
11. b, c (pp. 138–139)
12. a, b, c (pp. 136–137)
13. a (p. 129)
14. c, e (p. 129)
15. a (p. 139)
16. c, d (pp. 126–127)
17. b, c, d (pp. 128, 159–161)
18. a, d (p. 128)
19. c, e, f (p. 128)
20. c (pp. 128, 159)
21. a, c (pp. 157–158)
22. c, d (pp. 157–159)
23. a (p. 159)
24. b (p. 128)
25. a, d (p. 159)
26. b, d (p. 160)
27. c, d (pp. 160–161)

Index

*Page numbers printed in **boldface** type refer to tables or figures.*

QT interval prolongation. *See also*
   Conduction disturbance;
   Torsades de pointes
   antiarrhythmics and, **305**
   antibiotics and, **305**
   and antipsychotics, **18, 60,** 61
   cases, 340–344
   clozapine and, 60, 62
   delirium and, **16**
   kidney disease and, 73
   haloperidol and, 18, 19
   olanzapine and, 61
   phenothiazines and, 35, 61, 63
   quetiapine and, 61, 63
   risperidone and, 62
   SSRIs and, 53, 55
   tricyclic antidepressants and, **59**
   vasodilators and, **305**
   ziprasidone and, 21, 61, 63, 73
Quality of life
   HIV-associated dementia complex
      and, 182
   insomnia and, 193
   renal failure and, 78
Quazepam (Doral), **313**
Quetiapine (Seroquel). *See also*
      Atypical antipsychotics
   cardiovascular disease and, 61, 63
   delirium and, **19,** 21
   HIV-associated psychosis and, 185
   kidney disease and, 73
   obstetrics patients and, 155
   pulmonary disease and, 90
   sedative-hypnotic uses of, **314**
Quinidine, **6,** 55, 59, 65, **305**

Racial bias, and HIV, 195
Ranitidine (Zantac), 5, **6**
Rapport, with medically ill patients,
   10–11, 127, 233, 239
Rational suicide, 193
Reasoning, and decision-making
   capacity, **222–223**
Reassurance, and spiritual questions,
   239
Rebound insomnia, and delirium, 22
Recurrence
   of postpartum psychosis, 135–136,
      138
   of psychiatric disorders during
      pregnancy, 117
"Red flag" conditions, in irritable
   bowel syndrome, 101
Refusal, of medical treatment, 227,
   231. *See also* Termination
Regression, and spiritual issues,
   239

Rehabilitation programs, and
   cardiovascular disease, 52
Reitan-Indiana Aphasia Screening
   Test, 13
Relapse, obstetrics patients and
   prevention of, 117, 119, 122, 124,
   128, 138. *See also* Remission
Religion, and questions about suicide,
   248. *See also* Spiritual issues
Remission. *See also* Relapse
   of acute intermittent porphyria,
      108
   of asthma, 86
   eating disorders during pregnancy
      and, 123
Remote memory, and Korsakoff's
   syndrome, 37
Renal failure. *See* Kidney disease
Replacement therapy, for cobalamin
   deficiency, 111–112
ReproTox, **116**
Resilience, and medical problems,
   241–242, 252
Respirator-dependent patients. *See*
   Ventilated patients
Reverse anorexia nervosa, 167
Ribavirin, 202, 214, **215**
Risk-benefit analysis
   informed consent and, 227
   obstetrics patients and, 125
   psychopharmacology during
      pregnancy and, 125–126
Risk factors
   for bipolar disorder during
      pregnancy, **118**
   cardiovascular and use of
      antipsychotics, 60–62
   for delirium, 4
   for delirium tremens, **32**
   for depression before and after
      pregnancy, **118**
   for eating disorders during
      pregnancy, 123
   for HIV infection, **177,** 185–186
   for lithium-induced renal
      impairment, 75
   for pancreatic cancer, 107
   for postpartum depression, **118,**
      131, 133
   for postpartum psychosis, 135, 136
   for steroid-induced psychosis, 164–
      165
   for suicide in HIV patients, 193
   for torsades de pointes, **305**
Risperidone (Risperdal). *See also*
      Atypical antipsychotics
   alcoholic hallucinosis and, 40

cardiovascular disease and, 62
delirium and, **19,** 20
dementia-related behavioral
   problems and, 271
HIV-associated psychosis and, 184
kidney disease and, 73, **310**
obstetrics patients and, 155
organ transplantation and, 216
pulmonary disease and, 90, **92**
ritonavir and, 184
sedative-hypnotic uses of, **314**
steroid-induced psychiatric
   reactions and, 165
Ritalin, 216
Ritonavir (Norvir)
   HIV-associated psychosis and, 184
   psychotropic drugs and, 186, 187,
      188, 192
Romberg's sign, and gastrointestinal
   (GI) symptoms, 110
Rome II, criteria for irritable bowel
   syndrome, 101
Rule of two-thirds, 71, 72, 73
"Rum fits," 38

St. John's wort (*Hypericum perforatum*),
   281
Saw palmetto (*Serenoa repens*), **280**
Sceletium, **280**
Schizoaffective disorder, and
   obstetrics patients, **118,** 122, 128–
   129
Schizophrenia
   acute intermittent porphyria and,
      108
   alcoholic hallucinosis and, 40
   clozapine use during pregnancy
      and, 154
   delirium and, 2–3
   HIV and, differential diagnosis,
      175
   HIV psychosis and, 184
   high-risk sexual behavior and, 172
   obstetrics patients and, **118,** 122,
      128–129, 135, 139, 153, 154
   organ transplantation and, 212
   risperidone use during pregnancy
      and, 155
Scopolamine, **6**
Screening instruments
   for bipolar disorders, **323**
   of candidates for organ
      transplantation, 208–209
   for delirium, **12,** 12–14
   for depression during pregnancy,
      131
   for postpartum psychosis, 136